N Nicotinic Acid

O Ovral

P Penicillin
Periactin
Persantine
Potassium iodide
Prednisone
PUVA

Q Questran

R Ridaura
Rifampin

S Solatene
Synthroid

T Tetracycline
Thiabendazole

U Urinary anti-infectives

V Vaccines
Vitamin C
Vitamin E

W Weight Watchers

X X-ray
Xylocaine

Y Yearly review
Your interest and enthusiasm

Z Zinc
Zovirax

Ten Most Wanted Drugs

ADVANCED DERMATOLOGIC THERAPY

WALTER B. SHELLEY, M.D.
Professor of Dermatology

E. DORINDA SHELLEY, M.D.
Professor and Chief of Dermatology

*Division of Dermatology, Department of Medicine,
Medical College of Ohio, Toledo, Ohio*

W. B. SAUNDERS COMPANY
Philadelphia/London/Toronto/Mexico City/Rio de Janeiro/Sydney/Tokyo/Hong Kong

W. B. SAUNDERS COMPANY
Harcourt Brace Jovanovich, Inc.

The Curtis Center
Independence Square West
Philadelphia, PA 19106

Library of Congress Cataloging-in-Publication Data

Shelley, Walter B. (Walter Brown), 1917–
Advanced dermatologic therapy.

Bibliography: p.
1. Skin—Diseases—Treatment. I. Shelley, E. Dorinda. II. Title. [DNLM: 1. Skin Diseases—therapy. WR 650 S545a]
RL110.S54 1987 616.5′06 86-6638
ISBN 0-7216-1193-1

Acquisition Editor: John Dyson

Production Manager: Frank Polizzano

Manuscript Editor: Agnes Kelly

Indexer: Barbara Hodgson

Advanced Dermatologic Therapy ISBN 0-7216-1193-1

Last digit is the print number: 9 8 7 6 5 4 3 2

To

PETER

Here, my dear son, is a new book for you.

The authors and publisher cannot assume responsibility for any errors in dosage or drug which may have inadvertently entered this book. The reader is advised to check dosages, contraindications, untoward effects, and drug interactions in *Drug Information 86*, American Society of Hospital Pharmacists, Bethesda, MD, issued annually.

Acknowledgments

The Raymon H. Mulford Library of the Medical College of Ohio, the Alfred Taubman Medical Library of the University of Michigan, and the National Library of Medicine in Bethesda, Maryland, provided us with access to all of the scholars who have written of dermatologic therapy.

Georgiann Monhollen skillfully converted the entire manuscript from a nascent holograph to the final triumph of word processing.

Lorene Mehling marvelously minimized the administrative load for the divisional chief to permit time for writing.

John Dyson, medical editor at Saunders, guided us as well as the manuscript and illustrations through the intricacies of printing, proofing, and publication.

Lorraine Kilmer designed the format, typography, and setting in the elegant Saunders tradition.

To each, we bow in deep appreciation and admiration.

TELEPHONE (419) 381-3781

E. DORINDA SHELLEY, M.D.
WALTER B. SHELLEY, M.D.
MEDICAL COLLEGE OF OHIO
3000 ARLINGTON AVENUE
TOLEDO, OHIO 43699

DATE Jan 1, 1987

FOR New Ideas

℞

Read this book!

Sig: Use as directed
prn

REFILL
LABEL

E Dorinda Shelley, M.D.
Walter B. Shelley M.D.

Preface

Successful therapy is the goal of every office visit, clinical inquiry, and diagnostic test. Yet it is a goal not easily reached. This book has been written to offer assistance in reaching that goal. It provides a personalized data-bank of current and effective therapies as perceived by two clinicians engaged in daily practice.

We want this book to enhance your clinical expertise and enlarge your clinical mind. For some of you it will be an aide-memoire, while for others it will be an encounter with new ideas in therapy. But for all, we want this book to be useful.

The book has been written for the professional dermatologist, not the beginner—hence, the title. We assume that you have already made the correct diagnosis and are in quick search of the best therapeutic options. Accordingly, we have tried to present our data succinctly, alphabetized under diagnosis.

Furthermore, we have tried to be selective to avoid producing a mindless, computerized, multi-volumed encyclopedia of all the therapies in print. In making this book discriminant, we have biased it, hopefully in favor of success. We believe that our bias is not provincial, since our backgrounds range from the far East, at the University of Pennsylvania and Dartmouth Medical School, to the far West at Stanford University. Central to all this has been our experience in the Midwest at the Universities of Illinois, Missouri, and Minnesota and the Medical College of Ohio.

We have tried to bring you the best we could discern in referenced journals. Our annotated bibliographies speak to soundness, scope, and hazards. We have tried not only to introduce you to new therapy, but more importantly to give you the confidence to use these new ideas. Prescriptions not written by a timid physician are of no more value than prescriptions not filled by a noncompliant patient.

We have not covered ultra-rare skin disorders or described surgical techniques. We have avoided practice pearls, hints, kitchen recipes, and hallway tips. Nor have we belabored you with myriads of topical remedies and brand names.

We hope the format of this "prescriptionary" will allow you to rapidly scan and smoothly integrate these advanced dermatologic therapeutics with your experience. Finally, we have left space for you to jot down appealing new therapies. Use it to keep your book up to date. We will too.

WALTER B. SHELLEY
E. DORINDA SHELLEY

Contents

Principia Therapeutica

The chaos of therapy yields best to diagnostic and etiologic forces, modulated always by the severity of the disease. Ideally, all therapeutic decisions should be made on the basis of etiology. The ability to discern and eradicate a specific allergen or pathogen is the ideal. Lacking this, we seek a clinical diagnosis to bring order into our therapeutic decision making. Such a diagnosis opens a whole realm of specific and nonspecific therapy. It is the most commonly used guide into the network of patient treatment. It is indeed the guide for this dictionary of current treatment options.

However, the distinction between etiologic and diagnostic approaches to therapy is blurred or erased in actual practice. The clinical mind constantly oscillates between science and art. Observations, laboratory tests, and hypotheses may fail to find a specific cause for which specific treatment can be prescribed. It is in these instances that the diagnosis offers immense help by allowing the clinician to call upon his and his colleagues' experience in a well-defined area. It is a restrictive force that favors intelligent decision making.

The chaos of therapy is diminished not only by etiologic and diagnostic forces but also by the risk management factor. The physician is implicitly interested to make therapeutic decisions that do not burden the patient with an inappropriate risk. It is a sacred trust and sharply focuses one's thinking. Minor problems must not be treated with hazardous major drugs or procedures. Methotrexate should not be prescribed for psoriasis consisting only of scaling of the elbow or pitted fingernails. Accutane should not be considered for the patient with a giant comedone.

Conversely, the risk of the disease must be assessed and factored with the therapy. Major problems deserve major weapons, which invariably involve risk. Minor palliatives need not be considered in patients with major problems. Benzoyl peroxide gel is inappropriate for treating a rodent ulcer. Likewise, Synalar ointment is not the answer for the patient with tumor-stage mycosis fungoides. It is evident that matched consideration of the risk of therapy and the risk of the disease is a third force bringing order out of the chaos of chance selection of treatment.

Risk management demands considerable knowledge about the patient, the disease, and the drug. No therapeutic decision should be made without a careful history. This includes a detailed drug history:

Is the patient allergic to drugs?
Which ones?
What specifically was the nature of the reaction?
When did it occur and how long did it last?
Has that drug been given again?
What drugs have helped?
Which have had no effect?
Which made the problem worse?
Is the patient pregnant?
Are there drugs the patient fears?
Current medications?

Equally essential is full knowledge of the patient's health. Often the patient's adaptation to internal disease or diseases is so complete as to require specific questions. We prefer to do this face to face rather than having him fill out a questionnaire. Often this history time provides oblique glances into the patient's attitudes, background, and psychologic needs, which are invaluable in shaping the therapeutic regimen. It also allows the patient the opportunity to quietly, if not actively, assess the physician. It generally results in a more meaningful evaluation than the patient obtains from looking into a specialist or physician directory. Furthermore, it is a chance for the chemistries of the two agonists to react, both knowing that the reaction product should be a good one if long-term care and association prove necessary. We are reminded of the flow of appreciation of one of our patients who said, "Why, you are the first doctor to sit down with me!" Obviously, she had had only "curbstone" consultations elsewhere.

Knowledge of the particular skin problem the patient presents is equally important in making decisions with regard to therapy. Here again, diagnosis is the invaluable guide. It is the diagnosis that provides the physician with the greatest background on the risks the patient faces. Thus the lesion may be an insignificant vascular growth on the forehead, but when the diagnosis is angiosarcoma, heroic therapy must be contemplated. Nothing substitutes for experience, reading, and conferring with other specialists in making these risk judgments.

The third aspect of risk management is knowing your drug. How effective is it? Does it eradicate the cause? Obviously, we should take more risks with drugs that are curative than with those that are only a "blanket over the fire." Does the drug you have in mind interact significantly with a drug the patient is taking? Ketoconazole can easily elevate the blood levels of cyclosporin and convert it into a toxic drug when the two are given simultaneously. Does the drug have any known interference with the patient's other medical problems? Bactrim almost invariably induces a dermatitis medicamentosa in AIDS patients. Systemic corticosteroids elevate blood sugar in the diabetic. Erythromycin greatly increases blood levels of Theo-Dur, leading to theophylline toxicity.

Although common sense, judgment, and intuition are favorite descriptives for the successful therapist, we feel that these all operate through the vital force of knowledge. Know thy patient! Know thy disease! Know thy drug!

Shuster S: Loneliness of a long distanced reviewer. Br Med J 283:1443–1444, 1981.

"The only excuse for authorship, as distinct from a listing from a computer, is to give an opinion, a way of using things that will help the therapist through the chaos of crude fact."

Siemens HW: General Diagnosis and Therapy of Skin Diseases. Chicago, University of Chicago Press, 1958.

"Learn how to master a small, though sufficient, armamentarium and stick to it, instead of becoming a therapeutic butterfly that sips from one blossom today and tomorrow from another, never really familiar with anything."

Sutton RL, Waisman M: The art of medicine. Cutis 25:357–358, 1980.

—The physician's tone and comments must never be humiliating, derogatory, patronizing, or hypercritical.
—Levity and flippancy are inexcusable. No disease is funny to the patient who has it.

—Before deciding on treatments, undress the patient sufficiently. Use a magnifying lens—touch the skin with your examining hand.
—Patients resent a hurried, impatient, uncommunicative, casual manner, no matter how scientifically superior the physician may be.

Rees RB: The art of dermatology. Cutis 23:625–631, 1979.

We believe in:
—generous free dispensing of samples and special medications
—answering the patient's questions
—rational use of irrational therapy for problems outside the pale of specific therapy
—smiling

Houston WR: The Art of Treatment. New York, Macmillan, 1936.

Some physicians practice psychotherapy (just) as Monsieur Jourdain wrote prose without being aware of it.

Blau JN: Clinician and placebo. Lancet 1:344, 1985.

"The doctor who fails to have a placebo effect on his patients should become a pathologist or an anesthetist."

Petrozzi JW: "Forceful" prescriptions in dermatology. Int J Dermatol 19:83, 1980.

Sell your prescriptions with vigor and enthusiasm.
The erosion of physician enthusiasm with time and experience accounts for loss of placebo effect.

Blackwell B: Drug therapy: Patient compliance. N Engl J Med 289:249–252, 1973.

Remember that up to one half of all the drugs prescribed are really not taken as directed.

Reiser DE, Rosen DH: Medicine as a Human Experience. Baltimore, University Park Press, 1985.

Help on how to forgive yourself for your mistakes.
Help on recognizing and accepting your personal limitations.

Cassell EJ: Talking With Patients. Vol. 1, The Theory of Doctor-Patient Communication; Vol. 2, Clinical Technique. Cambridge, MA, MIT Press, 1985, 223 pp; 200 pp.

Emphasizes value of learning what the patient senses to be the problem, what his worries are, and what an acceptable solution might be.

Zen and the Art of Patient Maintenance

One cannot treat a patient one does not have. Accordingly, essential to all dermatologic therapy is patient maintenance. Here are our meditations on the art of attracting, keeping, and helping patients.

Be Professional

—Sit down.
—Take time.
—Take notes (patients then know that you know).
—Listen carefully.
—Use a loupe.
—Use Wood's light.
—Measure, draw, photograph.
Patients still believe that your supercomputer brain needs assistance.
—Examine irrelevant as well as relevant areas.
This is your best chance for cancer screening. Malignant melanomas are not always a presenting complaint. We recently detected an unrecognized basal cell carcinoma on the upper eyelid that could be seen only when the eye was closed.
—Do KOH, skin tests, biopsy.
—Do blood tests.
Patients often feel the cause can be revealed by blood, urine, and other tests. Moreover, we have discovered more than a few cases of diabetes, hypothyroidism, and hyperlipemia this way.
—Train or select office staff to be courteous, interested, and friendly.

Be Reassuring

—Smile.
—Use the patient's name.
—Touch the patient.
—If it is not cancer, tell the patient at once.
—If it is hair loss and you do not foresee baldness, tell the patient. Allay unexpressed but real fears!

Be Confident

—Let your confidence show you have spent years in training.
—Add to your confidence by acquiring special skills or using special tools.
—Do not use treatments that make you feel uncertain or fearful.
—You can always help a patient in some way.

Be Informative

—Answer the patient's questions, but do not go too far. Some patients want to know only what to do to get well. Others want diagnosis, pathogenesis, prognosis, biology of disease, risks of therapy, statistics on cure rates, treatment for their wife's hand eruption, genetic counseling, and details of appointment hours, as well as how to get their parking ticket validated.

—If you do a blood test, culture, or biopsy, call or write results. Never assume that the patient will return for his next appointment. Never let the patient wonder, "Was the test all right?" Do not let him be annoyed by getting the bill but no "billet" from you.

—Write to the referring physician, the family physician, or both.

—We discourage patients from reading package inserts, the *Physicians' Desk Reference,* handouts, health books, etc., since most of these dramatize the rare idiosyncratic reaction. One of us saw a hospitalized patient die of anaphylaxis after being given two aspirin tablets. Two of our patients suffered fractures as they left our office, and one was killed in an automobile accident on her way to see us. Nonetheless, we still prescribe aspirin and make office appointments. There seem to be no risk-free options in life. Indeed, the patient should know the risk of not treating some lesions. One of our patients is a paraplegic because a large untreated acne cyst on his back ruptured into the spinal column.

Be Therapeutic

—Treat:

Do not just diagnose. It is not enough to say that it is poison ivy or dermatitis and it will heal by itself. Remember, your anxiety is over the diagnosis, but the patient's anxiety is over the treatment.

—Prescribe:

Patients expect a prescription drug, not something over the counter.

—Advise:

Be specific.

Can a drug be taken with meals?

How many times a day should an ointment be applied? Before or after the bath?

Is alcohol contraindicated?

Will the drug sensitize the patient to the sun?

—Tailor treatment to the patient:

Do not use the same treatment as before, unless indicated and requested. Adapt to the desires of the patient.

If the patient wants no cortisone, use no cortisone. Avoid systemic drugs in the elderly or pregnant patient whenever possible.

—Do not give up.

Patients rarely leave doctors who try harder!

Be Smart

—Do not promise too much.

The lawyers wait outside!

—Do not promise too little.

You will wait for the patient to return!

—Do not lose your cool.

Do not let a patient anger or intimidate you. Remember, illness makes children of us all!

—Do not forget that some patients are noncompliant.
Your prescription may never be filled. You may be competing with the barber (barbers were once surgeons).
—Do not let the patient leave without samples.
They are better than green stamps.

Be Impatient

—Share your patients' impatience. Expect some progress, visit by visit. Do not forget, the psoriatic epidermis replaces itself every four to seven days. Do not wait months for results. Switch treatment if you are certain nothing is happening. Objective evidence of new health—nail growth, for example—is simply obtained by measurement. If it does not occur with griseofulvin within a month, switch to ketoconazole.

Be Responsive

—To the patient who complains, "You don't spend any time with me."
Explain how lucky he or she is to be in a group where the doctor does not spend hours groping for the right treatment.
—To the patient who complains, "I've waited an hour."
Give him or her the very first appointment at the next office visit.
Explain that doctor's offices, unlike dental and legal offices, do not reserve and charge for a specific block of time. Overbooking is done at times because some patients do not honor appointments (since they are not charged for failing to show).
Prepare the patient to be prepared for doctors' office waits by having something to read, write, or think about. Also, it is good napping time.
Advise the patient that his tight scheduling of other commitments only leads to ulcers. Sometimes we feel we should have a sign in our waiting room that reads, "If you can't wait to see Doctor Shelley, you can't see Doctor Shelley."
—To the patient who continually complains, "Nothing you do helps."
Give him help in finding another doctor.
—To the patient who wants a "second opinion."
We do not welcome this and feel it is better that the patient get a second doctor. Difficult chronic skin diseases need continuity in physician care and guidance. But remember, some patients like and need a change! Do not chain them to you.

Be Resourceful

Two of our patient histories suffice.

One was a young man who came to our office with the flexural tendon sheath of his left wrist bared. He had purchased instruments at a surgical supply house and attempted to remove the long white "outer-space worms" that had entered his skin. He had already seen four different dermatologists in the space of a week. Each had referred him to a psychiatrist, but to no avail.

We discussed the "worms" with this patient and told him we would have him seen by one of our colleagues who had special experience in this area. We then phoned our consultant psychiatrist who predictably said, "Sure, send him over." Our reply was a demand, "You have to come here or he will see his sixth dermatologist tomorrow." The psychiatrist finally came, gave him an injection of "worm medicine" in our office, and then hospitalized him for proper treatment.

The second patient was a Christian Scientist with the blisters of pemphigus vulgaris over her entire body. Her religious faith forbade medical treatment, and her daughter was distraught with fear. The daughter managed to bring her mother to our office to see me as a friend, not as a doctor. Once there, I proceeded to ask the stoic pemphigus patient if she did not sense that her daughter, who was sobbing, was ill. Once she said that she did, I explained to her that her daughter needed medicine, but that strangely she (the patient) would have to take it. She consulted her Christian Science advisor, who approved as long as the medicine was not for her, but for her daughter's health. We then embarked on a successful long-term course of clearing her pemphigus with oral steroids. At each visit, it was the daughter who was examined, and as her reactive depression improved the dose taken by the mother was gradually reduced. Attention was never paid to the mother's bullae, only to her daughter's assessment of them.

Unusual therapeutic challenges require unusual maneuvers. Look for them and add zest to your practice.

Be Yourself

The longer we practice the more certain we are that, given a choice, patients search out their kind of doctor. Some patients are completely satisfied by the gruff, uncommunicative doctor. Others will go only to the insecure, hesitant young doctor who is "so nice." But, however you practice, whatever your style, if you know how to get your patients well, quickly and safely, you will need no Zen meditations.

Sneddon IB: Then and now. Clin Exp Dermatol 9:3–17, 1984.

An engrossing personal account of dermatologic therapy some 50 years ago, when the treatment could be far worse than the disease. The majority of patients preferred to keep their disorder and failed to return.

Robertson WH: Patient compliance and the short-term treatment regimen. Chemotherapy 28(Suppl 1):80–86, 1982.

To improve compliance:

—Show sincere interest in the patient's illness.
—Watch for personal preferences and idiosyncrasies and consider them in a sympathetic manner.
—Explain—how to use, how long.
—The shorter the treatment regimen the greater the compliance.
—Can the patient afford the cost? Consider proprietary drugs.
—Avoid the Hawthorne effect—of checking.
—Curb overcompliance.
—Walk a tightrope between Scylla of medical authority and Charybdis of medical indifference.
—For the patient who fears drugs, point out there are no risk-free options in life. Disease is risky.

Eraker SA, Kirscht JP, Becker MH: Understanding and improving patient compliance. Ann Intern Med 100:258–268, 1984.

An exquisitely detailed review (169 references) of an increasingly critical area.

To enhance patient compliance:

1. Select therapy that reflects the patient's preferences and past experience with drug intolerance and allergy.
2. Give instructions that are few in number, understandable, and suitably emphasized.
3. Educate the patient regarding the nature and significance of the disease and the drug used.

Cotterill JA: Dermatological games. Br J Dermatol 105:311–320, 1981.

Practice is much more interesting if you observe the games being played by doctors and patients:

Yes, but—

In this game therapeutic advice is accepted by the patient momentarily and then rejected as being impracticable for one reason or another.

Peasant—

Advice at a meeting concerning a patient presented comes forth in great volume from those more anxious to impress their colleagues than to help the patient.

Collusion—

Retreat from a clinical challenge and the patient by having colleagues assist in the clinical load.

NDCD syndrome of Shuster—

Middle-aged physicians produce therapeutic tricks that have worked once, but rarely, if ever, after.

The trick thus qualifies as a "normal distribution curve deficit" and blocks other physicians' skill in distinguishing chance from cause.

See article for 20 more games to play.

Siemens HW: General Diagnosis and Therapy of Skin Disease. Chicago, University of Chicago Press, 1958.

Over 100 pages of therapeutic advice, including the observation that the results of treatment for nonpaying patients, such as relatives, friends, and members of compulsory health insurance plans, are, on the whole, much worse than for those who pay the normal fees.

Barsky AJ III: Hidden reasons some patients visit doctors. Arch Intern Med 94:492–498, 1981.

To find out:

—Ask the patient what he imagines is the cause of his illness.
—Ask how the patient had hoped the doctor might help.
—Ask the dissatisfied patient: Did he want an STS or a screen for AIDS?
—Ask the patient who initiates a visit without any change in clinical status, "What are your current life stresses?" Some life crises are met by adopting a sick role.

Remember, some patients consult doctors for psychologic, social, and informational reasons.

Eraker SA, Politser P: How decisions are reached: Physician and patient. Arch Intern Med 97:262–268, 1982.

Patients with very minor symptoms often visit a physician because of the "regret phenomenon." Should the problem prove significant they do not want to regret their failure to seek help. Awareness of this must enter physician's decision regarding diagnostic tests and therapy.

Graves JE: Taking care of the hateful patient. N Engl J Med 298:883–887, 1978.

A few "hateful" patients kindle aversion, fear, despair, even malice in their doctors. They come in for dreaded stereotypes, and you must not deny or disown the feelings they arouse:

1. Dependent clingers
   Make unlimited demands of the physician, often with flattery.
   Must be told early of your limits of knowledge, skill, time, and stamina!
2. Entitled demanders
   Have equally profound needs, but use intimidation, devaluation, and guilt induction to push you beyond your limits. You must avoid debates with the patient. Simply reiterate the theme of acceptance—that the patient deserves and will get first-rate care.
3. Manipulative help rejecters
   Are "crocks" who return time and again to report "no help." When one symptom is relieved, another appears. Keep your distance, not too far, yet not too close. Assure them that they will get first-rate medical care.
4. Self-destructive deniers
   Are those who find pleasure in actively combating the physician's attempts to save their lives. If possible, secure psychiatric assessment for treatable depression. Avoid excessive affection or anxiety on your part.

Franks RD: The angry patient. Am Fam Physician 24(11):123–125, 1981.

To deal with covert as well as overt *expressions of hostility*:

—Allow the patient to have control over as many nonessential aspects of the problem as possible.
—Share your experience with other physicians to reduce your own feelings of hostility and frustration.
—Consider referral to a colleague.

Ouslander JG: Drug therapy in the elderly. Ann Intern Med 95:711–722, 1981.

—Manage without drugs as often as possible.
—Use smaller doses.
—Pay attention to impaired intellect, poor vision, and hearing when instructing the patient and labeling prescriptions.
—Check that the patient can afford and get prescriptions and can open the container.
—Monitor frequently for compliance, drug effects, reactions, and toxicity.
—Seek help of relatives, friends, visiting nurses, and pharmacists.

Naish JM: Problems of deception in medical practice. Lancet 2:139–142, 1979.

They exist. It is best to look upon the deceivers, cheats, self-mutilators, and child harmers not as patients but as fellow humans, poor deluded people trying to say something at a nonverbal level and to get some sort of payoff. Only then do we perceive and record the truth.

Lynfield YL: Choosing and using a vehicle. J Am Acad Dermatol 10:56–59, 1984.

A study of 29 volunteers established that an ounce of a cream, ointment, or lotion would cover the entire body when self-applied thinly. (Avoid prescribing too much, or it will stay on the clothing if not in the tube. In this regard, it is said that Heinz made his fortune from the catsup left on the plate!)

What to Do When You Don't Know What to Do, or the "Doctor in a Corner"

What do you do when the lodestone of diagnosis points to a specific treatment, but that treatment proves to be ineffectual? What do you do when your diagnostic lodestone points to no specific therapy? What do you do when you have no diagnosis, no lodestone?

Enlarge Your History Base

—Take a medical-student–type history, not one attuned to a specific diagnosis.
—Be sympathetic to the patient's views as to the cause or treatments used.
—Do not turn off valuable advice by indifference or by acting amused by the patient's naiveté or ignorance.
—Keep an open mind.
Remember, the patient may have an answer even if it is not in the medical literature.
—*Review* the drugs taken.
Drug eruptions are the great imitators, so it is impossible to cross-examine too often. We had one patient about to have a craniotomy who had failed to tell more than a score of doctors that she was taking vitamin A in medical dosage, because she did not think it was a medicine. Another patient was hospitalized five times for attacks of erythema multiforme, each induced by a laxative she "forgot" to mention until the last attack.
—Review the pets, their diseases. We have found a number of patients for whom treatment had to be directed toward the pet's mites or fleas, rather than the patient.
—What were the best treatments, the worst treatments?
—Get help from relatives, siblings, neighbors, others.
—Recheck occupation and all hobbies.
We saw a four-year-old girl with a facial eruption misdiagnosed as seborrheic dermatitis. Awareness that she was an equestrienne led to detection of tinea faciei and successful treatment. In another instance, a year had to pass before the mystery of a contact dermatitis was solved. Every year a grandfather encountered oak sawdust while making toy doll houses for Christmas.
—Keep probing.

Examine Skin on Subsequent Visits

—Never fail to check for tinea pedis, despite the patient's assertion that the feet are healthy. A lifetime of noninflammatory fungal scaling is always considered normal by the patient.
—Piecemeal examination of the skin is better accepted by most patients than a total body skin scan. In any event, encourage the patient to show you any skin sites that have even questionable lesions.
—Have the patient come in immediately if there is any real flare-up. Sometimes this is the only way to see the primary lesion and make the diagnosis. We

had one patient with bullous pemphigoid in whom we waited five months for a diagnostic lesion to appear.

Enhance Your Laboratory Data Base

Use tests to broaden your view of possible causes and hence of treatment. Some examples are:

RPR
ANA
ASO
CEA
IgE
Blood chemistry profile
T_3, T_4
Serum iron, zinc
Serum protein electrophoresis

Entertain New Skin Tests

—Biopsy
H & E, immunofluorescence
immunoperoxidase
electron microscopy (transmission and scanning)
culture
—KOH scales
if it scales, do a KOH culture
—Patch tests
scout tray, contactants, perfumes, shoe tray
—Intradermal
bacteria, mites, fleas, *Trichophyton, Candida,* tuberculin

Enter Home or Factory

On-site inspection is valuable. We recall visiting the home of a patient who had to be hospitalized two times for a severe contact dermatitis. All tests had been negative, but on seeing her kitchen in which everything was stainless steel, we discovered her cure—eliminating all contact with the stainless steel *polish* she had used. In another instance, it was the silk wall covering that caused chronic urticaria and fevers, never a suspect in the patient's mind. The physician's index of suspicion is enhanced in the patient's environment.

Enlist Your Colleagues' Help

Consultant review assists in treatment, especially in the fields of peripheral vascular disease, plastic surgery, endocrinology, and gastroenterology.

Talk to or write to people with special expertise. Send slides or photos.

Educate Yourself in the Library

Do a specific search of the last three years of *Index Medicus* listings under your diagnostic heading. Do not be afraid of foreign journals (they usually have English summaries). The cited articles will bring you a world-class symposium on treatment and are guaranteed to produce novel approaches.

Research your texts for ideas (see Introductory section, The Compleat Therapist's Bookshelf).

DRUG THERAPY

Wart treatment with anthralin. Flindt-Hansen H, et al. **Acta Derm Venereol (Stockh)** 1984;64(2):177-9

Treatment of localized scleroderma and lichen sclerosus with etretinate. Neuhofer J, et al. **Acta Derm Venereol (Stockh)** 1984;64(2):171-4

The cutaneous effects of glucocorticoids. Cooper TW, et al. **Adv Exp Med Biol** 1984;171:73-80 (49 ref.)

Rational use of topical corticosteroids. Sherertz EF, et al. **Am Fam Physician** 1984 Jan;29(1):262-6

Acute febrile neutrophilic dermatosis (Sweet's syndrome). Response to dapsone. Aram H. **Arch Dermatol** 1984 Feb; 120(2):245-7

Oral isotretinoin therapy. Use in a patient with multiple cutaneous squamous cell carcinomas and keratoacanthomas. Levine N, et al. **Arch Dermatol** 1984 Sep;120(9):1215-7

Response of transient acantholytic dermatosis to photochemotherapy. Paul BS, et al. **Arch Dermatol** 1984 Jan;120(1):121-2

Treatment of cutaneous sarcoidosis with isotretinoin. Waldinger TP, et al. **Arch Dermatol** 1983 Dec; 119(12):1003-5

Successful treatment of lichen nitidus [letter] Wright S. **Arch Dermatol** 1984 Feb;120(2):155-6

Variations in skin photosensitization during repeated oral 8-methoxypsoralen medication. Jansén CT, et al. **Arch Dermatol Res** 1983;275(5):315-7

Studies on the therapeutic effect of Wratizolin in selected dermatoses. Michałowski R, et al. **Arch Immunol Ther Exp (Warsz)** 1983;31(5):649-54

Clinical studies on the effectiveness of Wratizolin in the treatment of some dermatoses. Szarmach H, et al. **Arch Immunol Ther Exp (Warsz)** 1983;31(5):655-61

Results of Wratizolin treatment of selected skin diseases with particular reference to those of viral etiology. Wąsik F, et al. **Arch Immunol Ther Exp (Warsz)** 1983;31(5):645-8

Topical corticosteroids. Gambrill J, et al. **Aust Fam Physician** 1984 Jan;13(1):45-7 (10 ref.)

The effect on adrenal axis function of topically appli- betamethasone valerate ointment 0.1%. Fischer GO. **Australas J Dermatol** 1983 Apr;24(1):26-32

Benoxaprofen and the skin [editorial] Allen BR. **Br J Dermatol** 1983 Sep;109(3):361-4

PUVA treatment of scleromyxoedema. Farr PM, et **Br J Dermatol** 1984 Mar;110(3):347-

Two cases of distinctive chroni-

Engage Your Conscious and Subconscious in the Search for Therapy

Think, think, think!

Some of our best ideas come from being forced to think. Do not practice the "decerebrate" dermatology that Sam Shuster abhors. Make hypotheses and build therapy out of them; e.g., dermatitis herpetiformis in the sulfa-sensitive patient is a real challenge. By hypothesizing that cholestyramine, an ion-exchange resin, could block absorption of an offending allergen, we were able to conceive of and demonstrate its usefulness in dermatitis herpetiformis.

By viewing progressive, ascending telangiectasia as a vasodilation analagous to rosacea, we found that tetracycline and ketoconazole could be of real help.

The subconscious is equally valuable in catching dream sequences and allowing the mind to pole-vault into new therapeutic territories. But if the patient's problem never is allowed to enter your subconscious, do not expect miracles. We suspect it was our subconscious that allowed us to find the cure of nicotinic acid for the photosensitivity that had rendered one of our patients a complete sun recluse for seven years. Certainly there was no dermatitis, dementia, or diarrhea that would signal pellagra, although his history revealed a partial gastrectomy and generally poor diet.

Escape from the Therapeutic Paralysis of Diagnostic Overload

Making a diagnosis may be more satisfying intellectually than therapeutically. Downplay the diagnosis and focus on the real cause by asking four "What if" questions.

1. What if the actual cause is an infection?
   Look for foci of infection—otitis, pharyngitis, sinusitis, dental abscesses, cholecystitis, cystitis, vaginitis.
   If no direct evidence or clues are found, treat *empirically* with short two-week courses of systemic:

Erythromycin	Metronidazole
Tetracycline	Dapsone
Bactrim DS	Griseofulvin
Clindamycin	Ketoconazole

   Promote immune response enhancement with cimetidine, zinc, and iron.

2. What if the cause is an allergen?
   Trial elimination of *all* medicines. That includes cough drops, nasal sprays, laxatives, tranquilizers, and anything you can get in a pharmacy
   Insist on a trial of a monastic life with no pets, wool, dust, cigarettes, or *alcohol* of any kind.
   Trial vacation from work, home, hobby, or even climate

3. What if the skin problem reflects metabolic or systemic disease?
   Probe for evidence of an underlying problem that requires treatment.
   Secure blood profile, sedimentation rate, CRP, ANA, CEA, serum protein electrophoresis.
   Consider radiographic studies of chest and bowel and liver/spleen scan, as well as CAT scan and studies with ultrasound and NMR.
   Correct vitamin, dietary deficiencies.

4. What if the diagnosis is misleading?
   Consider and search for the great imitators:

sarcoidosis	leprosy
lupus erythematosus	drug eruption
syphilis	factitial dermatitis

Eventually, Be Adventuresome

—Use something new
Chance favors the therapist who will do something.
—Do not demand positive cultures and antibiotograms before prescribing an antibiotic.
The causal organism may not even grow in vitro.
—Do not wait for FDA approval of a drug for a specific indication.
The FDA's job is to protect the public; yours is to help your patient.
—Do not fear lawsuits.
After all, you can be sued as readily for doing nothing as for doing something.

Envoi

If you still do not know what to do next after reading this chapter, read it again. Remember, you are never in trouble if you know what to do next.

Berger SA: The use of antimicrobial agents for noninfectious diseases. Rev Infect Dis 7:357–367, 1985.

Don't limit your use of antimicrobials to proven infections, since many of these drugs are also effective anti-inflammatory agents as well as having action against the immune system.

Brody H: The lie that heals: The ethics of giving placebos. Ann Intern Med 97:112–118, 1982.

A lie is not necessary. The placebo effect comes from any physician-patient relationship that makes the illness understandable, that instills a sense of caring and support, and that increases a feeling of control over the course of the disease.

Aram H: Colchicine in dermatologic therapy. Int J Dermatol 10:566–569, 1983.

Use if for:
psoriasis
palmoplantar pustulosis
Behçet's dermatitis herpetiformis
collagen vascular disorders
vasculitis
Sweet's syndrome

Roenigk RK: Cutaneous cryosurgery. Minor Med 67:617–621, 1984.

Lists 29 diseases for which cryosurgery has been used.

Chow AW, Jewesson PJ: Pharmacokinetics and safety of antimicrobial agents during pregnancy. Rev Infect Dis 7:287–313, 1985.

Penicillins, especially ampicillin, are proven to be the safest antibiotics for use during pregnancy. Erythromycin is also free of teratogenicity and other adverse effects.

Cunliffe WJ, Miller AJ (eds): Retinoid Therapy. Boston, MTP Press, 1983.

The new retinoids will revolutionize dermatologic therapy.

Tkach JR: My quick route to a tough diagnosis. Medical Economics, July 8, 1985, pp. 101–107.

The specifics on how to use the National Library of Medicine data bank MEDLINE and thereby tap into the six million articles from 3200 biomedical journals dating back to 1966. It took 30 minutes to write his search strategy, 5 minutes at the computer, and he had what he wanted in abstracts immediately.

Dau P: Therapeutic plasma exchange: Dermatologic applications. Dermatol Clin 1:571–589, 1983.

Therapeutic plasma exchange has been shown to be helpful in the following:

1. Behçet's syndrome
2. Bullous pemphigoid
3. Dermatitis herpetiformis
4. Dermatomyositis
5. Herpes gestationis
6. Leprosy, Lucio's phenomenon
7. Pemphigus
8. Polychondritis
9. Porphyria cutanea tarda
10. Psoriasis
11. Pyoderma gangrenosum
12. Scleroderma
13. Systemic lupus erythematosus
14. Vasculitides

Kronick DA: The Literature of the Life Sciences: Reading, Writing, Research. Philadelphia, ISI Press, 1985, 219 pp.

A delightful survey of how to enter and use the world of knowledge awaiting you in books and journals: Limit your reading to the relevant. Keep a personal information file—notes, tear outs, copies.

Page EH, Wexler DM, Guenther LC: Cyclosporin A. J Am Acad Derm 14:785–791, 1986.

Cyclosporin A (Sandimmune, 300–450 mg/day, up to 10–20 mg/kg) has been shown to be helpful in the following:

1. Psoriasis
2. Pemphigus
3. Bullous pemphigoid
4. Behçet's disease
5. Dermatomyositis
6. Sézary syndrome (pruritus)

The drug acts by producing reversible suppression of both humoral and cell-mediated immunity. Blood levels must be monitored because of nephrotoxicity.

The Compleat Therapist's Bookshelf

The Drugs

McEvoy GK: American Hospital Formulary Service Drug Information 86. Bethesda, MD, American Society of Hospital Pharmacists, 1986.

Absolutely indispensable, comprehensive 1968 page analysis of all drugs used in the United States. Authoritative but unreferenced details on chemistry, stability, pharmacology, pharmacokinetics, uses, cautions, toxicity, drug interactions, laboratory test interferences, dosage, administration, and brand names of all available forms.

Reynolds JEF: Martindale: The Extra Pharmacopoeia, 28th ed. London, The Pharmaceutical Press, 1982.

Invaluable, highly referenced annotations on all aspects of drugs.

Bickers DR, Hazen PG, Lynch WS: Clinical Pharmacology of Skin Disease. London, Churchill Livingstone, 1984.

The formulae, chemistry, metabolism, and mode of action of all drugs used by dermatologists.

Mater JP, DeGroot AC: Unwanted Effects of Cosmetics and Drugs Used in Dermatology. 2nd ed. New York, Elsevier Science Publishing, 1985.

A standard reference updated.

Dukes MNG: Side Effects of Drugs. Annual 7. Amsterdam, Excerpta Medica, 1983.

Gives references and data on more than 61 drugs causing allergic skin reactions.

The Diseases

Madden S (ed.): Current Dermatologic Therapy. Philadelphia, WB Saunders Co., 1982, 637 pp.

More than 190 clinicians describe current approaches to more than 250 skin diseases.

Arndt KA: Manual of Dermatologic Therapeutics. 3rd ed. Boston, Little, Brown & Co, 1983, 347 pp.

A very popular practical manual of specific therapy with current costs of medication given.

Provost TJ, Farmer ER (eds): Current Therapy in Dermatology 1984–1985. St. Louis, CV Mosby Co., 1984, 279 pp.

Ninety-five clinicians present personal unreferenced essays on how they treat 88 skin diseases.

Rook A, Parish LC, Beare JM: Practical Management of the Dermatologic Patient. Philadelphia, JB Lippincott Co., 1986, 304 pp.

A distinguished international group of 82 dermatologists pair off to give a balanced account of how to treat 81 disorders of the skin.

Landow RK: Handbook of Dermatologic Treatment. Greenbrae, CA, Jones Medical Publications, 1984, 219 pp.

A personal introductory text on therapy.

Polano MK: Topical Skin Therapeutics. New York, Churchill Livingstone, 1984, 197 pp.

The classic on topical therapy of all kinds.

Pettit JHS, Parish LC: Manual of Tropical Dermatology. New York, Springer-Verlag, 1984, 260 pp.

How to treat 29 fungal, parasitic, and bacterial diseases that can travel from the tropics to your office.

Rook A, Dawber R: Disease of the Hair and Scalp. London, Blackwell Scientific Publications, 1984, 571 pp.

Authoritative, comprehensive, classic.

Baran R, Dawber RPR (eds): Diseases of the Nails and Their Management. London, Blackwell Scientific Publications, 1984, 469 pp.

If it's in the nails, it's in this book.

Alexander JO: Arthropods and Human Skin. New York, Springer-Verlag, 1984, 422 pp.

One of the great books in dermatology with exquisitely detailed therapeutic advice. We stand in admiration and awe of Alexander the Great.

The Disciplines

Epstein E, Epstein E Jr.: Skin surgery, 6th ed. Philadelphia, WB Saunders Co., 1987, 900 pp.

The Bible.

Schultz BC, McKinney P: Office Practice of Skin Surgery. Philadelphia, WB Saunders Co., 1985, 183 pp.

The practical.

Stegman SJ, Tromovitch TA: Cosmetic Dermatologic Surgery. Chicago, Year Book Medical Publishers, 1984, 198 pp.

The specialized.

Zacarian SA (ed): Cryosurgery for skin cancer and cutaneous disorders. St. Louis, CV Mosby Co., 1985, 329 pp.

The cold.

Goldschmidt H (ed): Physical Modalities in Dermatologic Therapy: Radiotherapy, Electrosurgery, Phototherapy. New York, Springer-Verlag, 1978, 290 pp.

The old.

Morison WL: Phototherapy and Photochemotherapy of Skin Disease. New York, Praeger Publishers, 1983, 151 pp.

The new.

Arndt KA, Noe JM, Rosen S (eds): Cutaneous Laser Therapy: Principles and Methods. New York, John Wiley & Sons, 1983, 241 pp.

The newest.

Frost P, Horwitz SN (eds): Principles of Cosmetics for the Dermatologist. St. Louis, CV Mosby Co., 1982, 367 pp.

The cosmetic.

Ratz JL: Lasers in Cutaneous Medicine and Surgery. Chicago, Year Book Medical Publishers, Inc., 1986, 142 pp.

The latest.

Sources and Resources

This is our whole skin catalogue.

Allergens

Therapeutic and diagnostics, intradermal insect, house dust, foods, molds, pollens (trees, grasses, weeds), venoms, epidermals, smuts, and individual requirements.

Hollister-Stier Laboratories
Box 3145
Spokane, WA 99220
(509) 489-5656

Bacterial Vaccines

General

Ribi Immuno Chem Research, Inc.
P.O. Box 1409
Hamilton, MT 59840
(406) 363-6214

Mixed Respiratory Vaccine

Hollister-Stier Laboratories
Box 3145
Spokane, WA 99220
(509) 489-5656

Staphage Lysate

Delmont Laboratories
P.O. Box AA
Swarthmore, PA 19081
(215) 543-2747

Cosmetics

Who's Who in Cosmetic Development. Cosmetics and Toiletries 99:29-63, 1984.

Names the companies, vice presidents, and products.

Hypoallergenic Cosmetics

Almay Inc.
P.O. Box 748
Apex, NC 27502
(919) 362-7422

Cover-up Cosmetics

Covermark by Lydia O'Leary
1 Anderson Avenue
Moonachie, NJ 07074
(201) 460-7713

Dermablend Corrective Cosmetics
P.O. Box 601
Farmingdale, NJ 07727
(201) 938-7272

Cotton Clothing

The Cotton Company
P.O. Box 631
Chattanooga, TN 37401
(800) 421-4548

Janice Corporation
198 Rt 46
Budd Lake, NJ 07828
(800) JAN-ICES

Cotton Gloves

Photography supply shops stock these.

Cryosurgery

Frigitronics of Connecticut, Inc.
770 River Road
Shelton, CT 06484
(800) 243-2974

Drug Samples

Physicians' Desk Reference, 40th ed., 1986.
Medical Economics Co., Inc.,
Oradell, NJ 07649.

See Manufacturers' Index, pp. 1–24, for phone numbers.

Electrolysis Equipment

Lucy Peters International, Ltd.
150 East 58th Street
New York, NY 10155
(212) 486-9740

This whole system is available to the doctor on a franchise basis.

Electrosurgical Equipment

Ellman International Mfg.
1135 Railroad Avenue
Hewlett, NY 11557
(800) 835-5355

Elmed, Inc.
60 West Fay Street
Addison, IL 60101
(312) 543-2792

Bovie Products
Sybron Corporation
P.O. Box 23245
Rochester, NY 14692
(716) 385-7800

Flotation Support (Decubitus ulcer)

Support Systems International, Inc.
4349 Corporate Road
Charleston Heights, SC 29405
(803) 747-8002

Jobst Institute, Inc.
653 Miami Street
Toledo, OH 43605
(419) 698-1611

UHI Corporation
2464 Mariondale Avenue
Los Angeles, CA 90032
(213) 227-6161

Foundations and Groups for Patient Help and Information

American Academy of Dermatology
1567 Maple Avenue
Evanston, IL 60201
(312) 869-3954

Dermatology Foundation
1563 Maple Avenue
Evanston, IL 60201
(312) 328-2256

Dystrophic Epidermolysis Bullosa Research Association, Inc. (DEBRA)
2936 Avenue W
Brooklyn, NY 11229

Gluten Intolerance Group
Elaine Hartsock, Ph.D.
P.O. Box 23053
Seattle, WA 98102

Herpes Resource Center
American Social Health Assoc.
Palo Alto, CA
(415) 328-7710

Lupus Foundation of America
11921 A Olive Road
St. Louis, MO 63141
(314) 872-9036

National Alopecia Areata Foundation
P.O. Box 5027
Mill Valley, CA 94941

National Ichthyosis Foundation
Belmont, CA
(415) 591-1653

National Lupus Foundation
5430 Van Nuys Boulevard
Suite 20
Van Nuys, CA 91404

National Neurofibromatosis Foundation
70 West 40th Street
New York, NY 10018
(212) 869-9034

National Pediculosis Association
P.O. Box 149
Newton, MA 02161
(617) 969-5623

National Psoriasis Foundation
6415 S.W. Canyon Court
Suite 200
Portland, OR 97221
(503) 297-1545

National Self-Help Clearinghouse
City University of New York
33 West 42nd Street
New York, NY 10036

National Tuberous Sclerosus Association, Inc.
P.O. Box 159
Laguna Beach, CA 92652
(312) 869-3954

Skin Cancer Foundation
475 Park Avenue, South
New York, NY 10016

United Scleroderma Foundation
P.O. Box 350
Watsonville, CA 95077
(408) 728-2202

General Supplies

Dermatologic Lab and Supply Company
201 Ridge Avenue
Council Bluffs, IA 51501
(800) 831-6273 for catalogue, e.g.,
- 33-gauge needles
- KOH 20 per cent in DMSO
- Anagen hair dye
- Fungal culture media
- Monsel's solution
- Cotton glove liners
- Sealskin psoriasis suits
- 40 per cent urea paste for nail removal
- Methotrexate
- Evening-primrose oil
- Potassium permanganate

Lasers

Coherent Medical, Inc.
3270 West Bayshore Road
Palo Alto, CA 94303
(415) 858-2250

Xanar, Inc.
2868 Janitell Road
Colorado Springs, CO 80906
(303) 576-7050

Literature Search

—Index Medicus at your Medical Library

—MEDLINE
Medlars Management Section
8600 Rockville Pike
Bethesda, MD 20209
(800) 638-8480

—Derm R_x (therapy data) on-line computer
American Academy of Dermatology
1567 Maple Avenue
Evanston, IL 60201
(312) 869-3954

Occlusive Wear

Nylon Wear

Sleep Sauna
404 Westview
Elkins Park, PA 19117
(215) 635-3922

Occluwear Vinyl Occlusive Suits

Simmons Company
P.O. Box 3193
54 Shallowford Road
Chattanooga, TN 37404
(615) 622-1308

Sealskin Psoriasis Suits

Dermatologic Lab and Supply Company
201 Ridge Avenue
Council Bluffs, IA 51501
(800) 831-6273

Instruments

Mill-Bilt Equipment Company
2145 West Central Avenue
Toledo, OH 43606
(419) 472-7292

Roboz Surgical Instrument Company
1000 Connecticut Avenue, N.W.
Washington, DC 20036
(202) 393-1234

Diogenes Surgical Instruments, Inc.
P.O. Box 149
Staten Island, NY 10304
(212) 667-6021

They sell The Hand Engine.

Robbins Instruments, Inc.
2 North Passaic Ave.
Chatham, NJ 07928
(201) 635-8972

Precision Dermatological Instruments, Inc.
1440 South State College Boulevard
Anaheim, CA 92806
(714) 533-6811

George Tiemann & Company
21-45th Road
Long Island City, NY 11101
(212) 361-2012

Miltex Instruments Company
6 Ohio Drive
Lake Success, NY 11042
(516) 775-7100

Iontophoresis

R.A. Fischer Company, Inc.
517 Commercial Street
Glendale, CA 91203
(818) 241-1178

General Medical Company
1935 Armacost
Los Angeles, CA 90025
(213) 820-5881

Patch Test Kits and Supplies

Standard, Fragrance, Vehicle, and Preservative

Dermatology Services, Inc.
P.O. Box 192
Evanston, IL 60204

Screening Sets and Individual Allergens, Including Vegetation and Trees

Hollister-Stier Laboratories
Box 3145
Spokane, WA 99220
(509) 489-5656

Photobiologic Equipment

Derma Control, Inc.
P.O. Box 28
Dolton, IL 60419
(312) 841-4240

Elder Pharmaceuticals, Inc.
705 East Mulberry Street
P.O. Box 31
Bryan, OH 43506
(800) 537-4294

R.A. Fischer Company, Inc.
517 Commercial Street
Glendale, CA 91203
(818) 241-1178

National Biological Corporation
1532 Enterprise Parkway
Twinsburg, OH 44087
(800) 338-5045

Ultralite Enterprises, Inc.
277 Industrial Park Drive
Atlanta, GA 30245
(800) 241-7506

Uvatec, Incorporated
13135 Ventura Blvd.
Suite 306
Studio City, CA 91604
(818) 995-6071

Waldmann Lighting Company
1714 S. Wolf Road
Wheeling, IL 60090
(312) 520-1060

Photographic Equipment

Lester A. Dine, Inc.
100 Milbar Avenue
Farmingdale, NY 11735
(516) 454-6100

International PhotoMed Corporation
3800 W. El Segundo Blvd.
Suite 202
P.O. Box 354
Hawthorne, CA 90250–0354
(800) MD-PHOTO [637-4686]

Prescriptions: Unusual Compounding

Pharmacists Specializing in Dermatologic Compounding and Mail Order Business

Barclay Prescription Pharmacy
18th and Spruce Streets
Philadelphia, PA 19103
(215) 735-1410

Cambridge Chemists, Inc.
702 Madison Avenue
New York, NY 10021
(212) 838-1884

Custom Dermatologic Compounding
3601 S.W. Second Avenue
Gainesville, FL 32607
(904) 377-5200

Shoes, Sensitizer-Free

The Alden Shoe Company
Taunton Street
Middleboro, MA 02346
(617) 947-3926

Dermapedic shoes.

Walk-in Shoe Co.
Schuylkill Haven, PA 17972
(717) 385-0100

Rubber-free box toes.

For other companies see:

Fisher AA: Contact Dermatitis, 3rd ed. Philadelphia, Lea & Febiger, 1986.

Support Stockings and Other Support Devices, Including Venous Pressure Gradient

Jobst Institute, Inc.
Box 653
Toledo, OH 43694
(419) 698-1611

Surgical Gloves, Hypoallergenic

Allerderm Laboratories
P.O. Box 931
Mill Valley, CA 94942
(415) 381-0106

Elastryn gloves.

Wig Maker for Children's Wigs

Beau Velle
114 East Second Street
Covington, KY 41011
(606) 291-3211

UVL Protective Glasses and Screens

Yorktowne Optical Company, Inc.
Industrial Park
P.O. Box 276
Emigsville, PA 17318
(800) 233-1990

Recreational Innovations
P.O. Box 159
South Lyon, MI 48178
(313) 769-5565

Solar Screen Transparent
Window Coverings
53-11 105th St.
Corona, NY 11368

Noir sunglasses.

Your Own Diagnostic Lab

Belsey R, Baer D, Sewell D: Laboratory test analysis near the patient. Opportunities for improved clinical diagnosis and management. JAMA 255:775–786, 1986.

Provides detailed data on addresses and phone numbers of 65 company sources for laboratory equipment and supplies for doing tests in your own office:

urinalysis test systems
blood cell counters
sedimentation rate systems
coagulation tests systems
chemistry analyzers
pregnancy tests
microbiology culture systems
immunodiagnostic systems

Acanthosis Nigricans

Retin-A
Accutane
Periactin
Ortho-Novum

Here is a marker for internal disease, calling for consultation with the endocrinologist and internist. The majority of patients have either an endocrine disease or a tumor secreting an ectopic epidermotropic peptide. All will benefit from identification and definitive treatment of the underlying cause. This may range from surgical treatment of polycystic ovaries to gastrectomy for adenocarcinoma of the stomach.

If the cause is not found or cannot be corrected, symptomatic treatment with topical Retin-A cream or systemic Accutane may be tried. In some instances Periactin has been found to be helpful. In most idiopathic cases obesity is a common finding and may presage the late development of diabetes. Programs for weight loss are appropriate, but are no magic therapeutic wand. The patient should be cautioned that scrubbing the areas will not remove the thickened epidermis but will only accentuate the problem.

All in all, acanthosis nigricans calls for early and continuing endocrinologic study, as well as early and continuing monitoring for the presence of tumors. To do less is to ignore the call of acanthosis nigricans for help.

Brown J, Winkelmann RK: Acanthosis nigricans: A study of 90 cases. Medicine 47:33–51, 1968.

A comprehensive survey underscoring the need for searching out and eliminating the cause: In 20 of the 90 cases endocrine disease was demonstrable, 17 were associated with malignant disease, 6 were familial, 2 were due to nicotinic acid, and the rest remained unexplained, except for obesity.

Rigel DS, Jacobs MI: Malignant acanthosis nigricans: A review. J Dermatol Surg Oncol 6:923–927, 1980.

Gastric carcinoma was present in 55 per cent of the 227 cases of acanthosis nigricans reported in the literature to be associated with internal malignant disease. Secretion of hormones by a tumor is thought to cause the skin changes.

Flier JS: Case records of the Massachusetts General Hospital. N Engl J Med 306:1537–1544, 1982.

Case report of a 15-year-old black girl with acanthosis nigricans and virilization associated with hyperthecosis and type A insulin resistance. Acanthosis nigricans is a marker for a subset of women with hyperandrogenism and marked insulin resistance, as demonstrated by the presence of very high levels of plasma insulin (with or without diabetes). Ten of 200 patients with hyperandrogenism had acanthosis nigricans in addition to hirsutism. All were overweight and had polycystic ovaries, but none showed diabetes or virilization. The skin change was not attributable to elevated androgen levels,

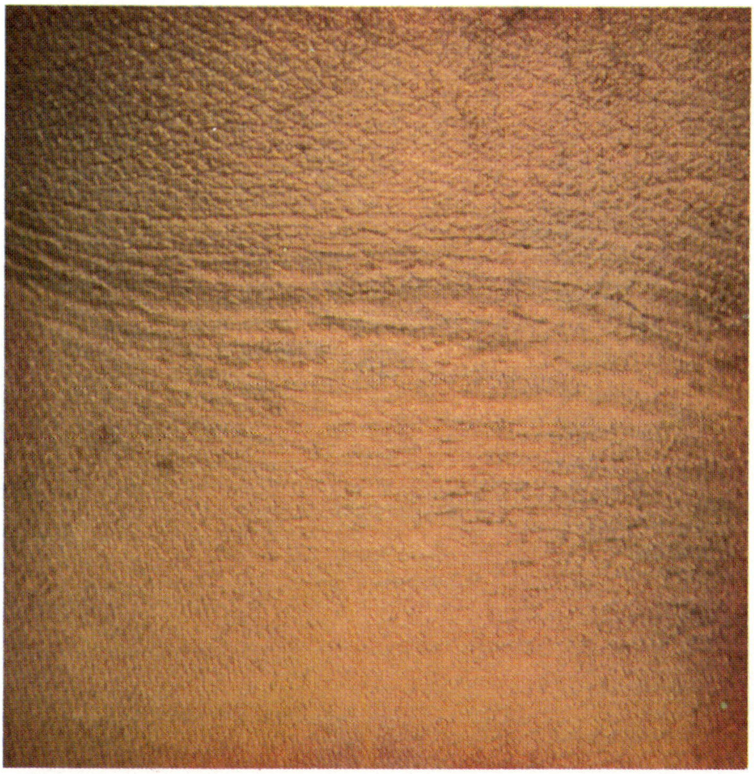

but was associated with insulin resistance and high plasma insulin levels. It might reflect the role of insulin as a nonspecific growth factor.

Sturner RA, Denning S, Marchase P: Acanthosis nigricans and autoimmune reactivity. JAMA 246:763–765, 1981.

Acanthosis nigricans may predate a variety of classic autoimmune diseases, such as systemic lupus erythematosus, scleroderma, and insulin-resistant diabetes (type B, i.e., with autoantibodies to insulin receptors). Long-term follow-up is advisable.

Nordlund JJ, Lerner AB: Cause of acanthosis nigricans. N Engl J Med 293:200, 1975.

Crude bovine pituitary extract injections bid for six weeks induced reversible mild acanthosis nigricans experimentally in one subject, suggesting that an unidentified peptide secreted by the pituitary or underlying neoplasm (ectopic hormone production) may be responsible for this disease.

Field JB, Johnson P, Herring B: Insulin-resistant diabetes associated with increased endogenous plasma insulin followed by complete remission. J Clin Invest 40:1672–1683, 1961.

Acanthosis nigricans, insulin-resistant diabetes, and polycystic ovarian disease present for three years showed spontaneous remission in an 18-year-old black woman.

Randle HW, Winkelmann RK: Steroid-induced acanthosis nigricans in dermatomyositis. Arch Dermatol 115:587–588, 1979.

Three cases occurring one to 16 years after the start of steroid treatment. One case did not involute until 10 years after the steroid was stopped.

Curth HO: Acanthosis nigricans following use of oral contraceptives. Arch Dermatol 111:1069, 1975.

One case in which acanthosis nigricans developed in a patient after 10 years of taking oral contraceptives and disappeared five years after the contraceptive was discontinued.

Banuchi SR, Cohen L, Lorincz AL, Morgan J: Acanthosis nigricans following diethylstilbestrol therapy: Occurrence in patients with childhood muscular dystrophy. Arch Dermatol 109:545–546, 1974.

Two brothers receiving diethylstilbestrol (5 mg/day) developed acanthosis nigricans after seven months. Do estrogens play a role in the development of acanthosis nigricans?

Elgart ML: Acanthosis nigricans and nicotinic acid. J Am Acad Dermatol 5:709–710, 1981.

A 21-year-old man developed acanthosis nigricans after six months' treatment with nicotinic acid, 2 to 4 gm/day, for schizophrenia. Complete endocrinologic and cancer work-up was normal. The lesions cleared gradually within three months of the stopping of the nicotinic acid.

Givens JR, Kerber IJ, Wiser WL, Andersen RN, Coleman SA, Fish SA: Remission of acanthosis nigricans associated with polycystic ovarian disease and a stromal luteoma. J Clin Endocrinol Metab 38:347–355, 1974.

Benign acanthosis nigricans can occur in association with:

Cushing's disease
acromegaly
Stein-Leventhal syndrome
Laurence-Moon-Bardet-Biedl syndrome
Prader-Willi syndrome
diabetes mellitus
congenital lipodystrophy

Cites case of 17-year-old girl with acanthosis nigricans, hirsutism, and amenorrhea in whom Ortho-Novum 2 mg (**norethindrone** 2 mg and **mestranol** 0.1 mg) induced complete remission of acanthosis nigricans and suppression of hyperandrogenism.

Bar RS, Muggeo M, Roth J, Kahn CR, Havrankova J, Imperato-McGinley J: Insulin resistance, acanthosis nigricans, and normal insulin receptors in a young woman: Evidence for a postreceptor defect. J Clin Endocrinol Metab 47:620–625, 1978.

Report of a 15-year-old girl with acanthosis nigricans, polycystic ovarian disease, and marked insulin resistance. Ovarian wedge resection resulted in improvement of acanthosis nigricans, onset of menses, and normalization of peripheral levels of androgens but not of insulin resistance, suggesting that separate factors are responsible for acanthosis nigricans and insulin resistance.

Estrogen therapy resulted in initiation of menses and improvement of acanthosis nigricans in two other patients with type A insulin resistance, without alteration of insulin resistance.

Imperato-McGinley J, Peterson RE, Sturla E, Dawood Y, Bar RS: Primary amenorrhea associated with hirsutism, acanthosis nigricans, dermoid cysts of the ovaries, and a new type of insulin resistance. Am J Med 65:389–395, 1978.

Acanthosis nigricans in a 15-year-old girl with amenorrhea and hirsutism diminished following excision of 80 per cent of ovarian tissue. Plasma androgen levels also returned to normal. One year later the acanthosis nigricans became worse, as plasma testosterone and androstenedione increased.

Levin SR, Hofeldt FD, Becker N, Wilson CB, Seymour R, Forsham PH: Hypersomatotropism and acanthosis nigricans in two brothers. Arch Intern Med 134:365–367, 1974.

In two brothers with acromegaly and very elevated growth hormone levels there was little change in the acanthosis nigricans after pituitary surgery, despite a drop in growth hormone levels.

Hage E, Hage J: Malignant acanthosis nigricans—a para-endocrine syndrome? Acta Derm Venereol 57:169–172, 1977.

Acanthosis nigricans subsided in a 71-year-old woman when her gastric carcinoma was excised, despite metastases. Enterochromaffin-like tumor cells of the APUD series of endocrine cells were present, which presumably secreted polypeptide or amino hormones that possibly were responsible for the acanthosis nigricans.

Curth HO: Malignant acanthosis nigricans. Arch Dermatol 102:479–481, 1970.

Remarkable example of acanthosis nigricans persisting for years after excision of a leiomyoma of the stomach and squamous cell carcinoma of the bladder, and nephrectomy for transitional cell carcinoma of one kidney. Later excision of an adenocarcinoma of the sigmoid colon was followed by immediate disappearance of the acanthosis nigricans. No recurrence in subsequent 5 years in an 89-year-old man.

Moral: To achieve cure you must excise the responsible hormone-secreting tumor, not just any tumor.

Hellerstrom S: Zur Kenntnis der Acanthosis nigricans. Weitgehende Rückbildung der Hauterscheinungen nach Kastration. Acta Derm Venereol 14:86–98, 1933.

A classic case of cure by castration a half-century ago: a 38-year-old patient with severe diabetes and with familial, juvenile acanthosis nigricans.

Katz RA: Treatment of acanthosis nigricans with oral isotretinoin. Arch Dermatol 116:110–111, 1980.

Accutane (2 to 3 mg/kg/day) for four months cleared acanthosis nigricans in a 33-year-old woman who also had hirsutism, irregular periods, obesity, and adult-onset diabetes. Stopping medication was followed in two months by full recurrence. Long-term maintenance required 2 mg/kg/day.

Montes LF, Hirschowitz BI, Krumdieck C: Acanthosis nigricans and hypovitaminosis A. Response to topical vitamin A acid. J Cutan Pathol 1:88–94, 1974.

Retinoic acid ointment 0.1% bid resulted in marked improvement of extensive acanthosis nigricans in two weeks and complete clearing in four weeks. A controlled study of one case (a teenage girl with familial syndrome: deafness, steatorrhea, bowel diverticula, loss of gastric motility, peripheral sensory nerve demyelinization, acanthosis nigricans, and hypovitaminosis A).

Greenwood R, Tring FC: Treatment of malignant acanthosis nigricans with cyproheptadine. Br J Dermatol 106:697–698, 1982.

Cyproheptadine (Periactin 4 mg tid) cleared acanthosis nigricans in three weeks in a 52-year-old man with adenocarcinoma of the stomach (treated four months previously with palliative gastrectomy).

Curth HO: Benign acanthosis nigricans. Arch Dermatol 91:412–413, 1965.

Simple subsection of lesions on the posterior area of the neck provided help to a 15-year-old white male with congenital acanthosis nigricans.

Tromovitch TA, Jacobs PH, Kern S: Acanthosis nigricans–like lesions from nicotinic acid. Arch Dermatol 89:222–223, 1964.

Nicotinic acid (4 gm/day) taken to lower the cholesterol level induced acanthosis nigricans after four months in a 42-year-old man with xanthomas. The acanthosis nigricans disappeared two months after the medication was stopped, then reappeared when therapy with it was reinstituted.

Katzenellenbogen I: Dermatoendocrinological syndrome due to diethylstilbestrol. JAMA 161:1695–1696, 1956.

Thirteen adults who handled diethylstilbestrol pellets made for caponizing cockerels and three children who presumably ingested poultry containing the drug developed acanthosis nigricans along with symptoms and signs of estrogen absorption. All signs disappeared two to three months after cessation of contact.

Crikelair GF, Cosman B: Histologically benign, clinically malignant lesions of the head and neck. Plast Reconstr Surg 42:343–354, 1968.

Dermabrasion of acanthosis nigricans lesions was helpful in a 14-year-old patient.

Sure, you can't turn sugar to gold, but you can give it a golden brown color using a little heat treatment. Help the patient accept reality by improving it.

Acne Vulgaris

Tetracycline	Vitamin A
Benzoyl peroxide	Accutane
Erythromycin	Dapsone
Clindamycin	Motrin

No treatment should be prescribed for an acne patient until you have a detailed history of prior treatment and its successes and its failures. To obtain this you cannot be a passive stenographer. You must query and cross-examine. You must ask directly about internal as well as external remedies. You must ascertain the details of the patient's cleansing routine. What is history at work and at home regarding exposure to greases, oils, and cosmetics? You must explore the patient's ideas as to what makes the acne worse, what helps. You must learn what worries him or his family regarding treatment. Does he want to avoid antibiotics? Is he hoping you will prescribe Accutane? You should discuss dietary habits. Do certain foods make the problem worse? Be alert to the patient's pet therapies. One of our patients recently found that the application of urine was helpful, so we were able to please her by prescribing urea lotion. It is extremely important in the initial and subsequent interviews to know your patient.

Acne treatment is best when it is specifically formulated on a personalized data base that includes both knowledge of the drugs available and knowledge of the patient. It is not likely that you will create patient bonding or any sense of excitement if you mindlessly write Desquam-X 10 for a patient who has used a variety of "oxy 10" OTC preparations with no help. The care and management of acne patients are an important part of any dermatologic practice. They must not sink into a "decerebrate" routine. With constant, mutual education of patient and physician it can be both stimulating and challenging. Nearly all of these patients deeply appreciate your intense personal interest in their facial well-being. If you please the patient, you have the "placebo effect" already working for you.

Although most of the patients we see have inflammatory acne, some show only comedones and noninflammatory papules. For these we advise the avoidance of greasy makeup, the frequent use of a soap such as Neutrogena acne-cleansing soap or Safeguard, and a trial with Retin-A cream 0.01 per cent. We recommend that the Retin-A cream be used sparingly on a trial patch initially, instructing the patient that it is not to be used if marked inflammatory change occurs. We do not prescribe it for atopic individuals or for patients with "sensitive" skin. We instruct the patient that several months may be required for obvious therapeutic benefits. If the patient has reached skeletal maturity we often prescribe Aquasol A (50,000 IU tid), pointing out that benefits will not be seen for six weeks.

In the more common inflammatory forms, a systemic antibiotic is a must. We prescribe Minocin (100 mg hs) unless the history we have taken would caution otherwise. We expect noticeable improvement in two weeks. If it has not occurred, our second-line antibiotic is erythromycin (250 mg qid). Again, this failing, we consider ampicillin (250 mg qid) or Bactrim DS (1 tablet hs). If all of these have failed or are contraindicated, we prescribe a short course of clindamycin (150 mg qid), advising immediate stopping if diarrhea ensues. Always we expect to see some lessening of tenderness and new lesions within a few weeks. If this occurs we persist with the drug for several months, gradually lowering the dosage. It is at times remarkable how low the dose of tetracycline can be and still be effective. We have had some patients who were able to lower the dose to 250 mg every seventh day, but not discontinue it without risking relapse. Recall that the sebaceous gland recycles every eighth day. Conversely, if tetracycline is not effective in a dosage of 1 gm/day, it may be prescribed as 2 gm/day with marked improvement in certain individuals.

Topically, we favor benzoyl peroxide in low percentage, such as Desquam-X 2.5 gel (2.5 per cent gel), increasing the strength as the skin acquires tolerance. It is also available in a face mask for 20-minute application (Neutrogena acne mask). We may alternatively or alternately use the topical clindamycin or erythromycin preparations (Cleocin T, A T S), always watching for signs of irritation from overtreatment. In the patient who cannot take antibiotics orally or who has severe cystic acne, we favor Vleminckx's solution compresses (diluted one to ten in very warm water 15 minutes once daily, wear rubber gloves, well-ventilated room). This is a sovereign remedy for those who will accept the malodor. A lesser version is Vlemasque, used as a facial mask for 20 minutes daily. Lastly, Akne-mycin ointment (erythromycin 2 per cent) is very helpful.

For the patient with severe inflammatory scarring or nodulocystic acne, the advent of the retinoids heralds a new era just as sulfanilamide did for patients with pneumonia. Accutane (13-*cis*-retinoic acid, or isotretinoin) is the first drug ever to consistently clear this type of acne. Furthermore, if given in adequate dosage (1.0 mg/kg, i.e., 40 mg bid, four to five months) it not only clears but cures the acne in a large percentage of patients. A second course may be required, but this again is all that is necessary. Since acne is a disease of abnormal keratinization and sebum secretion, this drug that inhibits sebum is remarkably specific. Patients are invariably grateful for the disappearance of the unpleasant seborrhea as well as the acne lesions. However, the side effects of cost, cheilitis, hyperlipidemia, and teratogenicity all enter into decision making in regard to Accutane. For patients in whom Accutane is not advisable, we generally prescribe Dapsone (100 mg/day), which is remarkably effective in combating severe cystic acne, although its hemolytic effect must be monitored.

Since acne is an inflammatory disease, it is not surprising that low-dose prednisone (5 to 10 mg/day) and dexamethasone (0.25 to 0.5 mg/day) and the nonsteroidal anti-inflammatory drugs (such as Motrin 600 mg qid) are beneficial. For women who are antibiotic resistant, the contraceptive Enovid-E (mestranol 100 μg and norethynodrel 2.5 mg) is sometimes dramatically effective. For the patient who has premenstrual flares of her acne, we advise the antihistamine Teldrin (chlorpheniramine). This is available without prescription and is taken for two weeks before each period (Teldrin 12 mg hs).

There are many peripheral approaches to acne treatment, often styled to the mutual pleasure of the patient and the doctor. We like to mechanically express any cosmetically dominant comedones (Schamberg extractor, narrow opening, microepisiotomy with No. 11 scalpel blade if difficult to express). We incise, drain, and sometimes pack large cysts. We like to inject very small amounts of Kenalog-10 suspension (dilute half strength to 5 mg/cc with saline) into selected cysts. We mourn the loss of that truly effective systemic antibiotic chloramphenicol, due to the risk-benefit consideration. We strongly advise no milk or nuts for our patients in their late teens or older, while always stressing a balanced diet and sensible rules of rest and recreation. Exam time is always a particularly hazardous period for acne flares, so we increase the antibiotic dosage at these times. We encourage patients to keep their hands off the acne by pointing out, "It belongs to somebody else."

Once the acne is gone, but the scars remain, we encourage patients to await the reconstruction of skin ("The red is the scaffolding for new skin"). In a few, dermabrasion is valuable, and in others collagen injections (Zyderm) may help. All of these are specialized procedures best known to those who employ them regularly. We hope that the prudent use of Accutane will obviate the need for them.

None of our approaches to acne is fixed or rigid. We like to improvise, to change, to learn from the patient and our colleagues. All in all, the care of acne patients has always been an adventure into every aspect of dermatologic management.

Frank SB (ed): Acne: Update for the Practitioner. New York, Yorke Medical Books, 1979, 280 pp.

Authoritative source for details on modern therapy: systemic antibiotics and topical **vitamin A acid**, **benzoyl peroxide**, **erythromycin**, **clindamycin**, and **tetracycline**.

Cunliffe WJ, Cotterill JA: The Acnes: Clinical Features, Pathogenesis and Treatment. Philadelphia, WB Saunders Co., 1975, 306 pp.

Superb comprehensive survey of how to control acne with contraceptives, steroids, peeling agents, antibacterials, surgery, ultraviolet light, intralesional injections, and psychotherapy. Concerning the last, "It is quite possible to discuss at some length with a demanding, obsessional acne sufferer the improvement or otherwise of one particular papule."

Plewig G, Kligman AM: Acne: Morphogenesis and Treatment. New York, Springer-Verlag, 1975, 333 pp.

A visual delight of colored pictures and the best possible aid for teaching patients and oneself.

Don't forget that acneiform eruptions can be caused by:

- —iodides and bromides
- —isonicotinic acid hydrazide
- —corticosteroids and ACTH
- —vitamin B_{12}
- —phenytoin
- —trimethadione
- —phenobarbital

Reisner RM: An overview of acne treatment. *In* Frank SB (ed): Acne: Update for the Practitioner. New York, Yorke Medical Books, 1979, pp 114–120.

It is during the critical formative interchange of the first visit that the bonds of mutual trust and understanding are formed. Spend time. Explain the disease to the patient, as well as what can and cannot be done. You will need the patient's (and family's) understanding and cooperation in the months or years to come.

Marks R: Acne: Advice on Cleaning Your Skin. New York, Arco Publishing, 1984.

For the patient who asks, "What can I read?"

Litt JZ: McDonald's acne. Arch Dermatol 110:956, 1974.

Acne was due to hot grease and cooking oil exposure of teenagers working in fast-food hamburger shops. It appeared suddenly (often in summer) and cleared dramatically when the job ended. Do you know what your patient is doing?

Kenyon FE: Psychosomatic aspects of acne. Br J Dermatol 78:344–351, 1966.

Explain to your patient that temporary exacerbations may occur following emotional stress.

Eady EA, Holland KT, Cunliffe WJ: The use of antibiotics in acne therapy: Oral or topical administration? J Antimicrob Chemother 10:89–115, 1982.

A monographic review of everything you could want to know about antibiotics and acne. Front-line attack is **tetracycline** orally and **clindamycin** topically. Includes extensive discussion of the following antibiotics:

oral		topical	
	—tetracycline		—tetracycline
	—erythromycin		—erythromycin
	—clindamycin		—clindamycin
	—co-trimoxazole (Bactrim, Septra)		—chloramphenicol

Lane P, Williamson DM: Treatment of acne vulgaris with tetracycline hydrochloride: A double-blind trial with 51 patients. Br Med J 2:76–79, 1969.

Statistically significant benefit from **tetracycline** (250 mg bid) for three months.

Hubbell CG, Hobbs ER, Rist T, White JW: Efficacy of minocycline compared with tetracycline in treatment of acne vulgaris. Arch Dermatol 118:989–992, 1982.

This six-month double-blind study of 49 patients with grade 2 and grade 3 acne found that both drugs were safe and effective. After six weeks, clearing occurred in twice as many patients in the **minocycline** (Minocin 100 mg/day) group as in the **tetracycline** (500 mg/day) group.

Nordin K, Hallander H, Fredriksson T, Rylander C: A clinical and bacteriological evaluation of the effect of sulphamethoxazole-trimethoprim in acne vulgaris, resistant to prior therapy with tetracyclines. Dermatologica 157:245–253, 1978.

Bactrim (**sulfamethoxazole** 400 mg and **trimethoprim** 80 mg bid) produced excellent results in 79 per cent of 42 patients after 6 to 18 weeks.

Shore RN: Usefulness of ampicillin in treatment of acne vulgaris. J Am Acad Dermatol 9:604–605, 1983.

A gram a day kept the acne away in 100 patients.

Cunliffe WJ, Cotterill JA: Clindamycin as an alternative to tetracycline in severe acne vulgaris. Practitioner 210:698–700, 1973.

Clindamycin (150 mg/day) gave marked improvement within one month in 90 per cent of a group of 67 patients.

Leyden JJ: Choice of antibiotics: Management of antibiotic-resistant acne. *In* Frank SB (ed): Acne: Update for the Practitioner. New York, Yorke Medical Books, 1979, pp 198–205.

For the patient with inflammatory acne who fails to respond to antibiotics: Use the Wood light to examine the tongue for yellowish green fluorescence to confirm compliance in taking **tetracycline**. Use Wood light to examine the nose and paranasal area for coral red follicular fluorescence to rule out malabsorption or noncompliance. Review history for:

1. Use of cosmetics, topical corticosteroids, anticonvulsants, systemic steroids
2. Acute emotional stress with concomitant seborrhea

3. Leaning on or squeezing acne areas
4. How and how often the patient washes

Shalita AR, Cunningham WJ, Leyden JJ, et al: Isotretinoin treatment of acne and related disorders: An update. J Am Acad Dermatol 9:629–638, 1983.

Isotretinoin (Accutane), the A bomb for acne, used in more than 200,000 patients by mid 1983, will result in dramatic clearing and often permanent remission of severe inflammatory acne when given in a dosage of 1.0 mg/kg/day for four to five months. Lower dosages risk relapse. Watch for musculoskeletal aches, pancreatitis, and pseudotumor cerebri, as well as liver function abnormalities and elevated triglyceride levels.

Cunliffe WJ, Jones DH, Holland KT, et al: 13-Cis-retinoic acid in acne—Mechanism of action. *In* Cunliffe WJ, Miller AJ (eds): Retinoid Therapy. A Review of Clinical and Laboratory Research. Boston, MTP Press, 1984, pp 255–266.

Accutane works effectively against four etiologic factors in the pathogenesis of acne:

1. Reduces sebum production
2. Reduces ductal hyperkeratinization
3. Reduces inflammation
4. Reduces bacterial flora indirectly

Kligman AM, Mills OH Jr, Leyden JJ, et al: Oral vitamin A in acne vulgaris. Preliminary report. Int J Dermatol 20:278–285, 1981.

By three to four months, one half of a group of 136 patients receiving 300,000 to 400,000 U/day of water-solubilized **vitamin A** (retinol) showed an excellent response. The dose was then reduced to a maintenance level, and control continued. Relapse occurred within a few months of stopping treatment. Side effects included headache, cheilitis, xerosis, and minor nose bleeds.

Darley CR, Moore JW, Besser GM, et al: Low dose prednisolone or oestrogen in the treatment of women with late onset or persistent acne vulgaris. Br J Dermatol 108:345–353, 1983.

In a study of 38 women, four months of treatment with either **prednisolone** (2.5 mg each morning, 5.0 mg each evening) or **ethinyl estradiol** (30 μg/day) coupled with **medroxyprogesterone acetate** (5 mg on days one to seven of each calendar month) gave significant improvement. The steroid acted by suppressing ACTH-dependent androgen secretion, while the estrogen effectively increased the serum sex hormone–binding globulin that binds (and thereby sequesters) androgen.

Hindson C, Lawlor F, Wacks H: Benoxaprofen for nodular acne. Lancet 1:1415, 1982.

Dramatic involution of acne nodules of the chest, back, abdomen, and buttocks was seen in 17 males taking the nonsteroidal anti-inflammatory agent **benoxaprofen** (600 mg/day for 1 month). A second one-month course was given to some patients after an interval of one month. Must watch for photosensitivity, onycholysis, and jaundice.

Wong RC, Kang S, Heezen JL, et al: Oral ibuprofen and tetracycline for the treatment of acne vulgaris. J Am Acad Dermatol 11:1076–1081, 1984.

Another example of help from a nonsteroidal anti-inflammatory drug: Motrin (**ibuprofen** 600 mg qid) was as effective as **tetracycline** (250 mg qid) in treating moderately severe acne in this double-blind study of 60 patients. When used conjointly over a two-month course, Motrin and tetracycline were significantly more effective than either alone.

Michaëlsson G: Oral zinc in acne. Acta Derm Venereol (Suppl 89):87–93, 1980.

Zinc (45 mg elemental zinc tid with food) was of value in the treatment of severe inflammatory acne.

Verma KC, Saini AS, Dhamija SK: Oral zinc sulphate therapy in acne vulgaris: A double-blind trial. Acta Derm Venereol 60:337–340, 1980.

Zinc sulfate (600 mg/day for three months) in a double-blind study of 56 patients resulted in definite improvement in 58 per cent of the patients. Serum vitamin A levels rose significantly in zinc-treated patients. Reviews conflicting data of literature.

Marynick SP, Chakmakjian ZH, McCaffree DL, Herndon JH Jr: Androgen excess in cystic acne. N Engl J Med 308:981–986, 1983.

In 59 women and 32 men with recalcitrant acne, serum levels of dehydroepiandrosterone sulfate were elevated (in women, measure at midmorning seven days after start of menstrual cycle). To lower this, **dexamethasone** (0.5 mg daily) or the oral contraceptive Demulen (**ethynodiol diacetate** 1 mg and **ethinyl estradiol** 50 μg daily) or both were given. Over a six-month period 97 per cent of women and 81 per cent of men had resolution or marked improvement of their acne.

Check JH: Improvement of intractable acne in a man following testosterone suppression using danazol. Cutis 26:393–394, 1980.

Danazol (200 mg qid) suppressed severe antibiotic-resistant acne in a 25-year-old man. Treatment was continued for more than a year, with a moderate flare of acne during a six-week period when the drug was stopped.

Goodfellow A, Alaghband-Zadeh J, Carter G, et al: Oral spironolactone improves acne vulgaris and reduces sebum excretion. Br J Dermatol 111:209–214, 1984.

Although topical antiandrogens are not helpful, the systemic antiandrogen **spironolactone** (200 mg/day for three months) was effective therapy in a double-blind study of 36 patients with severe acne. Use is limited in males because of gynecomastia and impotence associated with long-term treatment.

Hammerstein J, Meckies J, Leo-Rossberg I, et al: Use of cyproterone acetate (CPA) in the treatment of acne, hirsutism and virilism. J Steroid Biochem 6:827–836, 1975.

Acne and seborrhea responded dramatically within three months in women taking the following "reverse sequential regimen" of contraceptive:

—**cyproterone acetate** (100 mg/day) from days 5 to 14 of menstrual cycle
—**ethinyl estradiol** (50 μg) from days 5 to 25 of menstrual cycle

Hirsutism greatly improved in six to nine months. All symptoms of virilism reappeared after the medication was terminated unless an oral contraceptive containing a derivative of **17-acetoxyprogesterone** was given. (A low-dose oral contraceptive, Diane [cyproterone acetate 2 mg and ethinyl estradiol 50 μg in each pill], is available in many countries and is very effective in acne, seborrhea, and androgenic alopecia. See next reference for details.)

Hammerstein J, Moltz L, Schwartz U: Antiandrogens in the treatment of acne and hirsutism. J Steroid Biochem 19:591–597, 1983.

Spironolactone and **cyproterone acetate** (100 mg daily, decreased eventually to 10 to 50 mg daily), which inhibit both androgen production and androgen binding at receptors, were markedly helpful in the treatment of 71 acne patients, but required three to six months of treatment for noticeable benefit. Must exclude androgen-producing tumors prior to treatment. Do not give to pregnant women or males with severe acne unless all other treatments have failed.

Cunliffe WJ, Holland KT: The effect of benzoyl peroxide on acne. Acta Derm Venereol 61:267–269, 1981.

Benzoyl peroxide (5 per cent) in either gel (PanOxyl gel) or lotion (Benoxyl-5 lotion) reduced bacterial flora and surface-free fatty acids in a double-blind study of 48 acne patients over a period of several months.

Burke B, Eady EA, Cunliffe WJ: Benzoyl peroxide versus topical erythromycin in the treatment of acne vulgaris. Br J Dermatol 108:199–204, 1983.

In a double-blind study of 94 patients, **erythromycin** lotion (1.5 per cent) and **benzoyl peroxide** gel (5 per cent) were equally effective in significantly reducing the number of inflammatory acne lesions. However, benzoyl peroxide had the added advantage of also reducing the number of noninflamed lesions.

Shalita AR, Smith EB, Bauer E: Topical erythromycin *v* clindamycin therapy for acne: A multicenter, double-blind comparison. Arch Dermatol 120:351–355, 1984.

Both solutions were effective, and the results were comparable in patients with moderate acne. Of 74 patients treated with **erythromycin** solution (1.5 per cent bid), 73 per cent showed excellent or good responses at 12 weeks, while 62 per cent of 80 patients treated with **clindamycin phosphate** solution (1 per cent bid) showed the same results.

Chalker DK, Shalita A, Smith JG, Swann RW: A double-blind study of the effectiveness of a 3% erythromycin and 5% benzoyl peroxide combination in the treatment of acne vulgaris. J Am Acad Dermatol 9:933–936, 1983.

The combination of **erythromycin** (3 per cent) and **benzoyl peroxide** (5 per cent) (Benzamycin) in a gel was superior to the use of either alone in 165 subjects who applied the medications twice a day for 10 weeks.

Tucker SB, Tausend R, Cochran R, Flannigan SA: Comparison of topical clindamycin phosphate, benzoyl peroxide, and a combination of the two for the treatment of acne vulgaris. Br J Dermatol 110:487–492, 1984.

Topical **clindamycin** (1 per cent solution bid) and **benzoyl peroxide** (5 per cent gel bid) were equally effective. A single daily application of benzoyl peroxide gel in the morning and clindamycin in the evening gave the same results, but helped prevent irritation.

Wechsler HL, Kirk J, Slone J: Acne treated with a topical tetracycline preparation: Results of a one-year multi-group study. Int J Dermatol 17:237–242, 1978.

Topical **tetracycline HCl** in an ethanol-water solution with n-decyl methylsulfoxide (Topicycline) was shown to be helpful in treating inflammatory acne, but not comedonal or cystic acne. The multicenter study of 105 patients over a one-year period eliminated seasonal and other variables.

Knutson DD, Swinyer LJ, Smoot WH: Meclocycline sulfosalicylate: Topical antibiotic agent for the treatment of acne vulgaris. Cutis 27:203–210, 1981.

Use of an **oxytetracycline** derivative in a cream base (Meclan cream 1 per cent bid) resulted in more than a 50 per cent reduction of papules and pustules after 11 weeks in 82 per cent of 351 patients (double-blind study).

Heel RC, Brogden RN, Speight TM, Avery GS: Vitamin A acid: A review of its pharmacologic properties and therapeutic use in the topical treatment of acne vulgaris. Drugs 14:401–419, 1977.

Comprehensive review of **tretinoin** (Retin-A family—retinoic acid, vitamin A acid). Used topically in a cream, gel, or solution, it gives slow improvement in comedonal acne over a two- to five-month period in 75 per cent of patients. The cream and gel forms are less irritating than the alcoholic solution, but all may cause erythema and desquamation in the first month of use. Must avoid mucous membranes and the angles of the nose. Also minimize sun exposure and avoid excessive washing. Order of potency:

1. 0.05 per cent alcoholic solution
2. 0.025 per cent alcoholic gel
3. 0.1 per cent cream
4. 0.05 per cent cream (least potent)

Mills OH Jr, Kligman AM: Assay of comedolytic activity in acne patients. Acta Derm Venereol 63:68–71, 1983.

Retin-A (0.05 per cent solution) reduced the comedone count by 75 per cent in two months, whereas **salicylic acid** solution (5 per cent) reduced it by 40 per cent. In contrast, comedones were unaffected by topical benzoyl peroxide (10 per cent), clindamycin (1 per cent), or sulfur (5 per cent).

Hurley HJ, Shelley WB: Special topical approach to the treatment of acne: Suppression of sweating with aluminum chloride in an anhydrous formulation. Cutis 22:696–703, 1978.

Aluminum chloride hexahydrate (6.25 per cent in absolute ethyl alcohol, Xerac AC) is antibacterial and also effective in reducing the sweat that contributes to bacterial colonization. An open study of 141 patients showed it to be especially valuable in treating inflammatory acne of the back.

Shalita AR: Treatment of mild and moderate acne vulgaris with salicylic acid in an alcohol-detergent vehicle. Cutis 28:556–561, 1981.

A study of 49 patients showed significant reduction in inflammatory lesions and open comedones after one month of treatment with Stri-Dex medicated pads (0.5 per cent **salicylic acid**). This is another useful nonprescription item, in addition to the multiple **benzoyl peroxide** formulations available over the counter.

Milstein HG: 5-Fluorouracil as an aid in management of acne and melasma. J Am Acad Dermatol 4:97–98, 1981.

Efudex cream (5 per cent **5-fluorouracil** bid for two weeks) was observed to be of benefit in control of acne.

Durr NP, Orentreich N: Epidermabrasion for acne: The polyester fiber web sponge. Cutis 17:604–608, 1976.

Use of the "BUF-PUF" to abrade away rough surfaces gave 33 per cent of 285 patients a subjective feeling of improvement. (To paraphrase a song, "I'm going to rub that 'acne' right out of my skin.")

Graham GF: Cryosurgery in the treatment of acne. *In* Epstein E, Epstein E Jr (eds): Skin Surgery, 5th ed. Springfield, Ill., Charles C Thomas, 1982, pp 889–904.

Acne lesions involute within three to four days of treatment with a freezing spray of liquid nitrogen. Cryosurgery is a useful adjunctive measure for management of inflammatory and scarring lesions of acne but not comedones.

Lowney ED, Witkowski J, Simons HM, Zagula ZWJ: Value of comedo extraction in treatment of acne vulgaris. JAMA 189:1000–1002, 1964.

Unilateral expression of open and closed comedones clearly revealed it to be of cosmetic value in the majority of 32 patients. It particularly prevented the development of inflamed lesions on the forehead and helped patients with superficial acne. It did not help cystic acne.

Parish LC, Witkowski JA: The enigma of acne therapy: The acne abscess. Am J Med Sci 254:769–776, 1967.

Intralesional steroids, including **triamcinolone diacetate** (Aristocort intralesional 25 mg/ml) and **betamethasone acetate** (Celestone Soluspan 6 mg/ml) gave complete resolution of acne cysts in about four out of five instances in a study of 234 acne "abscesses" in 85 patients. Use of a tuberculin syringe and 27-gauge needle was superior to a Dermo-jet. Each cyst was injected to the point of distention.

Parrish JA, Strauss JS, Fleming TS, Fitzpatrick TB: Oral methoxsalen photochemotherapy for acne vulgaris. Arch Dermatol 114:1241–1242, 1978.

PUVA (three times/week for two months) given to seven patients with moderately severe acne caused no clinical improvement, but the "tan" made lesions less obvious.

Mills OH Jr, Kligman AM: Drugs that are ineffective in the treatment of acne vulgaris. Br J Dermatol 108:371–374, 1983.

Authors provide a GWAA (Generally Worthless Against Acne) list of 73 drugs and procedures, based on 20 years of their own "eyes-wide-open" observation of acne therapy. Surprises include topical chloramphenicol.

Crounse RG: The response of acne to placebos and antibiotics. JAMA 193:906–910, 1965.

A disturbing double-blind cross-over study comparing the effects on acne of **tetracycline, dimethylchlortetracycline,** and a placebo showed a marked placebo response. Each patient (14 males, 31 females) received each medication for four weeks, and results were evaluated weekly. Duration of study—12 weeks.

Burks JW: Dermabrasion and Chemical Peeling. Springfield, IL, Charles C Thomas, 1979, 236 pp.

For the scars that result when treatment fails or is not sought, surgical dermabrasion is of real value.

Fulton JE: Dermabrasion by diamond fraises revolving at 85,000 revolutions per minute. J Dermatol Surg Oncol 4:777–779, 1978.

Modern-style dermabrasion using Freon 12 for topical anesthesia, continuous lukewarm compresses for two to three days after surgery, and **erythromycin** ointment (1 per cent) for postoperative care.

Klein AW: Implantation techniques for injectable collagen: Two and one-half years of personal clinical experience. J Am Acad Dermatol 9:224–228, 1983.

Shallow saucer-shaped supple acne scars respond best to injectable collagen (Zyderm collagen implant). Recommends horizontal superficial intradermal injections 1/8 inch apart with maximum distention. Improvement persists for more than two and a half years, but "touch-ups" may be needed every six months to maintain full correction.

Remington BK: The Ligmaject for injection of triamcinalone acetonide and collagen. J Dermatol Surg Oncol 10:444, 1984.

A neat cartridge-style, 30-gauge needle unit for injection of collagen into atrophic scars or of steroids into hypertrophic scars and cysts. This special type of syringe was developed for intraligamentary anesthesia by the dental profession. Available from Healthco Dental Company, distributors in North America.

Cunliffe WJ, Clayden AD, Gould D, Simpson NB: Acne vulgaris—Its aetiology and treatment. A review. Clin Exp Dermatol 6:461–469, 1981.

Up to 30 per cent of teenagers develop acne severe enough to need medical treatment. Often a minimum of six months' treatment is needed to produce reasonable improvement. Enthusiasm for treatment, both by the patient and the doctor, is the essential ingredient for success.

Farber GA, Burks JW, Hegre AM, Brown GR: Football acne—An acneiform eruption. Cutis 20:356–360, 1977.

Inflammatory acne under the chin strap of the helmet appears early in the football season. Topical acne cleansers (such as Neutrogena acne-cleansing soap or pHisoHex) and astringents (such as Seba-Nil) used three times a day help decrease morbidity. The most effective treatment is the removal of the chin strap after football season.

Patients like doctors who like them.

Acrodermatitis Chronica Atrophicans

Penicillin
Tetracycline
Streptomycin
Chloroquine

Although Lennkof had demonstrated spirochetes in biopsy specimens of this disease as early as 1948 and penicillin had been shown to be effective, such therapy was considered empiric until recently when erythema chronicum migrans was also shown to be spirochetal in origin. Today penicillin is perceived as the rational treatment for acrodermatitis chronica atrophicans and is given in a dosage identical to that for syphilis. In those instances of penicillin hypersensitivity, alternate use of erythromycin or tetracycline should be equally curative. However, none of these treatments has any effect on the atrophy once this has occurred.

Prophylaxis consists of avoidance of exposure to ticks, since it is their bite that transmits the pathogenic spirochete.

Thyresson N: The penicillin treatment of acrodermatitis atrophicans chronica (Herxheimer). Acta Derm Venereol 29:572–621, 1949.

The classic reference study of 57 cases demonstrating curative effect of **penicillin** (400,000 U/day for two weeks). The fact that the inflammatory element disappeared, but atrophy was not reversible, argues for early institution of treatment.

Frithz A, Lagerholm B: Acrodermatitis chronica atrophicans, erythema chronicum migrans and lymphadenosis benigna cutis—spirochetal diseases? Acta Derm Venereol 63:432–436, 1983.

A triad of penicillin-responsive diseases due to previously unrecognized or unacknowledged spirochetes.

Steigleder GK: Ixodes-ricinus-Spirochäten: wahrscheinlich Ursache der Acrodermatitis Chronica Atrophicans Herxheimer. Dtsch Med Wochenschr 109:3–5, 1984.

Penicillin or **tetracycline** is specific treatment for this disease, which is due to a tick-borne spirochete.

Ludwig E: Über die Wirksamkeit der Antibiotica Streptomycin und Tetracyclin bei der Behandlung der Acrodermatitis atrophicans Herxheimer. Arch Klin Exp Dermatol 201:495–506, 1955.

Streptomycin and **tetracycline**—two antibiotics of proven value.

Huff SE: Acrodermatitis chronica atrophicans: Report of a case treated with chloroquine phosphate (Aralen). Arch Dermatol 72:132, 1955.

Although never given penicillin, a 64-year-old woman showed complete resolution of her lesions (thin pseudosclerodermatous plaques on arms and legs) in six months after taking **chloroquine** (250 mg tid for one week, bid for one week, then once daily).

Never underestimate the power of the body to heal.

Acrodermatitis Enteropathica

Zinc sulfate
Zinc oxide paste

Significant therapy never remains as an isolated report. A striking example of this was Moynahan's discovery that acrodermatitis enteropathica responds to oral zinc sulfate. He reported this in a letter to the *Lancet* in 1974. The 1976 *Index Medicus* listed 15 confirmatory studies, and by 1978 a comprehensive review stated that zinc was unequivocally the treatment of choice for this lethal disease.

And so it is. The thread of observations since acrodermatitis enteropathica was delineated in the 1930s is one of zinc. Mother's milk was beneficial (because of its available zinc). The drug Diodoquin was helpful (a chelate that carried zinc across the gut membrane barrier), and zinc oxide paste favored healing (cutaneous absorption of the vital zinc ion).

All of the patients have had their lives changed and have been given their first chance to reach and enjoy adulthood as a result of zinc sulfate. And as a sequel there is now clinical awareness of the essential nature of this metallic ion in the function of a score of critical cell enzymes. The expanding role of zinc is also being recognized in the pathogenesis of strange dermatitides and resistant infections and in the maintenance of the normal immune response. Most recently there has been recognition of skin changes due to zinc deficiency in patients receiving hyperalimentation and in alcoholics.

Zinc sulfate has all the attributes of an ideal drug: rapidly effective, safe, nonallergenic, available without prescription, and cheap. It should be prescribed for all infants with the signs of acrodermatitis enteropathica or any variant thereof. Furthermore, zinc deficiency should be sought in all patients with dietary aberrations, recalcitrant infections, or erosive disease. This is readily done by determinations of the zinc level, and therapy should be undertaken when appropriate. Public awareness of the essential nature of zinc (even in acne) and its availability in health stores as well as drug stores diminishes the chance of seeing hypozincemic patients. However, the need continues for surveillance of the zinc status of patients in your practice whose problem could be due to a depressed immune capability.

With attention to this, acrodermatitis enteropathica, already an endangered species of disease, should become extinct.

Nelder KH, Hambidge KM, Walravens PA: Acrodermatitis enteropathica. Int J Dermatol 17:380–387, 1978.

Zinc sulfate (50 to 200 mg/day PO with food) is the sovereign remedy, eliciting this timetable of response in the affected infant:

1 to 2 days	behavior improves less irritable takes naps easier to manage

2 to 3 days	normal appetite appears diarrhea abates
2 to 3 weeks	hair growth obvious hair color darkens
3 to 4 weeks	photophobia disappears (zinc allows utilization of vitamin A)
6 to 8 weeks	surge in body growth
8 to 12 weeks	mental ability improves

Moynahan EJ: Acrodermatitis enteropathica: A lethal inherited human zinc-deficiency disorder. Lancet 2:399–400, 1974.

The first note of the dramatic response of nine children to **zinc sulfate** (150 mg/day in divided doses—give with fruit juice).

Dillaha CJ, Lorincz AL, Aavik OR: Acrodermatitis enteropathica: Review of the literature and report of a case successfully treated with Diodoquin. JAMA 152:509–512, 1953.

Discovery of the first specific drug for this disease was an exercise in serendipity. A $2\frac{1}{2}$-year-old girl was initially diagnosed as having epidermolysis bullosa, and the Diodoquin was suggested as a treatment for candidiasis. (No longer available in the United States.)

Aggett PJ, Delves HT, Harries JT, Bangham AD: The possible role of Diodoquin as a zinc ionophore in the treatment of acrodermatitis enteropathica. Biochem Biophys Res Commun 87:513–517, 1979.

Partition studies showing that zinc may be carried across biologic membranes by binding to the chelate Diodoquin.

Aggett PJ, Delves HT, Thorn JM, et al: The therapeutic effect of amphotericin in acrodermatitis enteropathica: Hypothesis and implications. Eur J Pediatr 137:23–25, 1981.

A nine-year-old girl with acrodermatitis enteropathica failed to improve while taking oral **zinc sulfate**. Complete remission was achieved by giving supplemental **amphotericin B** lozenges (10 mg qid for 5 days). Presumably amphotericin promoted absorption of zinc by increasing cell permeability.

Oleske JM, Westphal ML, Shore S, et al: Zinc therapy of depressed cellular immunity in acrodermatitis enteropathica. Am J Dis Child 133:915–918, 1979.

Hyperalimentation-induced acrodermatitis enteropathica and depressed cellular immune response completely resolved in a 4-year-old girl after treatment with **zinc sulfate** (660 mg PO daily).

Ohlsson A: Acrodermatitis enteropathica: Reversibility of cerebral atrophy with zinc therapy. Acta Paediatr Scand 70:269–273, 1981.

Computed tomography showed increased growth of brain (probably due to improved myelination) occurring within two months of institution of zinc therapy (**zinc sulfate** 150 mg/day). Case report of a six-month-old boy, stressing importance of early diagnosis and treatment of acrodermatitis enteropathica.

Steger JW, Izuno GT: Acute zinc depletion syndrome during parenteral hyperalimentation. Int J Dermatol 18:472–479, 1979.

Large oral doses of calcium lactate, short-bowel syndrome, low serum albumin, and long-term intravenous hyperalimentation led to zinc deficiency and subsequent lesions of acrodermatitis enteropathica in a 55-year-old man with adenocarcinoma of the colon. **Zinc sulfate** (20 mg IV/day) resulted in improvement in 72 hours.

Ølholm-Larsen P: Untreated acrodermatitis enteropathica in adults. Dermatologica 156:155–156, 1978.

A 33-year-old man with an undiagnosed papulopustular eruption of the face, dermatitis of the ankles, and depression had received marginal help from a nature healer with a diet rich in beans and vitamins containing zinc 2.5 mg. Excellent response to oral **zinc sulfate** (400 to 800 mg/day).

A 40-year-old woman with depression, muscle rigidity, and a history of flaring of skin lesions during pregnancy improved greatly with zinc sulfate (200 mg tid).

Brenton DP, Jackson MJ, Young A: Two pregnancies in a patient with acrodermatitis enteropathica treated with zinc sulfate. Lancet 2:500–502, 1981.

Zinc is necessary to prevent fetal malformations and must be supplemented during pregnancy in those patients whose children are obligate heterozygotes and may not have normal placental zinc transport. Documents safety of **zinc sulfate** (300 mg/day) during two pregnancies in a patient with this rare autosomal disease. Serum zinc levels fell dramatically during pregnancy, even with the zinc supplementation.

Krieger I, Evans GW: Acrodermatitis enteropathica without hypozincemia: Therapeutic effect of a pancreatic enzyme preparation due to a zinc-binding ligand. J Pediatr 96:32–35, 1980.

Picolinic acid, a bidentate chelating ligand (similar to Diodoquin) present in the pancreatic enzyme Viokase (3 to 4 teaspoons daily = 6.75 to 9.08 gm/day), was presumed responsible for enhancement of zinc absorption and marked improvement in a 12-month-old girl with chronic diarrhea and perianal erythema. **Zinc sulfate** (45 mg elemental zinc daily) was later necessary to maintain clearing. The pancreatic enzyme is also known as Pancreatin in the United States.

Whitmore CW: Probable acrodermatitis enteropathica treated with nystatin (Mycostatin). Arch Dermatol 79:594, 1959.

Nystatin in zinc oxide emulsion applied locally and nystatin (100,000 U qid) given orally produced remarkable clearing in one week in a three-year-old black child.

Parra CA, Smalik AV: Percutaneous absorption of zinc in acrodermatitis enteropathica. Dermatologica 163:413–416, 1981.

Diaper dermatitis in an eight-month-old baby girl was treated twice a day with 25 per cent **zinc oxide** paste (Lassar's paste—25 per cent zinc oxide, 25 per cent starch, 50 per cent petrolatum). Result: Complete control of acrodermatitis enteropathica for over 1½ years. Mechanism: absorption through skin of essential zinc ion.

Has the patient really come to see you about something other than his "chief complaint"? Explore.

Acrodermatitis of Hallopeau

Corticosteroids Antibiotics Methotrexate Nitrogen mustard

Persistence helps with this disease. It is essential that the therapist be persistent, resourceful, and optimistic, or the patient will leave and the disease will continue its chronic course. Our empiric program of attack is initially the use of Diprosone ointment coupled with a systemic antibiotic such as Bactrim DS (one tablet hs). If a response is not evident in a week, we employ a series of topical agents (Loprox cream, Silvadene cream, Fototar, Anthra-derm) in sequence, hunting for the right key. Systemically, Nizoral, Accutane, and Flagyl are given on a trial basis. If this series is without effect, Dapsone (100 mg/day) is given, again on a short trial basis. In the severe cases we use Kenalog (40 mg IM) every three weeks. This invariably helps, but we rarely give the injection more than three times. Our ultimate weapon is methotrexate (25 mg IM or 2.5 mg orally once a day).

The diverse factors that trigger this amazingly recalcitrant disease reaction pattern range from yeast to bacterial sensitization, and in many individuals, it may represent the mystery of focal psoriasis that follows trauma. All this attests to the need for ingenuity and persistence on the part of the therapist.

White MI, Main RA: The treatment of Hallopeau's acrodermatitis. Arch Dermatol 115:235–236, 1979.

A 63-year-old man developed pustules on the fingers of one hand after injuring one finger with a hammer. He received dramatic help within 12 hours, using topical **neomycin** (0.5 per cent) and **nystatin** (100,000 U/gm) in a potent topical steroid cream (**clobetasol propionate** 0.05 per cent bid) applied under occlusion. He had failed to respond to systemic Bactrim and **cloxacillin** as well as topical nitrogen mustard soaks. With the topical cream (Dermolate NN cream—not available in the United States), pustulation stopped and nails regrew.

Arnold HL Jr.: Treatment of Hallopeau's acrodermatitis with triamcinolone acetonide. Arch Dermatol 114:963, 1978.

Use of **triamcinolone acetonide** suspension (60 mg IM, repeat in two weeks) is a very helpful approach.

McDonald RA, Lowe NJ: Mutilating acrodermatitis continua (Hallopeau's acrodermatitis). Arch Dermatol 114:1385–1386, 1978.

Prednisone proved to be the best treatment for this 53-year-old man with psoriasis, mutilation of fingers and toes, and a pustular eruption of the hands and feet. He had no help over 10 years with compresses, local steroids, topical antibiotics, systemic antibiotics, sulfapyridine, zinc sulfate, tar, and light therapy. A severe rebound flare developed after prednisone was stopped.

Lever WF: Acrodermatitis continua (Hallopeau): Effect of treatment with sulfapyridine. Arch Dermatol 49:273–277, 1944.

Early report on specific effectiveness of **sulfapyridine** (3 gm/day). The patient was a 51-year-old woman who had the problem on her thumb for six years. The pustules cleared in a few weeks but recurred whenever sulfapyridine was discontinued.

Konrad K: Acrodermatitis continua suppurativa Hallopeau: Behandlung mit methotrexat. Hautarzt 21:119–123, 1970.

An example of the disease controlled by **methotrexate** (50 mg/week, single oral dose). Recurrence whenever methotrexate was stopped during a $1\frac{1}{2}$-year-period of observation of this 71-year-old patient.

Leigh IM, Gold SC: Acrodermatitis of Hallopeau. Br J Dermatol 101 (Suppl 17):41–42, 1979.

Case report of a 50-year-old man with remarkable glove- and sock-like crusts and pustules and dystrophic nails lifted off by lakes of pus. Although pustules contained *Staphylococcus aureus*, flucloxacillin did not influence pustulation. These authors view the disease as a form of psoriasis, which responded to the new antimitotic drug, **razoxane** (250 mg bid for three days/week). (This piperazine derivative of the chelating agent EDTA is experimental and not available in the United States.)

Notowicz A, Stolz E, Heuvel NVD: Treatment of Hallopeau's acrodermatitis with topical mechlorethamine. Arch Dermatol 114:129, 1978.

For 14 years a 42-year-old woman had acrodermatitis of the fingertips resistant to radiation, tar, fluorinated steroids, and methotrexate soaks. The condition cleared with nitrogen mustard compresses (10 mg/60 ml water bid for two weeks, then 10 mg/120 ml water once daily and later twice a week). **Halcinonide** 0.1 per cent (Halog cream or ointment) was also applied once daily after compression. The skin returned to normal except for the absence of nails, and treatment was continued for seven months.

Baran R: Hallopeau's acrodermatitis. Arch Dermatol 115:815, 1979.

A 55-year-old woman with acropustulosis of one finger of 25 years' duration had complete clearing in one month by local application of **ethylester retinoid solution** (0.075 per cent for 1 week, then 0.05 per cent for 3 weeks).

The force of coincidence decreases in inverse proportion to the number of cures.

H. W. Siemens

Acrodynia

BAL
Penicillamine
Corticosteroids
Avoidance of mercury

Once a common disease, acrodynia is now a rarity. This has happened as a result of Warkany's discovery in 1945 that acrodynia is a form of mercury poisoning. As that seminal observation became public knowledge, mercury disappeared from the teething powders, the ointments, the felt hats, and the preservatives for wood, first by prudence and later by law. With the removal of mercury from the environment, acrodynia became a disease largely of the past. There are still sporadic cases from accidental mercury exposure, but preventive measures remain the best treatment for this most painful disease.

Treatment of the disease itself calls for identification and immediate elimination of exposure to mercury. The element is excreted from the body gradually, but this can be greatly accelerated by giving either penicillamine (250 mg qid) or BAL (5.0 mg/kg/day IM) for a short course. Both of these compounds act by chelating the residual tissue mercury and thereby mobilizing it for rapid excretion with these carrier drugs.

Warkany J: Acrodynia—Postmortem of a disease. Am J Dis Child 112:147–156, 1966.

A classic biography of a disease due to an idiosyncratic reaction to mercury, formerly an essential element in babies' teething powders. Tells story of how acrodynia was conquered without grants, foundations, or research institutes by one man's discovery that mercury was the cause. Profuse sweating and swollen, red, cold, clammy, desquamating hands and feet were the most characteristic symptoms.

McNeil NI, Issler HC, Olver RE, Wrong OM: Domestic metallic mercury poisoning. Lancet 1:269–271, 1984.

Spilling of a half-pint of mercury onto furniture and carpets in a home resulted within a few days in acrodynia in the father and daughter and nephrotic syndrome in the mother, but no symptoms in the son. Successful treatment involved relocation of the family, **penicillamine** (1 gm/day for 1 to 3 weeks), and replacement of the floor and walls of the room before the family moved back.

Matheson DS, Clarkson TW, Gelfand EW: Mercury toxicity (acrodynia) induced by long-term injection of gammaglobulin. J Pediatr 97:153–155, 1980.

Acrodynia developed in a 20-year-old man with agammaglobulinemia who had received 40 to 50 mg of mercury in the Merthiolate preservative used in gamma globulin injections given over 15 years. Treatment with **penicillamine** (2 gm/day) increased urinary excretion of mercury, but no mention is made of the effect on his photophobia, flushed cheeks, or pink pruritic scaly palms and soles.

Meme JS, Brown JD, Kagia J, et al: Mercury poisoning as a cause of acrodynia in Kenya children—A preliminary report. East Afr Med J 58:641–649, 1981.

Fungicides and pesticides used in agricultural areas were the presumed sources of mercury causing acrodynia (pink disease) in 110 children. Abdominal pain, tachycardia, profuse sweating, swollen itchy hands and feet, photophobia, ataxia, and squatting posture were common findings. Severe burning pain sometimes led to chewing off of painful fingers. Multiple courses of BAL and months in hospital were required.

Harris PF: Pink disease. Am J Dis Child 112:165, 1966 (reprinted from Br Med J 1:977, 1966).

Beware of teething powder. In this case a 21-month-old boy had used a teething powder (Steedman's, containing 26.7 per cent mercury) for over a year. The preventive measure was confiscating a gross of these packets at the grocer shop in England that at this late date was still selling this banned item.

Feldman GV: Pink disease. Am J Dis Child 112:165, 1966 (reprinted from Br Med J 1:977, 1966).

Beware of mercurial ointments applied to diaper rash—the cause of two cases of acrodynia.

Prediger V: Auslösung einer Akrodynie durch Aufnahme von Saatbeizmitteln. Monatsschr Kinderheilkd 124:36–37, 1976.

Acrodynia due to tooth powder in a five-year-old boy showed improvement within a week of eliminating the powder and starting **cortisone** therapy (2 mg/kg).

Magrizos C, Remogna M, Leo D, Pilotti G: Osservazioni su di un caso di acrodinia: Intossicazione mercuriale, iperreninemia, iperaldosteronemia. Minerva Pediatr 34:925–928, 1982.

Acrodynia in a two-year-old boy after ingestion of an antihelminthic containing a mercury compound cleared after three months of therapy with **D-penicillamine** and supplemental vitamin B_2, B_6, B_{12} therapy.

Bai KI, Sastry VN, Rao MD, Rao GK: Acrodynia (a case report). Indian Pediatr 16:81–82, 1979.

Prednisolone (5 mg tid), **tetracycline** (250 mg tid), and **vitamin B complex** (2 cc IM daily) were used successfully in the treatment of acrodynia in an eight-year-old girl with pink hands and feet for three days. Although extreme pain was gone in one week, gangrene in the terminal phalanges necessitated amputation of several fingers. Probable source of mercury: native medicine for purgation.

McEvoy GK (ed): American Hospital Formulary Service: Drug Information 86. Bethesda, MD, American Society of Hospital Pharmacists, 1986, pp 1485–1487, 1491–1495.

Two chelating compounds for removal of mercury:

1. BAL in oil, 100 mg/ml (British anti-Lewisite, **dimercaprol**) given in deep IM injection
   Dose (adult): 5 mg/kg IM initially, then 2.5 mg/kg IM bid for 10 days
   Dose (infants and children): 3 mg/kg IM q4h for two days, then q6h for one day, then q12h for seven or eight days.
2. **Penicillamine** (Cuprimine) 250 mg tablets:
   Dose: 250 mg qid (may empty contents of capsule into 15 to 30 ml pureed fruit or juice).

A smile is the best placebo.

Actinic Reticuloid

Solbar plus	Systemic steroids
Diprolene ointment	Nitrogen mustard
Chloroquine	Azathioprine

Few skin diseases lead a man to suicide, but this is one. Years of severe inexplicable sunlight reactions, and scores of disappointing remedies eventuate in deep reactive depressions. These patients with lichenified erythematous plaques of the face and hands and episodes of erythroderma need heroic treatment both to lift them from depression and to abort their steady progression into a cutaneous lymphoma. Nearly all have had the broad spectrum sun screens (Solbar Plus), powerful topical steroids (Diprolene ointment), systemic steroids, and chloroquine.

The time has come for either topical nitrogen mustard or azathioprine (Imuran 150 to 200 mg/day). If it is not that, they are faced with retreat into a black hole of total despair or total darkness. Either way, there can be no sunshine in their lives.

Ive FA, Magnus IA, Warin RP, Wilson Jones E: "Actinic reticuloid": A chronic dermatosis associated with severe photosensitivity and the histological resemblance to lymphoma. Br J Dermatol 81:469–485, 1969.

This severe persistent photosensitivity of unknown cause leads to thickening and ridging of exposed skin, simulating a lymphoma both clinically and histologically. The photosensitivity extends throughout the ultraviolet light spectrum into the visible rays.

The 10 elderly male patients reported here did not respond to topical steroids, sun barrier creams, oral **chloroquine**, **nicotinic acid**, or Grenz ray therapy. The only way to clear the eruption was to confine the patient to a room devoid of natural light and administer systemic steroids. Relapse occurred on re-exposure to sunlight. The ensuing reactive depression was of such severity that 5 of the 10 patients attempted suicide, but only one attempt was fatal.

Marx JL, Vale M, Dermer P, et al: Actinic reticuloid. Arch Dermatol 118:672–675, 1982.

A 58-year-old man with actinic reticuloid showed some improvement by avoiding sunlight, using sun screens (**oxybenzone-dioxybenzone** [Solbar] over **cinoxate-methyl anthranilate** [Maxifil]) and applying **betamethasone valerate** (Valisone ointment 0.1 per cent bid). **Beta-carotene** (180 mg/day) had no effect.

Haynes HA, Bernhard JD, Gange RW: Actinic reticuloid: Response to combination treatment with azathioprine, hydroxychloroquine, and prednisone. J Am Acad Dermatol 10:947–952, 1984.

A 59-year-old man with intractable actinic reticuloid and circulating Sézary cells responded favorably over six weeks to combination therapy with **aza-**

thioprine (Imuran 125 mg/day), **hydroxychloroquine** (200 mg bid), and **prednisone** (40 mg/day).

Protection from UVA and UVB while driving was secured by installing a clear plastic film inside the car windows (E-Z Bond protective film, Solar Screen Transparent Window Coverings, 53-11 105th St., Corona, NY 11368).

Volden G, Falk ES, Wisloff-Nilssen J, et al: Successful treatment of actinic reticuloid induced by whole-body topical application of mechlorethamine. Acta Derm Venereol 61:353–354, 1981.

Topical **nitrogen mustard** (10 mg in 50 ml water, applied to the entire skin once daily for one month) greatly increased tolerance to outdoor light in a 69-year-old man with a four-year history of actinic reticuloid. Two weeks after the treatment was stopped he could tolerate one hour of sunlight.

The therapist walks a tight rope between faith and skepticism, but should he fall, let it be toward faith.

Actinomycosis

Penicillin G	Minocin
Ampicillin	Surgical drainage
Clindamycin	Surgical debridement
Erythromycin	

It is hard to find an antibiotic that is not effective in the treatment of this disease. The causal bacteria, *Actinomyces israelii* and colleagues, are surprisingly sensitive to nearly all antibiotics. Yet the disease is hard to cure. This seems to stem from (1) the patient's immunologic tolerance of this anaerobe as a normal commensal within the oral cavity—an "old friend" that becomes an opportunistic invader and, hence, a pathogen; (2) the dense fibrotic wall surrounding the invading colonies that impedes delivery of antibiotics; (3) the gluelike polysaccharide coating that surrounds the "sulfur granule" colonies and again impedes drug entry.

The therapeutic approach is to use a very high dosage of a well-tolerated inexpensive antibiotic for very long periods. Specifically, the answer is most often penicillin G (10 to 20 million U IV daily for three weeks, then 5 million U/day orally for six months). Less intensive therapy may lead to recurrence. In the event of penicillin sensitivity, clindamycin and minocycline are alternates of proven worth.

Correction of dental problems is equally essential, since a periapical cyst or abscess is often the entry point for the actinomycetes. Simple surgical drainage may suffice, but if bone has been involved, surgical debridement is necessary also. More radical surgery may be necessary in some systemic forms.

A search for predisposing factors such as diabetes mellitus, steroids, neoplasm, or sinusitis may reveal other areas requiring therapeutic measures. From the prophylactic standpoint, avoidance of trauma, good dental care, and routine penicillin therapy after dental extractions will reduce the chance of those normal symbionts of our oral cavity becoming pathogens.

Actinomycosis remains much more of a challenge in recognition than in treatment. But once the therapeutic option is made, keep on treating for a long, long time. Remember, the antibiotic is on its own, with none of the usual help from the patient's immune system (which remains relatively indifferent to whether the actinomycetes are growing on the inside or outside).

Richtsmeier WJ, Johns ME: Actinomycosis of the head and neck. CRC Crit Rev Clin Lab Sci 11:175–202, 1979.

The ultimate reference with everything you could want to know.
Principles of therapy:
- High-dosage antibiotic over a long period
- Surgical drainage, debridement, and excision

Drug of choice:
- **Penicillin** (10 to 20 million U/day IV for three weeks); then

Penicillin V (3.2 to 4.8 million U/day PO for six months, e.g., Pen·Vee K 500 mg [800,000 U] 4 to 6 tabs daily); **probenecid** (Benemid) advisable

Alternates of proven value:

ampicillin	**lincomycin**
cephalosporin	**minocycline**
chloramphenicol	**stilbamidine**
clindamycin	**tetracycline**
erythromycin	**vancomycin**
isoniazid	

Robbins TS, Scott SA: Actinomycosis: The disease and its treatment. Drug Intell Clin Pharm 15:99–102, 1981.

Actinomyces israelii and related species are gram-positive anaerobic, non—acid-fast, filamentous bacteria that may normally grow in the mouth. Following dental extraction or in presence of carious teeth, large numbers enter tissue and establish colonies, which for a long time may escape the attention of the patient or the doctor.

Wallace RJ Jr, Musher DM: Actinomycosis: An update. Int J Dermatol 16:185–187, 1977.

The presenting skin lump and draining sinuses in the jaw, chest wall, or perirectal area call for a search for intraoral or visceral lesions.

Martin MV: The use of oral amoxycillin for the treatment of actinomycosis: A clinical and *in vitro* study. Br Dent J 156:252–254, 1984.

Ten patients with oral and cervical actinomycosis were successfully treated with oral **amoxicillin** (500 mg qid for six weeks) and surgical drainage. A study of 89 strains of *Actinomyces* showed the minimal inhibitory concentration (MIC) to be always below 0.8 μg/ml for amoxicillin, whereas it was 0.05 to 6.0 μg/ml for **benzylpenicillin**. Because of unpredictable absorption, use of oral **penicillin** may not lead to high enough serum values to reach the MIC for some isolates, so that IM or IV injections are preferable. Oral amoxicillin is more convenient for outpatients.

King JW, White MC: Pulmonary actinomycosis. Rapid improvement with isoniazid and rifampin. Arch Intern Med 141:1234–1235, 1981.

Isoniazid (300 mg/day) and **rifampin** (600 mg/day) (combined as Rifamate, 2 caps daily one hour before a meal) gave prompt improvement within two weeks in a 30-year-old man with pleural effusions, nightsweats, and fever. Treatment was switched to IV **penicillin** for two weeks after the diagnosis of pulmonary actinomycosis was established by open lung biopsy. Cure was achieved after 18 months of oral **penicillin V** (500 mg q6h).

van Marion WF, Thompson J, Mouton RP, et al: Successful single antibiotic therapy in Actinomyces septicemia and liver abscess. Infection 10:287–289, 1982.

In a 36-year-old man, cure of actinomycosis was achieved with two months of daily continuous IV **penicillin** (24 million U/day). Unusual aspects of this report:

1. The organism was probably of exogenous origin, i.e., the mouth of a deer that the patient had inspected for dental age. The organism could have penetrated the skin through several small knife wounds incurred while eviscerating the animal.
2. The organism was *Actinomyces bovis*.
3. No surgery was required.

Stenhouse D, MacDonald DG, MacFarlane TW: Cervico-facial and intra-oral actinomycosis: A 5-year retrospective study. Br J Oral Surg 13:172–182, 1975.

A study of 39 cases showed that the acute type rapidly resolves after extraction of any associated dental focus, incision and drainage of the facial swelling, and a three-week course of penicillin.

Perna E, Liguori R, Petrone G, Mannarino E: Actinomycotic granuloma of the gasserian ganglion with primary site in a dental root. J Neurosurg 54:553–555, 1981.

A two-year mystery of episodic right trigeminal area pain in a 25-year-old man was solved by demonstration of an actinomycotic granuloma in the right gasserian ganglion.
Source: periapical actinomycotic osteitis of the right third inferior molar tooth
Organism: *Actinomyces israelii*

Weese WC, Smith IM: A study of 57 cases of actinomycosis over a 36-year-period. A diagnostic "failure" with good prognosis after treatment. Arch Intern Med 135:1562–1568, 1975.

Actinomycosis continues to elude clinicians: Only 4 of these 57 cases had been correctly diagnosed at the time of the patient's admission to a university hospital. Organisms must be found either in biopsy material or in anaerobic cultures. Sulfur granules are not specific for actinomycosis.

The secret of the care of the patient is in caring for the patient.
FRANCIS W. PEABODY

Adiposis Dolorosa (Dercum's disease)

Lidocaine IV	Excision
Tocainide	Liposuction
Mexiletine	

The magic bullet here is lidocaine. Within minutes of a single intravenous dose of lidocaine, these patients note the disappearance of pain that has spoiled their lives for years. One therapist noted that his patient was observed to smile for the first time in 20 years. And the pain does not return for 2 to 12 months. True, the lipomas remain, and pains of other origin are unaffected, but the wonderful relief patients experience is something they thought could be achieved only by magic.

It is exciting to learn that an orally absorbed analogue of lidocaine, mexiletine (Mexitil), has the same remarkable effect as intravenous lidocaine. In this regard, another analogue, tocainide (Tonocard) might also provide a magic pain killer for Dercum's disease that could be given orally.

Atkinson RL: Intravenous lidocaine for the treatment of intractable pain of adiposis dolorosa. Int J Obes 6:351–357, 1982.

An exquisitely referenced classic article on this problem of painful adipose tissue that generally affects obese, asthenic, emotionally disturbed, postmenopausal women.

In this report a 48-year-old woman had three years of complete pain relief of adiposis dolorosa with injections of **lidocaine** IV (Xylocaine 200 mg in 60 ml 5 per cent dextrose) at intervals of 2 to 12 months. Her angina and diabetic neuropathy pain were not affected. Lidocaine is thought to alter the central nervous system, although the mechanism of pain relief remains uncertain.

The following therapeutic failures in the literature are cited:

- acetanilid
- ACTH
- aminoacetic acid
- aspirin
- codeine
- colchicine
- prostigmine
- tetraethylammonium chloride
- thyroxine
- local injections of:
  - chloroform
  - histamine
  - iodine
  - lidocaine
- epidural anesthesia
- local excision
- diathermy
- weight loss

Juhlin L: Longstanding pain relief of adiposis dolorosa Dercum after i.v. infusion of lidocaine. J Am Acad Dermatol 15:383–385, 1986.

Under careful supervision as recommended by anesthesiologists, high-dose intravenous **lidocaine** (100 mg IV, followed by an infusion of lidocaine 4 mg/ml saline given at a rate of 1 ml/kg/hour, total dose 1.3 gm/day for 4 days) gave a 60-year-old woman three weeks of complete relief from the pain she had suffered for 20 years. A second and third series of infusions each gave two months of freedom from pain. Placebo infusions were without effect, as were the following treatments given over the prior two decades:

- weight reduction
- transducer neural stimulation
- thyroxine
- nicotinic acid
- carbamazepine (Tegretol)
- oxyphenbutazone (Oxalid)
- aspirin
- indomethacin (Indocin)
- clofazimine
- penicillin
- prednisone
- sulfonamides
- alprenolol
- amitriptyline (Elavil)
- diazepam (Valium)
- chlorpromazine (Thorazine)
- zinc
- vitamin A
- prostaglandin E_1 IV
- surgical excision

Iwane T, Maruyama M, Matsuki M, et al: Management of intractable pain in adiposis dolorosa with intravenous administration of lidocaine. Anesth Analg 55:257–259, 1976.

Control of pain in a 48-year-old Japanese woman was achieved with **lidocaine** (400 mg IV infusion over 35 minutes every other day). However, the pain relief in this patient was of only 10 hours' duration.

Petersen P, Kastrup J, et al.: Treating the pain of Dercum's disease. Br Med J 288:1880, 1984.

Lidocaine (200 mg IV once every month) controlled severe pain in an 84-year-old woman with Dercum's disease of the thighs and knees. **Mexiletine** (Mexitil 50 mg tid PO) was equally effective. (In the United States, also try **tocainide**, Tonocard, 400 mg tid PO.)

Kutalek SP, Morganroth J, Horowitz LN: Tocainide: A new oral antiarrhythmic agent. Ann Intern Med 103:387–391, 1985.

Tocainide has essentially the same chemical structure as **lidocaine**, but unlike this parent compound, it is 100 per cent bioavailable when given orally. (Reasonably well-tolerated in oral dosages of 400 to 600 mg q8h, it should prove valuable in treating lidocaine-responsive patients, such as those with Dercum's disease.)

Lemont H, Picciotti J, Pruzansky J: Dercum's disease. J Am Podiatry Assoc 69:389–391, 1979.

Excision of painful lipomas from the knee area of a 62-year-old woman gave relief from lancinating pain and restored ability to walk comfortably. The pain may have been caused by intermittent fat compression of nerves. Thickened capillaries with microthrombi were found in the excised fat.

Boller R: Die novocainbehandlung des morbus Dercum. Klin Wochenschr 13:1786–1789, 1934.

Six patients were helped by multiple daily injections of 30 to 40 ml of **procaine** (0.2 to 0.4 per cent) directly into the pain sites.

Palmer ED: Dercum's disease: Adiposis dolorosa. Am Fam Physician 24(11):155–157, 1981.

Prednisone (20 mg/day) was helpful for a 42-year-old retired female nurse with "painful universal obesity" and numerous tender lipomas.

Listen to the patient, and he will listen to you.

Alopecia

Eliminate drug	Biotin
Reassurance	Zinc
Minoxidil	Cyproterone acetate
Fluorouracil	Surgery

First look for a cause. Nothing is more reassuring to the patient than pinpointing an antecedent event that not only accounts for an otherwise alarming telogen effluvium but promises regrowth. And nothing is more curative than identifying and eliminating a drug, such as a beta-blocker, responsible for the hair loss.

Do not limit your inquiry to the history. Examine the scalp. Be alert to the possibility of an underlying *Trichophyton tonsurans* infection, trichotillomania, syphilis, lupus erythematosus, or diffuse alopecia areata. Twist the hairs vigorously to assess their fragility. Many women complain of hair loss that is simply breakage of the hair shaft weakened by permanents, hair straighteners, and hot-comb treatments. Check the root strength by plucking. If more than 20 per cent of hairs tested come out, it is likely to be an anagen or telogen effluvium.

Use the microscope for more clues. Identify the phase of the hair cycle in which the hairs are being lost. Is it the anagen loss of toxic drugs or chemicals? Or is it the common telogen loss? Take a biopsy. Although rarely, we have found diffuse hair loss of the scalp to be due to clinically occult syringomas, pemphigus, and yeast folliculitis.

Turn to the clinical laboratory for further help. A health profile is essential. This should include ANA, RPR, thyroid function, sedimentation rate, and serum iron determinations. Keep searching for clues. The treatment of alopecia, like that of urticaria, is best done by the one who meticulously studies the patient for specific entry points for therapy. Bear in mind that the hair follicle is the most rapidly dividing cell line in the body. Given this mitotic rate, it is uniquely vulnerable to a myriad of factors, whether a crash diet, a death in the family, or a toxin.

The patient comes with the diagnosis of alopecia. It is for you to confirm it. Our assessment of hair loss (as well as hair growth) is primitive compared to our sophisticated technology for blood cell counts. It is well, however, to have the patient bring total daily combings for your inspection. If the loss is less than 50 hairs a day, the problem may be more one of anxiety than alopecia. If the loss is in the hundreds, it points to anagen or telogen effluvium. Once hair loss is confirmed, it is for you to secure the data on which to base your therapy.

But what if, like a fever, it still remains of undetermined origin? There are two biochemical entry points we use. One is biotin, the other zinc. We ask the patient to take biotin (OTC, 1000 μg tid). This is taken for a period of at least four months. If it is ineffective, as determined by the patient's count of hair lost during shampooing, we prescribe zinc (zinc sulfate 220 mg tid, with food) for a few months. Each of these approaches is empiric, but biotin and zinc have well-recognized roles in the metabolic pathways of rapidly metabolizing cells. More importantly, in our experience more than an occasional patient has shown a gratifying response to these simple approaches.

Much of the alopecia we see is of known origin—the insidious, steady, patterned physiologic loss of scalp hair. Genetically determined and androgen dependent, it is inexorable and accepted by most. But some patients continue to search for the hair of their youth. We can now offer them something better than wigs and hair pieces. Hair transplants and scalp reductions of bald areas have proven valuable in selected patients. And now the use of topical agents to stimulate senescent follicles has entered a new phase. The potent antihypertensive vasodilator minoxidil (Loniten) is the most popular. It is not available, or approved, for local use, but thousands of patients are trying it in an extemporaneous prescription of crushed tablets in propylene glycol (1 to 5 per cent) applied twice a day to balding areas. At present, only about one in ten patients shows a cosmetically noticeable response. But it is currently the darling of hair tonics.

As long as hair remains an index of youth and disease, every case of alopecia deserves evaluation, appropriate specific therapy, and an elixir of hope.

Pinkus H: Alopecia. Clinicopathologic correlations. Int J Dermatol 19:245–253, 1980.

This complete review of all causes of alopecia stresses the need for scalp biopsy (with elastic stains) to detect an unsuspected basis such as hamartoma or metastatic carcinoma. An unwashed dirty scalp gives the best clinical information. The patient should be instructed not to shampoo for seven days and to collect all fallen- and combed-out hair during that week, placing each day's harvest into a separate labeled envelope for inspection in the office.

Levantine A, Almeyda J: Drug induced alopecia. Br J Dermatol 89:549–553, 1973.

Is the patient taking or receiving:

- vitamin A
- amphetamines
- allopurinol
- iodine
- thiouracil
- trimethadione
- levodopa (L-dopa)
- gentamicin
- salicylates
- anticoagulants
  - heparin
  - coumadin
- antimetabolites
  - colchicine
  - hydroxyurea
  - cyclophosphamide
  - methotrexate
  - vincristine
- anticholesterol agents
  - clofibrate (Atromid-S)

Is there exposure to thallium?

Has she stopped oral contraceptives?

Maguire HC: Drug-induced alopecia. Am Fam Physician 19(1):178–179, 1979.

Is the patient receiving:

- beta-blockers
- lithium
- androgens
- doxorubicin
- x-ray

Duff P, Mayer AR: Generalized alopecia: An unusual complication of danazol therapy. Am J Obstet Gynecol 141:349–350, 1981.

Androgens, whether of intrinsic or extrinsic origin, promote hair loss. Danazol, a derivative of 17-alpha-ethinyl testosterone, is used to treat endometriosis and fibrocystic disease of the breast.

A 25-year-old woman with endometriosis received danazol (Danocrine 400 mg bid for seven weeks), and within five weeks there was distinct hair loss. This progressed to complete alopecia of the scalp, axillae, and pubis by the ninth week. Regrowth began six weeks after danazol was stopped and was complete by six months.

Khalsa JH, Graham C, Jones JK: Cimetidine-associated alopecia. Int J Dermatol 22:202–204, 1983.

Cites over 100 cases of alopecia associated with cimetidine therapy.

Goette DK, Odom RB: Profuse hair loss. Arch Dermatol 111:930, 1975.

Sudden weight loss (34 pounds in two months) due to crash dieting in two women was associated with marked telogen hair loss. Other causes of telogen effluvium were ruled out: high fever, surgery, anesthesia, childbirth, and emotional stress. R_x: food, food, glorious food.

Dahlin PA, George J, Nérette J-C: Telogen effluvium: Hair loss after spinal cord injury. Arch Phys Med Rehabil 65:485–486, 1984.

Sudden loss of scalp hair occurred in a 26-year-old man four months after complete spinal cord injury (C5) due to an automobile accident. Regrowth was complete seven months later, except for a permanent area of diffuse occipital loss. Diagnosis: psychogenic telogen effluvium.

Poma PA: Pressure-induced alopecia: Report of a case after gynecologic surgery. J Reprod Med 22:219–221, 1979.

A 35-year-old woman who underwent tubal repair lasting 5¼ hours developed a 5- by 4-cm seroma on the parietal scalp on the right, evident the day after surgery. After one month this area had been replaced by complete alopecia. Regrowth began three months after surgery and was later complete. There were 87 other examples in the literature due to ischemia from prolonged constant pressure, which can be prevented by changing the position of the head every 30 minutes during the period of unconsciousness. Permanent alopecia may also occur and is directly related to the period of head immobilization.

Kosanin RM, Riefkohl R, Barwick WJ: Postoperative alopecia in a woman after a lengthy plastic surgical procedure. Plast Reconstr Surg 73:308–309, 1984.

In a 44-year-old woman, it took six months for hair to regrow in an area of alopecia (similar to alopecia areata) over the vertex, which followed 9¼ hours of anesthesia needed for breast surgery. Initial signs, present on the third postoperative day, included redness, tenderness, swelling, serous exudate, and crusting. Sudden hair loss occurred on the sixth postoperative day.

Hochberg Z, Gilhar A, Haim S, et al.: Calcitriol-resistant rickets with alopecia. Arch Dermatol 121:646–647, 1985.

An inborn error in cytoplasmic and nuclear receptors for calcitriol (1,25-dihydroxyvitamin D_3) was associated with alopecia and rickets in four children of two kindred. Both conditions were totally resistant to all therapy with vitamin D and calcitriol analogues. The role of chronic hypocalcemia in alopecia is difficult to evaluate, as only occasional patients with hypoparathyroidism and hypocalcemia develop alopecia.

Snyder RA, Crain WR, McNutt NS: Alopecia mucinosa: Report of a case with diffuse alopecia and normal-appearing skin. Arch Dermatol 120:496–498, 1984.

A scalp biopsy detected occult alopecia mucinosa as the cause of extensive noncicatricial alopecia in a 69-year-old man. Interestingly, his hair regrew spontaneously without treatment during the subsequent nine months.

Martin J, Ross JB: Alopecia totalis as a presentation of cutaneous metastasis (alopecia neoplastica). Int J Dermatol 22:487–489, 1983.

A 69-year-old woman allowed her physician to examine only her alopecic scalp. Biopsy disclosed metastatic carcinoma. Only later did she admit to having widespread tumors of the skin. R_x: **Tamoxifen** (Nolvadex), an antiestrogen.

Rees RB: The art of dermatology. Cutis 23:625–631, 1979.

It is a kindness to attempt to manage a patient's problem of idiopathic hair loss instead of turning her away with the disappointing remark that you cannot help her.

Vanderveen EE, Ellis CN, Kang S, et al: Topical minoxidil for hair regrowth. J Am Acad Dermatol 11:416–421, 1984.

Five normotensive patients with androgenic alopecia were treated with topical **minoxidil** (1 to 5 per cent in a base of 20 per cent water—30 per cent propylene glycol—50 per cent alcohol; apply bid for 12 months; cover area with petrolatum after the evening application). Three of five patients showed some new hair growth, but this was appreciable in only one. Fifteen alopecia areata patients showed no response.

Rietschel RL, Madorsky DD: Male pattern alopecia regrowth following topical fluorouracil therapy. JAMA 238:1149, 1977.

A 45-year-old man with male pattern baldness had multiple actinic keratosis of the scalp, treated for three weeks with Efudex solution (2 per cent once daily) followed by **triamcinolone** cream (0.5 per cent applied 10 minutes later). The triamcinolone cream (0.5 per cent) alone was continued for another three weeks. After five months, appreciable growth of terminal hair had occurred in an area that had been bald for 10 years. Possibly the potent topical steroid normalized the vascular supply to the hair follicles.

Sweetman L, Surh L, Baker H, et al: Clinical and metabolic abnormalities in a boy with dietary deficiency of biotin. Pediatrics 68:553–558, 1981.

An 11-year-old retarded boy who ate two raw eggs a day for five years developed total hair loss and a generalized erythematous scaly eruption. These were reversed by **biotin** (1 mg/day). Raw eggs contain avidin, a protein that binds with essential biotin, resulting in biotin deficiency.

Smit AJ, Hoorntje SJ, Donker AJM: Zinc deficiency during captopril treatment. Nephron 34:196–197, 1983.

Captopril (Capoten 50 mg tid) resulted in loss of hair and taste within two months in a 60-year-old man with hypertension. Despite continued use of captopril (known to chelate zinc ions), taste and hair returned to normal within weeks of taking oral **zinc** (400 mg/day).

Seidman M, Westfried M, Maxey R, et al: Reversal of male pattern baldness by minoxidil. A case report. Cutis 28:551–553, 1981.

Minoxidil (20 mg bid for 10 months) induced complete regrowth of scalp hair in a 30-year-old black man with male pattern hair loss since age 24. He also had hypertension and chronic renal disease necessitating hemodialysis since age 26.

Fenton DA, English JS, Wilkinson JD: Reversal of male-pattern baldness, hypertrichosis, and accelerated hair and nail growth in patients receiving benoxaprofen. Br Med J 284:1228–1229, 1982.

Benoxaprofen (600 mg/day), a nonsteroidal anti-inflammatory drug, induced photosensitivity, onycholysis, and new hair growth in the bald scalps of two men after five and nine months respectively. One woman receiving the same dose showed an increase in scalp hair growth after four months.

Mortimer CH, Rushton H, James KC: Effective medical treatment for common baldness in women. Clin Exp Dermatol 9:342–350, 1984.

Since baldness in women reflects subtle androgen excess, the antiandrogen **cyproterone acetate** (50 mg daily for 10 days of each menstrual cycle) and **ethinyl estradiol** (40 μg/day for 21 days) was tried in three women with diffuse hair loss of 2 to 23 years' duration. After six months, each had an increase in hair density and thickness. One woman also recovered from severe depression associated with hair loss. Each patient had a decrease in plasma testosterone level.

Unger WP: New concepts and techniques in hair transplantation and alopecia reduction. J Dermatol Surg Oncol 10:937, 1984.

The introduction to a 60-page issue on surgical approaches to alopecia cites the following advances:

micrografts at hair line
improved donor harvesting
tissue expansion prior to alopecia reduction
free scalp flaps
minireductions

Howard N, Stenner RW: An improved "ice-cap" to prevent alopecia caused by Adriamycin (doxorubicin). Br J Radiol 56:963–964, 1983.

Although chemotherapy with Adriamycin invariably produces alopecia, this was totally prevented in 35 patients who received 201 such injections. The method involved wearing an ice cap on the scalp to constrict blood vessels and reduce the concentration of Adriamycin in that area. The rubber ice cap, which is commercially available in England (Camp Ltd., Winchester), was worn starting 30 minutes prior to treatment and until 45 minutes after therapy was concluded. After storage in the freezer, the cap is applied over wet hair covered by a wet cotton cap and is then covered by an insulating fleece-lined bonnet.

Graeber CW, Lapkin RA: Metoprolol and alopecia. Cutis 28:633–634, 1981.

An 18-year-old man with hypertension and chronic glomerulonephritis developed severe diffuse alopecia six to eight weeks after starting Lopressor (metoprolol 50 mg bid). Scalp biopsy showed telogen effluvium. Regrowth of scalp hair began two months after all beta-adrenoceptor blocking agents had been discontinued.

If you can imagine it might help, it might!

Alopecia Areata

Anthralin	Oral
Phenol	Intramuscular
Liquid N_2	PUVA
Corticosteroids	Contact allergens
Topical	Minoxidil
Intralesional	

Never consider alopecia areata to be a trivial cosmetic problem unworthy of your best therapeutic efforts. Even a patch of baldness no larger than a quarter is extremely disquieting to a patient who deserves to know that it is not a sign of cancer or internal disease and, furthermore, that it is not contagious. In its acute form, just as in urticaria, the prognosis is generally excellent. In the chronic form, present for months, the prognosis (as in chronic urticaria) is guarded. It is essential to stress that the "hair-growth switch" has been turned off, but that the "equipment" is in no way damaged, even in extensive and recurrent cases. Once the switch is turned back on, complete hair growth will occur.

The patient should be given calm, truthful reassurance, since this disease can be triggered by emotional shock and perpetuated by the profound anxiety it engenders in the patient. Only a subtle, persistent, noninflammatory T cell infiltrate around the dormant hair follicles keeps the switch from going back to the "on" position. With the growing awareness that the T cell population can reflect the emotional status of the patient, there is every reason to give the patient with alopecia areata understanding and sympathetic emotional support, as well as appropriate direct therapy.

Any assistance that can be given to the patient in correlating the onset of the hair loss with a dramatic psychic stress has a salutary effect. Awareness of a self-limiting cause is reassuring to both the patient and physician. A careful, cautious, probing history may reveal unrecalled precipitating factors. This is especially true for children whose hidden fears and disturbances can rarely be verbalized. One of our patients developed marked, but self-limiting, alopecia areata shortly after engine failure in the plane in which she was flying across the Atlantic. Another experienced hair loss soon after the ferry boat she was on capsized in the Hudson River. Simple knowledge of the significance of these nonrecurring "triggers" was of great therapeutic benefit.

For the ordinary example of idiopathic acute alopecia areata we prescribe Diprolene ointment to be applied sparingly each night to the affected sites. If at one month the hair follicle pits remain empty, we ask the patient additionally to apply 1 per cent anthralin cream for 20 minutes before showering. Should the process be extending we give Kenalog 40 mg intramuscularly at intervals of three weeks for three doses. Again, we must see evidence of hair growth within a month or two.

 We tend to avoid using intralesional steroids, except at patient request, when

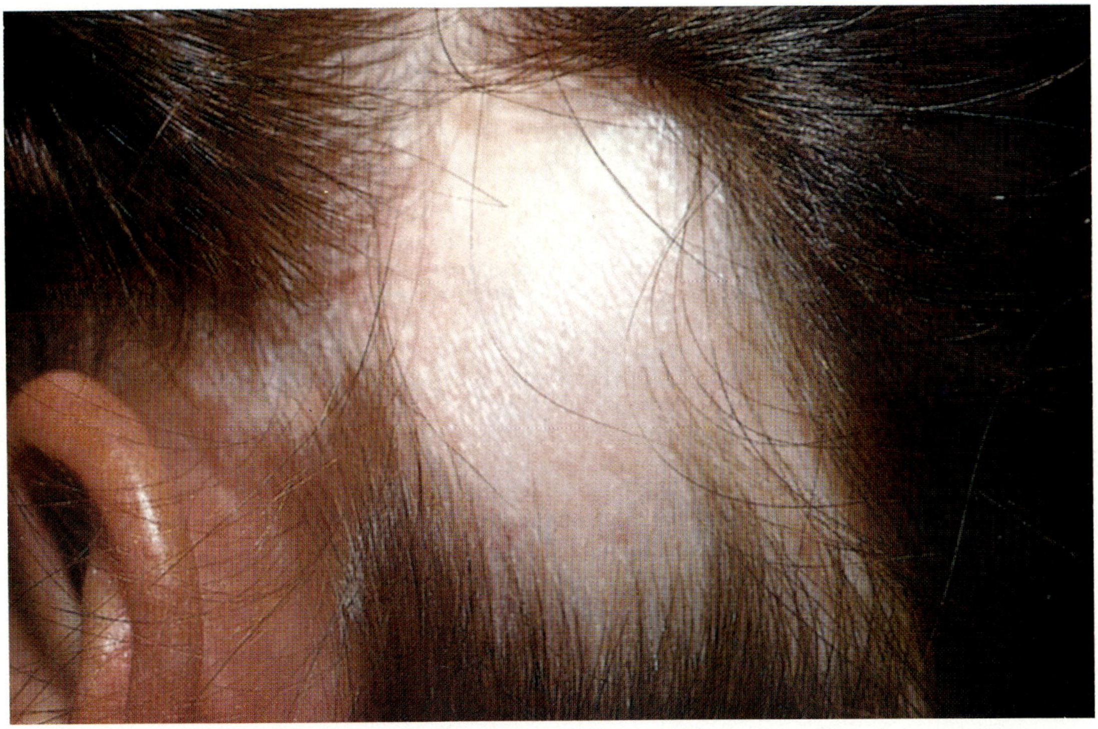

we will inject triamcinolone acetonide suspension (diluted to 2.5 or 5 mg/ml). This may be especially appreciated by the patient with eyebrow hair loss.

We have also used the induction of contact dermatitis with dinitrochlorobenzene with benefit in a few selected patients. Remarkably, in one patient the induction of sensitization on the arm with only one application was followed rapidly by good hair regrowth on the scalp.

Alopecia areata is a disease in which further knowledge of its immune basis should lead to specific therapy. At present we can only rejoice in the palliation we seem to provide for patients with this strange disorder of the hair cycle.

Mitchell AJ, Krull EA: Alopecia areata: Pathogenesis and treatment. J Am Acad Dermatol 11:763–775, 1984.

A splendid interpretative review of current palliative therapies and their rationale. 158 references.

Jillson OF: Alopecia. I. Alopecia areata. Cutis 31:262–273, 1983.

When to treat:

If hair loss continues for more than a few months
If no regrowth occurs after hair loss stops

Advocates nonspecific inflammatory approach:

Phenol (saturated solution): Paint on and neutralize with alcohol after area turns white. Repeat every two weeks.
Salicylic acid (0.6 gm) + **anthralin** (0.6 gm) in white petrolatum (qs ad 30.0 gm): Apply daily and wash off after 20 minutes.

OR

Erythema doses with Kromayer UV lamp

Directions for local injection of steroids:

Use **Triamcinolone acetonide** (5 mg/ml).
Inject multiple areas with 0.1 ml, but no closer than 1.0 cm.
Inject just under epidermis (like intradermal skin test).
Expect growth of pigmented hairs in four weeks (two weeks in eyebrows).

Ralfs I: Treatment of alopecia areata. Int J Dermatol 20:168–170, 1981.

Comprehensive survey of treatments from aloe to zinc, with steroids the most popular. Associated conditions included atopy, autoimmune disorders (with organ-specific autoantibodies), and prehypertension (family history of hypertension).

Gip L, Lodin A, Molin L: Alopecia areata: A follow-up investigation of outpatient material. Acta Derm Venereol 49:180–188, 1969.

Questionnaire survey of 133 patients seen over a five-year-period revealed nearly 50 per cent had regrowth in six months and 75 per cent by five years. Relapse was close to 40 per cent. Localization at onset did not influence either healing tendency or relapse frequency. No systemic or intralesional steroids were used.

Arnold HL: Alopecia areata: Prevalence in Japanese and prognosis after reassurance. Arch Dermatol 66:191–196, 1952.

Best treatment is reassurance. Only 7 of the author's 55 patients with recent onset of alopecia areata failed to show spontaneous regrowth within three months.

Wolf D, Wolf R: Simultaneous alopecia areata in two siblings. J Am Acad Dermatol 11:897–898, 1984.

The importance of sympathetic understanding and reassurance is documented by a case report of two sisters (ages four and nine years) in Israel who simultaneously developed alopecia areata six days after their mother left for an overseas vacation. Regrowth began within two weeks of awareness of the emotional facet of the problem.

Montes LF: Topical halcinonide in alopecia areata and alopecia totalis. J Cutan Pathol 4:47–50, 1977.

Halog cream (**halcinonide** 0.1 per cent) applied twice a day (with or without Saran wrap occlusion) in 10 patients was associated with full regrowth of hair in 6 to 18 months. Application was limited to 60 gm/month. After hair regrew, the amount of cream was gradually reduced and stopped without significant hair loss.

Fisher DA: Systemic steroids for treatment of alopecia areata. Arch Dermatol 113:1731–1732, 1977.

In a dozen patients success using intralesional steroid, followed by intramuscular **betamethasone valerate** every other week if necessary. Good regrowth by four months, at which time steroid is discontinued.

Frentz G: Topical treatment of extended alopecia: Intralesional steroid—Kromayer lamp. Dermatologica 155:147–154, 1977.

Intralesional steroid injections (triamcinolone acetonide 5 mg/ml given by jet injector once monthly for two to four treatments) inhibited spontaneous hair regrowth in three of six patients six to nine months after completion of treatment. Tissue atrophy may have been responsible despite lack of visible signs.

Michalowski R, Kuczynska L: Long-term intramuscular triamcinolone-acetonide therapy in alopecia areata, totalis, and universalis. Arch Dermatol Res 261:73–76, 1978.

Kenalog IM (40 to 80 mg initially once weekly, then gradually spaced to every six weeks), was given over 4 to 18 months. Average total dose 900 mg. Among 11 patients, it induced complete remission in three, some improvement in five, but no change in three. Alopecia areata regularly reappeared within six weeks of stopping injections.

Winter RJ, Kern F, Blizzard RM: Prednisone therapy for alopecia areata: A follow-up report. Arch Dermatol 112:1549–1552, 1976.

Reexamination of 18 patients 15 months after discontinuation of alternate-day **prednisone** therapy showed that the improvement noted initially was never sustained. Significant side effects were also common.

Burton JL, Shuster S: Large doses of glucocorticoid in the treatment of alopecia areata. Acta Derm Venereol 55:493–495, 1975.

Pulse therapy (**prednisolone** 2 gm single IV dose or 0.5 gm PO for five days) helped only 4 of 35 patients with severe chronic alopecia areata or alopecia totalis. Patients given prednisolone IV were kept at rest in the hospital for one week. Relapse occurred in some after six months.

Schmoeckel C, Weissmann I, Plewig G, Braun-Falco O: Treatment of alopecia areata by anthralin-induced dermatitis. Arch Dermatol 115:1254–1255, 1979.

Anthralin ointment (0.2 to 0.8 per cent in petrolatum or other base) was applied once daily for several months to maintain marked erythema and mild itching. Cosmetically acceptable regrowth of hair occurred in 18 of 24 patients with alopecia areata. Growth was initially seen after five to eight weeks. Only two of eight alopecia totalis patients responded similarly.

Lassus A, Kianto U, Johansson E, Juvakoski T: PUVA treatment for alopecia areata. Dermatologica 161:298–304, 1980.

UVA (1 to 9 J/sq cm) in ascending dosage 2 hours after 0.6 mg/kg 8-MOP orally twice a week for two to five months induced excellent regrowth in 26 of 41 patients. More importantly, only two of these had recurrence within 6 to 12 months.

Claudy AL, Gagnaire D: PUVA treatment of alopecia areata. Arch Dermatol 119:975–978, 1983.

PUVA (three times a week for up to six months) induced 90 per cent hair regrowth in 11 of 17 patients. Three showed later relapse.

van der Schaar WW, Sillevis Smitt JH: An evaluation of PUVA-therapy for alopecia areata. Dermatologica 168:250–252, 1984.

Only 9 of 30 patients in this study showed significant hair growth following PUVA three times per week with total body irradiation (total: 300 J/sq cm in 65 exposures over eight months). Eight of these nine lost the hair again once treatment was stopped (mean 7.7 months).

Happle R, Cebulla K, Echternacht-Happle K: Dinitrochlorobenzene therapy for alopecia areata. Arch Dermatol 114:1629–1631, 1978.

An immunotherapeutic adventure in treating a presumed autoimmune disease by maintaining a chronic contact dermatitis. Patients were deliberately sensitized to DNCB (**dinitrochlorobenzene**) (2 per cent in acetone) applied unilaterally one time to the scalp. Subsequent unilateral weekly applications of 0.1 per cent solution induced local hair growth in 89 per cent of the 90 patients. Peribulbar round-cell infiltrates were increased on the treated side.

de Prost Y, Paquez F, Touraine R: Dinitrochlorobenzene treatment of alopecia areata. Arch Dermatol 118:542–545, 1982.

Seven of 42 patients had complete and lasting hair growth following 3 to 15 months of **dinitrochlorobenzene** treatments (DNCB 0.01 to 33 per cent weekly in acetone or daily in cream). Interestingly, during the study six patients lost their contact sensitivity to the DNCB, but it was restored by giving the H_2 blocker **cimetidine** (Tagamet 1 gm daily for one month). Painful cervical adenopathy was almost constant. Stop treatment after 10 weeks if contact dermatitis or hair regrowth has not developed.

Swanson NA, Mitchell AJ, Leahy MS, Headington JT, Diaz LA: Topical treatment of alopecia areata: Contact allergen vs primary irritant therapy. Arch Dermatol 117:384–387, 1981.

Specificity of DNCB (**dinitrochlorobenzene**)-induced allergic contact dermatitis therapy was shown by response rate: Control group with irritant dermatitis induced by croton oil ointment showed 0 per cent hair growth; in DNCB group, 63 per cent grew hair.

Rhodes EL, Dolman W, Kennedy C, Taylor RR: Alopecia areata regrowth induced by *Primula obconica*. Br J Dermatol 104:339–340, 1981.

The primula leaf, another contact sensitizer, was used to stimulate hair growth. Five patients showed response in one to two months. Blistering was a problem.

Case PC, Mitchell AJ, Swanson NA, et al: Topical therapy of alopecia areata with squaric acid dibutyl ester. J Am Acad Dermatol 10:447–451, 1984.

A nonmutagenic alternative to DNCB (**dinitrochlorobenzene**) topical immunotherapy: Sensitize by application of **squaric acid dibutyl ester** (2 per cent in acetone) to scalp or forearm. Then with an appropriate dilution (usually 0.1 per cent in acetone applied three times weekly), maintain low-grade dermatitis of areas for four months. If patient develops tolerance to antigen, use Tagamet (**cimetidine** 300 mg tid for one month) to restore sensitivity. There was excellent regrowth in 11 of 21 patients (with greater than 30 per cent scalp involvement). Five additional patients could not be sensitized.

Giannetti A, Orecchia G: Clinical experience on the treatment of alopecia areata with squaric acid dibutyl ester. Dermatologica 167:280–282, 1983.

Advise avoidance of use of **dinitrochlorobenzene**, since it is mutagenic, cross-reacts with **chloramphenicol**, and may be an occupational hazard (algicide in water systems). The authors sensitize and treat with **squaric acid dibutyl ester** (up to 0.8 per cent in acetone applied once weekly). In 26 longstanding cases, good regrowth occurred in five and moderate growth in seven. Must continue treatment or hair will fall out in two to six months. Side effects included posterior cervical lymphadenopathy (12 cases), intense itching (15 cases), and a diffuse eczematous reaction of face and arms (3 cases).

Happle R, Hausen BM, Wiesner-Menzel L: Diphencyprone in the treatment of alopecia areata. Acta Derm Venereol 63:49–52, 1983.

Sensitization with **diphencyprone** (2 per cent in acetone, 1 to 2 ml applied once to one half of the scalp) was followed by similar applications of 0.1 per cent solution in acetone on the fourteenth and twenty-first days. Further weekly applications required adjustment of concentrations (1.0 to 0.0001 per cent) to maintain a mild eczematous reaction without blistering or oozing. A potent new contact allergen, more stable than squaric acid, was effective when used over 4 to 17 months. Control patients using the primary irritants anthralin, croton oil, and sodium lauryl sulfate showed no regrowth.

Machonko T, Grabowski T: Leczenie lysienia plackowatego plynnym. Azotem Przeg Derm 68:607–609, 1981.

Liquid N_2 applied with cotton applicator twice a week induced complete regrowth of hair in 5 of 20 patients with alopecia areata; 12 more showed partial response.

Scully K, Forsey RR: Hair regrowth following hemodialysis. Can Med Assoc J 128:1145, 1983.

Hemodialysis (twice weekly) in a 44-year-old man with alopecia totalis for four years was followed by the rapid appearance of normal hair growth over his scalp, eyebrows, eyelashes, and beard. Impressive photographs show the patient at the eight-month checkup. Renal failure was due to massive vesicoureteric reflux.

Weiss VC, West DP, Fu TS, et al: Alopecia areata treated with topical minoxidil. Arch Dermatol 120:457–463, 1984.

Of 48 patients treated topically with the antihypertensive vasodilator **minoxidil** (1 per cent solution in vehicle containing 70 per cent alcohol, 20 per cent water, 10 per cent propylene glycol) 11 grew cosmetically acceptable hair beginning after two months of therapy. The solution was applied twice a day with a glass rod to only one side of the scalp. White petrolatum was applied over the application at bedtime. Minoxidil may act as an immunomodulator, as the perifollicular lymphocytic infiltrate disappeared after treatment.

Fenton DA, Wilkinson JD: Topical minoxidil in the treatment of alopecia areata. Br Med J 287:1015–1017, 1983.

After six months in a double-blind study, **minoxidil** (1 per cent lotion or ointment bid) induced a cosmetically acceptable amount of hair in 16 of 30 patients, with regrowth beginning at six weeks. Topical nitroglycerin, a vasodilator, was without effect. Suspect that arteriolar vasodilatation (induced only by minoxidil) rather than venous vasodilatation is required. Androgen stimulation is not involved. No side effects.

De Weert J, Temmerman L, Kint A: Alopecia areata: A clinical study. Dermatologica 168:224–229, 1984.

Study of 100 cases: Prognosis worse if patient is atopic, has a positive family history of alopecia areata, or has autoantibodies (ANA, parietal cells, thyroid, smooth muscle, microsomes). Treatment of foci of infection found in 37 patients was no help.

Friedmann PS: Unsuccessful treatment of alopecia areata with dapsone. Br J Dermatol 104:597–598, 1981.

Dapsone (100 mg/day for three months) had no effect in a study of 22 patients. This demonstrates that neutrophil function is not critical in the pathogenesis of alopecia areata.

Ead RD: Oral zinc sulfate in alopecia areata—A double-blind trial. Br J Dermatol 104:483–484, 1981.

In this study, zinc sulfate (220 mg bid for three months) had no effect in 42 subjects, in contrast to an earlier favorable report.

Galbraith GMP, Thiers BH, Fudenberg HH: An open-label trial of immunomodulation therapy with inosiplex (Isoprinosine) in patients with alopecia totalis and cell-mediated immunodeficiency. J Am Acad Dermatol 11:224–230, 1984.

Inosiplex (50 mg/kg/day for 14 days, then 3 days/week for six months) induced significant hair regrowth in seven of nine patients with alopecia totalis and associated defects in T lymphocyte function. (Investigational drug—immunopotentiator—enhances T cell function. Mild hyperuricemia is the only side effect.)

Heyl T: Tick bite alopecia. Clin Exp Dermatol 7:537–542, 1982.

Hair loss resembling alopecia areata (with a few exclamation point hairs) may develop rapidly after a tick bite on the scalp. Look for ulcer at the bite site in the center of the alopecia. Hair regrows spontaneously.

Martin ES: Treatment of alopecia areata profiting from "natural" allergy to nickel. Arch Dermatol 120:1138–1139, 1984.

A 24-year-old women with an eight-month history of steroid-unresponsive alopecia areata was found on patch testing to be exquisitely sensitive to nickel sulfate. Daily application of 1 per cent $NiSO_4$ in petrolatum produced visible hair regrowth in five weeks and a normal full complement of 3-cm-long hair by four months. The applications were then discontinued. At eight months the scalp appearance was almost normal.

The patient's pessimism must always be diluted with the physician's optimism.

Angioedema

Antibiotics
Stanozolol
Amicar
C1 INH concentrate

Most patients with recurrent angioedema deserve the same careful study and treatment as does a patient with recurrent urticaria. Indeed, many have associated hives, and the angioedema is simply a severe focal example. A search must be made for trigger factors such as aspirin, vibrations, and exercise, as well as systemic disease (e.g., lymphoma, lupus, or bowel disease). Dental trauma has also been reported to induce attacks.

In striking contrast to the commonplace idiopathic angioedema is the rare hereditary form. Here, treatment has been directed by knowledge of its precise biochemical basis: the absence or functional impairment of the serum protein that inhibits activation of the complement system. Significantly, these patients do not have urticaria, but are at grave risk of airway obstruction and death. With a mortality of 30 per cent, it is little wonder that these individuals avoid the hazards of dental care, since dental trauma is the best known trigger for attacks. They all must be instructed about the hazards of physical trauma, including surgery.

The patient with mild attacks or the one who may go for years without attacks does not need the long-term therapy necessary for those with severe or frequent attacks. This therapy now centers on anabolic hormones to stimulate the synthesis of proteins—specifically, the synthesis of C1′esterase inhibitor. Currently, stanozolol (Winstrol 5 mg twice a week) is the most popular. It has replaced the early use of androgen (methyltestosterone) and its analogue, danazol (ethinyl testosterone). The other avenue for long-term therapy has been use of the antifibrinolytic agent aminocaproic acid (EACA, epsilon-aminocaproic acid), since the blood clotting process is integral to activation of the complement cascade. Aminocaproic acid (Amicar) must be given in large doses (8 to 10 gm/day) to achieve success, but for some patients the protection they receive is worth the trouble and expense.

To us it appears likely that the intravascular release of bacterial antigens known to occur during dental care is of great significance in initiating coagulation and thereby the complement cascade. Accordingly, prophylactic antibiotics may be helpful. The classic prophylactic treatment, however, has been the administration of either aminocaproic acid for at least three days prior to surgery or two units of fresh frozen plasma one day prior to surgery. This plasma serves as the temporary source of the needed C1 esterase inhibitor.

It is the acute attack, however, that has been the life-threatening problem that rarely responds to the invariably employed corticosteroids, antihistamines, and epinephrine. An exciting new development and singularly effective therapy has resulted from the purification and concentration of the esterase inhibitor itself. Within 15 minutes of giving this new isolate (1000 to 2000 U IV over a 10-minute

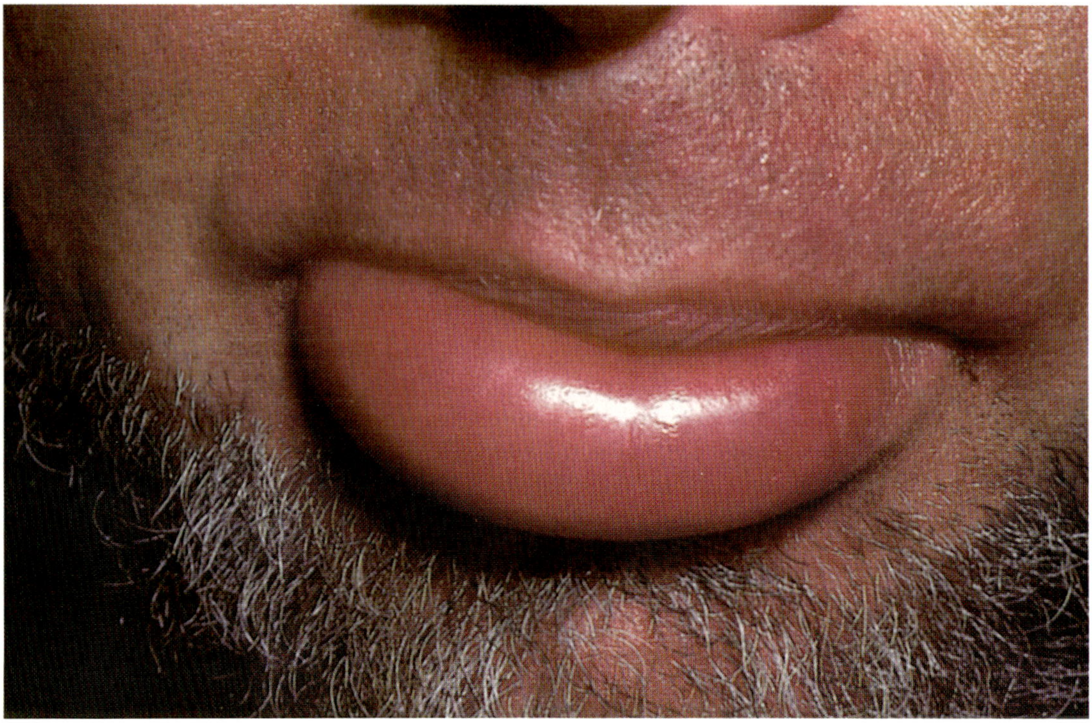

period) the edema of the mucosa abates and the laryngeal airway is restored to normal without tracheostomy. This is a major advance and should save lives once the product is available. It will also eliminate the need for narcotics in the emergency room treatment of these patients during their intensely painful abdominal attacks.

This C1 INH concentrate is an "orphan" drug that will have no trouble finding a home with this family of hereditary angioedema patients. In its absence, we would suggest that steroid pulse therapy (Medrol 1 g IV over 10 minutes) be considered for immediate relief.

Kaplan AP: Angioedema. N Engl J Med 310:1662–1664, 1984.

Recurrent angioedema is a vexing problem, since 90 per cent of cases are idiopathic and therapy is only palliative.

Frank MM, Gelfand JA, Atkinson JP: Hereditary angioedema: The clinical syndrome and its management. Ann Intern Med 84:580–593, 1976.

Their 30 patients had symptoms for an average of 21 years before diagnosis was made by finding low levels of either C4 or C1 esterase inhibitor activity, or both. Emotional upsets and trauma (e.g., tonsillectomy, dental manipulation, accidents) precipitated attacks in at least half of the patients. Provides detailed data on prophylactic treatment with long-term antifibrinolytic (**epsilon-aminocaproic acid** 15 gm/day) and androgen (**methyltestosterone** 10 mg tid) compounds.

Mortality was 30 per cent before the advent of therapy, and treatment of acute attacks is still not very satisfactory, requiring **epinephrine**, steroids, antihistamines, and airway support. Severe abdominal pain responds to narcotics.

Sweet LC, Jackson CE, Yanari SS, Yott JB: Danazol therapy in hereditary angioedema. Henry Ford Hosp Med J 28:31–35, 1980.

Danazol (Danocrine—**ethinyl testosterone**—100 to 200 mg/day) gave 11 patients freedom from attacks. Initial dose of 200 mg bid for two months was tapered by 50 mg bid every two months to reach the minimal effective dose.

Hosea SW, Santaella ML, Brown EJ, et al: Long-term therapy of hereditary angioedema with danazol. Ann Intern Med 93:809–812, 1980.

Danazol was more effective in higher doses (100 per cent at 600 mg/day), but may cause headaches, masculinization, and microscopic hematuria. Study of 69 patients over a six-year period. Must monitor long-term toxicity.

Warin AP, Greaves MW, Gatecliff M, et al: Treatment of hereditary angioedema by low dose attenuated androgens: Disassociation of clinical response from levels of C1 esterase inhibitor and C4. Br J Dermatol 103:405–409, 1980.

Two androgens, **danazol** (200 mg bid → 200 mg qod and **stanozolol** (5 mg daily → 5 mg q 2 to 10 days), provide effective long-term therapy by stimulating synthesis of critically lacking protein, C1 esterase inhibitor. Study of nine patients with this autosomal dominant disease.

Agostoni A, Cicardi M, Martignoni GC, et al: Danazol and stanozolol in long-term prophylactic treatment of hereditary angioedema. J Allergy Clin Immunol 65:75–79, 1980.

Attacks were prevented with 17α-alkylated androgens. Gave **danazol** (600 mg/day) intermittently (five days on and five days off) for the first month, then slowly tapered to minimum effective dose. No menstrual or liver abnormalities occurred. Treatment time—8 to 25 months. Alternative: **stanozolol** (4 to 12 mg/day).

Sheffer AL, Fearon DT, Austen KF: Clinical and biochemical effects of stanozolol therapy for hereditary angioedema. J Allergy Clin Immunol 68:181–187, 1981.

Stanozolol, an inexpensive anabolic steroid with 30:1 anabolic androgenic ratio, was given to 27 patients. All cases were controlled with 0.5 to 2 mg/day. Side effects: menstrual abnormalities and virilization (4/15 females) and elevated CPK level (5 males).

Bergamaschini L, Cicardi M, Tucci A, et al: C1 INH concentrate in the therapy of hereditary angioedema. Allergy 38:81–84, 1983.

Acute attacks can now be managed by intravenous administration of **C1 INH concentrate**, which gives a 70-fold increase in concentration over plasma. Nine patients were successfully treated by administration of 1100 to 2200 U of this concentrate over a 10-minute period.

Gadek JE, Hosea SW, Gelfand JA, et al: Replacement therapy in hereditary angioedema: Successful treatment of acute episodes of angioedema with partly purified C1 inhibitor. N Engl J Med 302:542–546, 1980.

An intravenous lyophilized plasma concentrate containing **C1 inhibitor** (prepared by American Red Cross and NIH) gave prompt alleviation of symptoms in eight patients with acute attacks. Androgen analogues were of no use in acute attacks, and frozen plasma introduces the risk of viral transmission.

Schreiber AD, Zweiman B, Atkins P, et al: Acquired angioedema with lymphoproliferative disorder: Association of C1 inhibitor deficiency with cellular abnormality. Blood 48:567–580, 1976.

Recurrent attacks of laryngeal edema similar to hereditary angioedema in a 73-year-old man were linked to abnormal lymphoid cells that may have interacted with the complement system (decreased C1, C2, C4, and undetectable C1 INH).

Smitz S, Legros J-J, Le Maire M: Naloxone, itch, asthma, urticaria and angioedema. Ann Intern Med 97:788–789, 1982.

A single patient had singular sustained relief from her chronic angioedema and urticaria following a single IV infusion of the opiate **naloxone** (Narcan 1.6 mg/hour for four hours).

Gleich GJ, Schroeter AJ, Marcoux JP, et al: Episodic angioedema associated with eosinophilia. N Engl J Med 310:1621–1626, 1984.

Four cases of a new entity: severe angioedema, urticaria, fever, weight gain, and leukocytosis with enormous eosinophilia. Responds to **prednisone** therapy (30 to 60 mg/day for three to four days during attacks).

Wener MH, Metzger WJ, Simon RA: Occupationally acquired vibratory angioedema with secondary carpal tunnel syndrome. Ann Intern Med 98:44–46, 1983.

No help from Benadryl, Atarax, or nonsteroidal anti-inflammatory drugs for this 32-year-old patient with swelling, itching, and pain in his hands, who had to avoid using the lawn mower, motorcycle, and air drill. Carpal tunnel release on one hand greatly relieved pain and paresthesias (due to secondary compression neuropathy) and enabled the patient to return to work.

Patterson R, Mellies CJ, Blankenship ML, Pruzansky JJ: Vibratory angioedema: A hereditary type of physical hypersensitivity. J Allergy Clin Immunol 50:174–182, 1972.

Avoidance of vibrators, massages, vigorous rubbing with towels, and cold weather helps prevent symptoms of this rare dominant condition. Deep urticarial lesions form within minutes at site of vibration or friction, followed by flushing and headache.

Highet AS, Felix RH: Vibratory urticaria. Br J Dermatol 105(Suppl 19):40–41, 1981.

Walking, running, bicycle riding on a bumpy path, and a vibratory massage belt triggered erythema, heat, itch, light-headedness, and collapse (on one occasion) in a 31-year-old woman. Symptoms were reduced by taking **mebhydroline** (Fabahistin 50 mg—not available in the United States) prior to exertion.

Lewis J, Lieberman P, Treadwell G, Erffmeyer J: Exercise-induced urticaria, angioedema, and anaphylactoid episodes. J Allergy Clin Immunol 68:432–437, 1981.

Symptoms of cholinergic urticaria, periorbital swelling, or giant urticaria began within 15 minutes of starting exercise. There was no elevation of plasma histamine, and systemic antihistamines were not effective. No successful prophylactic therapy. If patient insists on exercising, he should use the buddy system and carry an anaphylaxis treatment kit with **epinephrine** for self-administration.

Newton JA, McGibbon DH, Marsden RA: Leucocytoclastic vasculitis and angiooedema associated with inflammatory bowel disease. Clin Exp Dermatol 9:618–623, 1984.

Purpuric skin plaques and angioedema were the presenting signs of inflammatory bowel disease in two men, ages 61 and 68 years. In one patient the condition cleared with **colchicine** (250 μg tid), but relapsed twice when the drug was stopped. In the other control was obtained with **salazosul-**

fapyradine (**sulfasalazine**—Azulfidine 1 gm tid), which is broken down to sulfapyridine in the gut.

Cohen SH, Koethe SM, Kozin F, et al: Acquired angioedema associated with rectal carcinoma and its response to danazol therapy. Acquired angioedema treated with danazol. J Allergy Clin Immunol 62:217–221, 1978.

A 69-year-old man had recurrent laryngeal edema and decreased levels of $C\bar{1}$ INH, CH_{50}, C4, and $C\bar{1}$ (but normal C3) before and after surgical removal of a rectal carcinoma. **Danazol** (200 mg tid, then decreased to once daily) stopped the attacks, corrected the complement levels, and increased the $C\bar{1}$ esterase inhibitor level. Acquired angioedema has previously been associated with lymphomas and leukemia (complement pattern: decreased $C\bar{1}$, C2, C4, $C\bar{1}$ INH).

Sullivan TJ, Yecies LD, Shatz GS, et al: Desensitization of patients allergic to penicillin using orally administered β-lactam antibiotics. J Allergy Clin Immunol 69:275–282, 1982.

β-Lactam antibiotics include **penicillin**, semisynthetic penicillins, and **cephalosporins**. Help is available for patients faced with life-threatening infections (bacterial endocarditis, *Pseudomonas* sepsis) vs. possible fatal allergic reactions from antibiotics; 30 such patients were successfully desensitized with either oral **penicillin G** or **carbenicillin**.

Side effects: urticaria in nine, nephritis in one. All patients had positive skin tests to penicillin skin test reagents (benzylpenicillin G, penicillic acid, penicilloyl-polylysine, or carbenicillin).

Directions for desensitization:

Initial dose (oral): penicillin G (100 units) OR carbenicillin (60 μg)
- Give each oral dose with 50 ml water.
- Give progressively doubled dose every 15 minutes.

Doses
- Dose 1 to 13—oral: 100 U → 400,000 U
- Dose 14 to 16—subcutaneous: 200,000 to 800,000 U
- Dose 17—intramuscular: 1,000,000 U

Start IV antibiotics 15 minutes after last desensitization dose.

If you didn't ask about drugs, you didn't take a history.

Anthrax

Phenoxymethyl penicillin
Tetracycline
Erythromycin

Dutz W, Kohout-Dutz E: Anthrax. Int J Dermatol 20:203–206, 1981.

This occupational disease of livestock workers in semiarid countries and woolsorters in textile factories occurs as either a necrotic eschar or massive subcutaneous edema with blisters, resembling a second-degree burn or erysipelas. The anthrax bacillus is readily found in blister fluid.

Bacillus anthracis is eliminated by any of the following therapeutic regimens:

- **phenoxymethyl penicillin** (500 mg q6h for seven days)
- aqueous **procaine penicillin G** (600,000 U IM bid for five days)
- **tetracycline** (0.5 gm q4h for seven days)
- **erythromycin** (0.2 gm q4h for seven days)
- **sulfadiazine** (3 gm stat, then 1 gm q4h for seven days)

These antibacterial agents prevent dissemination of the bacteria and sterilize skin lesions within 24 hours. Dying and dead bacteria, however, continue to release endotoxin that can be lethal in cases of bacteremia. No antitoxin is available. Toxemia requires supportive therapy with **hydrocortisone sodium succinate** (Solu-Cortef 100 to 200 mg IV daily) plus maintenance of fluid and electrolyte balance. Oral steroids are also given in tapering dosage.

Prophylaxis for professionally exposed persons consists of:

Vaccination
(0.5 ml every two weeks for three doses)
booster every six months for three doses
then annual vaccination

If you're too busy to see your "detail reps," you're too busy.

The less we know what to do, the more we write about what to do.

Aphthous Stomatitis

Dapsone	Colchicine
Steroids	Zinc
Tetracycline	Elimination diet
B_{12}, folic acid, iron	

No malady has spawned more treatments. Ranging from Alka-Seltzer to zinc, each treatment has enthusiastic advocates, but none has universal acclaim. Our personal advocacy is for tetracycline compresses. We achieve success by having the patient apply directly over the ulcers soft cotton handkerchief packings soaked in freshly made tetracycline suspension (250 mg in 30 ml lukewarm water) for 15 minutes three times a day prior to eating. This greatly alleviates the pain and usually induces complete healing of the ulcers within three days. Future attacks are aborted by the same treatment used at the first sign of an erosion.

Such treatment is not practical for pharyngeal ulcerations, nor does it provide such dramatic success in the immunocompromised patient. We do not use it in the patient with tetracycline sensitivity, in children, or when candidiasis coexists. We feel it acts by killing pathogenic bacteria and also by interfering with the immune recruitment of inflammatory cells. Note that the concentration exceeds that used in antibiotic sensitivity testing. As an alternate, we have also employed ampicillin, but in much lower concentrations.

Such an approach is satisfactory in the minor forms of aphthous stomatitis, but the major forms require more. In these instances, malnutrition often intervenes, since eating is so painful that the use of viscous Xylocaine (lidocaine 2 per cent viscous solution) for topical anesthesia becomes necessary. In addition to nutritional deficiencies, we look for Behçet's disease, Crohn's disease, gluten enteropathy, periodic neutropenia, and factitial or dental trauma. Rough dentures as well as new fillings come under surveillance. We undertake a serious elimination diet beginning with a 48-hour fast and adding one food at a time every 48 hours. In this way we found one of our most severely affected patients to be milk sensitive. Elimination of all milk and milk products was curative. Another patient was challenge sensitive to cola drinks. Although such food sensitivities are rarely the cause, finding one is finding the cure for a disabling and unremitting problem.

We listen to the patient for clues. We instruct him in turn to avoid trauma to the mucosa, since this is the most common trigger. Even a stiff toothbrush can be the culprit. We do not need to tell him of the pain of acidic foods. We ask the patient to keep a diary—Do the attacks occur premenstrually? Does stress cause attacks? Could buccal biting or ragged teeth be implicated? If facilities are available we recommend leukocyte function testing.

Finally, we use systemic antibiotics, dapsone, ketoconazole, and now acyclovir for short trials, as aphthous ulcers are but a reaction pattern to varied origins. Rarely an injection of Kenalog (40 mg IM) is also necessary to give temporary help. The search for the right therapeutic key cannot be abandoned. We look for that key as long as these patients will look with us. The agony of their aphthae is a driving force for both of us.

Antoon JW, Miller RL: Aphthous ulcers—A review of the literature on etiology, pathogenesis, diagnosis, and treatment. J Am Dent Assoc 101:803–808, 1980.

Comprehensive review tabulating 20 treatment modalities. They recommend **betamethasone** emollient directly to the ulcer, **tetracycline** and **lidocaine** rinses, and multivitamin, **iron**, and **zinc** supplements. Minor trauma precedes 75 per cent of all aphthae. All patients should be observed for Reiter's syndrome, Behçet's syndrome, gastrointestinal diseases, neutropenias, and allergies.

Rostas A, McLean DI, Wilkinson RD: Management of recurrent aphthous stomatitis: A review. Cutis 22:183–189, 1978.

Tetracycline topically is the treatment of choice for mild to moderately severe aphthous stomatitis. Viscous **lidocaine** 2 per cent relieves pain. Cyclic estrogens are helpful in recurrent premenstrual aphthosis.

Aphthous ulceration. J R Soc Med 77:1–3, 1984.

Approximately 20 per cent of the population has these ulcers at some time. Most patients will not have a correctable cause. Smoking appears to inhibit the ulcers, as does pregnancy. Stress, minor trauma, and foods that release histamine appear to aggravate the ulcers. Possibly significant is an L-form of *Streptococcus sanguis* often isolated from the ulcers, which may be inappropriately handled by the patient's immune systems.

Convit J, Goihman-Yahr M, Rondon-Lugo AJ: Effectiveness of dapsone in Behçet's disease. Br J Dermatol 111:629–630, 1984.

Dapsone is also an effective treatment for severe recurrent oral aphthae.

Rogers RS III: Recurrent aphthous stomatitis: Clinical characteristics and evidence for an immunopathogenesis. J Invest Dermatol 69:499–509, 1977.

Clinical studies on therapeutic efficacy are hard to conduct because of the variable duration and frequency of lesions and the reduction of pain associated with the covering of the ulcer by the fibromembranous slough.

Tyldesley WR: Stomatitis and recurrent oral ulceration: Is a full blood screen necessary? Br J Oral Surg 21:27–30, 1983.

Yes! Of 398 patients with oral ulcerations who had full blood screens, 75 (18.8 per cent) had one or more hematologic abnormalities:

42 low folate levels (serum, red cells or both)
26 iron deficiency
19 low B_{12} levels

Note also that four had celiac disease, four had pernicious anemia, and one had Crohn's disease.

Wray D, Ferguson MM, Mason DK, et al: Recurrent aphthae: Treatment with vitamin B_{12}, folic acid, and iron. Br Med J 2:490–493, 1975.

Among 130 patients screened hematologically, 23 (17.7 per cent) had one or more deficiencies:

15 iron deficiency
7 folic acid deficiency, B_{12} deficiency
5 B_{12} deficiency

Specific replacement therapy cleared the condition in 15 of these patients and improved it in 8 others. Only 33 of the remaining 107 patients experienced improvement or remission with local symptomatic treatment (**zinc chloride/zinc sulfate** mouthwash plus topical steroids). Among the 23 patients with deficiencies, four had addisonian pernicious anemia, seven had malabsorption syndrome (including five with gluten enteropathy), and four had other gastrointestinal problems.

Ferguson MM, Wray D, Carmichael HA, et al: Coeliac disease associated with recurrent aphthae. Gut 21:223–226, 1980.

Only two of 50 patients with recurrent aphthae had celiac disease, but in these two the disease cleared within one month of eliminating gluten from their diet. Both had low folate levels and pathognomonic jejunal biopsy findings. No aphthae appeared during a two-year follow-up.

The authors feel that all patients with recurrent aphthae should be screened for folate, vitamin B_{12}, and iron deficiency. If a depressed level of whole blood folate is found (as in eight patients in this series), it is reasonable to perform a jejunal biopsy to look for celiac disease (yield: two of eight in this study).

Wray D, Graykowski EA, Notkins AL: Role of mucosal injury in initiating recurrent aphthous stomatitis. Br Med J 283:1569–1570, 1981.

Test puncture wounds in oral mucosa were made by suture placement, tenaculum penetration, and hypodermic needles. Aphthous ulcers were induced at 26 sites in 13 of 30 patients with a history of aphthous stomatitis. No lesions were induced in 15 controls.

Hay KD, Reade PC: The use of an elimination diet in the treatment of recurrent aphthous ulceration of the oral cavity. Oral Surg 57:504–507, 1984.

Seventeen patients with aphthae embarked on a cereal-free and fruit-free elimination diet (Rowe) for six to eight weeks. Results: five dropped out, five had remission, and seven had no change. Specific causal food allergens identified in four patients:

milk-cheese
wheat
tomatoes
figs

The latent period was usually 24 to 48 hours. Previous foods implicated as precipitating factors had included coffee, chocolate, potato, nuts, citrus fruits, and gluten.

Pimlott SJ, Walker DM: A controlled clinical trial of the efficacy of topically applied fluocinonide in the treatment of recurrent aphthous ulceration. Br Dent J 154:174–177, 1983.

An extemporaneous preparation of **fluocinonide** (0.05 per cent ointment combined with equal weight of Orabase) applied to ulcers five times a day for six weeks significantly decreased the size and duration of ulcers in 18 of 20 patients, as compared with the control base. The number of new ulcers remained unchanged.

Yeoman CM, Greenspan JS, Harding SM: Recurrent oral ulceration: A double-blind comparison of treatment with betamethasone valerate aerosol and placebo. Br Dent J 144:114–116, 1978.

Betamethasone valerate aerosol (1 puff of 100 μg q4h) was helpful in 11 of 14 patients with minor aphthae, especially for lesions in inaccessible sites. It does not alter the serum cortisol levels.

Graykowski EA, Kingman A: Double-blind trial of tetracycline in recurrent aphthous ulceration. J Oral Pathol 7:376–382, 1978.

Since an L-form of streptococcus inhabits aphthous ulcers, they used **tet-**

racycline suspension (250 mg/5 ml [1 teaspoon] tid—hold in mouth two minutes, then swallow) for treatment. Double-blind data indicated that this regimen reduced the size, duration, and pain of ulcers in 25 patients studied for 20 weeks.

Gatot A, Tovi F: Colchicine therapy in recurrent oral ulcers. Arch Dermatol 120:994, 1984.

In four patients with recurrent aphthous ulcers for many years clearance occurred following treatment with **colchicine** (0.6 to 1.2 mg/day). One patient needed it only for five days preceding each menstrual period; another patient was cured after one month; and the two others needed long-term dosage.

Bowers PW, Powell RJ: Effect of thalidomide on orogenital ulceration. Br Med J 287:799–800, 1983.

In three patients with treatment-resistant aphthous stomatitis the condition cleared with **thalidomide** (200 mg bid for five days, then 200 mg/day), but a maintenance dose was required or relapse occurred. Neuropathy and teratogenesis remain serious important side effects of this drug, and informed consent is necessary prior to its use.

Genvo MF, Faure M, Thivolet J: Traitement de l'aphtose par la thalidomide et la colchicine. Dermatologica 168:182–188, 1984.

Thalidomide (200 to 300 mg/day) with or without **colchicine** (2 to 3 mg/day) was given to 25 patients with aphthosis, including 13 with Behçet's disease. Major improvement was noted in all groups, with rapid healing, rapid reduction in pain, and no new outbreaks of ulcers with a maintenance dose of thalidomide (50 to 100 mg/day alone or with colchicine 1 mg/day). There was rapid recurrence within a few weeks after the end of treatment. In the Behçet's patients, ocular symptoms, arthritis, and superficial nodular phlebitis as well as the skin aphthae quickly disappeared.

Rosenthal S: Does phenelzine relieve aphthous ulcers of the mouth? N Engl J Med 311:1442, 1984.

Three patients were cleared of recurrent aphthous ulcers by Nardil (**phenelzine sulfate**—usual starting dose 15 mg tid). This monoamine oxidase inhibitor antidepressant requires dietary avoidance of cheese, yogurt, herring, sausage, liver, broad beans, beer, wine, yeast, chocolate, and caffeine. Relapse occurred on stopping the drug.

Schulkind ML, Heim LR, South MA, et al: A case report of the successful treatment of recurrent aphthous stomatitis with some preparations of orally administered transfer factor. Cell Immunol 84:415–421, 1984.

A careful double-blind study of one 14-year-old boy with disabling recurrent aphthous stomatitis demonstrated some effectiveness of two of four different transfer factor preparations given orally (0.25 ml once weekly). Transfer factor is prepared by freeze-thawing normal buffy coat 10 times and filtering the lysate through dialysis tubing. Presumably transfer factor would help correct impaired immunity to an as-yet-unidentified common virus.

Merchant HW, Gangarosa LP, Glassman AB, Sobel RE: Zinc sulfate supplementation for treatment of recurring oral ulcers. South Med J 70:559–561, 1977.

Serum zinc determinations in 32 patients with recurrent aphthous ulcers showed that 14 patients had low levels (<110 μg/dl). All nine patients with low serum zinc levels who were given **zinc sulfate** (220 mg tid with food) showed 50 to 100 per cent reduction in frequency of attacks of oral ulcers. Only three of eight patients with initial zinc levels above 110 μg/dl improved with zinc supplementation.

Wray D: A double-blind trial of systemic zinc sulfate in recurrent aphthous stomatitis. Oral Surg 53:469–472, 1982.

No therapeutic effect of zinc sulfate (220 mg tid for 12 weeks) on aphthous stomatitis could be demonstrated once 25 patients and the physician were "kept in the dark."

Potts AJC, Frame JW, Batemen JRM, Asquith P: Sodium cromoglycate toothpaste in the management of aphthous ulceration. Br Dent J 156:250–251, 1984.

Despite the known anti-inflammatory effect of cromoglycate, its use in a toothpaste (4 per cent cromoglycate bid for three minutes for 12 weeks) was without effect on the number, size, duration, pain, or frequency of aphthous ulcers in 30 patients participating in a double-blind cross-over trial.

Less is more.

MIES VAN DER ROHE

What this patient needs is a doctor.

EUGENE STEAD

Atopic Dermatitis

Environmental control	Atarax
Emollients	PUVA
Topical steroids	Cetaphil
Erythromycin	

Nowhere in dermatologic therapy is environmental control more important than in the management of atopic dermatitis. This is a disease that responds directly to the control of external irritants and allergens. All of these patients have an exquisite IgE-mediated pruritus. It is this pruritus that in turn mediates the dermatitis, for without scratching there is no atopic dermatitis. It is the incessant rubbing, clawing, scratching, and tearing at the epidermis that produces the epidermal trauma and a cascade of secondary inflammatory intermediates. In its minimal form it is simply patches of dry skin following subclinical eczema. In its maximal form it is the dreaded exfoliative dermatitis.

Our scheme for environmental control centers on an intelligent parent or patient, who is aware of the need for constant surveillance and control of the personal environment. We begin by emphasizing control of the temperature, humidity, and dust content of the air. The room temperature must be kept on the cool side, as heat dramatically increases the number of itch sensory impulses transmitted by the intraepidermal nerve endings and induces sweating. In skin that has postinflammatory poral closure, the potential for miliaria is great, which magnifies the pruritus and inflammation induced by the original IgE-induced epidermal reaction. The development of miliaria is common in atopic infants whose mothers are particularly prone to place them in a tropical environment by overdressing them and covering them with too many blankets.

The humidity must be kept above 40 per cent to keep the already dry atopic skin from becoming completely dehydrated. A humidifier is essential in many homes with hot-air heating. With respect to dust, we stress a monastic life, with bare floors and absence of wool carpets, blankets, and drapes, and frequent vacuuming while the atopic patient is out of the house. We also ask that insecticides, deodorant sprays, and perfumes not be used.

Other sources of air pollution, including cigarette smoke, animal dander, and house dust mites, must be identified and minimized, if not eliminated. We seek to prevent attacks by not permitting chrysanthemum plants, live Christmas fir trees, or paints or varnish in the patient's home. Cats, dogs, and birds are particularly hazardous to the atopic child, and children on the farm are at especial risk. The craving for pets can be assuaged with fish, turtles, or other aquatic specimens. Inhalant allergens take on an increasing importance for the child around two years of age. Some of these are identifiable as seasonal, making an appropriate vacation remarkably beneficial.

For the young adult who still has significant atopic dermatitis, we strongly caution against choosing an occupation that requires exposure to dusts or antigenic

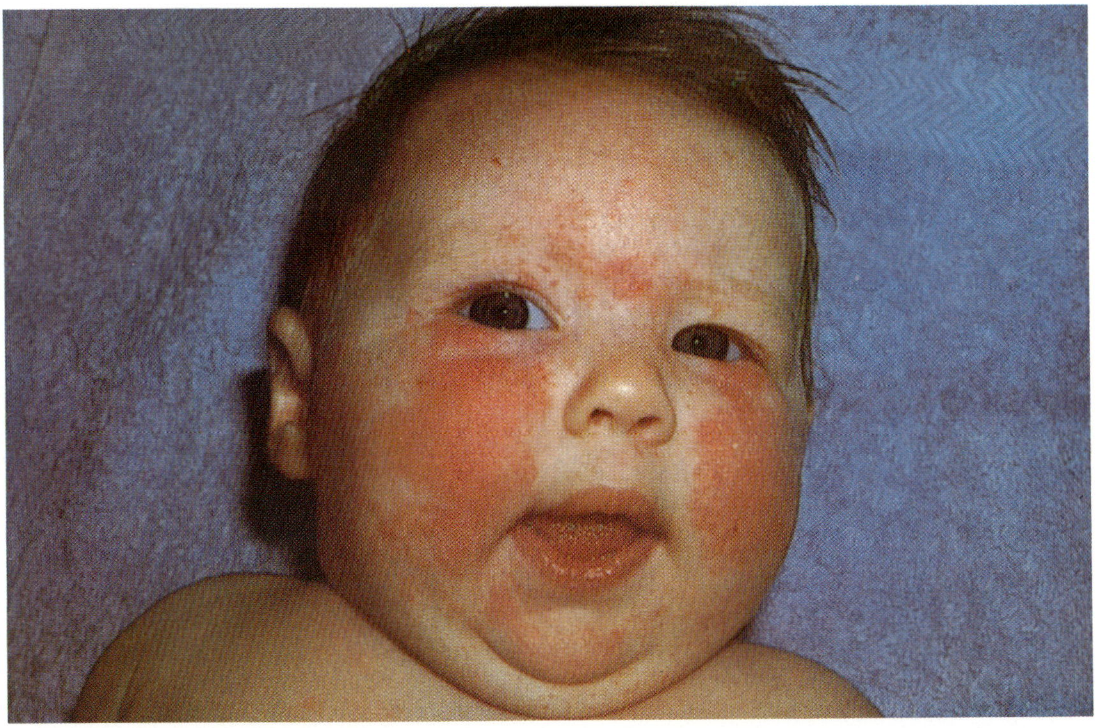

chemicals or frequent handwashing or bathing. The role of the environment was vividly documented by one of our severely atopic patients we sent to the Virgin Islands. Within 48 hours his pruritus was gone and his skin gradually became completely normal for the first time in his life. He remained on the Islands for more than two years with no problem, but upon returning home to Philadelphia for a Christmas reunion, he required emergency treatment within three days. His pruritus and atopic dermatitis had returned full force and remained so until he returned to the Islands. We have often urged similarly affected atopic patients to give their skin a trial of environmental change. Since its value is apparent within a few days, serious decisions concerning relocation can be made rapidly.

Another area of environmental control centers on contactants. The atopic infant often has a facial rash due to contact with foods such as tomatoes or citrus fruits. Feeding must be immediately followed (or even interrupted) by facial cleaning with copious water flushes, done by hand without washcloth or soap. Equally important is the avoidance of new, rough clothing. All-cotton, well-washed clothing is the safest. Wool is the worst, with its innumerable harpoon-like barbs. The child must not be allowed to play on rough upholstery or floor rugs. A few minutes of even gentle rubbing of the itchy skin on a rug can bring about weeks of dermatitis. The price of a healthy skin is indeed diurnal vigilance.

Control of the internal environment is also important. The single most important aspect of this is protection of the infant's intestinal tract from potential allergens. Many believe that solid foods should be avoided for the first six months in any child with atopic parentage. We simply tend to have them avoid eggs and cow's milk. Tampering with the diet can be hazardous, and elimination of foods, followed by challenge, is fraught with the danger of anaphylaxis. Our golden rule is to respect (and eliminate) the foods for which the atopic child has a real and sincere dislike. Often this dislike stems from occult gastrointestinal reactions that may be a harbinger of skin problems to come.

Still another aspect of internal environmental control is the avoidance of excessive physical activity leading to hyperthermia and sweating. The atopic individual remains a victim of sweat retention and miliaria whether the stimulus comes from without or within. It is this same deranged sweat mechanism that calls for a degree of emotional calm and hence absence of autonomic activation of these same glands. It is a goal more easily identified than reached with a screaming infant, but at the very least the parent will be more understanding of the burst of itch and redness the infant sustains. In the older individual, emotional control more often can be attained as the mature atopic patient learns how to keep his family, boss, and job from getting into his skin via the emotionally activated sweat gland. But then there is always a visit to the dentist! Here, xylocaine has been invaluable.

Given the best environmental control possible, one still has to use topical and systemic measures. Topically, we prescribe Synalar ointment (0.025 per cent) to be applied after the shower. If this is not tolerated because of the petrolatum base, we suspect it is being applied too liberally and we reinstruct the patient (who does not need to use it as though preparing to swim the English Channel). We also use Hytone cream (hydrocortisone 1 per cent), particularly in children. The stronger corticosteroids are saved for attacks on foci of real resistance.

Our major systemic measure is erythromycin (250 mg qid). This regularly reduces the pruritogenic, yet clinically inapparent, colonization of dermatitic skin by *Staphylococcus aureus.* We continue this dosage for several weeks, slowly reducing it, but recognize that long-term treatment—for months—is often necessary. We are also alert to the possibility of eczema herpeticum, which should respond well to acyclovir (200 mg, five times a day for 10 days). Another systemic weapon is ketoconazole (200 mg/day) for the atopic patient with yeast colonization.

Atopic dermatitis remains one of our most common challenges, but one so highly diversified as to call for uncommon efforts in history taking, patient instruction, and overall assistance in environmental control. It is the "scratch" that will not go away without a lot of digging on your part.

Hanifin JM: Basic and clinical aspects of atopic dermatitis: A review. Ann Allergy 52:386–395, 1984.

Ten Commandments:

1. Take short cool showers only.
2. Use soap only in intertriginous areas.
3. Avoid situations, environments, and exercises that induce sweating.
4. Avoid lanolin, fragrances, preservatives, **neomycin**, **benzocaine**.
5. Apply topical **corticosteroid** ointment or cream to affected areas within 8 minutes of showering.
6. Use Burow's compresses (1:30) for weeping lesions.
7. Use **erythromycin** or **dicloxacillin** systemically for secondary bacterial infection (five days of treatment is usually sufficient).
8. Watch for food sensitivity factors (present in 20 per cent of children with atopic dermatitis).
9. Avoid jobs that require handwashing or subject the skin to physical or chemical trauma.
10. Consider hospitalization.

Roth HL, Kierland RR: The natural history of atopic dermatitis: A 20-year follow-up study. Arch Dermatol 89:209–214, 1964.

Over half of 492 patients had associated asthma, hay fever, rhinitis, urticaria, or migraine headaches, as well as a family history of atopy. The usual time of onset of atopic dermatitis was at the age of four months. Of patients with severe atopic dermatitis, 13 per cent developed cataracts, in contrast to 4 per cent with mild disease. Factors most helpful in treatment included relaxation, temperate climate, and topical and systemic steroids. Avoidance of nervous tension, cold climate, perspiration, and primary irritants helped greatly. Hyposensitization therapy helped only 5 per cent of patients.

Rajka G: Atopic Dermatitis. Philadelphia, WB Saunders Co, 1975, 165 pp.

The master reference. Places emphasis on the value of vacationing in or moving to a different climate.

Engman MF, Weiss RS, Engman MF Jr: Eczema and environment. Med Clin North Am 20:651–663, 1936.

Classic demonstration in a two-year-old child that skin bandaged to prevent scratching and rubbing remained clinically normal despite intense itch induced by oral challenge with a known wheat allergen. The authors also note that plant pollens (such as ragweed) that float through the air may aggravate eczema.

Krafchik BR: Atopic dermatitis. Pediatr Clin North Am 30:669–685, 1983.

A thoughtful review stressing the value of:

- A humidifier in the bedroom during dry months
- 100 per cent cotton clothing (The Cotton Company, PO Box 631, Chattanooga, TN 37401; phone 1-800-421-4548)
- Atarax at bedtime to promote hours of peaceful sleep
- Avoidance of detergent, bleach, and fabric softeners in laundering clothing

Verbov J: Atopic dermatitis. Practitioner 223:820–825, 1979.

More thoughts:

1. Keep the fingernails short and clean.
2. Use mitten coverings for hands to prevent scratching.
3. **Urea** cream (10 per cent) and **coal tar** in **zinc oxide** paste are useful alternates to steroids.
4. Be alert to the possibility of eczema herpeticum.
5. Occasionally a short course of systemic steroids is necessary for the uncontrollable flare.

Oakes RC, Cox AD, Burgdorf WHC: Atopic dermatitis: A review of diagnosis, pathogenesis and management. Clin Pediatr 22:467–475, 1983.

Scratch tests and desensitization are of no therapeutic value. If parents need the therapy of diagnostic tests, order a serum IgE and a CBC, looking for eosinophilia.

Intensive treatment of acute dermatitis at home should include:

- Cool wet dressings (Burow's solution, normal saline, or tap water) applied with old T-shirts or cotton sheets for 20 to 30 minutes four to six times daily
- Tepid baths with bath oil added 10 minutes after start of bath (to allow hydration of keratin)
- Topical steroids (**triamcinolone** 0.025 per cent cream or ointment) applied while skin is still wet
- Systemic antibiotics
- Sedation with antihistamines

Roberts DLL: House dust mite avoidance and atopic dermatitis. Br J Dermatol 110:735–739, 1984.

Regular vacuum cleaning of carpets, curtains, and bedding, coupled with the use of a plastic mattress cover, reduces the house dust mite population. In an eight-week open study of 18 patients with severe atopic dermatitis, 15 definitely showed concurrent clinical improvement. It may be possible to control house dust mites in the home by using a fungicide spray to destroy *Aspergillus penicilloides*, on which the mite feeds.

Champion RH: Atopic sensitivity to algae and lichens. Br J Dermatol 85:551–557, 1971.

In five patients with atopic dermatitis, flare occurred from both inhalation and contact with green algae and lichens (which contain algae in symbiosis with fungi). Prick tests with suspensions of a lichen or alga (25 per cent by volume in saline + 0.5 per cent phenol + centrifugation or filtration) helped show which patients would benefit from specific desensitization.

Tuft L: Importance of inhalant allergens in atopic dermatitis. J Invest Dermatol 12:211–219, 1949.

House dust, pollens (especially ragweed), wool, animal dander, silk, and cooking odors are potent inhalant allergens causing flares of atopic dermatitis.

Hatch KL, Maibach HI: Textile fiber dermatitis. Contact Dermatitis 12:1–11, 1985.

The protein fibers wool and silk aggravate atopic dermatitis both as inhalants and by direct contact with the skin.

Atherton DJ: Breast feeding and atopic eczema. Br Med J 287:775–776, 1983.

Lactating mothers of infants at risk for atopy should keep their intake of cow's milk and eggs low. Mothers should breast feed their infants exclusively for four months and continue supplementary breast feeding for one year.

Kajosaari M, Saarinen UM: Prophylaxis of atopic disease by six months total solid food elimination: Evaluation of 135 exclusively breast-fed infants of atopic families. Acta Paediatr Scand 72:411–414, 1983.

Food allergens remain a significant cause of atopic dermatitis in infants. The authors identified the following specific offenders in their series:

eggs	strawberries
citrus fruits	cow's milk
fish	peas
tomato	chocolate

Avoidance of all solid food for the first six months of life is advisable, since 35 per cent of the group receiving solids early developed atopic dermatitis, in contrast to 10 per cent getting only mother's milk.

Metcalfe DD: Food allergens. Clin Rev Allergy 3:331–349, 1985.

Food allergens are often found to be water-soluble glycoproteins that resist heat, proteases, and denaturants and thus resist degradation during food preparation and digestion.

There is no evidence to support benefit from either injection immunotherapy or oral desensitization in the treatment of food allergy.

Individuals allergic to specific foods are well advised to avoid other closely related foods in the same plant or animal family. For instance, a table of common food groupings reveals these relationships:

Osteichthyes
- sardine
- trout
- salmon
- whitefish

Gramineae
barley rye
corn wheat
oats rice

Drupaceae
almond apricot
plum cherry
peach

Solanaceae
white potato
chili pepper
tomato

Pomaceae
apple
pear

Liliaceae
garlic
onion
asparagus

Leguminosae
beans peanuts
pea soybean

David TJ: Anaphylactic shock during elimination diets for severe atopic eczema. Arch Dis Child 59:983–986, 1984.

Dislike for a food is a helpful clue concerning food allergy. Four patients developed anaphylactic shock upon reintroduction of a single food (soya, chicken, corn, cow's milk). Note that such reactions usually occur within minutes, but may be delayed up to 10½ hours. Cites example of year-old baby in the hospital who reacted by vomiting to a cow's milk challenge, so that it was stopped. Eight hours later he was found dead in his crib. Ideally, children undergoing food challenge should be hospitalized and observed for 12 hours after the challenge.

Van Asperen PP, Lewis M, Rogers M, et al: Experience with an elimination diet in children with atopic dermatitis. Clin Allergy 13:479–485, 1983.

Dietary manipulation in older children (ages 2 to 12 years) with chronic atopic dermatitis offers only limited long-term therapeutic gains. In only 2 of 29 children could responsible foods be identified (cheese, eggs, vegemite, and beans). Short-term improvement was seen in 7 of 13 children completing the two-week elimination diet.

Reed ML, Koehler PB: A usage-safety study of two new, dry skin formulations in patients with atopic dermatitis. Cutis 32:180–184, 1983.

Two formulations with high concentrations of petrolatum (Vaseline dermatology formula lotion or cream applied two to four times/day for four weeks) were found to be pleasing and effective treatment for the atopic patient's universal complaint of dry skin.

Queille C, Pommarede R, Saurat J-H: Efficacy versus systemic effects of six topical steroids in the treatment of atopic dermatitis of childhood. Pediatr Dermatol 1:246–253, 1984.

Potent topical steroids such as **betamethasone dipropionate** 0.05 per cent (Diprosone cream) or **halcinonide** cream 0.1 per cent (Halog cream) give a rapid marked therapeutic effect when applied once daily without occlusion, but in children this is accompanied by a fall in the level of plasma cortisol. Consider the advisability of alternate-day applications.

Lupton ES, Abbrecht MM, Brandon ML: Short-term topical corticosteroid therapy (halcinonide ointment) in the management of atopic dermatitis. Cutis 30:671–675, 1982.

Halog ointment (**halcinonide** 0.1 per cent applied tid), evaluated in a double-blind paired comparison study of 214 patients with atopic dermatitis, proved to be excellent in 64 per cent of patients, whereas the placebo base gave comparable help in only 24 per cent.

Roth HL: Pathophysiology and treatment of atopic dermatitis. Int J Dermatol 16:163–178, 1977.

Do not put children on an elimination diet with a stock list of allergenic foods, as guilt over occasional indiscretions may have long-lasting effects.

Don't forget that 5 per cent liquor carbonis detergens (LCD) in a bland vehicle is of value. **Ichthammol** (1 to 3 per cent) in **zinc oxide** paste with Tween 80 (10 per cent) is also helpful.

Group psychotherapy helped patients accept the disease and brought them reassurance.

Frosch PJ, Schwanitz HJ, Macher E: A double blind trial of H_1 and H_2 receptor antagonists in the treatment of atopic dermatitis. Arch Dermatol Res 276:36–40, 1984.

Neither the combination of Chlortrimeton (4 mg qid) and Tagamet (400 mg qid) nor Chlortrimeton alone gave any more help for itching or the overall dermatitis than a placebo in this study of 18 patients. Each treatment period lasted four weeks.

Foulds IS, MacKie RM: A double-blind trial of the H_2 receptor antagonist cimetidine, and the H_1 receptor antagonist promethazine hydrochloride in the treatment of atopic dermatitis. Clin Allergy 11:319–323, 1981.

In 20 young adults with atopic dermatitis, there was no significant treatment advantage in adding **cimetidine** (Tagamet 400 mg tid) to **promethazine hydrochloride** (Phenergan 50 mg tid). Cimetidine alone also offered no advantage over Phenergan.

Klein GL, Galant SP: A comparison of the antipruritic efficacy of hydroxyzine and cyproheptadine in children with atopic dermatitis. Ann Allergy 44:142–145, 1980.

Atarax (1.25 mg/kg tid—maximum 30 mg tid) was superior to Periactin (0.25 mg/kg tid—maximum 6 mg tid) in a one-week double-blind study of 20 children. The only other treatment used during the study was Lubriderm cream (applied three times a day for lubrication).

Dahl MV: *Staphylococcus aureus* and atopic dermatitis. Arch Dermatol 119:840–846, 1983.

A fully referenced review of the inapparent, usually present, and often ignored *Staphylococcus aureus* colonization of atopic dermatitis. These bacteria may aggravate the dermatitis and prevent resolution. Systemic or topical antibiotic therapy is frequently followed by clinical improvement.

Leyden JJ, Marples RR, Kligman AM: *Staphylococcus aureus* in the lesions of atopic dermatitis. Br J Dermatol 90:525–530, 1974.

Most patients with atopic dermatitis experience long-term colonization with coagulase-positive *Staphylococcus aureus* (14×10^6 organisms/sq cm in exudative forms), despite the absence of clinical signs of infection. Systemic **erythromycin** (250 mg qid) or topical **neomycin** (1 per cent cream bid) produced a profound decrease in the numbers of bacteria present and subsequent clinical improvement in 24 patients studied.

Leyden JJ, Baker DA: Localized *Herpes simplex* infections in atopic dermatitis. Arch Dermatol 115:311–312, 1979.

Herpes simplex infections, localized to areas of atopic dermatitis, were demonstrated by viral cultures in 10 children with low-grade fever and discrete vesicles or punched-out ulcers within areas of dermatitis. Recurrent attacks were associated with active herpes labialis in other family members or close friends (another indication now for oral **acyclovir** therapy).

White I, Blatchford N: The treatment of secondary bacterial infections in atopic eczema with miconazole plus hydrocortisone. Br J Clin Pract 37:215–216, 1983.

In over half of 19 patients with severe atopic eczema and secondary infection, a cream containing **miconazole** 2 per cent (active against gram-positive bacteria) and **hydrocortisone** 1 per cent eradicated surface bacterial overgrowth (including *Staphylococcus aureus*) after two weeks of use.

Washington JA II, Wilson WR: Erythromycin: A microbial and clinical perspective after 30 years of clinical use (first of two parts). Mayo Clin Proc 60:189–203, 1985.

A comprehensive review of the drug most commonly prescribed for atopic patients notes the unique and remarkable concentration of **erythromycin** achieved within the polymorphonuclear leukocytes, as well as its broad antimicrobial spectrum.

Caputo RV: Recent advances in pediatric dermatology. Pediatr Clin North Am 30:735–748, 1983.

Do not prescribe **erythromycin** for atopic individuals if **theophylline** is already being given. In one week of conjoint therapy the serum theophylline levels may rise 40 per cent, resulting in toxic theophylline reactions. Other antibiotics such as **tetracycline**, **cephalosporins**, and **penicillin** do not do this. If erythromycin must be used because of penicillin allergy, decrease the dosage of theophylline by at least 25 per cent and monitor serum theophylline levels (toxic if greater than 20 μg/ml).

Wright S, Burton JL: Oral evening-primrose-seed oil improves atopic eczema. Lancet 2:1120–1122, 1982.

Evening-primose–seed oil capsules (two to six capsules bid for 12 weeks), each containing the essential fatty acids linoleic acid 360 mg and gamma-linolenic acid 45 mg, resulted in 30 to 43 per cent improvement in pruritus and scaling in 99 atopic dermatitis patients in this double-blind controlled cross-over study. Children improved less than adults, possibly because of lower dosage.

Molkhou P, Waguet J-C: Food allergy and atopic dermatitis in children: Treatment with oral sodium cromoglycate. Ann Allergy 47:173–175, 1981.

Food allergies in 35 children with atopic dermatitis were proven by dietary elimination and challenge, radioallergosorbent tests (RAST), and human basophil degranulation tests.

Common food allergens included:

egg (28)	fish (4)
cow's milk (27)	orange (4)
chocolate (15)	nuts (1)
cereals (11)	

Oral **sodium cromoglycate** for one to three months (100 mg/day for several days, then 200 mg/day, occasionally 300 to 600 mg/day) helped 23 children have almost complete clearing of skin lesions while tolerating a normal (unrestricted) diet.

Daugbjerg PS, Bach-Mortensen N, Østerballe O: Oral sodium cromoglycate treatment of atopic dermatitis related to food allergy. Allergy 39:535–541, 1984.

Despite a series of uncontrolled testimonials for therapy with this mast cell blocker, a carefully controlled trial with 34 patients found oral cromolyn (200 to 1600 mg/day) to be of no help.

Sannwald C, Ortonne JP, Thivolet J: La photochimiotherapie orale de l'eczéma atopique. Dermatologica 159:71–77, 1979.

Nine of 11 atopic patients showed improvement of 80 per cent or more with PUVA, but maintenance treatment was successful in only three of these.

Scholtz JR: Management of atopic dermatitis. Calif Med 102:210–216, 1965.

Do not tell patients not to scratch.

The author's program, now known as the Scholtz regimen, was successful in 14 patients with severe atopic eczema previously requiring systemic steroids for control. The program is designed to preserve the natural lipid surface film, avoid sweating, and control skin infection.

Treatment regimen:

Discontinue systemic steroids.
Stop bathing or washing—no hot baths or showers; ocean swimming is OK.
Cetaphil (lipid-free lotion) cleansing daily—gently wipe off or leave to dry.
Soap and water "spot cleansing" only of fingers, toes, axillae, groin, and perianal areas (if free of dermatitis).
No greasy or lipid lubricants.
Systemic antibiotics for 10 to 12 days.
Topical steroids—**fluocinolone acetonide** 0.01 per cent in **propylene glycol** (Synalar solution) 15 to 20 ml daily was preferred—alternates: fluocinolone acetonide cream (Synalar cream) or **triamcinolone acetonide** cream (Kenalog, Aristocort).
Vitamin A (50,000 IU/day for 6 months)—use in adults.
Thyroid extract USP (30 to 60 mg/day)—given to potentiate the vitamin A.
Antihistamines for a few days to control pruritus.
Stop exercise and sun exposure until skin has improved enough to see sweat on the skin surface.

Scholtz JR: Atopic dermatitis. Arch Dermatol 115:110, 1979.

An updated version: the three greatest measures for controlling atopic dermatitis are simply these:

1. Reduce sweating by avoiding
   - Hot baths
   - Exercise
   - Emotional stimuli
2. Use systemic antibiotics to reduce the bacterial population on dermatitic skin.
3. Use topical corticosteroids in nongreasy bases.

Millikan LE: Atopic dermatitis: Clinical spectrum and approach to treatment. Postgrad Med 76:139–146, 1984.

A fully informed parent or patient is an essential part of successful, long-term management of this chronic disease.

Recommendations:

Avoid systemic steroids unless the patient is disabled from work.
Use bath oils containing tar.
Avoid harsh soaps—use a soap substitute or superfatted soap.
Use topical steroids, antihistamines, and lubrication.
Consider using tar plus ultraviolet light (Goeckerman treatment).

Uehara M, Takada K: Use of soap in the management of atopic dermatitis. Clin Exp Dermatol 10:419–425, 1985.

Ninety-two per cent of 130 patients with atopic dermatitis who had been using topical corticosteroids but avoiding soap for one month to eight years experienced considerable improvement in their skin lesions within one week of adding common toilet soap to their total body bathing routine. The improvement was sustained and continued use did not lead to dry skin, thus belying the view that soap is harmful for the atopic.

It may be an indiscretion to leave your patient's next appointment to his discretion.

Don't expect patients to criticize a medication. Prescribe or dispense only a small amount. You'll know it's effective when they *request more.*

Atrophie Blanche

Antibiotics
Aspirin-Persantine
Heparin
Procardia
Trental

While these residual white scars of cutaneous infarcts are not susceptible to treatment, therapy may prevent new lesions resulting from sporadic occlusion of vessels in the middle and deep dermis and also hasten healing of ulcerations. The causes of the continuing painful vasculitis are multiple and often unknown. Treatment has centered on altering the clotting mechanism by inhibiting platelet thrombus formation or stimulating endogenous fibrinolytic activity.

Although clotting in the peripheral vessels is the known cause of atrophie blanche, the systems controlling clotting and bleeding are delicately balanced, so that major interference using anticoagulants or fibrinolytic agents (streptokinase or urokinase) risks bleeding (e.g., gastrointestinal tract, intracranial). New fibinolytic drugs may deserve a trial.

Milstone LM, Braverman IM, Lucky P, Fleckman P: Classification and therapy of atrophie blanche. Arch Dermatol 119:963–969, 1983.

A thoughtful complete review. Rule out arterial or venous insufficiency, abnormal serum proteins, Raynaud's disease, and collagen-vascular disease. Consider bedrest, debridement, and systemic antibiotics.

Drucker CR, Duncan WC: Antiplatelet therapy in atrophie blanche and livedo vasculitis. J Am Acad Dermatol 7:359–363, 1982.

Aspirin (325 mg tid) and **dipyridamole** (Persantine) (75 mg qid) produced rapid pain relief and healing of vasculitic ulcers in seven patients after two to seven months. Elastic stockings, silver nitrate cautery, and topical and systemic steroids had given only temporary relief.

Aspirin inhibits prostaglandin synthesis critical in platelet aggregation, and dipyridamole inhibits platelet function. They act together to prevent thrombosis in small vessels.

Kern AB: Atrophie blanche: Report of two patients treated with aspirin and dipyridamole. J Am Acad Dermatol 6:1048–1053, 1982.

Aspirin (325 mg bid) and **dipyridamole** (50 mg tid) healed ulcers in two patients within two to four weeks. At least six months of treatment was necessary to prevent recurrences.

Jetton RL, Lazarus GS: Minidose heparin therapy for vasculitis of atrophie blanche. J Am Acad Dermatol 8:23–26, 1983.

Subcutaneous **heparin** (5000 U every third day) produced complete remission in three months in a 28-year-old man. This heparin dosage did not alter the clotting, prothrombin, or partial thromboplastin times. With heparin reduction to every fourth day, a small ulcer appeared, which cleared on resumption of the more frequent dose. Clearing had previously occurred with **phenformin** (50 to 100 mg) and **ethylestrenol** (2 to 6 mg daily), but phenformin has not been available in the United States since 1977. **Prednisone** (40 mg/day) produced some improvement, but was poorly tolerated. Previous unsuccessful classic treatments over 16 years included:

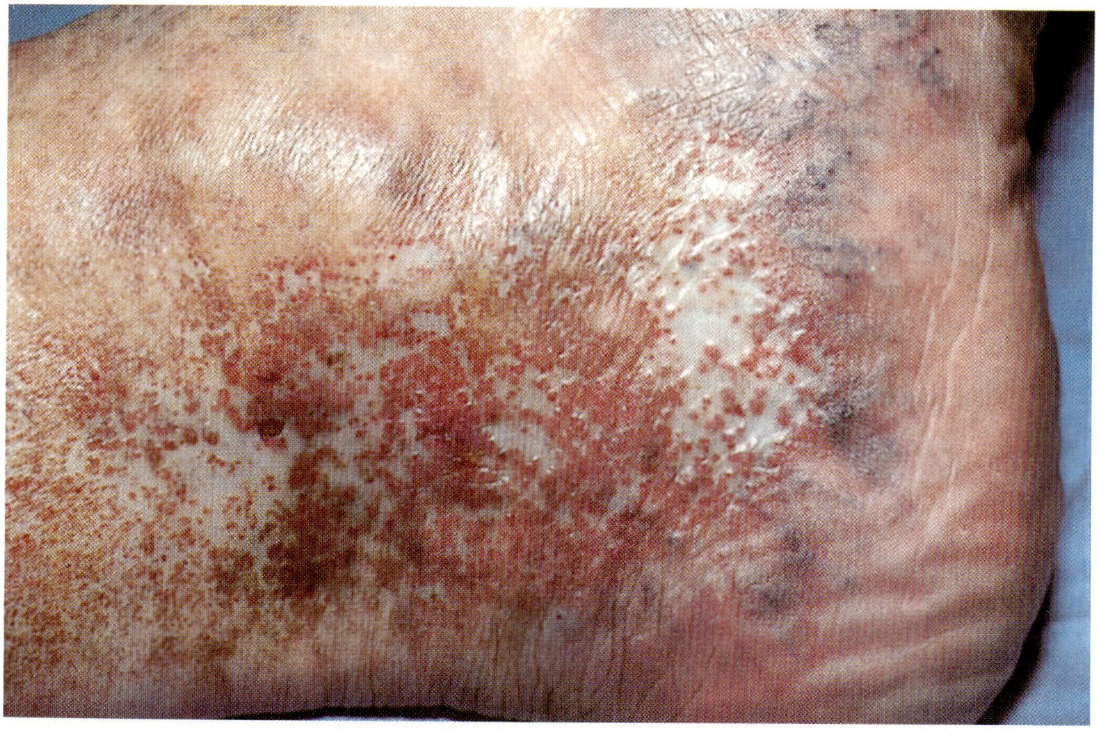

aspirin-Persantine	Motrin
colchicine	nicotinic acid
Dapsone	potassium iodide
erythromycin	

Cunliffe WJ, Menon IS: The association between cutaneous vasculitis and decreased blood fibrinolytic activity. Br J Dermatol 84:99–105, 1971.

Nine of ten patients with atrophie blanche were successfully treated with conjoint **phenformin** and **ethylestrenol**.

Gilliam JN, Herndon JH, Prystowsky SD: Fibrinolytic therapy for vasculitis of atrophie blanche. Arch Dermatol 109:664–667, 1974.

Five cases responded favorably to **phenformin** (50 mg bid) and **ethylestrenol** (2 mg bid). Painful ulcers healed with one to four months. Two patients developed amenorrhea from the androgenic effect of ethylestrenol.

Purcell SM, Hayes TJ: Nifedipine treatment of idiopathic atrophie blanche. J Am Acad Derm 14:851–854, 1986.

Nifedipine (Procardia, 10 mg tid, on long-term basis) was effective therapy in one patient. Acting as a calcium channel blocker, it induces arterial vasodilation. Thus, it is also of use in Raynaud's phenomenon and urticaria pigmentosa.

Sauer GC: Pentoxifylline (Trental) therapy for the vasculitis of atrophie blanche. Arch Dermatol 122:380–381, 1986.

Pentoxifylline (Trental, 400 mg tid) induced healing of ulcers and reduced induration and tenderness in six patients with atrophie blanche. The drug acts by lowering blood viscosity and by improving erythrocyte flexibility, thereby enhancing the cutaneous blood flow.

The most valuable by-product of experience is confidence.

Autoimmune Progesterone Dermatitis

Estradiol Premarin Oophorectomy

Shelley WB, Preucel RW, Spoont SS: Autoimmune progesterone dermatitis: Cure by oophorectomy. JAMA 190:35–38, 1964.

For five years a 27-year-old woman had had an extensive pruritic vesiculobullous eruption resembling dermatitis herpetiformis clinically and erythema multiforme histologically. It showed exacerbations premenstrually and on challenge with progesterone (20 mg PO). It had not responded to **sulfapyridine**, corticosteroids, **griseofulvin**, or antihistamines. A **progesterone** desensitization program (0.1 mg/day with 0.1-mg-daily increments for 10 days) greatly worsened the dermatitis, while **estinyl estradiol** (Estinyl 0.05 mg tid) to inhibit ovulation suppressed the lesions. The ultimate cure was oophorectomy.

Hart R: Autoimmune progesterone dermatitis. Arch Dermatol 113:426–430, 1977.

In five of seven women, cyclic treatment with **conjugated estrogens** (Premarin 1.25 mg/day for 21 days) resulted in remission. All cases were characterized by the recurrence of skin lesions (urticaria, dyshidrosis, or erythema multiforme) 5 to 10 days prior to menses and a positive progesterone skin test.* Enovid-E therapy was not helpful.

---

* Progesterone skin test: aqueous progesterone suspension (100 mg/ml)—dilute with normal saline to 0.1 mg/ml, 0.01 mg/ml, and 0.001 mg/ml. Inject intradermally and read the three tests at 48 hours.

It is better to try a doubtful remedy than to try none.
HIPPOCRATES

Balanitis

Antibiotics topical	Ketoconazole
Antibiotics systemic	Circumcision
Clotrimazole	

The treatment of balanitis is essentially the treatment of infection. Nowhere on the skin are conditions more optimal for the growth of organisms, as the foreskin forms a "culture tube" around the glans penis. If it is not regularly everted and cleansed, bacteria and yeasts of all types flourish, and their toxins induce both balanitis and posthitis. Thus, congenital phimosis and indifferent hygiene favor these inflammatory changes. Interestingly, the urethra exposed to the same pathogens and opportunistic flora generally remains free of disease because of the automatic flushing and cleansing that occur during urination.

Although cultural studies may be indicated in recalcitrant cases of balanitis, we generally proceed directly to a treatment program that centers on good gentle washing of the glans with the foreskin retracted. We recommend an antibacterial soap such as Dial and emphasize the need for careful rinsing. Monistat-Derm or Spectazole cream is applied sparingly after each washing. This is generally curative. We do not use topical steroids because of their atrophogenic potential.

In more severe cases we prescribe $KMnO_4$ compresses or soaks (used immediately after formulation with $2\frac{1}{2}$ grains to a quart of tap water, 15 minutes bid). This is used in conjunction with a systemic antibiotic for one week, such as erythromycin (250 mg qid), ampicillin (500 mg qid), or metronidazole (250 mg tid). If the balanitis is of yeast origin and severe, we prescribe Nizoral (200 mg/day for one week).

All patients with balanitis should have a serologic test for syphilis as well as a health profile to detect diabetes or other predisposing conditions. Of equal importance is a careful examination of the oral mucous membrane for the presence of lichen planus, cicatricial pemphigoid, or Behçet's disease. General inspection of the skin allows detection of minor forms of psoriasis, seborrheic dermatitis, or Reiter's syndrome, to which the patient may be indifferent or of which he may be unaware. Furthermore, a biopsy may, on rare occasions, be significant in detecting plasma cell balanitis or an underlying malignant or atrophic process masquerading as balanitis. The possibility of a contact sensitivity or irritant reaction should also be ruled out. Finally, a good drug history rules out a drug eruption.

Recurrent examples deserve investigation and possible treatment of sexual partners since vaginitis or infection elsewhere is a significant source of infectious balanitis. Always, however, the most satisfactory prophylactic measure is circumcision, since this eliminates the favorable environment for this disease.

Cree GE, Willis AT, Phillips KD, Brazier JS: Anaerobic balanoposthitis. Br Med J 284:859–860, 1982.

Infection (nonspecific, bacterial, candidal, and herpetic) accounted for 95 per cent of 104 cases of balanitis. Spread by vaginal or orogenital intercourse, as well as the hands-mouth-penis route. Does not occur in circumcised individuals. In 31 of 104 there was anaerobic erosive balanitis with penile ulceration, foul-smelling discharge, and a mixed and motile bacterial flora. This responded rapidly to **metronidazole** (200 mg tid for five days) and **clotrimazole** ointment (1 per cent) topically.

Kinghorn GR, Jones BM, Chowdhury FH, Geary I: Balanoposthitis associated with *Gardnerella vaginalis* infection in men. Br J Vener Dis 58:127–129, 1982.

In a series of 194 cases of balanitis, 14 were due to *Gardnerella vaginalis* (formerly *Corynebacterium vaginale*) infection. All were in uncircumcised patients, with phimosis and poor hygiene contributory. (No comment on treatment, but this organism is commonly sensitive to **erythromycin**.)

Brook I: Group B beta-hemolytic streptococci causing balanitis. South Med J 73:1095, 1980.

Abundant streptococci were present on the swollen red glans of a 28-year-old man and also in a cervical culture from the patient's wife. Complete clearing with **ampicillin** (500 mg q6h for 10 days).

Masfari AN, Kinghorn GR, Duerden BI: Anaerobes in genitourinary infections in men. Br J Vener Dis 59:255–259, 1983.

The predominant organism in 79 patients with balanoposthitis was *Bacteroides* spp. Underscores the need for bacterial cultures and antibacterial therapy.

Petrozzi JW, Erlich A: Pseudomonal balanitis. Arch Dermatol 113:952–953, 1977.

A teaching example of balanitis in a 29-year-old, unresponsive to Mycolog cream and Fungizone lotion, was cured by cool saline compresses, **gentamicin sulfate** cream (Garamycin), and circumcision after cultures revealed *Pseudomonas aeruginosa.* Long-term administration of topical steroids, antibacterial, and anticandidal therapy probably led to colonization by *Pseudomonas* spp. The authors emphasize the need for laboratory and clinical study to rule out contact reaction, trauma, venereal diseases, tuberculosis, and amebiasis, as well as staphylococcal, streptococcal, and trichomonal infections.

Waugh MA, Evans EGV, Nayyar KC, Fong R: Clotrimazole (Canesten) in the treatment of candidal balanitis in men: With incidental observations on diabetic candidal balanoposthitis. Br J Vener Dis 54:184–186, 1978.

Clotrimazole cream 1 per cent (e.g., Lotrimin bid for three weeks) was curative in 98 per cent of 138 men with candidal balanitis. Note that 11 per cent had diabetes mellitus!

Waugh MA: Clinical presentation of candidal balanitis—Its differential diagnosis and treatment. Chemotherapy 28(Suppl 1):56–60, 1982.

Advises:

1. Wash twice daily.
2. Copper sulfate solution (aqueous compress 1:500 bid)
3. **Nystatin** cream (Mycostatin) or **clotrimazole** cream (Lotrimin, Mycelex) bid for two weeks
4. Consider **ketoconazole** (Nizoral 200 mg bid for one to three weeks).
5. Treat partner if there is yeast vaginitis or candidasis elsewhere.

Chakraborty AK, Dutta AK: Herpetic balanoposthitis. Indian J Dermatol 26:15–23, 1981.

Of 113 cases of balanoposthitis 81 per cent were due to infection, with 20 per cent of these due to *herpes simplex.* For herpetic balanitis, use **idoxuridine** drops 0.1 per cent (Stoxil q2h day and night for three days, followed by reduction in frequency of application for an additional seven days).

Peutherer JF, Smith IW, Robertson HH: Necrotising balanitis due to a generalised primary infection with *herpes simplex* virus type 2. Br J Vener Dis 55:48–51, 1979.

Idoxuridine (5 per cent in dimethyl sulfoxide tid for five days) gave rapid improvement in a 37-year-old, who also had disseminated lesions of herpes simplex.

Powers RD, Rein MF, Hayden FG: Necrotizing balanitis due to herpes simplex type 1. JAMA 248:215–216, 1982.

Suggests **acyclovir** therapy. Need to be aggressive since urethral stricture may ensue.

Lejman K, Starzycki Z: Syphilitic balanitis of Follmann developing after the appearance of the primary chancre. A case report. Br J Vener Dis 51:138–140, 1975.

A giant primary chancre of the coronal sulcus and subsequent balanitis due to astonishing swarms of spirochetes within the epidermis healed in six days following **procaine penicillin** (600,000 U IM each day for 32 days).

Farkas J: Balanitis medicamentosa erythematosa, bullosa, erosiva et ulcerosa combustiformis als Erscheinung eines fixen Arzneimittelexanthems. Dermatol Monatsschr 162:250–253, 1976.

Four cases of fixed-drug balanitis were not cured until the offending drugs were stopped (amidopyrine, ketophenylbutazone, oxyphyllin, and tetracycline, respectively).

Brown ST: Tetracycline balanitis: Fixed drug reaction. JAMA 227:801, 1974.

Three cases were cured by stopping tetracycline. In each case, rechallenge with tetracycline caused recurrence of lesions within a few hours.

Finnerty EF: Dermatitis artefacta of the genitals. Cutis 18:199–200, 1976.

"Dermatitis erotica" in a 40-year-old male was likely due to multiple cigarette burns. Successful treatment: cold boric acid soaks (10 minutes tid) and 3 per cent **iodochlorhydroxyquin** in 1 per cent **hydrocortisone** lotion (Vioform-hydrocortisone).

Sonnex TS, Dawber RPR, Ryan TJ, Ralfs IG: Zoon's (plasma-cell) balanitis: Treatment by circumcision. Br J Dermatol 106:585–588, 1982.

Two biopsy-proven cases that failed to respond to local steroids, antifungals, and antiseptics were rapidly cured by circumcision.

Ferrándiz C, Ribera M: Zoon's balanitis treated by circumcision. J Dermatol Surg Oncol 10:622–625, 1984.

Seven patients with plasma cell balanitis, each of which was negative on bacteriologic study, were permanently cured by circumcision.

Michalowski R: Balano-posthites a Trichomonas: A propos de 16 observations. Ann Dermatol Venereol 108:731–738, 1981.

Erosive lesions of the glans penis and foreskin occurrred in 16 of 46 patients with trichomoniasis. The infection was favored by a long foreskin. Phimosis was the dominant complication. Treatment with **metronidazole** for 10 days cleared the lesions.

If the patient is you, try a placebo or two.

Balanitis Xerotica Obliterans

Corticosteroids
Testosterone ointment
Circumcision
Surgery

This strange, atrophic, and at times premalignant lesion appears to be a subset of lichen sclerosus et atrophicus with only penile lesions. Its course is insidiously slow, but its presence calls for conjoint dermatologic and urologic care, since stenosis of the meatus may occur.

Our initial care for the mucocutaneous lesions that may start as no more than perimeatal erythema is the regular daily use of a mild topical steroid such as hydrocortisone (Hytone 1 per cent ointment). Testosterone propionate ointment (2 to 3 per cent in Vaseline or petrolatum base) at bedtime is then added. Hyperkeratotic excrescences are removed by superficial subsection (Gillette Super Blue Blade). Tears and infection are treated with erythromycin (250 mg qid for five days).

Frequently, circumcision must be undertaken. If interference with the urinary stream occurs, meatotomy or meatoplasty must be considered.

In all instances, careful long-term surveillance is necessary, and appropriate biopsy must be done if changes occur that in any way suggest malignancy. Few patients ever want less.

Poynter JH, Levy J: Balanitis xerotica obliterans: Effective treatment with topical and sublesional corticosteroids. Br J Urol 39:420–425, 1967.

Presenting complaint in a 34-year-old man: Tearing of foreskin during intercourse.

℞:

Circumcision.

Injection sublesionally of 2 ml **triamcinolone acetonide** (5 mg/cc Kenalog-10 diluted in equal parts with 1 per cent Xylocaine) q3 weeks for four times was superior to **fluocinolone acetonide** cream (Synalar) under plastic occlusion.

Pasieczny TAH: The treatment of balanitis xerotica obliterans with testosterone propionate ointment. Acta Derm Venereol 57:275–277, 1977.

Four patients had considerable improvement after three to four months and cure in one to two years following the daily application of **testosterone propionate** (2.5 per cent in water-miscible base bid). Advises avoidance of atrophogenic topical corticosteroids.

Khezri AA, Dounis A, Dunn M: Balanitis xerotica obliterans. Br J Urol 51:229–231, 1979.

Study of 20 patients in whom the disease was controlled by circumcision, regular meatal dilatation, meatotomy followed by regular dilatation, and meatoplasty (in advanced cases).

Campus GV, Ena P, Scuderi N: Surgical treatment of balanitis xerotica obliterans. Plast Reconstr Surg 73:652–657, 1984.

Based on experience with 32 patients, the authors recommend topical corticosteroids (**betamethasone 17-valerate** cream 0.1 per cent) for one to two months in the initial stages. Progressive phimosis, fissures, and erosions of the glans and prepuce call for modified circumcision. Likewise, meatal stenosis and scar adhesions call for meatoplasty, excision of scleroatrophic tracts, and full-thickness skin grafting. This gave the majority of patients complete resolution of their major symptoms (burning, itching, painful erection with secondary impotence, and urinary disorders). There were no recurrences over a four-year observation period.

Rosemberg SK, Jacobs H: Continuous wave carbon dioxide treatment of balanitis xerotica obliterans. Urology 19:539–541, 1982.

First case to have lesions vaporized by laser beams. Re-epithelialization required six weeks. Good result.

Ratz JL: Carbon dioxide laser treatment of balanitis xerotica obliterans. J Am Acad Dermatol 10:925–928, 1984.

Another success story for laser therapy in a 39-year-old man with a raw, erosive, exquisitely painful glans penis. Postoperative pain lasted three weeks, but by 12 weeks normal sexual function had been restored.

Neuhofer J, Fritsch P: Treatment of localized scleroderma and lichen sclerosus with etretinate. Acta Derm Venereol 64:171–174, 1984.

The European retinoid Tigason (0.5 mg/kg for 3 to 12 months) failed to have any effect on the course of the disease in three patients with balanitis xerotica obliterans. However, in two of three children with lichen sclerosus et atrophicus (juvenile genital type) clearing occurred.

Bart RS, Kopf AW: Squamous-cell carcinoma arising in balanitis xerotica obliterans. J Dermatol Surg Oncol 4:556–558, 1978.

Moh's chemosurgery following circumcision was successful in this case. Underscores the need for close follow-up of all these patients for early recognition and treatment of malignancy.

If the patient is young, let the medicine be pleasant to the tongue.

Behçet's Disease

Acyclovir	Levamisole
Corticosteroids	Thalidomide
Chlorambucil	Sabin vaccine
Colchicine	Plasmapheresis
Dapsone	

There are no pat answers to this disease. True, systemic steroids suppress the acute inflammatory reaction, but they cannot be given down through the years that this disease continues to attack the patient. Other immunosuppressants must be called upon. Chlorambucil (Leukeran) is currently a favorite. In addition, all methods of modulating the destructive forces of an ectodermal tissue turned upon itself must be considered and possibly tried. These include cyclosporine, colchicine, dapsone, and thalidomide. Methods of nonspecific alteration of the immune status, such as use of levamisole and use of the Sabin live oral polio vaccine, are also potentially useful. Plasmapheresis (when available) offers similar hope.

Today our first therapeutic trial would be with acyclovir (Zovirax 400 mg q4h for two weeks) in the hope that the herpes simplex virus may be pathogenic in some of these patients. A second weapon would be ketoconazole (Nizoral 200 mg or more each day) in the hope that yeast antigens might be significant in the pathogenesis of this mysterious disease. A third medication to try would be 13-*cis* retinoic acid (Accutane 40 mg bid), because the disease centers its destruction in the ectodermal lineage: the mucous membrane, eye, gut, and central nervous system.

Failing to see a response, we would fall back on Kenalog (40 mg IM every three weeks), coupled with chlorambucil (2 to 4 mg a day). Confronted with adverse effects, we would turn to successive trials with dapsone (100 mg/day), cimetidine (300 mg qid), and zinc (220 mg tid with food).

Always we have intensively treated the aphthous ulcers, which are indeed deep, necrotic, and at times purulent. We use tetracycline for direct packing of the ulcer base when accessible, using soft, fine-woven white cotton cloth soaked in tetracycline suspension (one 250 mg capsule emptied into one ounce of tap water, left in place for 15 minutes before each meal). Viscous xylocaine (Xylocaine 2 per cent viscous solution) is useful as a local anesthetic to relieve the pain. We have the patient take metronidazole (Flagyl 250 mg tid) to reduce secondary infection. If the ulcers persist, we prescribe dexamethasone elixir (one teaspoonful tid to be held in the mouth as long as possible, then swallowed).

Since oral aphthae often precede signs of ocular disease, early ophthalmologic consultation is required. Likewise, one must be alert to potential involvement of the central nervous system. Finally, skin tests are interdicted in view of the known tendency of these patients to develop an intense vasculitic reaction at the sites of needle punctures. Protection of normal skin from mechanical injury, particularly on the legs, also lessens the chance of erythema nodosum appearing.

Behçet's disease is a slow, insidious vasculitis that calls for an enterprising, empiric approach to therapy. Here is a disease in which chance favors the mind prepared to explore therapeutic options. Each of our new, powerful antiviral, antifungal, antibacterial, and anti-inflammatory drugs offers promise. Try them. You have the time, if you have the will. Be an opportunist, not an agnostic. Some day a pat answer will be found for this disease, but it won't be found by not looking.

Michelson JB, Chisari FV: Behçet's disease. Surv Ophthalmol 26:190–203, 1982.

A good review of this chronic multisystem disease that blinds one in four of its victims, paralyzes one in ten, and may kill through occlusive vasculitis of the central nervous system. The course is so unpredictable and intermittent as to make evaluation of therapy very difficult. Ninety-one references.

Wong RC, Ellis CN, Diaz LA: Behçet's disease. Int J Dermatol 23:25–32, 1984.

Another excellent review pointing out that systemic corticosteroids (**prednisone** 60 mg/day to start) are the mainstay of therapy, with **chlorambucil** (Leukeran 6 to 8 mg/day) added to enable tapering of steroids. Sixty-seven references.

Lehner T: Progress report: Oral ulceration and Behçet's syndrome. Gut 18:491–511, 1977.

For the treatment of the oral aphthae that invariably accompany and may precede the other manifestations of this disease:

Topical steroids—apply three to four times a day:
- **triamcinolone** (Kenalog 0.1 per cent in Orabase)
- **hydrocortisone sodium succinate** (2.5-mg tablet)
- **betamethasone valerate** (0.1-mg tablet)

Topical **tetracycline** four times a day:
- Suspend 250-mg capsule contents in 5 ml water, hold in mouth two minutes before swallowing.
- A combination capsule of tetracycline with **nystatin** (Mysteclin-F) may be used similarly to prevent candidiasis.

Systemic steroids
- **Prednisone** (40 mg daily for 7 to 10 days)

Prieto J, Suárez J, Civeira P: Acyclovir and Behçet's disease. Ann Intern Med 101:565–566, 1984.

Acyclovir (Zovirax 15 mg/kg/day IV in three divided doses for five days, then orally qid for 20 days) induced long-term remarkable involution of painful aphthae in a 36-year-old woman.

Betamethasone (1 mg/day) was discontinued just prior to starting acyclovir and was not required over the two-month follow-up period.

Firat T: Results of immunosuppressive treatment in Behçet's disease: Report of 55 cases. Ann Ophthalmol 10:1421–1423, 1978.

Azathioprine (Imuran 100 to 200 mg/day) or **cyclophosphamide** (Cytoxan 200 to 400 mg/day) coupled with **prednisolone** (10 mg/day) or **dexamethasone** (1 mg/day) produced complete clearing in 8 of 55 patients with Behçet's disease. There was marked improvement in another 26 patients, but little improvement in the remaining 21. Treatment at full dose was continued for two to six months, followed by half dose for at least another six months prior to cessation.

Sharquie KE: Suppression of Behçet's disease with dapsone. Br J Dermatol 110:493–494, 1984.

Dapsone (100 mg/day) improved the clinical status of all seven male patients to whom it was given. Notably, the pathergic response of these patients to a deep intradermal needle prick was suppressed during the period of dapsone therapy, but reappeared once the drug was stopped.

Pezzi PP, Gasparri V, De Liso P, Catarinelli G: Prognosis in Behçet's disease. Ann Ophthalmol 17:20–25, 1985.

In a 10-year follow-up study of 51 patients, **chlorambucil** (0.1 to 0.2 mg/kg/day) was effective therapy for the retinal vasculitis of Behçet's disease and was considered to be the first-choice immunosuppressant. It must be started at the first sign of retinal vasculitis (as observed with fluorescein angiography). It has low toxicity, but does induce irreversible azoospermia.

Tabbara KF: Chlorambucil in Behçet's disease: A reappraisal. Ophthalmology 90:906–908, 1983.

In this study of 10 men with Behçet's disease, **chlorambucil** (0.2 mg/kg/day) was not found to be helpful. The author advised that it not be given for more than six weeks, if at all.

Harper RM, Allen BS: Use of colchicine in the treatment of Behçet's disease. Int J Dermatol 21:551–554, 1982.

In one month, **colchicine** (0.6 mg bid) resulted in complete clearing in an 18-year-old girl who had had Behçet's disease for five years.

Aktulga E, Altac M, Muftuoglu A, et al: A double blind study of colchicine in Behçet's disease. Haematologica 65:399–402, 1980.

Colchicine (0.5 mg tid) in a double-blind study of 35 Behçet's disease patients showed no effect on aphthae or other signs of the disease.

Hamza M, Ayed K, Ben Ayed H: Treatment of Behçet's disease with levamisole. Arthritis Rheum 25:714–715, 1982.

Levamisole (150 mg/day or 150 mg/day for three consecutive days each week), an antihelmintic drug used for immunostimulation, alleviated oral and genital aphthosis in 17 of 22 patients with Behçet's disease.

Fishel B, Tager A, Fishel R, Yaron M: Poliomyelitis vaccine in the treatment of Behçet's syndrome. Arch Dermatol 116:1348, 1980.

Sabin poliomyelitis vaccine (5 drops orally, once a month for five months) completely cleared the oral and scrotal ulcerations and the neurologic symptoms of a 22-year-old man with Behçet's disease. The remission was complete during the following 2½ years, except for occasional joint pains and continuing uveitis.

Saylan T, Saltik I: Thalidomide in the treatment of Behçet's syndrome. Arch Dermatol 118:536, 1982.

In 22 patients with Behçet's disease, **thalidomide** (200 mg bid for 5 days, then 100 mg bid for 15 to 60 days) rapidly healed the aphthae and reduced their recurrence rate, but had no effect on the iridocyclitis. Eighteen patients had had the disease for more than 10 years and had been unresponsive to antihistamines, vitamins, steroids, colchicine, cyclophosphamide, and levamisole.

Side effects of thalidomide included somnolence, sweating, and headache.

Ffrench-Constant C, Wolman R, Geraint James D: Cyclosporin in Behçet's disease. Lancet 2:454, 1983.

Cyclosporine (10 mg/kg/day for 10 days) produced complete clinical remission in one week of all orogenital ulcerations and polyarthralgias in a 44-year-old Turkish man with Behçet's disease. When the drug was stopped because of rising creatinine levels, the symptoms were back in one week. Retreatment was immediately successful, although a trial of cyclosporine (5 mg/kg/day) was inadequate for long-term control.

Sanders MD, James DG, Graham E, et al: Cyclosporine in Behçet's disease. Lancet 2:454–455, 1983.

Another patient with Behçet's inflammatory eye disease (posterior uveitis and retinal vasculitis) showed prompt subsidence of inflammation when given cyclosporine (10 mg/kg/day for four months).

You B, Lardenet F, Schooneman F, et al: L'utilisation des échanges plasmatiques dans le traitment de la maladie de Behçet. Nouv Presse Med 12:1732, 1983.

Three of five patients with Behçet's disease received help with monthly plasma exchange therapy.

Kikuchi I: The effects of walnuts on Behçet's syndrome in two sisters. J Dermatol 12:290–291, 1985.

After eating seven to eight walnuts from Hawaii, a 30-year-old Japanese woman with Behçet's syndrome suddenly developed inflammation of the right knee that persisted for several months despite treatment.

Reference is made to other work showing that exacerbations of Behçet's syndrome may be associated with eating:

English walnuts	rice cakes
chocolate	oranges
tomatoes	

Jorizzo JL: Behçet's disease. An update based on the 1985 International Conference in London. Arch Dermatol 122:556–558, 1986.

Combinations of **prednisone** (1 mg/kg/day) and **azathioprine** are the mainstay of treatment for severe Behçet's disease. Alternate choices include **chlorambucil** (0.1 mg/kg/day tapered to as low as 2 mg/day), **cyclosporine**, and **thalidomide**.

The following were considered of little or no benefit: cyclophosphamide, penicillamine, acyclovir, and total lymphoid irradiation.

Don't think of the cost of the drug, think of its effectiveness.

Blistering Distal Dactylitis

Phenoxymethyl penicillin Erythromycin

McCray MK, Esterly NB: Blistering distal dactylitis. J Am Acad Dermatol 5:592-594, 1981.

Two youngsters with this distinct, superficial, tender bullous β-hemolytic streptococcal infection of the volar fat pad of the distal phalanx showed prompt response to incision and drainage, Burow's solution compresses, and a 10-day course of phenoxymethyl penicillin (**penicillin V**). **Erythromycin** is the alternate drug of choice.

It is nice to know how a drug works, but even nicer to know it does work.

Three failures erase the memory of your one success. One failure erases the memory of a success you read or heard about.

Bullous Pemphigoid

Corticosteroids	Azathioprine
Dapsone	Plasma exchange
Erythromycin	Cyclosporine

If you know how to treat pemphigus, you know how to treat bullous pemphigoid. Exactly the same drugs are used, but for pemphigoid the dosage is smaller and the treatment period is shorter. In both instances you are treating an autoimmune reaction against the epidermis. But in bullous pemphigoid the reaction is more limited, being against the anchoring basement membrane rather than the entire keratinocyte population.

In our initial assessment of a patient with bullous pemphigoid, we search for unusual triggering factors such as drugs, physical trauma, or an internal malignant tumor. Although the usual case is idiopathic, we have seen two older patients in whom surgical removal of adenocarcinoma of the colon was associated with cure of the pemphigoid. Elimination of drugs is an even simpler approach that occasionally succeeds. We are reminded of one patient who continued to have lesions until her Valium was discontinued.

Our treatment of choice is Kenalog 40 mg IM. It provides standardized controlled steroid dosage, not subject to the vagaries of underdosage and overdosage so common in older patients who form the bulk of the victims of this disease. We give 40 mg (IM) every three weeks, gradually lengthening the interval.

We have used alternate treatments in patients in whom osteoporosis, diabetes, or other contraindications to steroids exist. We always try dapsone (100 mg/day) or erythromycin (250 qid). Indeed, these may be used in conjunction with Kenalog. In the event of failure, the heavier artillery of immunosuppressants is brought in. We prefer Cytoxan (50 mg tid), but other possible choices include Imuran, methotrexate, and the T cell inhibitor, cyclosporine. Always, the dosage is regularly reduced as we search for maintenance levels. We strive for suppression, but not complete absence of lesions while the disease runs its course. The overriding consideration, as always, is to protect the patient from both the disease and the drug.

Bean SF, Fritz KA, Jordon RE: Bullous dermatoses. J Am Acad Dermatol 11:1151–1159, 1984.

Bullous pemphigoid
- is a relatively benign disease
- usually clears after five to six years
- shows remissions and recurrences
- has a variety of forms: vesicular, vegetating, erythematous, erythrodermic, and pruriginous
- responds best to corticosteroids

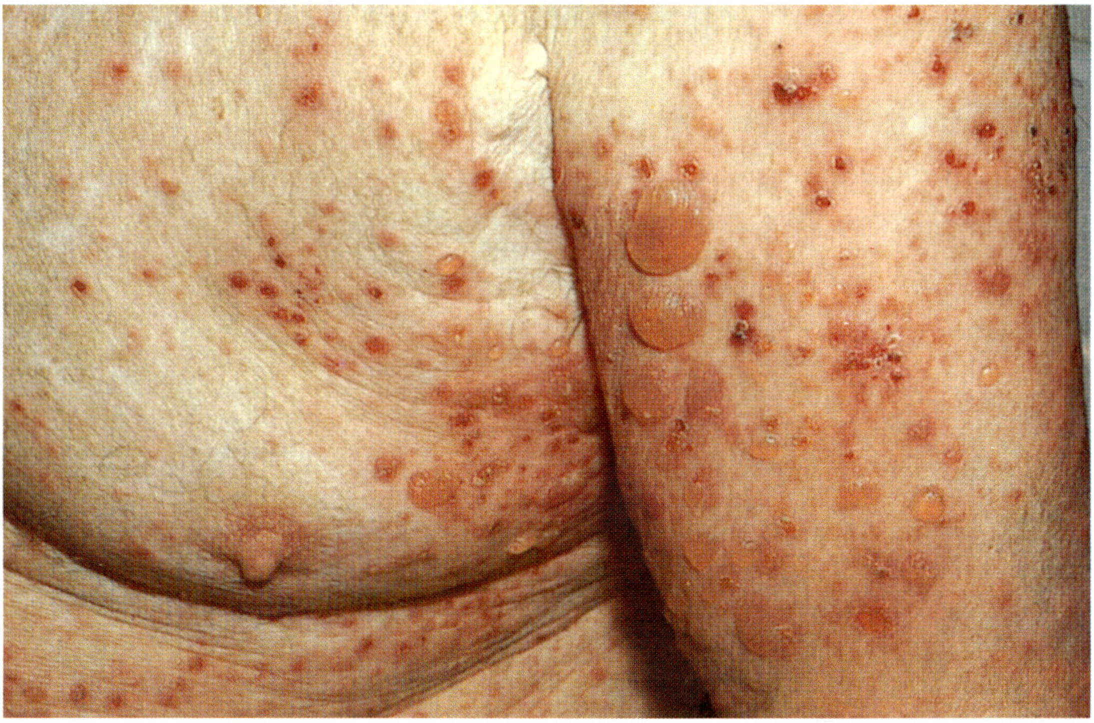

Kashihara M, Danno K, Miyachi Y, et al: Bullous pemphigoid-like lesions induced by phenacetin: Report of a case and an immunopathologic study. Arch Dermatol 120:1196–1199, 1984.

An immunologically proven example of **phenacetin**-induced bullous pemphigoid occurred in an 84-year-old man. **Betamethasone** (Celestone 3 mg/day) therapy cleared the eruption in one month. A later challenge with phenacetin (60 mg) reproduced the blisters in 12 hours. None of the other drugs he had taken had any effect on challenge.

Fellner MJ, Katz JM: Occurrence of bullous pemphigoid after furosemide therapy. Arch Dermatol 112:75–77, 1976.

Prednisone-responsive bullous pemphigoid in a 78-year-old woman was shown by challenge to be due to furosemide (Lasix). The bullae did not reappear until after 10 daily doses of Lasix (40 mg/day).

Dahl MGC, Cook LJ: Lesions induced by trauma in pemphigoid. Br J Dermatol 101:469–473, 1979.

Simply scratching the skin could induce linear blisters in three patients with bullous pemphigoid.

Thomsen K, Schmidt H: PUVA-induced bullous pemphigoid. Br J Dermatol 95:568–569, 1976.

PUVA therapy of psoriasis induced reappearance of bullous pemphigoid in a 57-year-old man who had had no lesions for six months. Rapid control was achieved with **prednisone** (100 mg/day) and **azathioprine** (200 mg/day).

Tanaka T, Ogino A, Ogura K, Nakagawa K: A case of bullous pemphigoid and transitional cell carcinoma of the bladder: Demonstration of a circulating factor reactive with basement membrane zone of skin and of bladder carcinoma. Arch Dermatol 119:704–705, 1983.

Bullous pemphigoid developed in a 54-year-old woman with transitional cell carcinoma of the urinary bladder and was controlled with **betamethasone sodium phosphate** (4 mg/day). Immunofluorescent evidence of a common antigen in basement membrane of epidermis and of transitional cell carcinomas suggested a direct relationship of the tumor and skin changes.

Stone SP, Schroeter AL: Bullous pemphigoid and associated malignant neoplasms. Arch Dermatol 111:991–994, 1975.

In an age-controlled study of 219 patients, the incidence of systemic malignant disease was no higher in patients with bullous pemphigoid (8 in 73) than in patients with psoriasis (10 in 73) or in patients with contact dermatitis (11 in 73). Extensive diagnostic studies for malignant neoplasms should be based on consideration of age, condition of the patient, and clinical findings rather than on the presence of bullous pemphigoid.

Chadwick JM, Downham TF II: Topical sulfadiazine silver for bullous pemphigoid. Arch Dermatol 114:803, 1978.

It was possible to avoid all internal treatment and successfully treat two patients with localized bullous pemphigoid using applications of **silver sulfadiazine** 1 per cent (Silvadene cream bid). This preparation is active against both gram-negative and gram-positive bacteria as well as yeast. Because of potential absorption, it should not be used on more than 10 to 20 per cent of the body area at one time. Use with caution in patients with glucose-6-phosphate dehydrogenase deficiency, liver or renal impairment, or hypersensitivity to sulfonamides or methylparaben.

Siegel J, Eaglstein WH: High-dose methylprednisolone in the treatment of bullous pemphigoid. Arch Dermatol 120:1157–1165, 1984.

Seven of eight hospitalized patients with active bullous pemphigoid (average age 74.5 years) received relief within 24 hours from **methylprednisolone sodium succinate** pulse therapy (Solu-Medrol 15 mg/kg IV over a one-hour period daily for three days). Subsequent oral **prednisone** (0.4 mg/kg = 28 mg/70 kg person) was required.

Person JR, Rogers RS III: Bullous pemphigoid responding to sulfapyridine and the sulfones. Arch Dermatol 113:610–615, 1977.

Of 41 patients with bullous pemphigoid, 5 were completely controlled with **sulfapyridine** (500 to 1000 mg qid). **Sodium bicarbonate** was given to alkalize the urine.

Fox BJ, Odom RB, Findlay RF: Erythromycin therapy in bullous pemphigoid: Possible anti-inflammatory effects. J Am Acad Dermatol 7:504–510, 1982.

Erythromycin (250 mg qid) greatly suppressed bullous pemphigoid in an 87-year-old woman, and intermittent erythromycin therapy was also helpful in a 4½-year-old girl. It may be used as a substitute for, or supplement to, corticosteroids.

Krain LS, Landau JW, Newcomer VD: Cyclophosphamide in the treatment of pemphigus vulgaris and bullous pemphigoid. Arch Dermatol 106:657–661, 1972.

Cyclophosphamide (100 to 150 mg/day) permitted gradual reduction in **prednisone** to small dosage (60 to 75 mg down to 10 mg/day) for two patients with bullous pemphigoid. Attendant side effects of prednisone (hirsutism, moon facies, diabetes mellitus, and depression) were thus eliminated.

Greaves MW, Burton JL, Marks J, Dawber RPR: Azathioprine in treatment of bullous pemphigoid. Br Med J 1:144–145, 1971.

Azathioprine (2.5 mg/kg/day) was given to 11 patients with bullous pemphigoid. In nine of these it was possible to completely stop **prednisone** therapy while continuing azathioprine alone. In the other two, the prednisone requirement was considerably reduced.

Burton JL, Harman RMM, Peachey RDG, Warin RP: A controlled trial of azathioprine in the treatment of pemphigoid. Br J Dermatol 99 (Suppl 16):14, 1978.

A 3-year-study of 25 patients showed that **azathioprine** (2.5 mg/kg/day) greatly reduced the need for **prednisone** and also improved the prognosis in 12 patients, as compared to prednisone used alone in 13 patients.

Ahmed AR, Maize JC, Provost TT: Bullous pemphigoid: Clinical and immunologic follow-up after successful therapy. Arch Dermatol 113:1043–1046, 1977.

A state of prolonged remission of bullous pemphigoid was achieved in 16 of 36 patients (ages 43 to 92 years) after 1 to 10 months of therapy. The authors found **azathioprine** (1.5 mg/kg/day) plus **prednisone** (15 mg/day) to be superior to prednisone alone (30 mg/day).

Downham TF II, Chapel TA: Bullous pemphigoid: Therapy in patients with and without diabetes mellitus. Arch Dermatol 114:1639–1642, 1978.

It is best to initiate treatment with both **methotrexate** (2.5 to 15 mg PO twice weekly or every other day) and **prednisone** (100 mg/day) if a patient with bullous pemphigoid also has diabetes mellitus. In this study of 34 patients, 38 per cent could not be controlled by steroid alone.

Roujeau J-C, Morel P, Dalle E, et al: Plasma exchange in bullous pemphigoid. Lancet 2:486–489, 1984.

A multicenter evaluation of 41 patients with pemphigoid demonstrated that plasma exchange (eight large volume exchanges over four weeks) was a useful adjuvant for reducing the **cortisone** requirement. Control of the disease was achieved with less daily **prednisolone** (0.52 mg/kg) in the plasma exchange group than in the group receiving prednisolone (0.97 mg/kg) only. However, plasma exchange remains costly and did not reduce the number of side effects from corticosteroids.

Thivolet J, Barthelemy H, Rigot-Muller G, Bendelac A: Effects of cyclosporin on bullous pemphigoid and pemphigus. Lancet 1:334–335, 1985.

Cyclosporine (cyclosporine, Sandimmune 6 mg/kg/day for two to three months PO), adapted to a plasma level of 80 to 180 μg/liter, cleared two patients of their bullous pemphigoid lesions within one month. No relapse occurred two months after stopping treatment.

Skeete M, Greaves MW: Juvenile bullous pemphigoid. Br J Dermatol 95 (Suppl 14):23–25, 1976.

A 12-year-old school girl with a sulfapyridine- and dapsone-resistant pruritic bullous eruption of 10 months showed indirect immunofluorescent basement membrane titers of 1:320. She required **prednisone** (500 mg/day) initially, which was gradually reduced to 50 mg/day over three months, and later to 20 mg/day.

Piamphongsant T, Chaikittisilpa S, Kullavanijaya P: Bullous pemphigoid in childhood: Report of three cases and a review of literature. Int J Dermatol 16:126–133, 1977.

Three patients (ages one, six, and eight years) showed excellent responses to **dapsone** (25 to 75 mg/day).

Sams WM, Jordan RE: Correlation of pemphigoid and pemphigus antibody titres with activity of disease. Br J Dermatol 84:7–13, 1971.

Although circulating pemphigus antibody titers can serve as a guide for therapy in pemphigus vulgaris, the pemphigoid antibody titers showed no correlation with disease activity in four patients and hence were not of value in assessing therapy.

Chorzelski TP, Maciejowski E, Jablonska S, et al: Coexistence of pemphigus and bullous pemphigoid. Arch Dermatol 109:849–853, 1974.

Prednisone was successful in controlling the cutaneous lesions in three patients who had both pemphigus and pemphigoid serum antibodies.

Jablonska S, Chorzelski TP, Beutner EH, et al: Dermatitis herpetiformis and bullous pemphigoid: Intermediate and mixed forms. Arch Dermatol 112:45–48, 1976.

The authors described nine unusual patients with clinical and immunofluorescent features of both dermatitis herpetiformis and bullous pemphigoid. Five responded to **sulfapyridine** or sulfones, and two to combined treatment with **prednisone**.

Beware if your competence/confidence ratio is below 1.0.

If the patient is pregnant, drugs are taboo.

Candidiasis

Clotrimazole	Nystatin
Miconazole	Loprox
Econazole	Ketoconazole
Haloprogin	

In times past the clinician's skill in distinguishing candidiasis, tinea, erythrasma, and intertrigo of the groin led to different modes of therapy. Today the imidazoles have eliminated the need for such clinical acumen. All four of these conditions are responsive to econazole and ketoconazole, the newest of the topical imidazoles.

Mycostatin had been the undisputed master antimicrobial for candidiasis until tolnaftate and haloprogin were introduced. Now the imidazoles combat not only yeast infections but also other superficial and deep fungal infections and some gram-positive bacterial infections. The newest member, ketoconazole, is water-soluble and can be given orally for systemic action. These compounds plus another new antifungal family of pyridone derivatives, represented by Loprox, spell revolutionary advances in control of this common infection of mucous membranes and moist intertriginous areas, including the fingerwebs and the angles of the mouth.

Such areas must be kept dry, in addition to having a thin coating of powerful antimicrobial applied. We generally use Spectazole, because its shotgun scatter of fire power includes the resistant *Trichophyton rubrum*. For candidal nail infections we employ ketoconazole (200 mg/day), which again attacks the dermatophytes as well.

Prevention centers on dryness in the intertriginous areas, reduction in sweating, and avoidance of tight garments.

Dramatic as the results have been in simple candidiasis, it is the treatment of mucocutaneous candidiasis in the immunocompromised individual that has been most gratifying. Ketoconazole has proved to be a wonder drug for these unfortunate patients. In some cases, simple topical imidazoles alone have been dramatically helpful. We also have been impressed by adjuvant therapy with zinc, accessory vitamins, and correction of iron deficiency. In all patients, however, long-term treatment for months to years is the rule.

Raab WPE: The Treatment of Mycosis with Imidazole Derivatives. New York, Springer-Verlag, 1980, 157 pp.

Detailed data on the treatment of candidiasis with **clotrimazole**, **miconazole**, **econazole**, and **ketoconazole**. All compounds were also equally effective against dermatophyte infections.

Jones HE: Therapy for superficial fungal infection. Med Clin North Am 66:873–893, 1982.

Oral thrush

Removal of precipitating factors (antibiotics, corticosteroids)

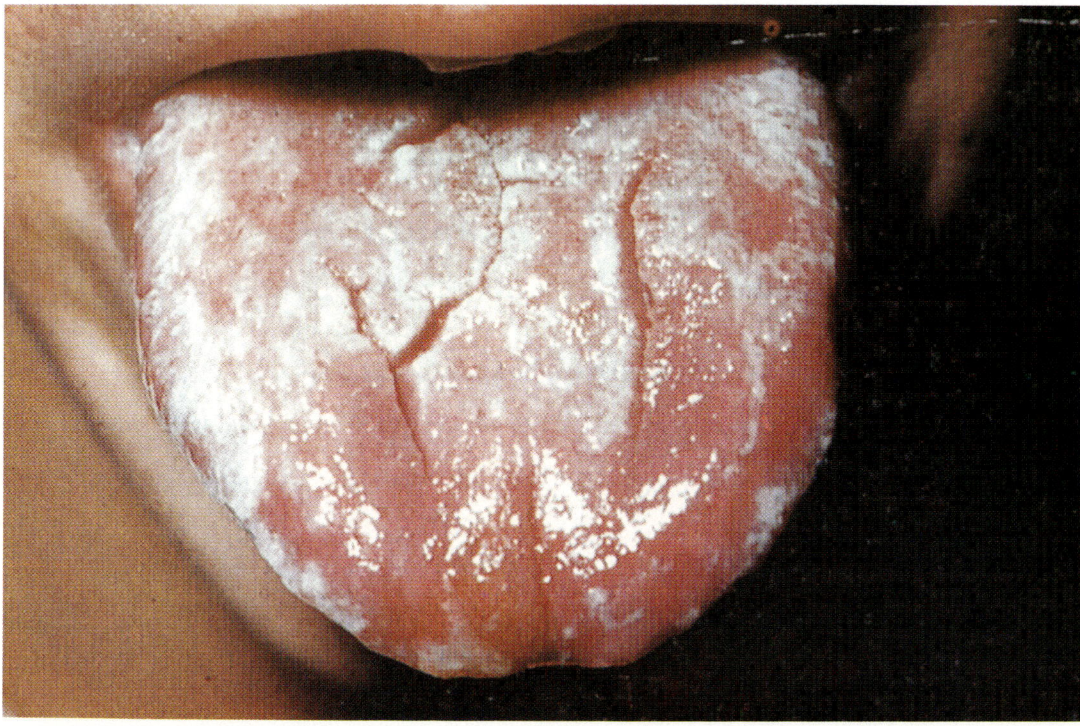

Oral **nystatin** suspension for 10 days (Mycostatin 5 cc tid—hold in mouth five minutes, then swallow)

Miconazole or **clotrimazole** cream—apply with toothbrush to buccal cavity

Ketoconazole (200 mg/day) for 10 to 14 days (can give as acidified solution to children)

Candidal intertrigo

Dry out area with heat lamp, fan, and powder

Topical nystatin or **imidazole**

Ketoconazole (200 mg/day) for 2 weeks

Combine antifungal with topical steroid cream or lotion to hasten relief

Candidal paronychia

Thymol 4 per cent in chloroform

Ketoconazole

Vulvovaginal candidiasis

Ketoconazole (400 mg/day) for five to seven days cures 90 per cent

Chronic mucocutaneous candidiasis

Ketoconazole (200 to 400 mg/day)

Systemic agents:

5-Fluorocytosine

(**flucytosine** [Ancobon 250 mg and 500 mg capsules])

Oral dosage (50 to 150 mg/kg/day) spread over 15-minute intervals to decrease nausea

Candida develops resistance in two weeks

Monitor CBC and renal function biweekly

Ketoconazole

Oral dosage (200 to 400 mg/day)

Contraindications—hepatic failure or (possibly) history of infectious hepatitis

Side effects in less than 10 per cent (nausea, pruritus, photophobia, gynecomastia)—hepatitis very rare

Monitor monthly chemistry profile

Amphotericin B
(Fungizone)
IV infusion over 6 hours—increase dosage slowly from 0.25 mg/kg/day to 0.65 mg/kg/day
Maximum in adult 30 to 50 mg/day
Contraindication—impaired renal function
Side effects—chills, fever, phlebitis
Decrease with **heparin** and **hydrocortisone** in infusion
Decrease with **aspirin** and antihistamine
Monitor weekly CBC, platelet count, UA, BUN, creatinine, potassium, and magnesium

Miconazole
IV infusion over 30 to 60 minutes one to two times daily
200 to 1200 mg/dose
Mix 20 mg ampule with 200 ml 0.9 per cent sodium chloride or 5 per cent dextrose
Indication—chronic mucocutaneous candidiasis and candida granuloma
Drug interaction—Coumadin (must increase dose)
Contraindication—severe electrolyte imbalance
Monitor electrolytes, CBC, serum lipids (altered by vehicle, PEG 40 castor oil)
Thrombophlebitis may necessitate central venous line

Munz D, Powell KR, Pai CH: Treatment of candidal diaper dermatitis: A double-blind placebo-controlled comparison of topical nystatin with topical plus oral nystatin. J Pediatr 101:1022–1025, 1982.

No statistical difference in results with or without oral **nystatin** (100,000 U/ml qid). Authors advise three weeks of treatment with nystatin cream (Mycostatin 100,000 U/gm qid) without any oral drug. Wash between each diaper change and do not use occlusive rubber pants.

Carter VH, Olansky S: Haloprogin and nystatin therapy for cutaneous candidiasis. Arch Dermatol 110:81–82, 1974.

Double-blind study of 67 patients found no difference in cure rate (80 per cent). **Haloprogin** cream 1 per cent (Halotex) was preferred, since it is effective against dermatophytes, in contrast to **nystatin** (Mycostatin) ointment 100,000 U/gm.

Guess W, Engley FB Jr, Blaylock WK, Shelley ED, et al: Topical antifungal drug products for over-the-counter human use: Establishment of a monograph. Fed Reg 47(56):12501–12506, March 23, 1982.

This detailed review discusses the safety and effectiveness of **nystatin** (100,000 U/gm).

Montes LF, Hermann HW: Clinical and antimicrobial effects of haloprogin cream in diaper dermatitis. Cutis 21:410–412, 1978.

Cure rate 100 per cent in one week when **haloprogin** cream 1 per cent (Halotex) was applied qid. Prior to therapy, *Candida albicans* was isolated from seven of eight babies studied.

Cullen SI: Cutaneous candidiasis: Treatment with miconazole nitrate. Cutis 19:126–129, 1977.

Of 30 cases 87 per cent were cured both clinically and mycologically with **miconazole nitrate** (2 per cent lotion applied bid for 14 days).

Puolakka J, Tuimala R: A comparison between oral ketoconazole and topical miconazole in the treatment of vaginal candidiasis. Acta Obstet Gynecol Scand 62:575–577, 1983.

Mycologic cure rate was the same (75 per cent) with either **ketoconazole** (200 mg/day for six days) or **miconazole** vaginal tablet (100 mg/day for 14 days). Women preferred oral therapy. Follow-up: one week after stopping therapy. Recurrent cases probably need longer course of ketoconazole to prevent relapses.

Rajan VS, Thirumoorthy T: Treatment of cutaneous candidiasis: A double-blind, parallel comparison of sulconazole nitrate 1% cream and clotrimazole 1% cream. Australas J Dermatol 24:33–36, 1983.

Clotrimazole (1 per cent cream bid for three weeks) cleared 16 of 18 cases. Follow-up: four weeks off treatment. Similar results with **sulconazole nitrate** (1 per cent cream applied once daily for three weeks).

Cullen SI, Rex IH, Thorne EG: A comparison of a new antifungal agent, 1 per cent econazole nitrate (Spectazole) cream versus 1% clotrimazole cream in the treatment of intertriginous candidiasis. Curr Therapy Res 35:606–609, 1984.

Double-blind study of 38 patients who applied creams to intertriginous areas twice daily for three weeks. Cure rates: **econazole** (Spectazole) 71 per cent, **clotrimazole** (Lotrimin) 61 per cent. Four weeks after stopping treatment 90 per cent of the econazole group and 73 per cent of the clotrimazole group remained cured. No statistical differences.

Symoens J, Moens M, Dom J, et al: An evaluation of two years of clinical experience with ketoconazole. Rev Infect Dis 2:674–687, 1980.

Results of treating 1104 patients with fungal diseases in many centers. Two weeks of oral **ketoconazole** (200 mg/day) eliminates *Candida* from the gastrointestinal tract. Give after meals, as absorption depends on gastric acidity (drug is transformed into hydrochloride salt). Anticholinergic drugs, antacids, or cimetidine may cause treatment failure. No evidence that more than one daily dose is helpful. Treatment recommendations with ketoconazole:

Vaginal candidiasis (400 mg/day) for three to five days
Oral thrush (200 mg/day) for one to two weeks
Chronic mucocutaneous candidiasis (200 mg/day) for five months (range 1 to 12 months)
Dermatomycoses (yeasts) (200 mg/day) for three weeks (range one to six weeks)
Prophylaxis of candidiasis in leukemia patients undergoing chemotherapy (200 mg/day) for one month (range up to 12 months)

Experience with 57 children (aged less than 1 year to 15 years)

- Dosage 2.6 to 7.7 mg/kg daily
- Highest dose given, 25 mg/kg daily for two months
- Median duration of treatment, one month
- Longest treatment, six months

Adverse effects

In 69 patients (11 per cent), none serious
Nausea and itching were most common
Headache, dizziness, constipation, diarrhea, somnolence, nervousness
Treatment was stopped in only 13 patients (2 per cent)

Montes LF, Soto TG, Parker JM, Ramer GN: Clotrimazole troches: A new therapeutic approach to oral candidiasis. Cutis 17:277–280, 1976.

All 12 patients with chronic oral candidiasis improved significantly by sucking on **clotrimazole** troches (10 mg or 50 mg each, 10 troches/day for 14 days).

Owens NJ, Nightingale CH, Schweizer RT, et al: Prophylaxis of oral candidiasis with clotrimazole troches. Arch Intern Med 144:290–293, 1984.

Clotrimazole lozenges (Mycelex 10 mg tid) were effective in preventing oropharyngeal candidiasis in patients with renal transplants or malignant neoplasms, but not leukemia. Continue treatment until steroids are tapered to 20 mg/day, antineoplastic therapy is stopped, or recovery from neutropenia occurs (WBC greater than 2000/cu mm).

Schechtman LB, Funaro L, Robin T, et al: Clotrimazole treatment of oral candidiasis in patients with neoplastic disease. Am J Med 76:91–94, 1984.

Clotrimazole troches (10 mg PO five times daily for 2 to 28 days) were retained in the mouth and allowed to dissolve over 15 to 30 minutes in saliva, which was swallowed. This effectively cleared and prevented esophagitis in five of six patients. Recommended as prophylaxis in high-risk patients who will be developing neutropenia or receiving steroids or broad-spectrum antibiotics. Cannot be used long term because of induction of hepatic microsomal enzymes, which accelerate catabolism of the drug.

Mansour A, Gelfand EW: A new approach to the use of antifungal agents in infants with persistent oral candidiasis. J Pediatr 98:161–162, 1981.

Insert **clotrimazole** (100 mg) or **nystatin** (100,000 U) suppository (or troche) into slit in tip of pacifier or nipple and give to infant four times a day as a "lozenge." Report of two cases unresponsive to oral nystatin (Mycostatin) suspension.

Abramovits W: Resistant oral candidiasis in an infant due to pacifier contamination. Clin Pediatr 20:393, 1981.

Surprising failure of **nystatin** oral suspension (500 units qid) to eliminate mucosal candidiasis in a three-month-old infant was traced to presence of yeast colonies inside the baby's rubber pacifier. The infection cleared within a week after use of the contaminated pacifier was stopped. Reminder to check IVs and indwelling catheters for eradication of candidiasis in all ages.

Graybill JR, Herndon JH, Kniker WT, Levine HB: Ketoconazole treatment of chronic mucocutaneous candidiasis. Arch Dermatol 116:1137–1141, 1980.

Thrush cleared in three to seven days in each of five patients taking **ketoconazole** (200 mg/day). Cutaneous lesions required several months of therapy, often at 400 mg/day.

Petersen EA, Alling DW, Kirkpatrick CH: Treatment of chronic mucocutaneous candidiasis with ketoconazole: A controlled clinical trial. Ann Intern Med 93:791–795, 1980.

Ketoconazole (200 mg/day) induced virtually complete regression of all mucosal, skin, and nail lesions within six months. Of 12 patients studied, one developed liver toxicity. Maintenance dose of 200 mg/day was required to prevent recurrence.

Horsburgh CR, Kirkpatrick CH: Long-term therapy of chronic mucocutaneous candidiasis with ketoconazole: Experience with twenty-one patients. Am J Med 74 (Suppl: Ketoconazole Symposium):23–29, 1983.

Success in all 21 patients. Mucosal lesions improved in 7 days, cutaneous lesions in 23 days, and nails in 92 days. Note endocrine abnormalities in eight patients: hypothyroid (four), hypoparathyroid (four), hypoadrenal (two).

In 19 of 20 cases of chronic mucocutaneous candidiasis, **ketoconazole** (200 to 400 mg/day for 1 to 15 months) resulted in clearing of all sites. After eight months, relapse in mouth was seen in five cases.

Hay RJ, Clayton YM: The treatment of patients with chronic mucocutaneous candidosis and *Candida* onychomycosis with ketoconazole. Clin Exp Dermatol 7:155–162, 1982.

Ketoconazole (200 mg/day) cleared 11 cases of candidal onychomycosis after a mean of 7½ months. Relapse in one case eight months later. Raynaud's phenomenon was present in five of 11 cases.

Pazin GJ, Nagel JE, Friday GA, Fireman P: Topical clotrimazole treatment of chronic mucocutaneous candidiasis. J Pediatr 94:322–324, 1979.

Without systemic therapy, two cases were kept clear using **clotrimazole** 1 per cent cream (Lotrimin) bid for over 20 months.

Lin C-Y: Treatment of chronic mucocutaneous candidiasis with 5-fluorocytosine. Ann Allergy 49:298–300, 1982.

In the absence of **amphotericin B**, oral **5-fluorocytosine** (200 mg/kg/day for four months) produced marked clinical improvement in an immune-deficient four-year-old girl. No alteration in immunologic abnormalities.

Kirkpatrick CH, Windhorst DB: Mucocutaneous candidiasis and thymoma. Am J Med 66:939–945, 1979.

Look for thymoma in adult-onset chronic candidiasis. Review of 27 patients. Check for associated systemic lupus erythematosus, hypogammaglobulinemia, and myasthenia gravis.

Higgs JM, Wells RS: Diffuse chronic mucocutaneous candidiasis: Report of two patients treated with topical clotrimazole and replacement of nutritional deficiencies. Guy's Hosp Rep 122:135–153, 1973.

Two children received significant benefit for oral candidiasis by adding iron (**ferrous fumarate** 200 mg tid), **vitamin A** (10,000 IU daily), and **pyridoxine** (10 mg tid) in an effort to correct low serum levels. Scalp lesions cleared in three weeks after excision of surface crusts (under sedation) followed by alternate-day treatment with topical **clotrimazole** and **salicylic acid** 15 per cent in emulsifying ointment.

Miles MR, Olsen L, Rogers A: Recurrent vaginal candidiasis: Importance of an intestinal reservoir. JAMA 238:1836–1837, 1977.

Among 98 young women with vaginitis, 51 harbored *Candida albicans* with 100 per cent correlation between the presence of *C. albicans* in the vagina and in the bowel. Approximately 35 to 50 per cent of humans harbor intestinal *C. albicans*, and it probably never leaves spontaneously. Vigorous treatment of the vagina alone will not cure the problem.

Rennie JS, MacDonald DG, Dagg JH: Iron and the oral epithelium: A review. J R Soc Med 77:602–607, 1984.

Cites increase in candidiasis in iron-deficient patients. Be sure to screen for iron deficiency.

Higgs JM, Wells RS: Chronic mucocutaneous candidiasis: Associated abnormalities of iron metabolism. Br J Dermatol 86 (Suppl 8):88–101, 1972.

Iron deficiency was present in 23 of 31 patients. Oral **ferrous fumarate** (200 mg tid for several months) or intravenous **iron** therapy (Imferon total dose) or both significantly improved 9 of 11 patients. Must monitor serum iron and iron-binding capacity as well as hemoglobin to assess correction of iron stores.

Achten G, Degreef H, Dockx P: Treatment of onychomycosis with a solution of miconazole 2% in alcohol. Mykosen 20:251–256, 1977.

This "nail varnish" was particularly helpful in clearing paronychial inflammation (53 per cent cure rate) and *Candida*-infected nails.

The placebo effect comes from the physician, not the prescription.

Cat-Scratch Disease

Margileth AM: Cat scratch disease: Nonbacterial regional lymphadenitis: The study of 145 patients and a review of the literature. Pediatrics 42:803–818, 1968.

Observations:

This is a benign and self-limited disease in most instances.

Aspiration of fluctuant purulent lymph nodes seen in 30 of the patients was immediately effective in relieving local pain in 27 of 28 cases. Reaspiration was required in 11 patients.

Forty-five trials of single and combined antimicrobials were ineffective in 40 patients.

Margileth AM, Wear DJ, Hadfield TL, et al: Cat scratch disease: Bacteria in skin at the primary inoculation site. JAMA 252:928–931, 1984.

This disease is now demonstrated to be due to small gram-negative pleomorphic bacilli that are not sensitive to the antibiotics used so far, e.g.:

minocycline (Minocin)
tetracycline (500 mg qid)
doxycycline (Vibramycin 100 mg bid)
cefadroxil (Duricef 1 gm/day)

The usual treatment consists of close observation and reassurance that the skin lesion and lymphadenopathy will subside spontaneously in two to five months.

Hadfield TL, Schlagel C, Margileth A: Stalking the cause of cat-scratch disease. Diagn Med 8:23–27 (Jan.) 1985.

Although seven deaths due to cat-scratch disease have been reported in the literature, in this group's experience with 2200 patients over 25 years there were no deaths. Conclusions:

Therapy:

Intervention is seldom required, as the lymphadenopathy will spontaneously subside.
Give analgesic as necessary.
Aspirate node if fluctuant (relieves pain).
A biopsy should not be done or a node excised (unless needed for diagnosis).
Antibiotics are no help.

Prophylaxis:

Declaw the cat.
Avoid cat bites and scratches.

If the patient is old, don't be bold. Keep your drugs to one or two and a low dose too.

Chancroid

Erythromycin Minocycline Bactrim DS

Gaisin A, Heaton CL: Chancroid: Alias the soft chancre. Int J Dermatol 14:188–197, 1975.

This comprehensive review concludes that the appropriate treatments for chancroid include:

First choice:
- **tetracycline** (500 mg q6h for 15 days)
- **sulfisoxazole** (Gantrisin 1 gm q6h for 15 days) (alone or in combination)

Alternates:
- **doxycycline** (Vibramycin 100 mg/day for 15 days)
- **co-trimoxazole** (Bactrim DS 4 tabs single dose)
- **cephalothin** (Keflin 500 mg q6h IV for 5 to 10 days)
- **kanamycin** (Kantrex 500 mg q12h IM for 5 to 14 days)
- **streptomycin** (500 mg q12h IM for 4 to 6 days)

Plummer FA, Nsanze H, D'Costa LJ, et al: Single-dose therapy of chancroid with trimethoprim-sulfametrole. N Engl J Med 309:67–71, 1983.

Trimethoprim-sulfametrole (eight tablets, i.e., 640 mg/3200 mg given as a single dose) proved to be as effective in eradicating chancroid ulcers and buboes as the same drug given in a dose of 160 mg/800 mg daily for five days. This double-blind study involved 107 infected male patients in Nairobi, and healing was seen within two weeks.

Ronald AR: Chancroid: Recent advances in treatment and control. Int J Dermatol 25:31–33, 1986.

In Kenya most isolates of *Haemophilus ducreyi* are now resistant to tetracycline, sulfonamides, and ampicillin. However, a 95 per cent cure rate was achieved with either erythromycin (500 mg qid for 10 days) or trimethoprim-sulfamethoxazole (one double-strength tablet bid for 7 days). All sexual contacts of men with chancroid should be treated with the regimen effective for the index patient.

Schmid GP: The treatment of chancroid. JAMA 255:1757–1762, 1986.

Effective new alternate treatments include (1) Augmentin (**amoxicillin** 500 mg and **clavulanic acid** 125 mg, tid for seven days) and (2) Rocephin (**ceftriaxone** 250 mg IM once).

While the ulcers heal rapidly, the buboes may continue to enlarge and become fluctuant, requiring aspiration through adjacent normal skin.

Physicians . . . should unite tenderness with steadiness, and condescension with authority, as to inspire the minds of their patients with gratitude, respect, and confidence.

Thomas Percival (1803)

Cheilitis

Eliminate contactants	Clotrimazole
Eliminate drugs	5-Fluorouracil
Topical steroids	Surgery

Success in the treatment of cheilitis rests on the discernment of the cause. Many examples are the result of undue exposure to wind, low humidities, and sun. Simple protection with Vaseline or a sun screen lipstick (RVPaba sun stick) will provide relief. In the more persistent cases, we use Synalar ointment 0.025 per cent as needed. The atopic individual is particularly prone to developing cheilitis and must be specially warned about the danger of environmental factors as well as seemingly innocent contactants.

Contact allergens unrecognized by the patient account for many examples. Sometimes the agent may be a photosensitizer, as in lipsticks, so that not only the contactant but the sun must be avoided. We instruct patients to eliminate all lipsticks, lip pomades, salves, toothpastes, lozenges, mouthwashes, denture adhesives, and candies, as well as routine dental visits, until the cheilitis is clear. They are cautioned against holding paper clips, bobby pins, and pens between their lips, and they must not lick envelope seals. A particular word of warning is also given concerning lip contact with citrus fruit rinds, such as sucking on oranges. Kissing lipstick-adorned lips is likewise forbidden.

Systemic drugs are also suspect. Indeed, cheilitis is seen in virtually every patient receiving Accutane, although it can be greatly ameliorated by taking vitamin E (400 IU tid).

If the cheilitis is of actinic origin and severe, we routinely use Efudex cream (5 per cent 5-fluorouracil). It is applied each night for two weeks, and we alert the patient to the severity of response necessary to achieve cure. Actinic cheilitis is so common that many patients receiving 5-fluorouracil systemically show cheilitis, as the drug selectively inflames all actinically damaged tissue.

Candidal cheilitis is often overlooked, but can readily be eliminated with topical anticandidal drugs such as clotrimazole (Lotrimin cream) or systemic ketoconazole.

For puzzling persistent cheilitis, we look to the possibility of a factitial origin. Many patients constantly suck their lips in an effort to relieve the dryness and scaling, which then becomes a self-perpetuating process. At times this is difficult to discern. We recall an example in which our nurse made the diagnosis because by chance she was on a bus where she observed one of our patients with chronic cheilitis continuously chewing, biting, and licking her lips. We have had two such patients in whom relief was obtained only after superficial subsection removal of the entire vermilion band of chronically inflamed tissue. This was done using a Gillette Super Blue Blade and local Xylocaine anesthesia, followed by hemostasis with Monsel solution.

Persistent unexplained edema of the lips always calls for expert dental search for and correction of any periapical abscesses or granulomas. A trial of systemic antibiotics is also valuable. A biopsy may disclose granulomatous change, which calls for more intensive measures (see *Cheilitis granulomatosa*).

Finally, all patients with persistent actinic cheilitis need continuing surveillance because of its premalignant nature.

Swerlick RA, Cooper PH: Cheilitis glandularis: A re-evaluation. J Am Acad Dermatol 10:466–472, 1984.

A comprehensive review of cheilitis with mucopurulent discharge from salivary ducts as a reaction pattern to chronic irritation of the lips. For the large group due to actinic damage, the authors recommend cryosurgery, vermilionectomy, chemosurgery, or chemotherapy (**5-fluorouracil**). Atopic cheilitis and factitial cheilitis are two other factors deserving specialized attention.

Volden G, Krokan H, Kauli G, Midelfart K: Phototoxic and contact toxic reactions to the exocarp of sweet oranges: A common cause of cheilitis. Contact Dermatitis 9:201–204, 1983.

Cheilitis occurs in people who suck on citrus fruits as a result of primary irritation and phototoxicity.

Angeline G, Vena GA: Allergic contact cheilitis to guaiazulene. Contact Dermatitis 10:311, 1984.

Presents five patients in whom cheilitis was due to sensitization to a component of toothpaste (guaiazulene). Other known causes include sensitivity to lipstick, dental preparations, and mouthwashes.

Duxbury AJ, Turner EP, Watts DC: Hypersensitivity to epimine containing dental materials. Br Dent J 147:331–333, 1979.

A 45-year-old man had three attacks of swollen upper lip, fever, and oral ulcerations starting within 24 hours of placement of a temporary Scutan crown. Scutan, an imine bisphenol-A derivative, produced a positive patch test. Impregum impression material also contains the same chemical and caused the same reaction.

Cronin E: Lipstick dermatitis due to propyl gallate. Contact Dermatitis 6:213–214, 1980.

Propyl gallate was the patch test–positive allergen common to a variety of lipsticks, each of which induced acute cheilitis within three days of application. Patch tests to the lipsticks themselves were repeatedly negative.

Hindson C: Phenyl salicylate (Salol) in a lip salve. Contact Dermatitis 6:216, 1980.

Cheilitis of the upper and lower lips for one month in a 25-year-old woman proved to be due to a lip balm she had used for more than five years. The offending allergen was found to be phenyl salicylate, recently added by the manufacturers without notice.

Hindson TC: Clarinettist's cheilitis. Br Med J 2:1295, 1978.

Three clarinetists developed occupational cheilitis on the median area of the lower lip in exact contact with the reed. Extensive patch testing was negative.

Shalita AR, Cunningham WJ, Leyden JJ, et al: Isotretinoin treatment of acne and related disorders: An update. J Am Acad Dermatol 9:629–638, 1983.

Accutane therapy induces cheilitis, which appears within a few days and persists throughout the entire period of use. Treatment: frequent application of an emollient such as petrolatum or a water-in-oil ointment. Prior hydration of the lips with warm water compresses is helpful. A corticosteroid ointment is indicated for more severe examples. Discomfort of fissures can be relieved by **lidocaine** ointment (3 or 5 per cent).

Price ML, MacDonald DM: Cheilitis and cobalt allergy related to ingestion of vitamin B_{12}. Contact Dermatitis 7:352, 1981.

A 60-year-old woman had a two-year history of recurrent swelling and crusting of the lips, exacerbated by wind and sun exposure. A positive patch test to cobalt led the authors to stop her vitamin B_{12} tablets (which contain cobalt), and cure resulted. Interestingly, a vitamin B_{12} patch test was negative.

Tangsrud SE, Golf S: Cheilostomatitis associated with propranolol treatment. Br Med J 2:1385–1386, 1977.

Two weeks after starting Inderal (120 mg/day) therapy a 65-year-old woman developed cheilitis and stomatitis. The problem did not clear until after the Inderal was stopped and promptly recurred within one week of daily oral challenge with the same dose of the drug.

Duxbury AJ, Ead RD, Turner EP: Erosive cheilitis related to prochlorperazine maleate. Br Dent J 153:271–272, 1982.

Challenge-proven Stemetil-induced erosive cheilitis responded to **betamethasone valerate** cream (Valisone 0.1 per cent tid) only after the oral drug used for treating vertigo was stopped.

Epstein E: Treatment of lip keratoses (actinic cheilitis) with topical fluorouracil. Arch Dermatol 113:906–908, 1977.

In a series of 12 patients, **fluorouracil** (Efudex solution 5 per cent tid for 9 to 15 days) was curative, with recurrence in only two individuals. Provides a medical alternative to surgical excision of the vermilion border of the diffusely actinically damaged lip. Recurrences were successfully treated with liquid nitrogen.

Cataldo E, Doku HC: Solar cheilitis. J Dermatol Surg Oncol 7:989–995, 1981.

Includes splendid color photographs showing variations in this condition.

Treatment:

- Avoidance of radiation therapy
- Efudex cream 5 per cent (apply 3 to 4 times a day for 14 days, then cover with petrolatum)
- Freezing
- Electrosurgery
- Dermabrasion
- Chemocautery
- Full-thickness (5 mm) excision of the affected vermilion, closed by advancement of labial mucosa, which has been undermined
- To protect lips, opaque sunshade cream containing 5 per cent **menthyl anthranilate** and 5 per cent **titanium dioxide** (A-Fil cream)

Jansen GT, Dillaha CJ, Honeycutt WM: Candida cheilitis. Arch Dermatol 88:325–329, 1963.

Erosive and granular forms of cheilitis in 15 patients showed splendid prompt response to antimonilial therapy (**nystatin** cream). Look for underlying diabetes and involvement of other areas (groin, perianal) with yeast infection.

Finnerty EF: Candidiasis of the lips. Cutis 18:236, 1976.

Nystatin cream (qid for three weeks) was curative, but Valisone cream and Neosporin ointment were without effect.

Thomas JR III, Greene SL, Dicken CH: Factitious cheilitis. J Am Acad Dermatol 8:368–372, 1983.

Must rule out infectious causes, contact dermatitis, and actinic cheilitis before factitious cheilitis is considered. Successful approaches for five patients:

First patient
Topical steroid (**hydrocortisone** cream 1 per cent) plus explanation of deleterious effect of licking lips.
Second patient
Topical steroid (hydrocortisone cream 1 per cent) and reassurance that it was not cancer.
Third patient
Sweitzer's wet dressings (**copper sulfate**, **zinc sulfate**, **camphor**, water) followed by 40 per cent **sulfur** in petrolatum, Burow's compresses (**aluminum subacetate**), and **neomycin**.
Fourth patient
Burow's compresses and 1 per cent hydrocortisone cream.
Fifth patient
Forty per cent sulfur in petrolatum, Burow's compresses, and psychiatric counseling.

Butterworth T, Leoni EP, Beerman H, et al: Cheilitis of mongolism. J Invest Dermatol 35:347–352, 1960.

Fifty-six cases were treated successfully with a six- to eight-week combined regimen consisting of systemic steroid (**hydrocortisone** 20 mg/day), vitamin A (25,000 U/day), and **thyroid** (2 grains/day). The three drugs had to be used together to heal the vertical fissures and hyperkeratosis. Relapse occurred when the drugs were stopped. An alternative treatment was **dexamethasone** cream (Decadron cream 0.1 per cent) applied frequently.

Haldar B: Cheilitis glandularis treated by injection of intralesional triamcinolone. Indian J Dermatol 21:53–54, 1976.

Considerable improvement occurred in a 42-year-old woman with a severe case of 12 years' duration following oral **tetracycline** (1 gm/day for six weeks) and weekly intralesional **triamcinolone** injections.

Tyldesley WR: Exfoliative cheilitis. Br J Oral Surg 10:357–359, 1973.

A 22-year-old man with this rare recalcitrant cheilitis that flares periodically failed to respond to **neomycin-bacitracin** ointment, fluorinated corticosteroids, **ichthammol**, and vitamin supplements. Valium (**diazepam** 2 mg tid) provided some help.

Brooke RI: Exfoliative cheilitis. Oral Surgery 45:52–55, 1978.

A 13-year-old girl was cured within a few days after rigorous cleaning of the mouth done under general anesthesia.

Morton ME, Ead RD: Granulomatous cheilitis: A report of three cases. Br Dent J 156:247–249, 1984.

All three patients were treated with steroids. One case cleared in nine months after short-term treatment with **prednisone** (30 mg/day for four days, then 15 mg/day for four days) followed by maintenance with Vioform-hydrocortisone ointment to the lips. The other two patients received intralesional **triamcinolone acetonide** (10 mg/ml 1 cc into each side of affected lip following local anesthesia). Such injections had to be repeated occasionally, as there was a tendency to relapse. Vioform-hydrocortisone ointment was used between injections.

Michalowski R: Munchausen's syndrome: A new variety of bleeding type—self-inflicted cheilorrhagia and cheilitis glandularis. Dermatologica 170:94–97, 1985.

Lacerations of the lip which were self-induced with a piece of thread were a major cause of a patient's cheilitis, which had defied therapy for 13 years.

Patients love to hear you use their name.

Cheilitis Granulomatosa (Melkersson-Rosenthal)

Antibiotics	Dental consultation
Intralesional steroid	Surgical resection
Immunosuppressant	

Mysterious, chronic, and disfiguring, these swollen lips represent a granulomatous inflammation of unknown cause. They may occur without other signs of disease or be an integral part of the rare Melkersson-Rosenthal syndrome (cheilitis, facial paralysis, and plicated tongue). At other times they herald the presence of Crohn's disease.

In any event, our solitary direct lead for therapy is the eradication of foci of infection. This relates specifically to dental foci or infection within the bowel.

Having established the diagnosis by biopsy, we seek active help from the dental surgeon to hunt for and eliminate any periapical abscesses or granulomas. Oral hygiene must be idealized and periodontic care superb. We also seek involvement with the otolaryngologist to clear any chronic sinusitis by medical or surgical means. Attention must likewise be paid to the gut to clear out apparent or inapparent foci of infection. We regularly order a complete gastrointestinal roentgenographic study, looking for diverticulitis, colitis, or tumor. Given no specific avenue of entry, we prescribe a series of antibiotics on a short-term trial basis. This includes erythromycin, ampicillin, Bactrim DS, metronidazole, and ketoconazole.

The next step is the injection intralesionally of triamcinolone acetonide (Kenalog-10, or Kenalog-40 if the weaker strength is not effective). A few patients may need plastic surgical excision or debulking of the enormously enlarged lips.

Worsaae N, Christensen KC, Schiødt M, Reibel J: Melkersson-Rosenthal syndrome and cheilitis granulomatosa:A clinicopathologic study of thirty-three patients with special reference to their oral lesions. Oral Surg 54:404–413, 1982.

A complete review stressing the elimination of dental foci of infection as the best treatment. Dramatically illustrated by a patient with swollen lips for two years cured by removing periapical inflammatory lesion of a lower first molar. The authors consider granulomatous swollen lips to be a monosymptomatic form of the Melkersson-Rosenthal syndrome.

Hornstein OP: Melkersson-Rosenthal syndrome: A neuro-muco-cutaneous disease of complex origin. Curr Probl Dermatol 5:117–156, 1973.

A monograph with overview of possible therapeutic maneuvers:

prednisone (40 mg/day for two to three weeks, then slowly taper to zero)
chloroquine
phenylbutazone
isoniazid (10 mg/kg for six to eight weeks)

pantothenic acid (6 gm/day) and **pyridoxine** (600 mg/day) conjoint therapy
intralesional corticosteroids
removal of foci of infection (tonsillar, dental)
surgical resection: debulking (deep wedge-shaped excision from mucosal side of lip)

Morton ME, Ead RD: Granulomatous cheilitis: A report of three cases. Br Dent J 156:247–249, 1984.

Two of three cases cleared with injections of **triamcinolone acetonide** 10 mg/ml (Kenalog-10, 1 ml in each side of affected lip after local anesthesia). The third case had cleared after 9 months following a short course of oral **prednisolone** (30 mg/day for four days, then 15 mg/day for four days) coupled with daily Vioform-hydrocortisone ointment (**iodochlorhydroxyquin** 3 per cent and **hydrocortisone** 1 per cent in petrolatum) locally.

The authors advise a work-up for Crohn's disease, including roentgenograms with a barium meal. If abdominal symptoms are present, sigmoidoscopy and rectal biopsy may be indicated.

Krutchkoff D, James R: Cheilitis granulomatosa: Successful treatment with combined local triamcinolone injections and surgery. Arch Dermatol 114:1203–1206, 1978.

Four months of biweekly injections of **triamcinolone acetonide** (10 mg/ml) resulted in 40 per cent reduction in lip size in a 45-year-old man who had granulomatous cheilitis for 15 years. Subsequent cheiloplasty and further steroid injections gave an excellent result, but the process recurred when injections were stopped. Maintenance injections were needed monthly.

White IR, Souteyrand P, MacDonald DM: Granulomatous cheilitis (Miescher). Clin Exp Dermatol 6:391–397, 1981.

Success was achieved by intralesional injection of **triamcinolone** (400 mg total, in four divided doses over three months) in a 30-year-old man with a five-year history of chronically swollen lips. The possibility of sarcoidosis and zirconium- or beryllium-allergic granulomas was ruled out through biopsy and skin tests. He had no evidence of Crohn's disease.

Brook IM, King DJ, Miller ID: Chronic granulomatous cheilitis and its relationship to Crohn's disease. Oral Surg 56:405–408, 1983.

Always check for Crohn's disease, but a swollen lip may precede this by years. Successful treatment in a 15-year-old boy with malabsorption syndrome centered on **azathioprine** (50 mg/day) plus vitamin B_{12} and folic acid supplementation.

Carr D: Granulomatous cheilitis in Crohn's disease. Br Med J 4:636, 1974.

A 14-year-old boy developed a swollen lower lip and right cheek nine years before radiologic evidence of Crohn's disease. He failed to respond to systemic antibiotics and topical steroid creams. Intralesional **triamcinolone** gave best results, but he also responded partially to **prednisone** (5 to 10 mg daily).

Madanes AE, Farber M: Danazol. Ann Intern Med 96:625–630, 1982.

Danazol, which inhibits sex steroid synthesis as well as sex steroid binding, gave some improvement in one patient with Melkersson-Rosenthal syndrome.

Neuhofer J, Fritsch P: Cheilitis granulomatosa (Melkersson-Rosenthal-Syndrom): Behandlung mit Clofazimin. Hautarzt 35:459–463, 1984.

In seven patients, **clofazimine** (100 mg/day for 10 days, then 100 mg two to four times a week for 2 to 12 months) completely suppressed attacks of lip swelling. However, persistent residual lip swelling due to inflammatory infiltrates responded incompletely. After drug withdrawal four patients remained free of symptoms for 5 to 45 months.

Stevens FA: Streptococcic infection of the "fibroedema" of Melkersson's syndrome. JAMA 156:223–224, 1954.

In one patient streptococcal vaccine therapy was helpful more than 30 years ago.

Rada DC, Koranda FC, Katz FS: Cheilitis glandularis: A disorder of ductal ectasia. J Dermatol Surg Oncol 11:372–375, 1985.

Vermilionectomy followed by mucosal undermining and primary closure gave functional and esthetic reduction of lip eversion and protrusion in a 64-year-old man with cheilitis glandularis of several years' duration. Prior to surgery he had prominent ductal orifices with salivary secretions on the protuberant lower lip mucosa.

As the patient's concern over disease rises, his concern over cost falls.

Consultants provide road maps, but you have to pick the route.

Chronic Bullous Disease of Childhood

Dapsone
Sulfapyridine
Corticosteroids

Babies' bullae that run in rings can be stopped with sulfones. The jewel-like clusters of tense vesicles favor the genital and perioral areas. Look for linear IgA at the basement membrane zone.

Marsden RA, Skeete MVH, Black MM: The chronic acquired bullous diseases of childhood. Clin Exp Dermatol 4:227–240, 1979.

An instructive review article that lets immunofluorescence light the path for the clinician down through the various bullae of babies and children.

Benign chronic bullous dermatosis of childhood:
Synonyms: juvenile dermatitis herpetiformis, juvenile pemphigoid
Treatment: first choice—**sulfapyridine**; alternates—oral corticosteroids, **dapsone**
Direct immunofluorescence: linear basement membrane zone IgA

Sweren RJ, Burnett JW: Benign chronic bullous dermatosis of childhood: A review. Cutis 29:350–352, 356–357, 1982.

These rosettes or circinate clusters of large tense bullae usually respond to **sulfone** therapy.

Marsden RA: The treatment of benign chronic bullous dermatosis of childhood, and dermatitis herpetiformis and bullous pemphigoid beginning in childhood. Clin Exp Dermatol 7:653–663, 1982.

Twenty children with chronic bullous disease of childhood had the sudden onset of bullae in rings and idiopathic exacerbations at two- to four-week intervals. Treatment included:

1. **Sulfapyridine** (0.25 to 3.0 gm/day for one week to seven years)
   Fifteen patients: complete clearing in four, partial clearing in seven, no clearing in two, intolerance in two
2. **Dapsone** (20 to 200 mg/day, up to 28 months)
   Thirteen patients: partial clearing in five, no effect in two
3. **Prednisolone** (1 to 15 mg/day)
   Helpful as supplement to sulfapyridine (three cases) and dapsone (four cases)
4. **Sulfamethoxypyridazine** (Lederkyn 0.5 to 1.0 gm daily)
   helpful in two cases not controlled with combinations of prednisolone and sulfapyridine or dapsone. (Not available in the United States.)

Rogers M, Bartlett B, Walder B, Cains G: Chronic bullous disease of childhood—Aspects of management. Aust J Dermatol 23:62–69, 1982.

Excellent response in five boys (ages 5 to 12 with subepidermal bullae and linear IgA in the basement membrane zone) to:

Sulfapyridine
  (250 mg tid)—two cases
  (1 gm tid)—one case
Dapsone
  (100 mg/day)—one case
  (50 mg/day)—one case

Esterly NB, Furey NL, Kirschner BS, et al: Chronic bullous dermatosis of childhood. Arch Dermatol 113:42–46, 1977.

Healing occurred in five days following sulfapyridine (65 to 68 mg/kg/day or 250 mg tid) given to two baby boys with this immune disorder. Maintenance doses of sulfapyridine (500 to 625 mg/day) were required, and sodium citrate 10 per cent (5 ml PO qid) was also given to alkalize the urine and thus decrease crystalluria.

Marsden RA, McKee PH, Bhogal B, et al: A study of benign chronic bullous dermatosis of childhood and comparison with dermatitis herpetiformis and bullous pemphigoid occurring in childhood. Clin Exp Dermatol 5:159–176, 1980.

In contrast to dermatitis herpetiformis (22 cases), one third of cases of benign chronic bullous disease of childhood (18 cases) went into remission.
histopathology:
  routine biopsy was of little help in distinguishing the three diseases
  immunofluorescence
    direct: linear IgA at basement membrane in 15 of 16 cases
    indirect: circulating IgA basement membrane zone antibody in 12 of 17 cases
treatment
  Sulfapyridine or **dapsone** controlled chronic bullous dermatosis of childhood within two to three days, but frequent dosage adjustments were necessary.
    dapsone (20 to 125 mg/day)
    sulfapyridine (250 mg to 3 gm/day)

Surbrugg SK, Weston WL: The course of chronic bullous disease of childhood. Pediatr Dermatol 2:213–215, 1985.

This childhood linear IgA dermatosis has a benign course with disease-free remissions and eventual lack of need for therapy. Reviews three patients who were able to discontinue therapy after two months to two years of **sulfapyridine** (60 to 90 mg/kg/day):
30-month-old boy: sulfapyridine (250 mg qid for two years)
4½-year-old girl: sulfapyridine (500 mg tid for two weeks, then tapered and stopped after two months)
30-month-old boy: sulfapyridine (250 mg tid for 13 months)

You are never in trouble if you know what to do next.
FRANCIS WOOD

Cicatricial Pemphigoid

Antibiotics	Azathioprine
Corticosteroids	Cyclophosphamide
Dapsone	

Make friends with these patients, as you will be seeing them for a long time. They need your help, not for months but for years.

Their disease is the mucosal analogue of bullous pemphigoid. The mucous membranes come off along the basement membrane zone just as the epidermis comes off in bullous pemphigoid. Both diseases also have mysterious autoimmune-driven forces that respond to the immunosuppressive therapy of corticosteroids, dapsone, and cyclophosphamide.

But there is a difference. Cicatricial pemphigoid scars, whereas bullous pemphigoid usually does not. Although the scarring pemphigoid may affect any mucosal surface, it is the ocular lesion that is most feared. The mucosal scarring in the eye insidiously and progressively leads to blindness in as many as one in four patients. This scarring must be averted, since once the fine subepithelial fibrous striae of the inner conjunctivae have turned to sheets of symblepharon, there is no turning back the hands of the clock. We have no techniques of lysing the constricting bands, and eye surgeons fear to cut the mucosa and face the hydra of new scars. Indeed, we have no antifibroblast therapy except for topical steroids, which must be used regularly, faithfully, and indefinitely.

But more than topical antifibroplasia measures are needed. These cicatricial pemphigoid patients require systemic therapy. Our preference, derived from long-term experience with more than a dozen patients, is dapsone (100 mg/day). If this is ineffectual we give prednisone (100 mg/day with gradual tapering). Usually we combine prednisone with either dapsone or cyclophosphamide (Cytoxan 150 mg/day) to reduce the maintenance level of steroid.

For oral mucosal lesions we prescribe dexamethasone elixir (Decadron elixir 0.5 mg/5 ml, one teaspoon to be held in the mouth for a few minutes, then swallowed). Skin lesions are best treated with a high-potency topical steroid (such as Diprolene ointment twice a day). Secondary infection, common on the scalp, calls for erythromycin (250 mg qid) and daily use of an antibacterial shampoo such as Ionil. Also be alert to possible lesions elsewhere, such as nasal, laryngeal, and anal sites.

Most of these patients are in the older age group, so that screening for malignant disease is valuable. We also check for occult infection and unusual drug associations. One of our patients had an associated genitourinary tract infection with *Escherichia coli*, and the bullous skin lesions were reproduced by an intradermal skin test to phenol-killed *E. coli*. Long-term treatment with ampicillin (2 gm daily) prevented new lesions. Even if no occult infection is found, we give short therapeutic trials with metronidazole, ketoconazole, and acyclovir.

Always the ophthalmologist must be a colleague in the care of these patients, particularly to evaluate visual function and watch for evidence of steroid intolerance, such as glaucoma or cataract. Once lid mobility or lacrimal function is compromised, the patient must use artificial tears. With scar-induced entropion, regular or permanent epilation of the eyelashes is essential to avoid scratching the cornea. In some patients corrective eyelid surgery may be advantageous.

Cicatricial pemphigoid varies from the trivial to the terrible, from the blister to blindness. It is a full-spectrum disease that requires full-spectrum care. Give it and you will have a friend for life.

Hardy KM, Perry HO, Pingree GC, Kirby TJ: Benign mucous membrane pemphigoid. Arch Dermatol 104:467–475, 1971.

Systemic corticosteroid such as **prednisone** (40 mg/day) or equivalent **triamcinolone** (Aristocort) is the best single treatment for this disease. In this Mayo Clinic study of 81 patients, 19 had skin involvement as well as mucous membrane lesions, and 21 became blind (17 in both eyes).

Schamberg IL, Decherd J: Benign mucous membrane pemphigoid. Arch Dermatol 107:449–450, 1973.

In a 70-year-old woman with scattered blisters (throat and trunk), painful red eyes, photophobia, and lacrimation, healing was slow, with eyelash epilation every two weeks (by an ophthalmologist) and **prednisone** (80 mg Monday-Wednesday-Friday).

It is difficult to call this disease benign, since it blinds 20 per cent of its victims by:

1. Entropion-induced trichiasis, which scars the cornea
2. Impaired motility of eyelids (and lacrimal function), which leads to dryness and thereby corneal keratinization
3. An inflammatory granulomatous vascularizing process resulting in corneal pannus

Rosenbaum MM, Esterly NB, Greenwald MJ, Gerson CR: Cicatricial pemphigoid in a 6-year-old child: Report of a case and review of the literature. Pediatr Dermatol 2:13–22, 1984.

A six-year-old black male had conjunctivitis, erosions of the oral and genital mucosa, hoarseness, dysphagia, recurrent vomiting, and weight loss. Upper airway obstruction due to a chronically inflamed and scarred epiglottis necessitated tracheostomy. The disease was controlled with **prednisone** (4 mg/kg/day) plus **dapsone** (2 mg/kg/day).

A masterful review with 46 references of a disease usually seen in the elderly.

Rogers RS III, Seehafer JR, Perry HO: Treatment of cicatricial (benign mucous membrane) pemphigoid with dapsone. J Am Acad Dermatol 6:215–223, 1982.

Using **dapsone** (100 mg/day), 20 of 24 patients with cicatricial pemphigoid had partial or complete control with mild to no inflammatory activity. Control was achieved in one month in 11 of the 20 patients. They start with low-dose dapsone (25 mg/day for three days) in hopes that the bone marrow can adapt, then slowly increase thereafter if needed (25 mg bid for three days, 25 mg tid for three days, 50 mg bid for three days, 125 mg/day for seven days, 75 mg bid).

A trial of dapsone for 12 weeks is warranted prior to starting long-term systemic corticosteroid or immunosuppressive drug therapy. **Sulfapyridine** was less efficacious.

Mondino BJ, Brown SI: Immunosuppressive therapy in ocular cicatricial pemphigoid. Am J Ophthalmol 96:453–459, 1983.

Although **azathioprine** (Imuran 1.5 mg/kg/day) or **cyclophosphamide** (Cytoxan 1.5 mg/kg/day) alone or in combination with **prednisone** (60 to 80 mg/day) helped, some "eyes" in this group of 57 patients progressed through symblepharon and ankyloblepharon. It is important to note that in the untreated group, the disease had a variable course, with some patients showing absolutely no disease progression.

Foster CS, Wilson LA, Ekins MB: Immunosuppressive therapy for progressive ocular cicatricial pemphigoid. Ophthalmology 89:340–353, 1982.

This collaborative, controlled, nonrandomized longitudinal cohort study of 26 patients with progressive cicatricial pemphigoid of the eyes had a protocol of **cyclophosphamide** (1 to 2 mg/kg/day) coupled with **prednisone** (80 to 120 mg/day for three weeks, then alternate-day therapy). Alopecia was experienced by 100 per cent of patients, and 78 per cent had macrocytic anemia; 14 of 15 patients who were immunosuppressed successfully for prolonged periods experienced cessation of episodic ocular inflammation and halting of progressive conjunctival cicatrization. However, vision improved in only two patients.

Person JR, Rogers RS III: Bullous and cicatricial pemphigoid: Clinical, histopathologic, and immunopathologic correlations. Mayo Clin Proc 52:54–66, 1977.

A study of 60 patients with cicatricial pemphigoid, some of whom were treated with combination steroids and **azathioprine**. Ocular lesions were helped by intralesional steroids. 112 references.

Herron BE: Immunologic aspects of cicatricial pemphigoid. Am J Ophthalmol 79:271–278, 1975.

In a 56-year-old woman with cicatricial pemphigoid, artificial tears and corticosteroid drops were valuable adjuvants to oral **triamcinolone** (Aristocort 80 mg/day). Injection of **triamcinolone acetonide** (0.5 ml three times) into the symblepharon did not reverse this scarring.

van Joost TH, Crone RA, Overdijk AD: Ocular cicatricial pemphigoid associated with practolol therapy. Br J Dermatol 94:447–450, 1976.

A 46-year-old man developed conjunctivitis leading to ocular cicatricial pemphigoid after $2\frac{1}{2}$ years of **practolol** therapy (600 mg/day) for angina. The process was aborted, but not reversed, by stopping the beta-blocker, practolol.

Greer KE, Beacham BE, Askew FC Jr.: Benign mucous membrane pemphigoid in association with internal malignancy. Cutis 25:183–185, 1980.

In a 47-year-old man with cicatricial pemphigoid for six months, radiation therapy of a newly discovered lung cancer had no effect on the mucosal lesions, which were controlled with **prednisone** (60 mg/day).

Hurley HJ: Benign mucous membrane pemphigoid. Arch Dermatol 107:449, 1973.

A most instructive case history:

1. Recurrent attacks in a young black man followed each episode of genitourinary infection.
2. He developed a specific bullous intradermal skin test reaction to *Escherichia coli* extract isolated from his urine. Intradermal tests with other bacterial antigens were negative.
3. The patient had bullae of the upper respiratory and gastrointestinal tracts, as well as cicatrizing eye changes and bullous and granulomatous skin lesions.
4. Laboratory studies showed a positive STS and LE test, and increased gamma globulins.
5. Death resulted from asphyxiation due to laryngeal lesions.

Therapy sails on the winds of diagnosis.

Darier's Disease

Aquasol A
Accutane
Retin-A
Surgery

This autosomal dominant disorder of keratinization has long been known to be somewhat responsive to water-solubilized vitamin A in dosages of 150,000 U/day. Larger doses have been more effective, but also more toxic. Our preference has been to prescribe Aquasol A 50,000 U tid. If there has been no response within 6 weeks, we switch to the new retinoid, Accutane, in a dosage of 40 mg bid. This is continued until either significant benefit is seen or six weeks have passed with no discernible improvement. The benefits of the vitamin A or Accutane are short term, and repeated courses are needed. Their potential toxicity militates against continuous long-term administration.

We instruct all of our patients to avoid suntanning, since many are photosensitive, as may be evident by the distribution of lesions. A sun screen with a 15 rating is often advisable. Even more important is alerting the patient that he has a depressed immunity as part of his disease. He must thus avoid direct contact with patients who have viral infections such as *Herpes simplex* or varicella. Fortunately the threat of vaccinia infections is gone, but the patient must remain alert to the hazard of other virus infections such as farmyard pox. Contact with patients with pyodermas is equally hazardous, although complications arising in this fashion are more amenable to therapy than the cutaneous viral infections.

We generally prescribe erythromycin for the treatment of secondary bacterial infections, ketoconazole if there is a secondary yeast infection, and oral acyclovir for herpetic infections. Topical Micatin cream and Silvadene cream have been of value prophylactically.

The results with topical therapy have been variable. Some patients are definitely helped by the use of retinoic acid cream or gel (Retin-A). Others find these preparations too irritating. In all instances a trial with the lowest concentration (or even diluted in a steroid cream) applied for only an hour is valuable. If the preparation is tolerated, increased dosage in both concentration and contact time can be tried.

In the most serious instances, removal of the epidermis and the most superficial dermis can produce permanent local cure. This may be done by dermabrasion, dermatome, or razor blade subsection. It is especially valuable in the management of facial lesions.

Dicken CH, Bauer EA, Hazen PG, et al: Isotretinoin treatment of Darier's disease. J Am Acad Dermatol 6:721–726, 1982.

A cooperative study of 104 patients at 19 medical centers proved Accutane (0.5 mg/kg/day, or more) to be very effective, but it did not induce long-term remissions; 70 per cent had improved significantly by four weeks, and 95 per cent by 16 weeks.

Thomas JR, Cooke JP, Winkelmann RK: High-dose vitamin A therapy for Darier's disease. Arch Dermatol 118:891–894, 1982.

Improvement of 50 to 80 per cent occurred in three patients following a two-week course of massive oral **vitamin A** dosage (1 million U/day). Side effects included drowsiness, headache, dry lips, and dry nose. Improvement was maintained for one year in two patients with follow-up.

Ayres S Jr: Darier's disease: Update on an effective new therapy. Arch Dermatol 119:710, 1983.

Instructive case report of a 26-year-old man with Darier's disease and photosensitivity who had only slight benefit from **vitamin A** (200,000 U/day for five years). Institution of conjoint therapy with **vitamin E** (1600 U/day) and vitamin A (100,000 U/day) gave essentially complete clearing of both problems within a few months, which was sustained during the following five years of this therapy (but relapse occurred if he lowered the dosage or stopped both vitamins).

Note: Inorganic iron interferes with absorption of vitamin E, so the patient should avoid reinforced white breads and cereals, female hormones, laxatives, and excessive polyunsaturated fatty acids.

Christiansen JV, Holm P, Møller R, et al: Treatment of dyskeratosis follicularis Darier with the retinoic acid derivative RO 10-9359 (Tigason). Dermatologica 163:164–168, 1981.

The new European retinoid **etretinate** (Tigason) is hailed as the most efficient treatment for Darier's disease. Modest dosage (25 to 50 mg/day to start, then 0.5 mg/kg body weight) controlled the disease with 50 per cent clearing in 29 patients studied for an 18-month period.

Löwhagen G-B, Michaëlsson G, Mobacken H, et al.: Effect of etretinate (RO 10-9359) on Darier's disease. Dermatologica 165:123–130, 1982.

Six of 17 patients receiving **etretinate** (Tigason 50 mg/day for two to six weeks) showed complete clearing and remissions of more than one month. Six others improved progressively over the 10-week treatment period, and five stopped because of side effects (severe itching and an isomorphic response due to dryness and excoriations). Systemic and topical antibacterial treatment enabled shortening of the treatment time and lowering of the dose of etretinate.

Sonnichsen N, Brenke A, Diezel W: Dyskeratosis follicularis vegetans (Morbus Darier)—Therapie mit dem aromatischen Retinoid RO 10-9359 (Tigason) in kombination mit systemischer photochemotherapie (Re PUVA). Dermatol Monatsschr 168:520–522, 1982.

A case report of a patient requiring supplemental PUVA, since the retinoid Tigason gave only partial relief.

Cohen IK, Kraemer KH, Peck GL: Cornifying Darier disease—A unique variant. II. Surgical treatment. Arch Dermatol 112:504–506, 1976.

Free-hand dermatome excision of the desired upper dermis and epidermis (followed by dermabrasion of deeper lesions) gave scars free of any lesions for more than four years. The lesions recur at once unless papillary dermis is removed. This patient's lesions had been indifferent to:

Vitamin A 500,000 U/day for three months
Retin-A ointment under occlusion
Steroid creams
Intralesional steroid injections
40 per cent urea soaks
Dinitrochlorobenzene (DNCB) topically
Lead oleate ointment

Dellon AL, Chretien PB, Peck GL: Successful treatment of Darier's disease by partial-thickness removal of skin. Plast Reconstr Surg 59:823-830, 1977.

Details of a surgical technique successful in three patients with three-year follow-up. The authors used a dermatome, free-hand knife, or dermabrasion to remove critical papillary dermis. Bleeding was controlled with deep dermal and subcutaneous infiltration of **epinephrine** 1:300,000. An alternate suggestion was made to use pressure sponges wrung out with 1:5000 epinephrine solution and held in place by manual pressure with a gauze pad.

Zachariae H: Dermabrasion in Darier's disease. Acta Derm Venereol 59:184–186, 1979.

Five patients were freed of lesions locally for more than $2\frac{1}{2}$ years following dermabrasion through the papillary dermis (deep dermabrasion). Wounds healed completely in two weeks.

Cipollaro VA, Shaps R: The treatment of Darier's disease: A comparison of superficial x-ray and Grenz ray therapy. Int J Dermatol 18:580–583, 1979.

Neither is recommended.

Jegasothy BV, Humeniuk JM: Darier's disease: A partially immunodeficient state. J Invest Dermatol 76:129–132, 1981.

These patients continue to show deficient immune T cell function despite good response to Accutane therapy and are thus at risk for severe progressive viral and bacterial skin infections.

Leroy D, Pedailles S, Maillard V, Freymuth F, Talel R, Deschamps P: Traitement par acyclovir d'un eczema herpeticum compliquant une maladie de Darier. Dematologica 167:212–216, 1983.

Acyclovir (15 mg/kg/day for five days) had an ameliorative effect on secondary herpes simplex infection in a 29-year-old woman with Darier's disease.

One therapist is worth a dozen diagnosticians.

Decubitus Ulcer

Nursing care	Benzoyl peroxide
Support systems	Metronidazole
Collagenase ointment	

It has been said that the bed is the most dangerous splint yet devised. And indeed, one of its dangers is the decubitus ulcer, resulting from necrosis of skin denied its blood supply by the unyielding bed splint. No malady is more preventable, and yet more inevitable, in the aged immobile patient lying for hours with a portion of skin squeezed by the unrelenting pressure of bone against bed. As many as 6 to 10 per cent of all nursing home residents develop bedsores, for who is there to reposition immobilized patients by precision clockwork every two hours, night and day? The skin cannot stand this circulatory-arrest trauma from compression of the body weight any more than a limb can survive an unattended tourniquet.

Prevention can be dismissed with the advice to move, or make the patient move, every two hours, or else be prepared to treat a skin infarct for two months. We must not think of the decubitus ulcer as a simple bed sore. It is the result of neglect, even for one night, with an infarct and slow subsequent slough of dead skin and subcutaneous tissue. Heel and elbow protector pads are helpful, as well as soft mattresses ("egg crate"), but short of having the patient "floating on air" in the Clinitron fluidized air bed, nothing relieves us of the responsibility of seeing to it that bony prominences not remain immobilized for hours in the bed splint.

But once the accident has happened, what to do? We favor intensified attention to spontaneous and assisted movement of the patient. No ulcer can heal if the new tissue remains compromised. We debride the dead leathery skin with collagenase ointment (Biozyme-C applied three times a day) and a Gillette razor blade for easy excision of islands of eschar. Infection is minimized by using benzoyl peroxide (10 per cent cream in the ulcer base once daily), with care being taken to keep it off the adjacent healthy skin. We rarely need systemic antibiotics unless the patient has a foul-smelling purulent ulcer, in which case metronidazole (Flagyl 250 mg tid) is used.

In extensive, recalcitrant ulcers, the possibility of a sinus tract or underlying osteomyelitis must be explored. Ulcers that have not healed in six months should be evaluated by a surgeon as to the possibility of skin grafting or covering the defect with a musculocutaneous flap.

Every decubitus ulcer patient must be restored to maximal good health. Hyperalimentation (enteral or parenteral) is essential to promote healing and induce fat cushioning for averting future pressure infarcts. We routinely prescribe iron (Feosol Spansules 1 tid), ascorbic acid (500 mg bid), and zinc (zinc sulfate 220 mg tid with food). These three medications are of vital importance in favoring the healing of ulcers.

But one element of even greater importance is patience. The doctor, the nurse, the family, and, most of all, the patient must recognize that filling in the ulcer will take a minimum of eight long weeks. There must be steady adherence to a standardized regimen of care. The temptation to try an assortment of home remedies or an arsenal of medical compounds should be resisted. Yielding only leads to frustration, if not irritation and sensitization. Progress comes week by week, not day by day. To expect more rapid healing is neither wise nor helpful. Spend time moving the patient, not fretting or watching. Remember, a "watched" ulcer never heals.

Roaf R: The causation and prevention of bedsores. *In* Kenedi RM, Cowden JM (eds): Bedsores Biomechanics. Baltimore, University Park Press, 1976, pp 5–9.

Nine clinical factors that place a patient at risk for decubitus ulcers:

poor health	impaired sensation
anemia	paralysis
infection	incontinence
shock	immobility
anesthesia	

All aspects for minimizing this risk are discussed in the 357-page report of the proceedings of a seminar on tissue viability and clinical applications held in Glasgow in 1975.

Rao DB, Sane PG, Georgiev EL: Collagenase in the treatment of dermal and decubitus ulcers. J Am Geriatr Soc 23:22–30, 1975.

Collagenase ointment (Santyl) applied once daily to decubitus ulcers was a useful debriding agent in 21 patients. Firm eschars were crosshatched to permit better penetration of the ointment.

Horsley JA: Preventing Decubitus Ulcers. New York, Grune & Stratton, 1981, 174 pp.

This pragmatic nursing research primer thoroughly evaluates known treatment and prevention methods of this preventable, piezogenic problem.

You name it, she evaluates it:

—from soap to silicone cream
—from electric lamp to hand vibrator
—from sawdust mattresses to air-fluidized beds

Parish LC, Witkowski JA, Crissey JT (eds): The Decubitus Ulcer. Chicago, Year Book Medical Publishers, 1983, 134 pp.

A third major reference source in which are listed 48 of the 2200 compounds known to have been recommended for the treatment of decubitus ulcers. Among the most valuable are the enzymes used in early debridement:

collagenase (Santyl ointment)
sutilains (Travase ointment)
trypsin (Granulex aerosol)
fibrinolysin and **desoxyribonuclease** (Elase ointment)
papain (Panafil ointment)

Le KM, Madsen BL, Barth PW, et al: An in-depth look at pressure sores using monolithic silicon pressure sensors. Plastic Reconst Surg 74:745–754, 1984.

Pressure sores begin in the deep tissue over bony prominences where the pressure is three to five times that found in the skin.

Shea JD: Pressure sores: Classification and management. Clin Orthop 112:89–100, 1975.

Treatment of pressure sores varies with their extent and depth:

Grade	*Anatomic Limit*	*Treatment*
I	Dermis	Local wound care
II	Subcutaneous fat	Local wound care
III	Deep fascia	Surgery
IV	No limit—into muscle, bone	Radical surgery
Closed	Deep fascia	Surgery

Reuler JB, Cooney TG: The pressure sore: Pathophysiology and principles of management. Ann Intern Med 94:661–666, 1981.

The four caveats of prophylaxis:

1. Avoid prolonged pressure over bony prominences (immobility)—"Where there is no pressure, there is no sore."
2. Avoid shearing forces (rapid elevation of the head of the bed).
3. Avoid frictional forces (rough patient handling across bed sheets).
4. Avoid moisture (from incontinence and perspiration).

Specific pointers on prevention:

1. Minimize friction.
    - Keep sheets loose, not restricting movement.
    - Remove particulate matter (food) from bed.
    - Lift patient instead of dragging.
    - Pat skin dry rather than rub it.
2. Control spasticity with medications, such as **diazepam** (Valium) 10 to 40 mg/day.
3. Prevent shearing forces.
    - Do not raise head of bed.
    - Use firm footboard if bed must be tilted.
    - Use sheepskin pads.
4. Moisture control
    - Sheepskin pads
    - Indwelling catheter
5. Pressure relief
    - Rotate patient every two hours—side to side, back to front.
    - Position with six or more soft pillows.
    - Use warning sensors and timing devices (go off if do not have 30 seconds of pressure relief every 15 to 30 minutes).
    - Do *not* use "donuts."
    - Alternate support surfaces:
        - Fluid support systems
        - Air support systems
        - Alternating pressure mattresses
        - Mud beds
    - For wheelchairs—flat support boards with specially molded thick foam-rubber cushions

Hendricks WM: Pressure ulcers. Ann Intern Med 95:239, 1981.

Patients in nursing homes most commonly have pressure ulcers on the heels, sides of the feet, and malleoli.

Management principles:

1. Accomplish local debridement with collagenase ointment and 10 per cent **benzoyl peroxide** lotion (Benoxyl-10).
2. Clean the tissue with **hydrogen peroxide** (3 per cent H_2O_2 bid, using cotton-tipped applicators and gauze dressings).
3. If base is dry: Use Polysporin ointment to prevent gauze dressing from sticking.
4. If base is moist: Use dextranomer (Debrisan) powder, which absorbs bacteria and four times its weight in fluid.

5. Surgical grafts are only rarely indicated.
6. Instruct nursing staff how to prevent pressure ulcers.

Nasar MA, Morley R: Cost effectiveness in treating deep pressure sores and ulcers. Practitioner 226:307–310, 1982.

In 9 of 12 elderly patients with decubitus ulcers, cost-effective treatment consisted of the use of a large-cell ripple mattress, ultraviolet light, and the application of a beaded, hydrophilic dextran macromolecular-chain wound-cleaning agent, Debrisan. The Debrisan was mixed 4:1 with sterile glycerol and applied twice a day initially, then once daily, and was removed carefully, using a syringe of saline. Recommended mainly for moist infected ulcers.

Yarkony GM, Kramer E, King R, et al: Pressure sore management: Efficacy of a moisture reactive occlusive dressing. Arch Phys Med Rehabil 65:597–600, 1984.

Daily wound care was eliminated by using DuoDerm hydroactive dressing (an inert polymer-containing moist gel dressing impermeable to O_2), applied to pressure ulcers only once weekly after cleansing of the base with H_2O_2 3 per cent and saline irrigation and careful drying of the wound. The dressing was applied to extend 3 cm beyond the ulcer margin. In 21 patients, 56 per cent of 25 recalcitrant pressure sores healed, or virtually healed, in an average of six weeks.

Gomolin IH, Brandt JL: Topical metronidazole therapy for pressure sores of geriatric patients. J Am Geriatr Soc 31:710–712, 1983.

In four patients, extemporaneous 1 per cent solution of **metronidazole** (250 mg tablet crushed in 25 ml sterile water, steam sterilized at 250°C for 30 minutes, applied in a gauze dressing q8h), eliminated the offensive odor and purulent discharge and stimulated remarkable granulation of deep pressure ulcers in areas of fecal soilage in 10 days.

Barron JJ, Jacobson WE, Tidd G: Treatment of decubitus ulcers: A new approach. Minn Med 68:103–106, 1985.

Five of six decubitus ulcers showing no response to conventional therapy healed within one month of applying low-intensity nongalvanic electrical energy to the ulcer margins. The Micro-Electro Medical Stimulation was given three times weekly for three weeks, using a pair of noninvasive probes placed circumferentially around the ulcer.

Sugarman B: Infection and pressure sores. Arch Phys Med Rehabil 66:177–179, 1985.

A refreshing, modern look at a seemingly prosaic area of medical care.

1. Pressure sores will develop in 50 per cent of all persons with spinal cord injury.
2. Failure of the sore to heal is noninfectious: continued pressure, malnutrition, heterotopic bone, vascular disease.
3. Osteomyelitis of the bone under the ulcer was present in 49 of 205 ulcers associated with spinal cord injury.
4. Use sinograms, CT scans, bone scans, bone biopsy, and aspiration for full evaluation of the nonhealing ulcer.

Sugarman B, Hawes S, Musher DM, et al: Osteomyelitis beneath pressure sores. Arch Intern Med 143:683–688, 1983.

Observations of subdecubitus ulcer osteomyelitis in nine instances:

1. X-ray examination detected the condition in only four.
2. Technetium ^{99m}Tc medronate bone scans were positive in all cases, but were also nonspecific.
3. Bone biopsy was diagnostic and often necessary to make the diagnosis.
4. Bone cultures showed anaerobic bacteria and gram-negative bacilli present. Sensitivity determinations were used to guide antibiotic therapy.

Buchanan DL, Agris J: Gluteal plication closure of sacral pressure ulcers. Plast Reconstr Surg 72:49–54, 1983.

Primary closure of gluteal pressure sores through excision followed by musculocutaneous flaps was used successfully in 19 of 21 paraplegic and quadriplegic patients. It was most useful if the defect was less than 8 cm in diameter.

McGregor JC: Surgical treatment of ischial pressure sores. J R Coll Surg Edinb 29:242–245, 1984.

In a retrospective 10-year study of 65 ischial pressure sores in 41 patients, smaller superficial sores were healed by conservative measures with no recurrence. However, after excision and direct closure of larger sores there was 25 per cent recurrence, and when flaps were used the recurrence rate was 36 per cent.

Prior to surgery the patient should receive general supportive measures, such as vitamins, high-protein diet, correction of anemia, and local treatment to reduce infection in the ulcer.

Abruzzese RS: Early assessment and prevention of pressure sores. *In* Lee BY (ed): Chronic Ulcers of the Skin. New York, McGraw-Hill Book Co, 1985, pp 1–19.

A cogent message from the nursing front:

1. One of the major reasons pressure sores form and heal slowly is that there is no consistency in assessment and treatment:

   Nurses have their own preferred remedy—so that different ointments, medications, dressings, or solutions may be used on the same ulcer every eight hours.

   Moreover, physicians may prescribe three different treatments in a single week.
2. Decubitus ulcers still heal slowly at best:

   Three to eight weeks is normal, and 16 weeks not rare.

   Have patience. Don't switch from air mattresses to foam padding to sheepskin. Such brownian movement is costly and discouraging.
3. Why the preventable will remain unpreventable until we have more nurses:

   It takes at least 20 minutes to gather the materials needed, walk into a patient's room, speak to the patient, lower the side rails, prepare the patient for turning and reposition with pillows, rub his or her back, change damp bed linens or gown, and straighten the bed covers. If 20 per cent of patients are at risk on a 40-bed unit (i.e., eight patients), there is a need for 160 minutes of nursing care every two hours both night and day.

Seiler WO, Allen S, Stähelin HB: Decubitus ulcer prevention: A new investigative method using transcutaneous oxygen tension measurement. J Am Geriatr Soc 31:786–789, 1983.

The noninvasive Clark oxygen electrode, which measures transcutaneous oxygen tension and anoxemia, enables immediate assessment of the efficacy of measures to prevent decubitus ulcers.

Dolezal R, Cohen M, Schultz RC: The use of Clinitron therapy unit in the immediate postoperative care of pressure ulcers. Ann Plast Surg 14:33–36, 1985.

The Clinitron (a bed of air-suspended fine glass beads that levitates the patient so that pressure on skin is so small [<32 mm Hg] as not to compress the capillary vessels) was useful in the postoperative care of 16 patients with decubitus ulcers.

Andersen KE, Jensen O, Kvorning SA, Bach E: Decubitus prophylaxis: A prospective trial on the efficiency of alternating-pressure air-mattresses and water-mattresses. Acta Derm Venereol 63:227–230, 1982.

Of 200 patients at risk for pressure sores, seven developed decubitus ulcers when left on an alternating-pressure air mattress. The same incidence occurred in a matched group of 200 on a water mattress. However, in the control group kept on the ordinary hospital mattress, the incidence of decubitus ulcers was tripled to 21 of 200 patients. Both patients and staff disliked the water mattresses, and many patients also disliked the air mattresses.

Berjian RA, Douglass HO, Holyoke ED, et al: Skin pressure measurements on various mattress surfaces in cancer patients. Am J Phys Med 62:217–226, 1983.

A statistical analysis of pressures measured while monitoring 28 bedfast patients on eight mattress surfaces revealed that the Mud Gel bed was rated the best for minimizing pressure on the skin.

The following mattress surfaces were evaluated:

Dynamic
- Alternating pressure pad[1]
- Lapidus (alternating pressure) mattress[2]

Static
- Cotton muslin sheet
- Cotton blanket
- Sheepskin (Derma-Care pad)[2]
- Egg crate pad, single layer[3]
- Egg crate pad, double layer[3]
- Mud gel bed[1]

Eccott H, Touey FI: Prevention of heel pressure sores. Lancet 1:875, 1980.

To make gutter splints to support the lower legs and prevent heel pressure sores:

1. Cut blocks of foam rubber from an old mattress to a suitable length to reach from the knee to just above the malleolus.
2. Hollow these out with a knife to accommodate the shape of the calf.

In use, the heel is left free over the splint, and the weight of the lower leg is borne by the whole length of the splint. No heel sores have occurred in three years of use.

Souther SG, Carr SD, Vistnes LM: Wheelchair cushions to reduce pressure under bony prominences. Arch Phys Med Rehabil 55:460–464, 1974.

Evaluation of 11 commercially available wheelchair cushions in a study of 10 subjects disclosed that the Jobst Hydro-Float cushion reduced pressure beneath the ischial tuberosities to a greater degree than the other cushions.

Garber SL, Krouskop TA: Wheelchair cushion modification and its effect on pressure. Arch Phys Med Rehabil 65:579–583, 1984.

Polyurethane foam, the most commonly used wheelchair cushion material, has to be form-tailored for the specific individual. There is no geometric design of universal superiority.

Taylor TV, Rimmer S, Day B, et al: Ascorbic acid supplementation in the treatment of pressure-sores. Lancet 2:544–546, 1974.

Manufacturers

1. Gaymar Industries, Inc.
1 Bank Street
Orchard Park, NY 14127
2. American Hospital Supply Corp.
1250 Waukegan Rd.
McGaw Park, IL 60085
3. Bio-Clinic Co.
1455 East Victoria Ave.
San Bernardino, CA 92408

In a double-blind controlled study of 20 surgical patients with pressure sores, **ascorbic acid** (500 mg bid for one month) significantly improved the rate of healing, with 84 per cent mean reduction in ulcer size compared to 42.7 per cent reduction in the placebo group.

Other important factors in treatment include correction of:

protein deficiency	ischemia
anemia	incontinence
prolonged direct pressure	

Stewart P, Wharton GW: Bridging: An effective and practical method of preventive skin care for the immobilized person. South Med J 69:1469–1473, 1475, 1976.

Bridging is accomplished through the proper positioning of pillows beneath the patient, allowing enough space between the bony prominences and the bed surface to freely pass a hand. It requires 8 to 10 pillows and is simple and inexpensive. Pillow placement for various positions is illustrated.

Denne WA: An objective assessment of the sheepskins used for decubitus sore prophylaxis. Rheumatol Rehabil 18:23–29, 1979.

Resilient natural sheepskins were the best interface for the prevention and management of decubitus ulcers because of their ability to absorb water vapor and keep the patient's skin dry. Polyester simulations of sheepskins were very poor at water vapor absorption and also produced the greatest friction.

Reswick JB, Rogers JE: Experience at Rancho Los Amigos Hospital with devices and techniques to prevent pressure sores. *In* Kenedi RM, Cowden JM, Scales JT (eds): Bedsore Biomechanics. Baltimore, University Park Press, 1976, pp 301–310.

Two special beds developed in Downey, California, particularly help recumbent patients:

1. Rancho flotation bed (mud bed). This contains fluid made twice as heavy as water by adding a colloidal suspension of pulverized barite (40 per cent) and a thixotropic clay, bentonite (10 per cent to 50 per cent water). The patient floats half submerged, with maximum pressures of 15 to 25 mm Hg at points of deepest submergence.
2. Polyflotation mattress (Scimedics, Inc., 16220 Gundry St., Paramount, CA). This large block of polyurethane foam (15 cm by 92 cm by 460 cm) has been cut with numerous transverse and longitudinal wedge-shaped slits, top and bottom. The cuts are concentrated in the sacral and heel areas and longitudinally in the trunk areas. The mattress is covered by a thin elastic sheet of polyurethane film. Maximum pressures range from 20 to 25 mm Hg.

Vetra H, Whittaker D: Hydrotherapy and topical collagenase for decubitus ulcers. Geriatrics 30:53–58 (Aug.) 1975.

In a neuropsychiatric hospital, daily hydrotherapy (40°C) and daily application of collagenase 0.5 per cent in petrolatum (Santyl ointment) cleared 80 per cent of 30 decubitus ulcers in an average of 37 days. Good granulation tissue was seen in all patients.

Rosenthal AM, Schurman A: Hyperbaric treatment of pressure sores. Arch Phys Med Rehab 52:413–415, 433, 1971.

Treatment of 18 patients with 38 pressure sores in a hyperbaric chamber (three atmospheres pressure, 2 hours daily, five days weekly) resulted in complete healing of 22 ulcers. The average number of treatments was 37 (range 14 to 60 days of treatment). Only 11 of 38 ulcers required surgical closure.

Presumably the hyperbaric chamber delivered more oxygen to the deeper tissues and stimulated healing.

If patients make you irritable, it's time for your *vacation.*

Delayed Pressure Urticaria

Aspirin
Indomethacin
Corticosteroids

Patients with this unusual form of urticaria seek relief not only for the swelling but also for the pain. This pain and the delayed onset of the urticaria suggest that mediators other than histamine are involved. Indeed, antihistaminic therapy is ineffective. The nonsteroidal anti-flammatory drugs such as aspirin and indomethacin deserve a trial, but the only truly effective therapy is systemic steroids. We favor Kenalog 40 mg IM given every three weeks for a few months.

Little is known concerning specific causes, so that empiric measures as well as comprehensive medical study must be undertaken in severe cases. All of these patients deserve the same meticulous analysis given to patients with chronic urticaria, although the final mediator pathway is entirely different. In this respect, we have cleared two cases with Nizoral (200 mg/day) given over an extended period.

Baughman RD, Jillson OF: Seven specific types of urticaria: With special reference to delayed persistent dermographism. Ann Allergy 21:248–255, 1963.

Among six patients with disabling delayed dermographism, several had tinea pedis, allergic drug reactions to mold products, and significant reactions to intradermal trichophyton and molds. Fungal allergens were thought to play a role, and hyposensitization was proposed as treatment along with systemic steroids (no results documented).

Sussman GL, Harvey RP, Schocket AL: Delayed pressure urticaria. J Allergy Clin Immunol 70:337–342, 1982.

In 17 patients, antihistamines had no effect on the pressure urticaria, but did control associated chronic urticarial lesions. Fever, chills, and arthralgias occurred in 78 per cent. Lesions were reproduced with 15 pounds of sandbags draped over the shoulder for 15 minutes. They appeared $6\frac{1}{2}$ hours after challenge, peaked at 9 hours, and resolved in 24 to 48 hours. Nonsteroidal anti-inflammatory drugs (**aspirin** 3900 mg/day, **ibuprofen** [Motrin], and **indomethacin** [Indocin]) were helpful in 80 per cent, but nearly all required **prednisone** (40 mg/day tapered to 5 to 15 mg daily after four months) to control pressure symptoms.

Ryan TJ, Shim-Young N, Turk JL: Delayed pressure urticaria. Br J Dermatol 80:485–490, 1968.

In 15 patients the condition was unaffected by antihistamines (**chlorpheniramine maleate** 8 mg q6h or **promethazine hydrochloride** 50 mg q8h), but was controlled with steroids (**prednisolone** 30 mg daily). Positive trichophyton reactions developed in 3 of 11 patients tested.

Estes SA, Yung CW: Delayed pressure urticaria: An investigation of some parameters of lesion induction. J Am Acad Dermatol 5:25–31, 1981.

In two patients, lesions produced experimentally with a pressure-testing device reached maximum size nine hours later, with tenderness, burning, and stinging. Each reaction site was refractory to additional stimuli for more than 48 hours.

Davis KC, Mekori YA, Kohler PF, Schocket AL: Late cutaneous reactions in patients with delayed pressure urticaria. J Allergy Clin Immunol 73:810–812, 1984.

Intradermal injections of the mast cell degranulation compound 48/80 (0.02 cc, 0.5 and 5.0 mg/ml) but not histamine (0.02 cc, 0.1 and 0.01 mg/ml) reproduced the disease in 10 patients.

It is a good thing for a physician to have prematurely gray hair and itching piles. The first makes him appear to know more than he does, and the second gives him an expression of concern, which the patient interprets as being on his behalf.

A. Benson Cannon

Delusions of Parasitosis

Orap
Inderal
Valium
Parnate

These patients are among the most interesting to come to your office. They bring you a wondrous array of flora and fauna from a subliminal fairyland. All this is accompanied by tales of lively worms, bugs, and sundry uncategorized creatures that dart in and out of the sweat pores, sleep in the hairs, and generally cause great havoc. Let them take you back to your childhood and, indeed, to the childhood of medicine when fantasy knew the cause of disease.

Generally these patients are strange, lonely, pleasant, and elderly, (maybe in their second childhood). They need individualized care and a physician who will listen, look, and "love." All are deadly serious in their delusion. One of our associates was awakened at 1:00 AM by such a patient, who excitedly exclaimed, "I've found them" and begged him to come immediately to his home. Responsive to the urgency in the patient's voice and nudged by curiosity, the physician went to the home to find several *Demodex* in full display under a microscope the patient had rented from a physicians' supply house.

It is important to look at their menagerie. We cured one patient of his delusion by showing him microscopically the actual knots in his hairs that he had perceived as parasites.

Some patients come only with graphic stories, not specimens. We recall an elderly gentleman who told us that every evening at exactly 6:00 PM hundreds of small undulating worms came out of his skin. We confidently told him to apply Aquaphor over his entire body at exactly 5:45 PM each day, and he would have no further trouble. No return appointment was scheduled, but several months later he reappeared, completely "cured." He came asking us "for a good bone doctor. They're now coming out of my bones at 6:00 PM every day."

Another of our patients, a young pharmaceutical chemist, was cured of his delusions of parasitosis simply by removing him from a laboratory where he was engaged in organic synthesis of psychotropic drugs. Another one of our patients, a young man with delusions of parasites localized to his scalp, was cured by treatment with the adrenergic beta-blocker, propranolol (Inderal 20 mg tid). It was possible to discontinue this after a few months with no recurrence.

It is apparent that paresthesias or even parasitic infection can initiate a delusional state in certain people. Causes such as diabetes mellitus, pellagra, xerosis, glass fibers, scabies, and *Cheyletiella* infestation must be ruled out, as well as drug ingestion or intolerance. Evaluation for organic brain disease, Alzheimer's disease, or schizophrenia is also important. Look for failing memory.

The vast majority of these delusional patients, however, prove to be an example of a monosymptomatic hypochondriacal psychosis. For all of these the new neuroleptic drug Orap (pimozide 2 to 12 mg once/day) is indicated. Discovered serendipitously 10 years ago, it is widely used in Europe with great success; it has just been released in the United States. It is no cure, but in many patients it reduces or eliminates the delusions while it is being taken. For the seriously affected patient who burns his furniture, tears out walls, calls in exterminators weekly, and visits literally dozens of doctors in search of help, pimozide is a marvelous "delusional parasitocide."

We believe in treating, not dismissing, these patients. We examine every specimen they bring, schedule regular appointments, and prescribe trial medications. It is important to note that we do *not* share the delusion, but rather we share the misery the patients have. We feel that interest, concern, and treatment for them does not reinforce a delusion that is already so profound as to lead to suicide.

These patients cannot easily be referred to a psychiatrist. They ignore or reject such advice, realizing at once that you do not have a grasp of their problem. "Who ever heard of a psychiatrist treating parasites?" And yet, the delusional state may indicate a serious psychosis that demands psychiatric attention. We recall a young man who came to our office displaying a large worm in his wrist, which had infected him from outer space. The "worm" was a flexural tendon of his left wrist that he had dissected free with a scalpel and hemostat. His history revealed that he had consulted four dermatologists that week. Each had seen the exposed tendons and referred him to a psychiatrist! We explained to the patient that we would get a parasitologist in consultation immediately. We then called the psychiatrist, who said, "Sure, send him over." Only by pressure did we get the psychiatrist to make an office call to *our* office. He came, the patient was given an injection of a "sleep-inducing parasitocidal" drug, then taken away by ambulance for institutionalization and definitive care. The moral: Don't send this type of patient to the psychiatrist, but send the psychiatrist to him!

The ultimate goal of therapy should be the disappearance of the delusion, not the patient.

Lyell A: Delusions of parasitosis. Br J Dermatol 108:485–499, 1983.

A superb questionnaire study of 282 patients with delusions of parasitosis treated by 216 physicians.

Observations:

Of 60 patients treated with **pimozide** (Orap 2 to 12 mg single dose daily) 44 showed good response; 16 failed to respond. Discontinuing the pimozide resulted in recurrence of the delusions.

In 13 others there was remission, in two as a result of being told they were deluded, in one by topical **malathion**.

Many were helped by a prescription for antidepressants and the use of emollients.

Five committed suicide.

Gould WM, Gragg TM: Delusions of parasitosis: An approach to the problem. Arch Dermatol 112:1745–1748, 1976.

A valuable source of therapeutic ideas for the dermatologic management of these patients who need, but always refuse, psychiatric care:

Be certain of the diagnosis.
Listen carefully to the patient's story.
Explore the patient's behavior response.
Establish good rapport.
Find an area in which you can help.
Reduce the patient's sense of isolation.

Consider the use of antianxiety drugs such as **diazepam** (Valium) or **chlordiazepoxide** (Librium)

Lyell A: Delusions of parasitosis. J Am Acad Dermatol 8:895–897, 1983.

Look for and eliminate the causes of paresthesia:

liver disease	dermatitis herpetiformis
kidney disease	alcoholism and toxic states
diabetes mellitus	vitamin B_{12} deficiency
cardiovascular disease	pellagra
lymphoma	drug reactions
anemia	arthropods
iron deficiency	glass fibers (environmental irritants)
peripheral neuritis	

Liebowitz MR, Nuetzel EJ, Bowser AE, Klein DF: Phenelzine and delusions of parasitosis: A case report. Am J Psychiatry 135:1565–1566, 1978.

Delusions of parasitosis may occur:
With use of psychostimulants:
- amphetamines
- **cocaine**
- **methylphenidate** (Ritalin)

With monosymptomatic hypochondriacal psychosis
With disease
- temporal lobe epilepsy
- schizophrenia
- delirium tremens

With monoamine oxidase inhibitor drugs as in the following report:

A young woman, after 18 weeks of therapy with **phenelzine** (Nardil 45 mg/day) for the syndrome of hysteroid dysphoria, developed the delusion that small black bugs were infesting her hair and body and coming out her pores. When phenelzine was discontinued, the visualization of bugs and the itching gradually subsided over a three-month period. Resumption of the phenelzine (15 mg/day) resulted in return of the delusions of parasitosis within 48 hours. Switching to a placebo in a single-blind fashion resulted in disappearance of the delusional state in several days.

Hamann K, Avnstorp C: Delusions of infestation treated by pimozide: A double-blind crossover clinical study. Acta Derm Venereol 62:55–58, 1982.

Delusions and pruritus abated slowly in 10 of 11 patients given oral **pimozide** (1 to 5 mg daily for six weeks). Patients are best treated by a dermatologist. The drug also can be given by injection. Side effects noted:
- fatigue (5)
- vertigo (4)
- depression (2)
- parkinsonian signs (2)

Munro A: Monosymptomatic hypochondriacal psychosis manifesting as delusions of parasitosis: A description of four cases successfully treated with pimozide. Arch Dermatol 114:940–943, 1978.

Instructive cases from the practice of the psychiatrist who discovered **pimozide** (2 to 8 mg/day) therapy for this disease. None of the patients ever admitted that their disease was psychologic, nor were they confronted with this fact.

Case 1: A 60-year-old woman had complained of mites crawling all over her body ever since finding some maggots in flour in her kitchen two years before. It was very difficult to persuade her to start medication, but she developed a sense of well-being after taking pimozide (4 mg/day for one month). She was being seen every three months and was symptom free as long as she continued the same dose.

Case 2: A 70-year-old man had complained for one year of a flea infestation coming from a pet canary. Results after starting pimozide:

4 mg/day for 3 weeks: no help
6 mg/day for 2 weeks: very helpful
12 mg/day: complete remission
The "imaginary flea count" correlated directly with the dose of pimozide.

Case 3: A 56-year-old woman complained of infestation with black bugs and white eggs on her skin ever since a mouse entered her house from the sewer five months before during sewer digging outside her house. Treatment with pimozide (6 mg/day) stopped the delusion but also made her lethargic, so that she stopped the drug. In three days the delusions returned, and she has required maintenance of 6 mg daily.

Case 4: A 29-year-old man with generalized itching following an attack of pubic lice was convinced he was infested with insects. Pimozide (2 mg/day for two months) cleared the delusion, but the patient considered it to be an insecticidal drug.

Roberts J, Roberts R: Delusions of parasitosis. Br Med J 1:1219, 1977.

Use of the monamine oxidase inhibitor, **tranylcypromine** (Parnate 10 mg qid) in combination with **trifluoperazine** (Stelazine 1 mg qid) resulted in complete removal of delusions in one week in a 58-year-old woman convinced that small bugs or worms had been crawling about in her gums for over two years. She had shown no response to prior electric convulsion therapy, **amitriptyline** (Elavil), trifluoperazine and **chlorpromazine** (Thorazine). The drugs and monthly office visits have kept the delusions away for nearly 10 years. The authors hope that, after the drug is stopped, she will not revert to coming to their house at all hours with her little packets.

Hopkinson G: Delusions of infestation. Acta Psychiatr Scand 46:111–119, 1970.

Electroshock therapy temporarily cured one woman with a depressive psychosis and delusions about spiders in her hair. The antidepressant **imipramine** (Tofranil) cured another woman with delusions of worms and lice burrowing into her skin.

Frankel EB: Treatment of delusions of parasitosis. J Am Acad Dermatol 9:772–773, 1983.

Advises:

"Confirm" that the patient has parasites.

Say you have precisely the medicine that will kill the bug through a particular odor that no bug or insect can withstand.

Dispense crude coal tar liquid (one capful in shallow tub used every two to three days)

It nearly always works. Should the bugs go into the nose or the bowels, increase the dose of crude coal tar in the bath (but stress that it should not be ingested).

Mack PJ: Hairy dentures: A monosymptomatic hypochondriacal psychosis. Br Dent J 158:50–51, 1985.

A 70-year-old man complained of continuous growth of hairlike threads from his acrylic dentures. **Pimozide** (Orap 2 mg/day) relieved the delusion in eight weeks. Later, complete replacement of the dentures was accomplished with no problems.

Alexander J O'D: Arthropods and Human Skin. New York, Springer-Verlag, 1984.

Management of delusions of parasitosis:

Be certain of the diagnosis.
Do not exaggerate the attempt to find parasites.
Take the patient seriously.
Do not directly refer the patient to a psychiatrist.

Offer relief for the skin irritation, but don't enter into the patient's system of delusion.

If delusions are toxic in origin or due to a vitamin deficiency, correct the cause.

The single best drug is **pimozide** (diphenylbutyl piperidine, a dopamine blocker). May get toxicity at doses over 8 mg daily (drowsiness, depression, parkinsonism, indigestion, torticollis, tardive dyskinesia, dry mouth, visual disturbances, incontinence).

Prognosis is poor in schizophrenia, especially with marked paranoia.

Physician: One upon whom we set our hopes when ill, and our dogs when well.

AMBROSE BIERCE

Dermatitis Herpetiformis

Dapsone	Gluten-free diet
Sulfapyridine	Colchicine
Azulfidine	Cholestyramine
Prednisone	Heparin

The dermatitis herpetiformis patient has the easy choice of drug therapy or the hard choice of dietary therapy. Since chronicity of the disease is measured in decades and jejunal enteropathy is often present, the patient should be actively involved in therapeutic decision making.

We instruct our patients concerning the immune nature of their disease and the critical role of gluten sensitivity. We likewise advise them that iodine and iodine-containing medicines or foods (seafood) can make their condition worse. Elimination of gluten from the diet is desirable to reduce both the severity of the disease and the need for drug therapy, but six months to several years is required for improvement. This "carrot" of relief is so far distant that only intelligent, well-informed patients will be sufficiently motivated to alter their dietary life styles. The patient who is serious about the diet cannot succeed with an indifferent cook (even Accent is verboten). The patient who regularly eats in restaurants or has only a mild form of the disease simply is not a candidate for rigorous dietary control. However, for the patient who wants a "cure," we recommend consultation with a hospital dietitian and the purchase and study of the cookbooks cited below.

We strongly advise strict elimination of seafood, iodine, wheat products, beer, and liquor. Corn and rice are safe pleasant substitutes.

Many patients elect the easy choice of dapsone therapy. We prescribe 100 mg a day, and monitor the resultant hemolytic anemia and methemoglobinemia with blood counts and clinical inspection of the lips and fingernails for cyanosis. Once control is established we attempt every few months to find a lower maintenance level of dapsone by careful reduction of dose. We do not aim for total suppression of lesions in our patients, but attempt to find a dose that gives them significant relief of pruritus. They must recognize that dapsone will have to be continued year in and year out, unless they follow the gluten-free diet or are in the lucky 10 per cent in whom spontaneous remission occurs.

Topical treatment has never been a prominent feature in our program because of the effectiveness of dapsone or its analogue, sulfapyridine, in suppressing the disease. To date, no drug has proven curative. Systemic steroids (Kenalog 40 mg IM) are often effective but give only three to four weeks of relief per injection.

Patients who are dapsone sensitive may benefit from cholestyramine as a substitute therapy. In these cases, vitamin supplementation is necessary.

Finally, recall that scabies may mimic dermatitis herpetiformis, so that all atypical cases deserve a careful trial of Kwell lotion topically.

Alexander JO: Dermatitis herpetiformis. Philadelphia, WB Saunders Co, 1975, 346 pp.

Classic encyclopedic monograph, including review of successful treatments of yesteryear: **nicotinic acid**, **heparin**, topical steroids, and arsenic.

Fry L: The treatment of dermatitis herpetiformis. Clin Exp Dermatol 7:633–642, 1982.

Dapsone (100 mg/day) is the drug of choice.

Side effects: Methemoglobinemia (children and elderly adults also risk angina from decreased oxygen-carrying capacity).

Hemolytic anemia—dose related (iron and folate deficiency from malabsorption may contribute)

Agranulocytosis (rare)

Headache

Lethargy, insomnia, depression

Peripheral neuropathy

Drug eruptions

Alternative drugs: **Sulfapyridine**, a short-acting sulfonamide (0.5 gm twice weekly to 4.0 gm/day): side effects—nausea, lethargy

Sulfamethoxypyridazine, the first of the long-acting sulfonamides (Kynex 0.5 to 1.0 g/day): side effect—skin rash

Diet, gluten free: must be strict to be helpful

consider restriction of milk and iodides

Remission rate without treatment: 10 per cent

Katz SI: Sulfoxone (Diasone) in the treatment of dermatitis herpetiformis. Arch Dermatol 118:809–812, 1982.

Sulfoxone sodium (Diasone 300 to 600 mg/day) was the first sulfone used for treating dermatitis herpetiformis. Its parent compound, **dapsone** (DDS, Avlosulfon), has largely replaced it.

Before prescribing dapsone, determine the CBC in all patients and the G6PD (glucose-6-phosphate dehydrogenase) level in Asians, blacks, and patients of Mediterranean descent. If the enzyme is absent, profound hemolysis occurs.

Follow-up: CBC every one to two weeks for three months, then every two months.

Give the patient a wallet medication card, since the blue gray of methemoglobinemia may puzzle emergency room physicians.

Tuffanelli DL: Successful pregnancy in a patient with dermatitis herpetiformis treated with low-dose dapsone. Arch Dermatol 118:876, 1982.

A patient who had taken **dapsone** (25 to 50 mg/day) for 16 years had a successful pregnancy, the dose being continued at the same level throughout pregnancy.

Sanders SW, Zone JJ, Foltz RL, Tolman KG, Rollins DE: Hemolytic anemia induced by dapsone transmitted through breast milk. Ann Intern Med 96:465–466, 1982.

The breast-fed infant of a mother given **dapsone** (50 mg/day) during and after pregnancy was found to have hemolytic anemia and dapsone in the serum at the six-week checkup.

Kazmierowski JA, Ross JE, Peizner DS, Wuepper KD: Dermatitis herpetiformis: Effects of sulfones and sulfonamides on neutrophil myeloperoxidase-mediated iodination and cytotoxicity. J Clin Immunol 4:55–64, 1984.

Dapsone specifically interferes with the biochemical functioning (iodination) and the cytotoxic properties of the patient's neutrophils.

Costello MJ: Sulfapyridine in the treatment of dermatitis herpetiformis. Arch Dermatol 56:614–628, 1947.

This seminal article pointed out that other sulfonamides (**sulfanilamide, sulfathiazole, sulfadiazine**) were not as effective as **sulfapyridine**. Pyribenzamine hydrochloride (**tripelennamine** 200 to 300 mg/day) may help a patient intolerant of sulfapyridine.

Andreozzi RJ, Nus DD: Dermatitis herpetiformis: Treatment with Azulfidine. Cutis 13:366–370, 1974.

Azulfidine (**salicylazosulfapyridine**), converted in the gut to sulfapyridine, is also effective.

Starting dose: 1 gm qid.

Lowney ED: Use of sulfasalazine in dermatitis herpetiformis in young people. Arch Dermatol 114:1553, 1978.

Advocates **sulfasalazine** (Azulfidine 500 mg qid) as being less toxic than **sulfapyridine**. May need 3 to 4 gm/day for control.

Schiffner JH: Therapy of childhood linear IgA dermatitis herpetiformis. J Am Acad Dermatol 6:403–404, 1982.

Prednisone (20 mg/day) induced dramatic clearing in a 20-month-old girl with dermatitis herpetiformis resistant to **dapsone** and **sulfapyridine**. Maintenance prednisone (20 mg/day or 30 mg every other day) was still required after two years, despite addition of sulfapyridine (0.5 to 1 gm/day).

Reunala T, Blomquist K, Tarpila S, Halme H, Kangas K: Gluten-free diet in dermatitis herpetiformis. 1. Clinical response of skin lesions in 81 patients. Br J Dermatol 97:473–480, 1977.

Of 81 patients on a gluten-free diet for 6 to 36 months 28 per cent were able to stop **dapsone** therapy completely; 93 per cent were able to lower the dose to one fifth of the former level after three years.

Reunala T, Kosnai I, Karpati S, Kuitunen P, Torok E, Savilahti E: Dermatitis herpetiformis: Jejunal findings and skin response to gluten-free diet. Arch Dis Child 59:517–522, 1984.

Jejunal biopsies (57 children, Finland and Hungary) showed villous atrophy in 89 per cent. Repeat biopsies (18 children, gluten-free diet for 21 months) showed marked improvement.

Treatment results: gluten-free diet (alone)—three cases cleared in three to six months.

dapsone + gluten-free diet—eight of 12 could stop dapsone after 11 months.

Fry L, Leonard JN, Swain F, Tucker WFG, Haffenden G, Ring N, McMinn RMH: Long-term follow-up of dermatitis herpetiformis with and without dietary gluten withdrawal. Br J Dermatol 107:631–640, 1982.

Seventy-eight cases of dermatitis herpetiformis were followed for 3 to 14 years: Only 14 per cent (5 of 36) of patients in the control regular diet group were able to stop drug therapy, in contrast to 71 per cent (30 of 42) on gluten-free diets. Time required—8 months to reduce dosage, 29 months to stop medications.

Ljunghall K, Scheynius A, Jonsson J, Schilling W, Forsum U: Gluten-free diet in patients with dermatitis herpetiformis: Effect on the occurrence of antibodies to reticulin and gluten. Arch Dermatol 119:970–974, 1983.

Gluten-free diet for one to four years in 51 cases of dermatitis herpetiformis resulted in complete disappearance of IgA and IgG gluten and reticulin antibodies.

Hartwig MS: Sticking to a gluten-free diet. Am J Nursing 83:1308–1310, 1983.

Gluten is in all grains except rice and corn. It is a protein providing elasticity to bread. Patients must avoid flour, beer, rye, scotch, bourbon, gin, and chocolate milk. (A Xerox copy of this article will be gratefully received by the patient.)

Powers M: Gluten-Free and Good, 2nd rev ed. St. Charles, Mo., Old Town Press, 1983.

For the serious patient, this is invaluable.

Wood MN: Coping with the Gluten-Free Diet. Springfield, Ill., Charles C Thomas, 1982.

Kitchen help for the dermatitis herpetiformis patient.

Hills HC: Good Food: Gluten-free. New Canaan, Conn., Keats Publishing, 1976.

Another low-priced volume of directions.

Pock-Steen O Ch, Niordson AM: Milk sensitivity in dermatitis herpetiformis. Br J Dermatol 83:614–619, 1970.

One patient (30-year-old woman) with malabsorption and colic developed dermatitis herpetiformis while on a gluten-free diet when milk was added. Numerous challenges confirmed this observation:

eliminate milk: lesions disappeared
add milk: lesions flared

Successful diet: Avoid both gluten and milk products.

Engquist A, Pock-Steen O Ch: Dermatitis herpetiformis and milk-free diet. Lancet 2:438–439, 1971.

Gluten caused dyspepsia and milk caused dermatitis in a 74-year-old man with dermatitis herpetiformis. Elimination of milk cleared skin lesions in one week (in contrast to the slow clearing with a gluten-free diet that occurs in most dermatitis herpetiformis patients).

Silvers DN, Juhlin EA, Berczeller PH, McSorley J: Treatment of dermatitis herpetiformis with colchicine. Arch Dermatol 116:1373–1374, 1980.

Colchicine (0.6 mg tid) gave significant help to three of four patients unable to tolerate **dapsone**, **sulfapyridine**, or a gluten-free diet. (Do not give during pregnancy.)

Shelley WB: Treatment of dermatitis herpetiformis with cholestyramine. Br J Dermatol 103:663–666, 1980.

Cholestyramine (Questran 4 gm tid), an ion exchange resin, controlled dermatitis herpetiformis in two sulfonamide-sensitive patients. Theory: May block absorption of gluten, iodine, or endotoxin critical to pathogenesis of dermatitis herpetiformis.

Fry L, Swain F, Leonard J, McMinn RMH: Disodium cromoglycate in dermatitis herpetiformis. Br J Dermatol 105:83–86, 1981.

No help. Eight patients took disodium cromoglycate (1.5 to 1.6 gm/day) for 6 to 11 months. Intestinal biopsies were unchanged.

Alexander JO: The treatment of dermatitis herpetiformis with heparin. Br J Dermatol 75:289–293, 1963.

Complete heparinization in patients with dermatitis herpetiformis hospitalized for coronary insufficiency stopped itching and lesions for seven days. Intermittent dosage of **heparin** (daily or twice weekly) also gave partial relief. Weekly heparin maintenance after complete heparinization was not tried. Dicumarol was not effective.

Bonus
- Eliminate methemoglobinemia by stopping **dapsone**
- Dermatitis herpetiformis was easier to control with dapsone after heparin therapy

Heparin dosage
- Day 1—10,000 U IV q6h
- Day 2—7,500 U IV or IM q6h
- Days 3 and 4—5,000 U IM q6h
- (Note: IM route is no longer recommended because of bleeding—deep subcutaneous [intrafat] injection is preferred.)
- Must monitor coagulation tests and prothrombin activity.

Campbell-D'Hue G, Estes SA: A Koebner phenomenon in dermatitis herpetiformis. J Am Acad Dermatol 9:767–768, 1983.

Lesions occurred around waist and beneath breasts in a 57-year-old woman after she wore tight-fitting undergarments.

Patients should be told to avoid such clothing.

Marsden RA: The treatment of benign chronic bullous dermatosis of childhood, and dermatitis herpetiformis and bullous pemphigoid beginning in childhood. Clin Exp Dermatol 7:653–663, 1982.

Dermatitis herpetiformis—24 cases

Start with **dapsone** (50 mg daily), but dose may have to be increased.
Start gluten-free diet.
In one 18-month-old control was obtained with **sulfapyridine** (0.25 gm/day) + gluten-free diet.
In one six-year-old better control was achieved while taking **co-trimoxazole** (Septra, Bactrim) prophylactically for urinary tract infection.

Bullous pemphigoid—six cases

Start with **sulfapyridine** (1 to 2 gm daily with increase to 2 to 3 gm after seven days).
Alternative: **dapsone** (100 to 500 mg/day)
May need **prednisolone** (20 to 30 mg/day) in addition.
Alkalinize urine in ill children taking **sulfapyridine** to prevent drug crystalluria; use **sodium bicarbonate** (2.5 to 4 gm PO q4h).

Benign chronic bullous dermatosis of childhood (IgA linear dermatosis of childhood)—20 cases

Treatment is the same as for bullous pemphigoid.
Look for large blisters in pelvic area.

Surbrugg SK, Weston WL: The course of chronic bullous disease of childhood. Pediatr Dermatol 2:213–215, 1985.

Sulfapyridine (60 to 90 mg/kg/day) cleared three cases in children, who could stop therapy after two months to two years.

Dosages: 250 mg tid (2 ½-year-old boy);
250 mg qid (3-year-old boy);
500 mg tid (5-year-old girl).

Dermatomyositis

Prednisone	Azathioprine
Hydroxychloroquine	Cyclosporine
Methotrexate	Plasmapheresis
Cyclophosphamide	Cancer screen

Dermatomyositis in adults speaks to us of cancer. The last three patients in whom we have made that diagnosis had demonstrable malignancy. In one, the dermatomyositis cleared when an underlying ovarian carcinoma was excised and reappeared with an inoperable recurrence two years later. The other two patients had adenocarcinoma of the colon and carcinoma of the lung, respectively. Neither could be surgically treated at the time of presentation, and both patients died of metastatic carcinoma. Thus we feel a sense of urgency for intensive cancer screening of all adult patients with dermatomyositis. The cancer becomes the first thing to find and treat. In this day of CAT scans, laparoscopy, CEAs, and NMRs, surely we can raise the level of association of dermatomyositis with identifiable malignant disease above its current level of about 20 per cent.

Our treatment of the dermatomyositis itself has centered on systemic steroids (prednisone 60 mg/day), avoiding the massive doses that induce steroid myopathy on top of the polymyositis. We have used chloroquine (250 mg/day) with success in treating the cutaneous changes that reflect photosensitivity or a lupus-like set of vascular lesions.

Over a period of months the prednisone can be gradually tapered, with the introduction of methotrexate (12.5 mg q12h for three doses once weekly) if necessary. These patients need bedrest and good nutritional support. For those in whom no cancer is found the prognosis is reasonably good, but for all patients a rapid rate of regression portends the best prognosis.

Here is a disease of unknown cause and capricious course. Yet its heliotrope eyelids, vague proximal muscle weakness, elevated CPK level, and Gottron's papules may be telling us of underlying cancer. Find it before it is too late.

Callen JP: Dermatomyositis. Dermatol Clin 1:461–473, 1983.

A definitive review with 100 references that covers all aspects of this collagen vascular disease of unknown origin. Therapy centers on:

- bedrest
- high-protein diet
- physical therapy
- corticosteroids (60 mg/day)
- antimalarial drugs
- **methotrexate**
- **cyclophosphamide** (2 to 4 mg/kg/day) (for children)

Bohan A, Peter JB, Bowman RL, Pearson CM: A computer-assisted analysis of 153 patients with polymyositis and dermatomyositis. Medicine 56:255–286, 1977.

An authoritative study showing that corticosteroids are the most widely accepted therapy of choice and **methotrexate** is the favorite steroid-sparing immunosuppressive.

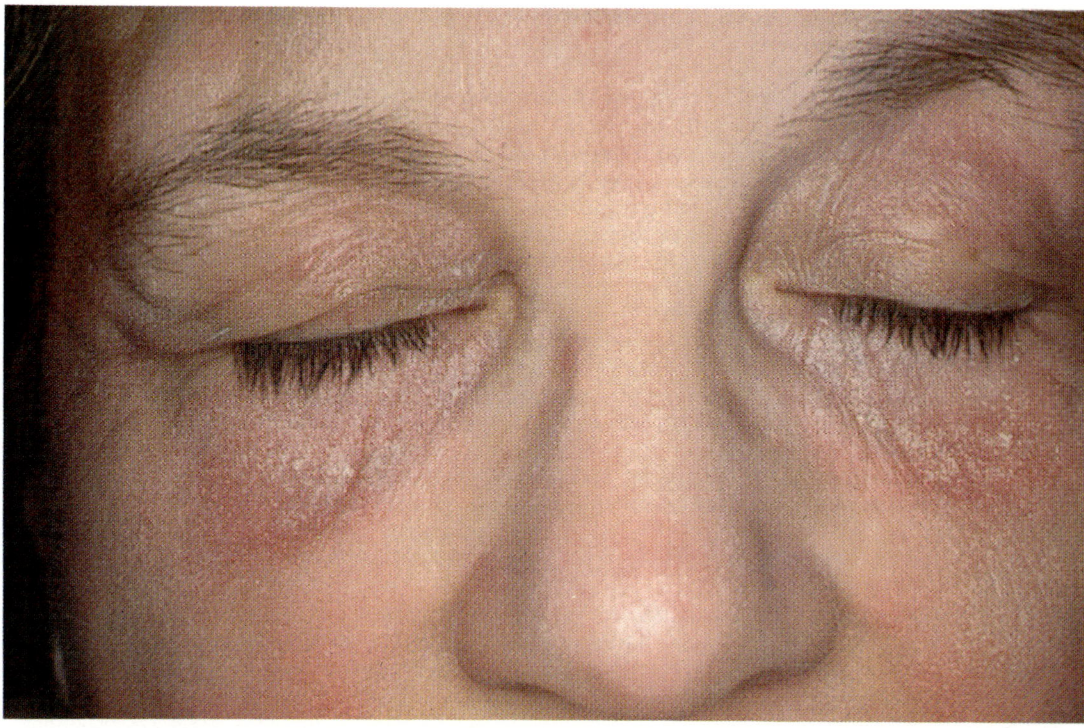

Steroid resistance was defined as failure to see improvement in either muscle strength or serum enzymes after prednisone (40 mg/day for four months) and indicates the need for an additional immunosuppressing drug.

Survival statistics show 87 to 91 per cent for the group, but only 46 per cent if there is associated malignant disease. This was seen in 8.5 per cent of all patients, but in 19.2 per cent of men over age 50 years.

Miller G, Heckmatt JZ, Dubowitz V: Drug treatment of juvenile dermatomyositis. Arch Dis Child 58:445–450, 1983.

In juvenile dermatomyositis without specific treatment:

One in three will recover in one year.
One in three will die within two years.
One in three will develop muscle atrophy, contractures, and calcinosis.
Spontaneous remissions and unexplained exacerbations are well known to occur in the course of the disease.

This study of 29 children concluded that treatment with low-dose **prednisolone** (1 mg/kg/day for one to two weeks followed by a reduction of 1.0 to 2.5 mg/week over six to nine months) was superior to higher doses of prednisolone (1 to 3 mg/kg/day for one to 15 weeks, with reduction over 12 to 84 months). The addition of **azathioprine** (2 to 4 mg/kg/day) in eight patients did not seem to make a difference in individual cases. Of the 29 patients, three died.

Metzger AL, Bohan A, Goldberg LS, et al: Polymyositis and dermatomyositis: Combined methotrexate and corticosteroid therapy. Ann Intern Med 81:182–189, 1974.

Of 22 patients receiving **methotrexate** (30 to 50 mg IV weekly, gradually decreased to two- to four-week intervals), 77 per cent showed normalization of CPK levels by 10 weeks, increased muscle strength by 13 weeks, and a reduction in required **prednisone** dosage (from 47 mg/day to 12 mg/day average) after 15 months.

Giannini M, Callen JP: Treatment of dermatomyositis with methotrexate and prednisone. Arch Dermatol 115:1251–1252, 1979.

A 67-year-old woman with **prednisone**-resistant (15 mg qid) dermatomyositis responded slowly over 2½ months to the addition of **methotrexate** (12.5 mg PO q12h for three doses once a week). It was possible to gradually decrease and stop the prednisone after three months. The condition has remained in remission with maintenance methotrexate (5 mg/week).

Woo TY, Callen JP, Voorhees JJ, et al: Cutaneous lesions of dermatomyositis are improved by hydroxychloroquine. J Am Acad Dermatol 10:592–600, 1984.

Although the myositis responds to corticosteroids or immunosuppressives or both, the cutaneous lesions may not respond. Seven patients whose cutaneous lesions had not responded were treated with supplemental **hydroxychloroquine** (Plaquenil 200 to 400 mg/day). There was a good response in all, with three of seven having total resolution of their skin lesions.

Zabel P, Leimenstoll G, Gross WL: Cyclosporin for acute dermatomyositis. Lancet 1:343, 1984.

Cyclosporin (3.0 mg/kg/day IV) temporarily reversed progressive myositis in a 15-year-old girl who had developed paralysis and dysphagia despite **prednisolone** and **azathioprine** therapy. However, she died of aspiration pneumonia.

Weiss VC, Serushan M: Kaposi's sarcoma in a patient with dermatomyositis receiving immunosuppressive therapy. Arch Dermatol 118:183–185, 1982.

Kaposi's sarcoma nodules developed on the feet of a 65-year-old Mexican woman with dermatomyositis who had been treated with **prednisone** (60 mg qod for 2½ years) and **azathioprine** (50 mg bid for four months). The Kaposi's lesions almost completely disappeared within two months of stopping the azathioprine. (We view this as the analogue of Kaposi's sarcoma seen in AIDS patients. DAIDS [drug-acquired immune deficiency syndrome] is thus one of the risks taken by all patients receiving immunosuppressants.)

Krain LS: Dermatomyositis in six patients without initial muscle involvement. Arch Dermatol 111:241–245, 1975.

In six patients there was an average delay of 18 months (2 to 50 months) before the diagnoses of contact dermatitis, polymorphous light eruption, trichinosis, atopic dermatitis, and erythroderma were abandoned for the correct diagnosis of dermatomyositis.

Prednisone (20 to 80 mg/day) resulted in fair to good improvement in five patients, but one patient with pulmonary fibrosis showed only a poor response. One child had a spontaneous remission and required no therapy.

Dau PC, Bennington JL: Plasmapheresis in childhood dermatomyositis. J Pediatr 98:237–240, 1981.

Plasmapheresis (1.5 liters/week for five months) dramatically cleared the muscles of heavy IgG and IgM deposits in vessel walls and was associated with progressive clinical improvement in a five-year-old girl with dermatomyositis. Concomitant therapy included **prednisone** (30 mg/day) and **chlorambucil** (4 mg/day).

Wojnarowska F: Dermatomyositis induced by penicillamine. J R Soc Med 73:884–886, 1980.

A 59-year-old woman with rheumatoid arthritis had previously developed adverse cutaneous reactions to gold and hydroxychloroquine. After about 6 months of **penicillamine** therapy (250 mg/day) she developed clinical and histologic evidence of dermatomyositis, which slowly abated once the penicillamine was stopped. There are two other such examples in the literature. Penicillamine may also induce pemphigus and systemic lupus erythematosus.

Callen JP, Hyla JF, Bole GG, Kay DR: The relationship of dermatomyositis and polymyositis to internal malignancy. Arch Dermatol 116:295–298, 1980.

Records of 27 patients with dermatomyositis revealed that seven had a demonstrable malignant tumor. The authors recommend a thorough history and physical examination, complete blood count, blood chemistries, stool guaiac test, urinalysis, and chest x-ray examination.

Callen JP: The value of malignancy evaluation in patients with dermatomyositis. J Am Acad Dermatol 6:253–259, 1982.

This complete review of the literature cites 329 cases of tumor associated with dermatomyositis.

Note:

One hundred and nine were in the breast or lung.

Many were not in areas or sites amenable to routine cancer search; e.g., one was an adenocarcinoma of the broad ligament discovered at autopsy.

The best kind of history-taking is at the same time the best kind of psychotherapy.

Erik Erickson

Dermographism

Hydroxyzine	Steroids
Chlorpheniramine	UVL
Cyproheptadine	Tolerance

As a special subset of urticaria, dermographism usually shows a splendid response to Atarax. At times, surprisingly low doses such as 25 mg taken at bedtime every other night are sufficient to suppress the tendency to enter the vicious itch-scratch cycle of dermographism. The patient should be instructed to find the critical minimal dose requirement for control of pruritus, since scratching is the major initiator of this form of physical "allergy."

The Atarax usually has to be given over long periods, but the patient can be encouraged by the fact that dermographism may disappear as mysteriously as it appears. Often it is the result of an occult antigen, just as in classic urticaria. Indeed, we feel that dermographism is the diminutive form of urticaria, with physical trauma being necessary to damage capillaries and allow antibody to come in contact with extravascular mast cells, with consequent histamine release. This occurs in many patients following penicillin injection. The sensitization is not sufficient to produce spontaneous lesions of urticaria, but does account for the scratch-induced hive. Accordingly, as penicillin is eliminated from the body, the dermographic state disappears.

Thus, all patients with severe dermographism need careful study and treatment as described in the section on urticaria. Particular attention to mild tinea pedis and yeast infections can be rewarding. Not all examples of dermographism are of immune origin. A biopsy may reveal occult urticaria pigmentosa. Sometimes we suspect that simple mast cell–capillary fragility may be responsible.

Since histamine released from the mast cell is the mediator, the use of antihistaminic agents is rational and effective. The new H_2 antihistamines have not proven to be particularly effective, but are useful adjuvants. Systemic steroids are reserved for patients whose dermographism is disabling and associated with urticaria.

Always, the patient can deplete the mast cell by vigorous toweling of the skin, but this gives only short time protection. More beneficial is tanning with ultraviolet light or sunlight, which reduces the tendency to dermographism and is a practical avenue of therapy.

Ostrov MR: Dermographia: A critical review. Ann Allergy 25:591–597, 1967.

A good review of a phenomenon that can be found in 5 per cent of the population and generally does not require treatment. It may follow allergic reactions to penicillin or other drugs or to poison ivy.

Greaves MW, Søndergaard J: Urticaria pigmentosa and factitious urticaria: Direct evidence for release of histamine and other smooth muscle contracting agents in dermographic skin. Arch Dermatol 101:418–425, 1970.

Demonstrates histamine as a major mediator of dermographism.

Matthews CNA, Kirby JD, James J, Warin RP: Dermographism: Reduction in weal size by chlorpheniramine and hydroxyzine. Br J Dermatol 88:279–282, 1973.

Double-blind study of 33 patients revealed that the majority had better control with **hydroxyzine** (Atarax 25 mg tid) than with **chlorpheniramine** (Chlor-Trimeton 4 mg tid).

Kaur S, Greaves M, Eftekhari N: Factitious urticaria (dermographism): Treatment by cimetidine and chlorpheniramine in a randomized double-blind study. Br J Dermatol 104:185–190, 1981.

Combination of **chlorpheniramine** (Chlor-Trimeton 4 mg qid) and **cimetidine** (Tagamet 400 mg qid) provided effective therapy, but neither alone gave more help than the placebo.

Mansfield LE, Smith JA, Nelson HS: Greater inhibition of dermographia with a combination of H_1 and H_2 antagonists. Ann Allergy 50:264–265, 1983.

Another confirmation of the value of combining **chlorpheniramine** (8 mg qid) with cimetidine (300 mg qid).

Garafalo J, Kaplan AP: Histamine release and therapy of severe dermatographism. J Allergy Clin Immunol 68:103–105, 1981.

Five patients had a good response to antihistamines, but the sixth patient had minimal relief until she took *both* **cyproheptadine** (Periactin 16 mg qid) and **diphenhydramine** (Benadryl 50 mg qid). Such massive dosage is unusual, but demonstrates the wide range of patient tolerance to drugs and the need for individualized care. Prior treatment with **aspirin**, **indomethacin**, and **cimetidine** had not been helpful.

Kaplan AP: Unusual cold-induced disorders: Cold-dependent dermatographism and systemic cold urticaria. J Allergy Clin Immunol 73:453–456, 1984.

Dermatographism and hives developed only when the skin was chilled in two patients and could be prevented by keeping the skin warm. Both patients had negative ice cube tests.

Illig L: Physical urticaria. Its diagnosis and treatment. Curr Probl Dermatol 5:79–116, 1973.

Dermographism (and other physically induced urticarias) may be successfully treated 40 per cent of the time with hypoglycemia treatment induced by insulin "shock" therapy (increasing doses of subcutaneous insulin [from 30 E up to 80 E] to the limit of coma, twice a week for two months). Give oral glucose as patient becomes drowsy.

Kalz F, Bower CM, Prichard H: Delayed and persistent dermographia. Arch Dermatol 61:772–780, 1950.

Iontophoresis of an antihistaminic drug, **pyranisamine maleate** (Neoantergen [not available in the United States] 5 per cent aqueous solution) gave local inhibition of dermographism for a few hours in one patient. He was also helped initially by histamine "desensitization" with intradermal injections of **histamine phosphate** (0.1 cc weekly, 1 : 10,000 initially with gradual increase to 1 : 1000 over several months).

Kalz F, Prichard H: Investigations of some side-effects observed in syphilitic patients treated with penicillin. Arch Dermatol 65:568–580, 1952.

Among 100 patients, persistent dermographia developed in 10 per cent after penicillin treatment. Intradermal injections of small increasing doses of **histamine phosphate** resulted in permanent relief of symptoms of follicular dermographism in two patients in whom antihistamines gave only temporary relief.

Rich WG: Dermographia. Br Med J 2:600, 1949.
Ultraviolet light therapy given every other day was beneficial to a nurse with dermographism.

Warin RP, Champion RH: Urticaria. WB Saunders Co, Philadelphia, 1974, 173 pp.
Vigorous toweling of skin to induce general whealing may give periods of relief for special occasions.

Pegum JS: Induced tolerance in physical urticarias. Br J Dermatol 93:473, 1975.
A patient with familial dermographism used a hair brush over his trunk and limbs each night to induce tolerance to mechanical trauma. As he put it, a brush for him was as good as a pill.

If a patient is unduly worried over a trivial lesion, review the medical history of family or friends.

Discoid Lupus Erythematosus

Diprolene ointment	β-Carotene
Intralesional steroids	Auranofin
Cryotherapy	Azathioprine
Chloroquine	Clofazimine
Hydroxychloroquine	Thalidomide
Atabrine	Excision
Dapsone	Cosmetics
Quinine	

Although only a small percentage of patients with discoid lupus erythematosus have or will develop systemic lupus, all patients with discoid lesions must be observed for this possibility. This includes a careful medical history, physical examination, and a battery of tests with special reference to antinuclear and anticytoplasmic autoantibodies. Evaluations should be repeated every six months while the discoid lesions remain active.

It is essential to know if flare of the patient's lesions is due to sunlight, as only a third are truly photosensitive. This group must guard against even erythemal dosage of sunlight and must strictly avoid the beaches, the sun at high noon, sunbathing in general, and the lure of a tropical cruise. They should regularly use a sun screen (SPF 15). All other patients with discoid lupus erythematosus should simply take ordinary precautions to avoid sunburn.

Minor limited lesions of discoid lupus erythematosus may be successfully treated with local applications of a powerful topical corticosteroid (Diprolene ointment twice a day). This can be coupled with the use of a cosmetic cover (Covermark), which hides the depigmented or hyperpigmented atrophic scars so disfiguring in black skin.

In more extensive or disseminated forms, systemic treatment with chloroquine (250 mg/day) is indicated and is generally our most effective treatment. We require an ophthalmologic baseline examination prior to initiating treatment and every six months during chloroquine therapy. Chloroquine retinopathy results from the ability of melanin to bind and retain chloroquine, with the cumulative total dose of chloroquine being the responsible factor. To counteract this, chloroquine should be stopped, if possible, during the low-intensity sunlight months of winter.

If chloroquine has not helped significantly within two months, we switch to hydroxychloroquine (Plaquenil 200 mg/day). If this fails, we try a combination of antimalarials: chloroquine 65 mg, hydroxychloroquine 50 mg, and quinacrine hydrochloride (Atabrine) 25 mg given in one capsule, once each day. While formerly available as Triquin, this now has to be made up by a pharmacist. It can be remarkably effective, with the active radical in all three drugs being 4-aminoquinoline. The precise mechanism of action remains unknown.

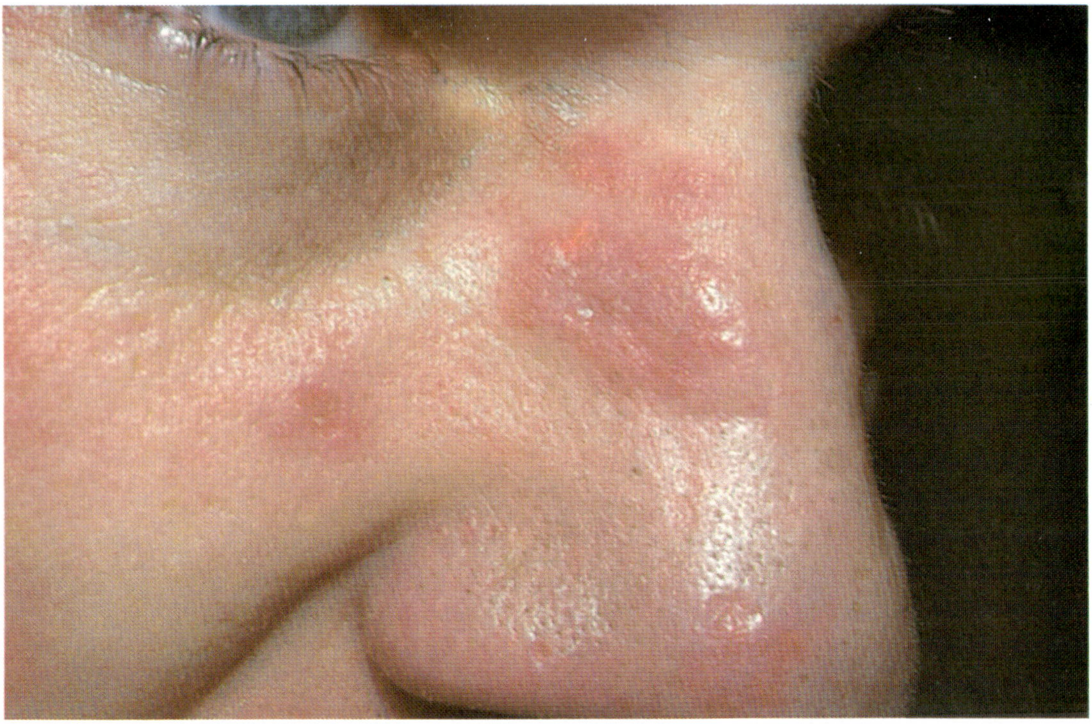

For localized recalcitrant lesions we inject Kenalog suspension (10 mg/ml, diluted with 2 per cent Xylocaine to half or quarter strength), and also occasionally use cryotherapy. In a few cases we have excised cosmetically disfiguring lesions after the disease has become quiescent.

Always, the patient must recognize that the disease scars. Success is measured in terms of elimination of the active inflammatory element, prevention of further scarring, and protection from developing the life-threatening systemic form.

Millard LG, Rowell NR: Abnormal laboratory test results and their relationship to prognosis in discoid lupus erythematosus: A long-term follow-up study of 92 patients. Arch Dermatol 115:1055–1058, 1979.

Approximately 66 per cent had abnormal laboratory tests over a 20-year period. The best predictors for development of disseminated discoid lupus erythematosus or systemic lupus erythematosus were:

ANA > 1:50 (speckled or homogeneous)
WBC < 5000/cu mm
Platelet count < 150,000/cu mm
False positive Wassermann reaction

Of the 92 patients with discoid lupus erythematosus:

6 developed systemic lupus erythematosus
19 developed disseminated discoid lupus erythematosus
42 had complete remission

Reymann F: Treatment of discoid lupus erythematosus with betamethasone-valerate cream 1 per cent. Dermatologica 149:65–68, 1974.

Over a 5-year period, 78 patients with discoid lupus erythematosus were treated with **betamethasone valerate** cream 1 per cent (Celestone valerate cream 1 per cent) bid. In 68 the disease was controlled well; 10 required chloroquine; none developed systemic lupus erythematosus.

Bjornberg A, Hellgren L: Treatment of chronic discoid lupus erythematosus with betamethasone-17, 21-dipropionate. Curr Ther Res 19:442–443, 1976.

Double-blind study of 16 patients with discoid lupus erythematosus showed that **betamethasone 17, 21-dipropionate** ointment 0.05 per cent (Diprolene) was superior to **betamethasone 17-valerate** ointment 0.1 per cent (Valisone). The more powerful the topical corticosteroid, the more effective it is in treating discoid lupus erythematosus.

Callen JP: Therapy of cutaneous lupus erythematosus. Med Clin North Am 66:795–805, 1982.

Of 40 patients treated with intralesional **triamcinolone acetonide** (2.5 to 4 mg/ml) 35 had good to excellent results.

Schiödt M: Local excision in the treatment of oral discoid lupus erythematosus. Acta Derm Venereol 58:274–276, 1978.

Excellent results with excision and primary closure of symptomatic lesions in oral mucosa in six of seven patients.

Kurwa AR, Evans AJ: Discoid lupus erythematosus treated by dermabrasion. Br J Dermatol 101 (Suppl 17):53–54, 1979.

Considerable improvement effected in one patient with hyperkeratotic indurated plaque on nose.

Dubois EL: Antimalarials in the management of discoid and systemic lupus erythematosus. Semin Arthritis Rheum 8:33–51, 1978.

The classic article with 157 references. Ninety-five per cent of patients show marked to moderate benefit from **chloroquine** (Aralen 250 mg/day). To minimize risk of ocular toxicity, do not exceed **hydroxychloroquine** 400 mg/day or chloroquine 250 mg/day (for patient weighing over 45 kg or 100 pounds).

Contraindications: psoriasis and myasthenia gravis.

Watch for bluish black pigmentation of shins, nails, palate, and sun-exposed areas.

All patients taking **chloroquine**, **hydroxychloroquine** (Plaquenil), or **amodiaquine** (Camoquin) should have an ophthalmologic evaluation before beginning the drug and every 4 months thereafter. Stop the drug if changes appear.

Bernstein HN: Chloroquine ocular toxicity. Surv Ophthalmol 12:415–447, 1967.

Too much chloroquine over long periods and your patient may note photophobia, flashes of light, blurred vision, and missing letters and words when reading. The state is largely irreversible and not treatable, so that it must be prevented by using minimal dosage, elimination of drug in winter, and immediately stopping it when the ophthalmologist detects early signs of retinopathy.

Buchanan RN Jr: Quinacrine in the treatment of discoid lupus erythematosus: A 5-year follow-up survey—Results and evaluation. South Med J 52:978–983, 1959.

Atabrine (**mepacrine**, **quinacrine** 200 mg/day) is an effective substitute for **chloroquine**. Five-year evaluation showed 30 of 32 patients experienced suppression of lesions. Retinopathy was not seen, but relapse was frequent on stopping the drug. Alert the patient that the skin will have a yellow hue.

Coburn PR, Shuster S: Dapsone and discoid lupus erythematosus. Br J Dermatol 106:105–106, 1982.

A new substitute for **chloroquine**: **Dapsone** (100 mg/day) for 1 to 4 months caused significant improvement in 9 of 11 patients.

Nurse DS: A reappraisal of oral quinine in discoid lupus erythematosus. Australas J Dermatol 13:55–59, 1972.

An old treatment, **quinine bisulfate** (300 mg bid) was effective in six of eight patients who could tolerate the drug. May help when **chloroquine** and **hydroxychloroquine** fail. Side effects: nausea, tinnitus, clouding of vision. Same formula as quinidine.

Harber LC, Bickers DR: Photosensitivity Diseases: Principles of Diagnosis and Treatment. Philadelphia, WB Saunders Co, 1981.

Although one in three patients with systemic lupus erythematosus is sensitive to sunlight, most patients with discoid lupus erythematosus show no photosensitivity.

Haeger-Aronsen B, Krook G, Abdulla M: Oral carotenoids for photohypersensitivity in patients with erythrohepatic protoporphyria, polymorphous light eruptions and lupus erythematodes discoides. Int J Dermatol 18:73–82, 1979.

β-Carotene (Solatene 75 to 250 mg/day) protected three of four photosensitive patients with discoid lupus erythematosus from flare due to sunlight.

Mackey JP, Barnes J: Clofazimine in the treatment of discoid lupus erythematosus. Br J Dermatol 91:93–96, 1974.

Clofazimine (Lamprene 100 to 200 mg/day) taken for three to six months caused improvement in 17 of 26 cases of discoid lupus erythematosus. The drug causes immunosuppression by depressing macrophage phagocytosis. Side effects: pink staining of the skin, hyperpigmentation of active lesions, keratosis pilaris, and xeroderma.

Not available in the United States.

Crovato F, Levi L: Clofazimine in the treatment of annular lupus erythematosus. Arch Dermatol 117:249–250, 1981.

Clofazimine (100 mg/day) cleared two cases of polycyclic, gyrate cutaneous lesions of lupus erythematosus that had shown no response to **prednisone** (60 mg/day) or Plaquenil (400 mg/day). Results in a few weeks.

Knop J, Bonsmann G, Happle R, Ludolph A, Matz DR, Mifsud EJ, Macher E: Thalidomide in the treatment of sixty cases of chronic discoid lupus erythematosus. Br J Dermatol 108:461–466, 1983.

Thalidomide (200 mg bid until marked clinical response, then 50 to 100 mg/day for three to five months) resulted in complete or marked regression of disease in 90 per cent of patients, but in 71 per cent there was relapse after stopping the drug. Side effect is neuropathy with distal paresthesias. Patient should avoid alcohol and potentially neurotoxic drugs.

Auerbach R, Weinstein GD: Occupational ultraviolet light and skin disease: Two case reports. Arch Dermatol 87:691–692, 1963.

Good detective work revealed that light from a fluorescent microscope over a period of 13 months was the cause of a single lesion of discoid lupus erythematosus on the left forearm of a female laboratory worker.

Lodin A: Discoid lupus erythematosus and trauma. Acta Derm Venereol 43:142–148, 1963.

Trauma is not a significant cause of discoid lupus erythematosus lesions. Specific local trauma (chemical burn, x-ray, frostbite, herpes zoster) antedated lesions in only 10 (2.2 per cent) of 458 cases.

Tsokos GC, Caughman SW, Klippel JH: Successful treatment of generalized discoid skin lesions with azathioprine: Its use in a patient with systemic lupus erythematosus. Arch Dermatol 121:1323–1325, 1985.

Azathioprine sodium (Imuran 100 mg/day) produced a rapid, dramatic resolution of discoid lesions that had been refractory to topical corticosteroids and high doses of oral hydroxychloroquine. Relapse occurred when the azathioprine was discontinued.

Dalziel K, Going S, Cartwright PH, et al: Treatment of chronic discoid lupus erythematosus with an oral gold preparation. Br J Dermatol 113:25–26, 1985.

Auranofin (Ridaura 6–9 mg/day for up to one year), a complex organic gold compound, produced marked improvement in 12 of 19 patients with discoid lupus erythematosus. In 5 others the improvement was definite, but less marked.

As a rule, disease as it stalks through the land cannot keep pace with the incurable vice of scribbling about it.

JOHN MAYOUR (1668)

Ecthyma

Systemic antibiotic	Benzoyl peroxide
Topical antibiotic	Urea compress

The virulence of the pathogenic beta-hemolytic streptococci in the lesions of ecthyma demands systemic antibiotic therapy, started as early as possible to minimize scarring. We generally prescribe erythromycin, but there is a whole cornucopia of effective alternatives. The usual case clears rapidly.

Topically, the most effective agent appears to be 10 per cent benzoyl peroxide gel applied precisely to the ulcer. For crusted lesions, aqueous urea compresses (20 per cent—20 minutes tid) are helpful, being both bactericidal and proteolytic.

In recalcitrant cases, bacteriologic culture and sensitivity studies are necessary. Awareness of immunologic depression from disease, drugs, or genetic factors alerts one to look for opportunistic organisms or rare pathogens that respond only to specific antibiotic treatment.

Since ecthymas represent secondary invasion of scratches and insect bites, first-aid treatment of such lesions with topical antibiotics (Neosporin ointment, Silvadene cream) can be of real prophylactic value.

Allen AM, Taplin D, Twigg L: Cutaneous streptococcal infections in Vietnam. Arch Dermatol 104:271–280, 1971.

Ninety per cent of ecthymas were due to group A beta-hemolytic streptococci colonization of minor abrasions or insect bites. Successful treatment included **procaine penicillin G** (600,000 U IM) followed by a 10-day oral course of either **phenoxymethyl penicillin potassium** (400,000 U qid, e.g., Pen-Vee K 250 mg qid) or **erythromycin** (250 mg qid).

Allen AM, Taplin D, Lowy JA, Twigg L: Skin infection in Vietnam. Milit Med 137:295–301, 1972.

Systemic tetracycline and topical antibiotics, with or without hexachlorophene scrubs, constitute *ineffective* treatment.

Turnbull D, Parry MF: Ecthyma-like skin lesions caused by *Staphylococcus aureus*. Arch Intern Med 141:689, 1981.

Oxacillin intravenously was required for four weeks to control infection in a patient with leukemia.

Kelly C, Taplin D, Allen AM: Streptococcal ecthyma treatment with benzathine penicillin G. Arch Dermatol 103:306–310, 1971.

Single injections of **benzathine penicillin G** (Bicillin 600,000 U IM) produced healing in one week in 100 per cent of the cases, whereas single injections of **procaine penicillin G** (600,000 U IM) cleared only 38 per cent in 2 weeks. Study of 66 cases.

Linder CW: Treatment of impetigo and ecthyma. Fam Pract 7:697–700, 1978.

Favors Bicillin (94 per cent cure rate in 72 children). Topical therapy found unnecessary.

Leyden JJ, Kligman AM: Rationale for topical antibiotics. Cutis 22:515–528, 1978.

Local antibiotics undoubtedly reduce bacterial load and are of prophylactic value.

Good records are a doctor's best friend in court.

Ecthyma Gangrenosum

Hospitalize
Gentamicin sulfate
Carbenicillin

This awesome life-threatening disease is usually the sign of *Pseudomonas aeruginosa* septicemia in an immunocompromised patient. It calls for immediate hospitalization and cultures of skin lesions and blood. The patient needs the full support of an intensive care unit, infectious disease specialist, and microbiology laboratory.

Intravenous aminoglycosides (gentamicin, tobramycin) and carbenicillin in high dosages, monitored by serum levels, are the first line of defense while awaiting laboratory confirmation and antibiotograms. Endotoxin and exotoxin formation by the causative gram-negative organisms contribute to hemorrhagic bulla formation at the sites of septic emboli and cause septic shock. Tachycardia, hypotension, leukopenia, jaundice, anuria, and paralytic ileus are problems to be anticipated. An underlying disease such as leukemia should also be expected.

Since the disease is truly a septicemia, it is not one for primary dermatologic management.

Solem LD, Zaske D, Strate RG: Ecthyma gangrenosum survival with individualized antibiotic therapy. Arch Surg 114:580–583, 1979.

Five children with burns and ecthyma gangrenosum received massive individualized dosages of **gentamicin sulfate** based on maintaining peak serum concentrations of 8 to 12 mg/ml immediately after one-hour infusions. Survival of 80 per cent was attributed to greatly exceeding the usual recommended gentamicin dosages (3 to 5 mg/kg/day). No ototoxicity or nephrotoxicity was observed. Treatment: IV gentamicin (15 to 30 mg/kg/day) and **carbenicillin** (300 to 900 mg/kg/day). Frequent monitoring of serum gentamicin levels is imperative for achieving therapeutic levels.

Anderson MG: *Pseudomonas* septicaemia and ecthyma gangrenosum. S Afr Med J 55:504–508, 1979.

Four case reports of infants, 50 per cent mortality. Aminoglycosides (**gentamicin**, **tobramycin**, **amikacin**) are best therapy, but resistance may develop.

Reed RK, Larter WE, Sieber OF, John TJ: Peripheral nodular lesions in *Pseudomonas* sepsis: The importance of incision and drainage. J Pediatr 88:977–979, 1976.

Incise fluctuant lesions and pack with gauze. Only by incising can one tell whether pus is present in deeply indurated, poorly marginated, erythematous nonfluctuant nodules. Local drainage was necessary for cure.

Mandell IN, Feiner HD, Price NM, Simberkoff M: *Pseudomonas cepacia* endocarditis and ecthyma gangrenosum. Arch Dermatol 113:199–202, 1977.

This gram-negative organism infected the cardiac tricuspid valve of a heroin addict. Oral Bactrim DS (**sulfisoxazole** 400 mg with **trimethoprim** 80 mg) and intravenous **polymyxin B sulfate** (50 mg) daily helped, but cure came only after surgical excision of the tricuspid valve.

Schackelford P, Ratzan SA, Sherarer WT: Ecthyma gangrenosum produced by *Aeromonas hydrophilia*. J Pediatr 83:100–101, 1973.

This uncommon gram-negative pathogen was aspirated from the solitary presenting lesion, a purplish nodule on the leg of a boy with leukemia, high fever, and vomiting. It cleared with IV **gentamicin** (5 mg/kg/day) for nine days and oral **chloramphenicol** continued for five days after hospital discharge.

Francis YF, Richman S, Hussain S, Schwartz J: *Aeromonas hydrophila* infection: Ecthyma gangrenosum with aplastic anemia. NY State J Med 82:1461–1464, 1982.

This time the aeromonads (gram-negative rods with polar flagellae that live in water) induced bacteremia in a 76-year-old woman with aplastic anemia. Death was due to septic shock. Probable source: backed-up toilet.

Fine JD, Miller JA, Harrist TJ, Haynes HA: Cutaneous lesions in disseminated candidiasis mimicking ecthyma gangrenosum. Am J Med 70:1133–1135, 1981.

Candida emboli produced rapidly developing necrotic pustules and ulcerations within indurated red plaques. Blood cultures and urine cultures remained negative for *Candida*, but pseudohyphae were identified in a skin biopsy specimen. Despite **amphotericin B** therapy, the patient died. (Today, **ketoconazole** would be indicated.)

Edmonds P, Suskind RR, MacMillan BG, Holder IA: Epidemiology of *Pseudomonas aeruginosa* in a burn hospital: Surveillance by a combined typing system. Appl Microbiol 24:219–225, 1972.

Sink drains were the major source of *Pseudomonas* in the intensive care unit—not the nursing personnel or other burn patients. Splashing of contaminated water from sinks to fomites was postulated. Whirlpools were also reservoirs. Sterilization of sink drains daily with hot water or formaldehyde was proposed.

Moral: Treat the sink as well as the patient!

Polk HC, Ward CG, Clarkson JG, Tephin D: Early detection of *Pseudomonas* burn infection: Clinical experience with Wood's light fluorescence. Arch Surg 98:292–295, 1969.

Blue-green fluorescence of *Pseudomonas aeruginosa* in burn wounds could be detected with a 100 watt Wood's light in a partially darkened hospital room two to three days prior to invasive sepsis. This enabled sharp demarcation for excision of grossly infected tissue and signaled the need for immediate systemic antibiotics (**polymyxin B** or **gentamicin sulfate**). Survival increased.

Baxter CR, Curreri PW, Marvin JA: The control of burn wound sepsis by the use of quantitative bacteriologic studies and sub-eschar clysis with antibiotics. Surg Clin North Am 53:1509–1518, 1973.

Multiple-needle (22-gauge) clysis delivered 25 ml of normal saline (0.85 per cent) with appropriate antibiotic into each 7.5-cm area of avascular subeschar space once daily. A pediatric graduated drip set was used.

If the cure comes slowly, so does the gratitude.

Eosinophilic Fasciitis

Prednisone Cimetidine

Rodnan GP, Schumacher HR (eds): Primer on the Rheumatic Diseases, 8th ed. Atlanta, Arthritis Foundation, 1983, pp 64–65.

In the great majority of examples, eosinophilic fasciitis appears to be a self-limited and uncomplicated disorder. Prednisone (10 to 15 mg/day) provides symptomatic relief and eliminates eosinophilia. It has no effect on the fibrosis and therefore is prescribed only in the early inflammatory phase. Complete or nearly complete resolution occurs after two to five years. Spontaneous remission has been observed in a number of instances. Recurrence is rare.

Kent LT, Cramer SF, Moskowitz RW: Eosinophilic fasciitis: Clinical, laboratory and microscopic considerations. Arthritis Rheum 24:677–683, 1981.

Eosinophilic fasciitis is distinguished from scleroderma by an excellent response to corticosteroids. This report describes two patients whose skin thickening disappeared following therapy with **prednisone** (20 mg bid for six weeks, then tapered over 14 months to 5 mg daily and 10 mg qod).

Additional medications that appeared to help included:

- **aspirin** (6 to 8 tablets daily)
- **hydroxychloroquine** (Plaquenil sulfate 200 mg bid)
- potassium para-aminobenzoate (Potaba 2 gm qid)

Solomon G, Barland P, Rifkin H: Eosinophilic fasciitis responsive to cimetidine. Ann Intern Med 97:547–549, 1982.

Brawny edema and induration of the skin in a 53-year-old man cleared within a few days of starting **cimetidine** (Tagamet 400 mg q6h), given for epigastric pain and a suspected ulcer induced by **prednisone** (20 mg daily for one year), which had controlled the induration. When the cimetidine was stopped one year later, the induration reappeared within three weeks. With resumption of cimetidine, there was dramatic improvement within 48 hours, and all of the physical findings were gone in one week.

Nonetheless, prednisone in low dosage remains the preferred treatment.

Diffuse fasciitis with eosinophilia spares the hands and feet and does not cause Raynaud's phenomenon, calcinosis, or visceral involvement. It usually begins acutely in autumn, frequently after physical exercise.

Laboratory findings:

Blood
- elevated erythrocyte sedimentation rate
- hypergammaglobulinemia
- eosinophilia
- increased serum eosinophilic chemotactic factor

Tissue
- inflammation of collagen bundles in deep fascia with perivascular plasma cells, lymphocytes, and occasional eosinophils

Patients who adore you today may abhor you tomorrow.

Epidermolysis Bullosa

Dilantin	Surgery
Antibiotics	Glutaraldehyde
Corticosteroids	Drysol
Physiotherapy	

Inherited diseases are notoriously difficult to treat. However, there is now an air of excitement about the therapy of the dystrophic form of this genetic disease. In 1978 Dilantin was first shown to dramatically enhance the adherence of the epidermis in these patients, and it has since proven to be specifically indicated for the severe scarring recessive dystrophic form. Significantly, the tear from simple mechanical trauma, common to all forms of epidermolysis bullosa, has a distinctive anatomy in this variant. It occurs below the epidermal basement membrane in an area abnormally rich in collagenase. In the simple type, in which the epidermal tear occurs within the epidermis, Dilantin has no effect. Nor does Dilatin offer promise for the third major type, the nonscarring (but at times lethal) junctional epidermolysis bullosa, in which separation occurs within the basement membrane itself. Accordingly, it has been surmised that Dilantin, a known collagenase inhibitor, is effective only in the dystrophic form in which collagenase specifically enters into the pathogenesis by degradation of the fibrils that anchor the epidermal basement membrane to the dermis.

The simplex and junctional types of epidermolysis bullosa remain without specific therapy, although in severe forms some therapists advocate corticosteroids. We have not been impressed by their efficacy. While Dilantin is regularly indicated in the treatment of dystrophic epidermolysis bullosa, it is not uniformly effective. Some patients show no response, whereas others get a significant reduction in the number and size of bullae (not total clearing). One point must be stressed. Dilantin cannot be prescribed on a simple basis like so many other drugs, but must be adjusted to maintain a serum level of at least 8 μg/ml. This necessitates careful serum monitoring of Dilantin concentrations in the initial stages of treatment.

We must look upon epidermolysis bullosa as a remarkably heterogeneous group of diseases in which the common theme is bulla formation due to mechanical force shearing the epidermis at the level of intercellular keratinocyte adhesion (simplex, type 1, dominant inheritance), or within the basement membrane (junctional, nonscarring type, recessive inheritance), or below the basement membrane (scarring, dermolytic, dystrophic type, recessive or dominant inheritance). There are numerous subsets in each of these three major categories making classification and prognosis difficult. At times one feels that aside from electron microscopic demonstration of the level of separation, epidermolysis bullosa is best subtyped by giving it the name of the patient affected.

In any event, all patients deserve the same gentle care of their delicately attached or delicately formed epidermis. The ones with the minor forms will learn to avoid 18-mile hikes, wrestling, and manual work. They learn of the protection cold gives their skin by inhibiting sweating. Hot weather work may produce blisters never seen in the cold seasons. The blisters of walking or working are greatly helped by nightly application of Drysol or 10 per cent glutaraldehyde to the palms or soles to reduce skin sweating and friction.

It is the infant or child with extensive areas denuded of epidermis who deserves your real help. Rare as it is (1:300,000 births), this lifelong problem demands full explanation to the parents, appropriate hospitalizations, and long-term supportive and adjunctive care. Classification aside, all need the same superb local skin care. Gentle handling of the infant is mandatory, and clothing must be soft and easy to put on. The parents soon learn the value of socks and mittens to reduce the trauma of rubbing or scratching. Adhesive tape and restraints must never be used. Bed linens must be soft and a Telfa sheet may be necessary to prevent sticking of the eroded skin. Blisters may be drained if large or enlarging or may be completely unroofed if infected.

Large areas of denudation may require dressings, such as Op-site. We often recommend Silvadene cream used as in burn cases (but not in very young infants, because of systemic absorption that the liver cannot yet handle). In most instances the erosions are left open to heal directly. Secondary bacterial infection may ensue and require systemic antibiotics. Cultures and sensitivity tests may aid in selection of the appropriate agent, but we generally start with erythromycin. Specific topical antibiotics may help, along with soothing compresses, to remove infected crusts. Always there must be awareness that what is used topically in extensive areas of denudation virtually becomes a systemic drug.

The mucosal attachment is also weak in these patients so that they often experience loss of mucosa within the oropharynx and esophagus (and probably the entire gastrointestinal tract) as a result of harsh or rough food. They need a soft diet with full complement of vitamins and minerals. Nursing is advisable or the use of large-orifice nipples. Moreover, the infant with extensive lesions experiences significant fluid and protein loss, as well as deficient food intake. Growth is impaired and hyperalimentation may be advisable in severe instances of malnutrition.

Hospitalization is necessary if more than 40 per cent of the skin surface is open, infection becomes extensive, or the child fails to gain weight. The parents must know this as well as the pediatrician. A number of clinics are available for specialized care and rehabilitation. The parents may also wish to secure further information and aid from DEBRA (2936 Avenue W, Brooklyn, NY 11229), a national organization dedicated to this disease.

Genetic counseling should be given to the parents or patient or both. This is best done by a geneticist who can also instruct them concerning the newly developing area of fetal skin biopsy for prenatal diagnosis of the serious forms of epidermolysis bullosa.

Most infants with extensive junctional-type epidermolysis bullosa die before reaching the age of two years. In contrast, the scarring dystrophic form of the disease threatens function more than life. These children may develop the mitten hand, ectropion, esophageal stenosis, and pyloric atresia, among other functional impairments. Here, plastic and other surgeons can do much in restoring function, if not grace, to the affected sites. Physiotherapy is indicated to keep the joints supple, and many require exceptional dental care because of the prevalence of cavities. Finally, one must always remain alert to the possibility of carcinomatous change in scars over the long term.

Moynahan EJ: The treatment and management of epidermolysis bullosa. Clin Exp Dermatol 7:665–672, 1982.

Authoritative review. Points out the value of corticosteroids in preventing blisters, esophageal and pharyngeal strictures, and conjunctival adhesions. Steroids also improve dentition and enable grafted skin to adhere more firmly. Specific recommendations:

Neonatal period
- *Breast feed* naked baby on parachute silk sheeting (and make clothes of same material).
- **Prednisolone** (40 to 60 mg/day for two to three days, then reduce dose by 5 mg/day to effective maintenance).
- Daily bath with emollient as substitute for soap.
- Leave blisters intact, but trim any rough edges to remove foci of infection.
- Avoid dressings.
- Eventually wean onto soft diet.
- Watch for anemia and sepsis.

Reconstructive hand surgery
- Premedicate for two to three days with prednisolone (50 to 60 mg daily).
- Maintain steroids for several days after surgery, then gradually reduce dosage.

Moynahan EJ: Epidermolysis bullosa dystrophica with severe deformity of hands and pharyngeal stenosis, relieved by cortisone. Proc R Soc Med 54:693–695, 1961.

A 14-year-old boy with difficulty in swallowing because of pharyngeal blisters improved dramatically after oral **cortisone** (300 mg/day for one week, then tapered over two months to 25 mg daily maintenance). Benefits included 50 per cent increase in body weight, control of blisters, and increase in lumen size of pharynx.

Advocates immediate treatment of newborn babies with "heroic doses" of steroids to suppress blisters (trial-and-error dosage).

Eisenberg M, Stevens LH, Schofield PJ: Epidermolysis bullosa—New therapeutic approaches. Aust J Dermatol 19:1–8, 1978.

Contrasts questionable help of past treatments for epidermolysis bullosa dystrophica (antimalarials, thyroid hormone, dietary supplements of **leucine**, **valine**, and **vitamin E**) with dramatic response to **diphenylhydantoin** (Dilantin 7 to 9 mg/kg/day) in two young children. Dilantan inhibited collagenase activity in vitro.

Stankler L: Home management of epidermolysis bullosa. Practitioner 210:411–412, 1973.

Specially padded bed, mittens, soft shoes, long trousers with ¼-inch foam rubber sewn inside knees, use no tape, care in handling, semisolid diet to prevent anal bleeding, glycerin suppositories for hard stools. Many suggestions about caring for babies and children. Puncture large blisters at two sites with a sterile needle and gently express fluid, but wait for a short period before doing this, as new blisters are very painful. Use cloth diapers washed in fabric softener. Protect fingers, toes, and knees with Elastoplast. Cover sharp objects with tape. Travel with first-aid kit.

Severin GL, Farber EM: The management of epidermolysis bullosa in children. Arch Dermatol 95:302–309, 1967.

Treatment of localized areas with a high-potency topical steroid, **fluocinolone acetonide** 0.2 per cent cream (Synalar-HP) applied at bedtime under plastic film occlusion cleared persistent bullous lesions in three to four days. Must watch for infection under occlusion. Lower concentration (0.025 per cent) of same cream was not effective.

Wodinsky HB: Cost analysis of the Kozak protocol as used in an Ontario hospital in the treatment of children with epidermolysis bullosa. Can Med Assoc J 130:715–717, 1984.

Empiric topical treatment (camomile tea baths, lotions, creams, compresses) and dietary restrictions (only freshly slaughtered beef or chicken, fresh ripe fruit) used in a biochemist's (Paul Kozak) private West Germany clinic were found to increase significantly the cost over regular hospitalization, largely because of the need for extensive nursing care. Inpatient stays ranged from 10 to 92 days for nine patients in the study. Parental involvement in nursing care could significantly decrease costs.

Haber RM, Ramsay CA, Boxall LBH: Assessment of a treatment for epidermolysis bullosa. Can Med Assoc J 131:10–14, 1984.

The Kozak therapy consists of special topical agents, oral vitamins, and a severely restricted diet. A study of 10 hospitalized patients demonstrated that the complex Kozak therapy protocol was helpful in 9, with a mean decrease of 76 per cent in numbers of blisters, less pain, and more rapid healing. Benefits were also seen in some outpatients. Recommends hospitalization two to three times a year for severely afflicted to receive intensive local treatment with topical antibiotics and good nursing and nutritional care. The Kozak diet was not felt to be essential. **Vitamins A**, **E**, **B_6**, **B_1**, **nicotinic acid**, **orotic acid**, and **glycine** were given orally.

Topical agents contained many ingredients, including steroids, **tetracycline**, **salicylic acid**, and **resorcinol**. Wet dressings with camomile tea were also used.

Haber RM, Ramsay CA, Boxall LBH: Epidermolysis bullosa: Assessment of a treatment regimen. Int J Dermatol 24:324–328, 1985.

Further details of the same Canadian study of the Kozak therapy:

Cleanse bullous areas daily with sunflower seed oil.
Incise blisters daily and treat q4h (while awake) with:

1. Camomile tea compresses (three teabags in 1 liter boiling water for 10 minutes, then cool). For a bath, add three liters of tea to a standard bath.
2. Ointment A (for bullae and erosions):
   Zinc oxide 8 per cent
   Bismuth subnitrate 8 per cent
   Tetracycline 2 per cent
   White petrolatum (base)
3. Ointment B (for flexures and crusts):
   Zinc oxide 4 per cent
   Bismuth subnitrate 4 per cent
   Tetracycline 2 per cent
   Betamethasone 17-valerate ointment 0.05 per cent
4. Lotion (for healed areas):
   Salicyclic acid 1.2 per cent
   Resorcinol 1.2 per cent
   Hydroquinone 1.2 per cent
   50 per cent alcohol (base)
5. Maintenance ointment (normal healed areas):
   Salicyclic acid 1.5 per cent
   Benzoic acid 1.5 per cent
   Hydroquinone 1.5 per cent
   Resorcinol 1.5 per cent
   Phosphoric acid 1.5 per cent
   Triamcinolone ointment (0.05 per cent) equal parts with Eucerin
   Heparin (adults only—500,000 U/kg ointment)

Mallory SB: Adjunctive therapy for epidermolysis bullosa. J Am Acad Dermatol 6:951–952, 1982.

Op-site dressings applied to denuded areas (and left in place as long as three weeks) promoted healing and relieved pain. Better than Silvadene cream or Polysporin ointment. Recommends use under ECG electrodes to prevent stripping off of epidermis.

Gould DJ, Condon P, Cunliffe WJ: Porcine dermis dressings in epidermolysis bullosa. Arch Dermatol 113:1456, 1977.

For a newborn baby, lyophilized porcine dermis (Ethicon Corethium) was rehydrated (10 minutes in normal saline solution at 25°C), cut to the shape of the defect, applied to denuded areas, and held in place with bandages moistened in saline. Repeated every two days on areas remaining denuded. Dermis absorbs onto blister base, sealing the wound. Helps increase rate of healing and decrease infection.

Michaelson JD, Schmidt JD, Dresden MH, Duncan C: Vitamin E treatment of epidermolysis bullosa: Changes in tissue collagenase levels. Arch Dermatol 109:67–69, 1974.

Dramatic rapid clearing of dystrophic epidermolysis bullosa lesions in three children receiving oral **vitamin E** (D-alpha-tocopherol 600 mg IU/day).

Unger WP, Nethercott JR: Epidermolysis bullosa dystrophica treated with vitamin E and oral corticosteroids. Can Med Assoc J 108:1136–1138, 1973.

Vitamin E (DL-alpha-tocopherol acetate 10,000 IU/day for seven weeks) was no help to this severely affected 12-year-old boy. Likewise, intermittent doses of **prednisone** (up to 120 mg/day) were not helpful and repeatedly allowed superinfection of blisters.

Fritsch P, Klein G, Auböck J, Hintner H: Retinoid therapy of recessive dystrophic epidermolysis bullosa. J Am Acad Dermatol 9:766–767, 1983.

Etretinate (20 mg/day) for seven months was no help to a 12-year-old girl. It was suggested that other retinoids with greater collagenase-inhibitory potency might be beneficial.

Cooper TW, Bauer EA: Therapeutic efficacy of phenytoin in recessive dystrophic epidermolysis: A comparison of short- and long-term treatment. Arch Dermatol 120:490–495, 1984.

In 14 of 22 patients there was at least a 40 per cent decline in the blister and crust count when they were given oral **phenytoin** (Dilantin 200 to 300 mg/day) for 8 to 99 weeks. The other eight were unresponsive. Phenytoin blood levels must be monitored so that a level of 8 to 10 μg/ml is achieved and maintained.

Wirth H, Nesch A, Ostapowicz B, Anton-Lamprecht I: Phenytoin therapy of recessive dystrophic epidermolysis bullosa (epidermolysis bullosa dystrophica, Hallopeau-Siemens, and epidermolysis bullosa dystrophica inversa). Z Hautkr 58:555–574, 1982.

Excellent results in six patients. The authors give details on management:

Dosage: 200 to 300 mg/day—maximum 600 mg/day
Check **phenytoin** levels at 7, 10, 13, 16 days
Weekly CBC
Monthly SMA 12
Trimonthly ANA
Yearly folic acid
Triennial x-rays (hands, feet, and esophagus)

Watch for serious side effects (e.g., Lyell's syndrome).

Bergfeld WF, Orlowski JP: Epidermolysis bullosa letalis and phenytoin. J Am Acad Dermatol 7:275–278, 1982.

Apparently ineffective in letalis type. Two infants died of pneumonia and sepsis two to six weeks after starting treatment with **phenytoin** (10 mg/kg/day).

Rogers RB, Yancey KB, Allen BS, Guill MF: Phenytoin therapy for junctional epidermolysis bullosa. Arch Dermatol 119:925–926, 1983.

A four-month-old boy improved (50 per cent reduction in blister formation) after two months of oral **phenytoin** (Dilantin 2 mg/kg/day gradually increased to 15 mg/kg/day). Serum level was maintained at 12 to 15 μg/ml. Flare within one week when treatment was interrupted. Death at age 17 months due to aspiration.

Schachner L, Lazarus GS, Dembitzer H: Epidermolysis bullosa hereditaria letalis: Pathology, natural history and therapy. Br J Dermatol 96:51–58, 1977.

Case report of a baby girl who survived 44 days with great help from **dexamethasone** (0.5 mg/day) until septicemia developed. Dermal-epidermal separation was seen in most tissues at autopsy. Example is cited in which a long-term survivor with the disease experienced remission during pregnancy and with daily Enovid-E therapy (**norethynodrel** 2.5 mg + **mestranol** 0.1 mg).

Skivolocki W, Harris BH, Boles ET: A new method for skin grafting a burned patient who has epidermolysis bullosa. Plast Reconstr Surg 53:355–357, 1974.

Do not use dermatome (epidermis will fragment).
Superficially incise borders of epidermal donor site.
Roll off epidermal sheet using two moistened cotton-tipped applicator sticks.
Unroll graft over burn site.
Secure with single layer of wide mesh gauze sutured over graft.
Treat donor and recipient sites with silver nitrate dressings (0.5 per cent).
Results: 90 to 100 per cent take of most grafts. Donor sites healed in two weeks without significant scarring.

Greider JL, Flatt AE: Care of the hand in recessive epidermolysis bullosa. Plast Reconstr Surg 72:222–227, 1983.

Repeated cycles of blistering produce scarring, contractures, and eventual encasement of digits in an "epidermal cocoon." Epidermal "degloving," full release of contractures, split-thickness grafts, and 14-day postoperative immobilization with Kirschner wires suspended from a traction bow result in some restoration of function. Wounds are covered only with antibiotic ointment. To prevent rapid recurrence of webbing, advises long-term use of Orthoplast splints with interdigital partitions. Observations on five children, ages 3 to 10 years.

Thawley SE, Black MJ, Dudek SE, Spector GJ: External auditory canal stricture secondary to epidermolysis bullosa. Arch Otolaryngol 103:55–57, 1977.

Stricture of canal resulted in conductive hearing loss as well as repeated episodes of otitis externa in a 24-year-old woman with epidermolysis bullosa simplex. Successfully treated by excision of scar and split-thickness skin grafting. Must avoid scrubbing skin in surgical preparation (prepare skin by spraying).

James I, Wark H: Airway management during anesthesia in patients with epidermolysis bullosa dystrophica. Anesthesiology 56:323–326, 1982.

Endotracheal intubation was used successfully in administering anesthesia to 33 patients with dystrophic epidermolysis bullosa. Facial bullae formed only nine times in 309 anesthesias. Avoid tape and shearing stress on face associated with use of face mask (unless unable to intubate). Use oral intubation with well-lubricated endotracheal tube one size smaller than usual.

There were no laryngeal or tracheal complications on 131 occasions when endotracheal intubation was used.

Fonkalsrud EW, Ament ME: Surgical management of esophageal stricture due to recessive dystrophic epidermolysis bullosa. J Pediatr Surg 12:221–226, 1977.

Established strictures of the esophagus are not responsive to steroid therapy, interfere with feeding, and pose a threat of squamous cell carcinoma. Mechanical dilatation may further injure the esophagus and lead to perforation.

℞: Excise the esophagus, replacing it with a segment of colon. Surgical wounds heal normally if pressure is minimized during preparation and operation. Total parenteral nutrition through a centrally placed Silastic catheter was useful postoperatively.

Shubailat G, Oumeish OY, Amr SS: Epidermolysis bullosa dystrophica triggered by sun exposure. Ann Plast Surg 10:239–243, 1983.

Beginning at the age of five years a girl from Jordan had noted that mild overexposure to sunlight produced bullae on the face and hands with resulting ectropion and scar contractures and deformities of the hands by age 17. Split-thickness skin grafts taken from protected areas and placed on the face were resistant to sunlight effects for five years.

Ponce-Nevarez E, Przybilla B: Bullöse skabies bei epidermolysis bullosa hereditaria dystrophica. Hautarzt 32:96–97, 1981.

In these patients the *Sarcoptes scabiei* produce bullae.

Matsuoka LY, Safai B: Resolution of epidermolysis bullosa following oophorohysterectomy. J Am Acad Dermatol 3:205, 1980.

Serendipitous surgical cure of 45 years of epidermolysis bullosa dystrophica continuously present since birth. Miracles can happen!

Löfberg L, Gustavii B: "Blind" versus direct vision technique for fetal skin sampling in cases for prenatal diagnosis. Clin Genet 25:37–41, 1984.

Fetal skin biopsy allows prenatal detection of serious hereditary epidermolysis bullosa. "Blind" sampling under local anesthesia often missed the target and was discontinued in favor of direct visualization. Under general anesthesia the uterus is exposed and two trocars with cannulas are introduced into the amniotic cavity, one for the needle scope and the other for the biopsy forceps. Few samples are needed, and the site of biopsy is controllable.

DesGroseilliers J-P, Brisson P: Localized epidermolysis bullosa: Report of two cases and evaluation of therapy with glutaraldehyde. Arch Dermatol 109:70–72, 1974.

Two patients with suprabasilar blisters of hands and feet in summer (Weber-Cockayne syndrome) were benefited by painting soles with 10 per cent **glutaraldehyde** (three times a week at bedtime). Must keep solution refrigerated and replace monthly. Disadvantages: yellow staining, irritation, and risk of sensitization.

Tkach JR: Treatment of recurrent bullous eruption of the hands and feet (Weber-Cockayne disease) with topical aluminum chloride. J Am Acad Dermatol 6:1095–1096, 1982.

Another approach to decreasing frictional shearing force and hence bulla formation is daily topical use at bedtime of Drysol (alcoholic solution of aluminum chloride hexahydrate 20 per cent). This avoids the problem with **glutaraldehyde** staining and sensitization as well as providing a product far more stable.

Gedde-Dahl T Jr: Sixteen types of epidermolysis bullosa: On the clinical discrimination, therapy and prenatal diagnosis. Acta Derm Venereol Suppl 95:74–87, 1981.

Superb review of all aspects. Electron-microscopic verification of the precise type of epidermolysis bullosa may point to the best therapy, as well as explain variable responses to both steroids and Dilantin. **Folic acid** supplement should be given during **phenytoin** therapy. The nonscarring herpetiform Dowling-Meara type of dominant epidermolysis bullosa, which regularly clears with high fever, is also helped by living in a hot climate, seaside bathing, and one-hour warm baths (32°C salt water).

Wechsler HL, Krugh FJ, Domonkos AN, et al: Polydysplastic epidermolysis bullosa and development of epidermal neoplasms. Arch Dermatol 102:374–380, 1970.

Watch out for development of squamous cell carcinoma in scars. Often difficult to tell from pseudoepitheliomatous hyperplasia until metastases develop. Remove surgically.

Furue M, Ando I, Inoue Y, et al: Pretibial epidermolysis bullosa: Successful therapy with a skin graft. Arch Dermatol 122:310–313, 1986.

This special localized form of epidermolysis bullosa present for eight years was cured by excision and grafting with skin taken from the patient's abdomen.

Management by committee is never successful and usually adds up to no management at all.

J. A. COTTERILL

Epidermolysis Bullosa Acquisita

Corticosteroids Imuran Methotrexate

Although this disease was named to indicate that it was an acquired form of epidermolysis bullosa, immunoelectron microscopy has disclosed it to be a form of bullous pemphigoid. The most effective treatment has been prednisone (60 mg/day), which can usually be tapered over a few weeks to a maintenance level (20 mg/day). Steroid-sparing immunosuppressants may be added, such as azathioprine (100 mg/day), cyclophosphamide (150 mg/day), or methotrexate (25 mg IM weekly). These are required for many months, but should be reduced periodically on a trial basis.

It is evident that the clinical assessment of bullous lesions may have to be supplemented by immunopathology before long-term hazardous therapeutic regimens are initiated.

Woodley DT, Briggaman RA, O'Keefe EJ, et al: Identification of the skin basement-membrane autoantigen in epidermolysis bullosa acquisita. N Engl J Med 310:1007–1013, 1984.

Immunoelectron microscopy reveals this to be a variant of bullous pemphigoid with circulating autoantibodies against a specific protein in the basement membrane. In both diseases the separation is within the basement membrane zone—in bullous pemphigoid (BP) above the lamina densa and in epidermolysis bullosa acquisita (EBA) below the lamina densa. When blisters form the BP antigen remains with the epidermis, whereas the EBA antigen stays with the dermis.

Gammon WR, Briggaman RA, Woodley DT, et al: Epidermolysis bullosa acquisita—A pemphigoid-like disease. J Am Acad Dermatol 11:820–832, 1984.

Recommend new name: *dermolytic pemphigoid* to emphasize resemblance to bullous pemphigoid and cicatricial pemphigoid. Review of five cases. Distinction between these may depend upon the ultrastructural location of IgG deposits and anti-BMZ antibodies with immunoelectron microscopy. Treatment: **prednisone** and **methotrexate**.

Richter BJ, McNutt NS: The spectrum of epidermolysis bullosa acquisita. Arch Dermatol 115:1325–1328, 1979.

Good results with Imuran (100 mg daily) and **prednisone** (80 mg/day tapered to 20 mg/day) over seven months. This 56-year-old black woman had a disease resembling cicatricial pemphigoid, with ocular, esophageal, and laryngeal scarring as well as an acquired scarring bullous eruption of skin.

Livden JK, Nilsen R: Acquired epidermolysis bullosa treated with a gold compound. Acta Derm Venereol 59:378–379, 1979.

Gold sodium thiomalate (Myochrysine 50 mg IM once weekly over nine months to total dose of 1000 mg) induced complete remission in a 20-year-old man who also had Crohn's disease. He had been nonresponsive to **prednisone** (40 mg/day) and **azathioprine** (150 mg/day). Start with weekly test doses of gold sodium thiomalate (10 mg IM, 20 mg IM, 20 mg IM).

Tan R: Epidermolysis bullosa acquisita. Br J Dermatol 97 (Suppl 15):46–48, 1977.

Check for concurrent enteritis, colitis, diabetes mellitus, occult malignant disease, myeloma, amyloid, porphyrins. No abnormalities were found in a 69-year-old man with dystrophic nails, milia, and hemorrhagic bullae.

Ray TL, Levine JB, Weiss W, Ward PA: Epidermolysis bullosa acquisita and inflammatory bowel disease. J Am Acad Dermatol 6:242–252, 1982.

Recommends rigorous search for inflammatory bowel disease (Crohn's disease and ulcerative colitis) as cause of EBA. Mild dysphagia or diarrhea may be overlooked. Search for immune complexes. Do immunofluorescence on skin biopsy.

The most important difference between a good and indifferent clinician lies in the amount of attention paid to the story of a patient.
FANQUHAR BUZZARD

Erythema Chronicum Migrans

Tetracycline
Penicillin
Erythromycin

Now that it has been established that this disease is due to a spirochete transmitted by *Ioxodes* ticks, the treatment schedules used for syphilis are entirely appropriate. A solitary annular lesion with central clearing and a red migrating border suggests the diagnosis, particularly if the patient has been camping recently or working in the woods. Other acute flu-like symptoms may include headaches, myalgias, arthralgias, low-grade fever, sore throat, nausea, and profound fatigue.

Asbrink E, Olsson I: Clinical manifestations of erythema chronicum migrans Afzelius in 161 patients: A comparison with Lyme disease. Acta Derm Venereol 65:43–52, 1985.

Based on experience with 132 patients, the best treatment is **phenoxymethyl penicillin** (penicillin V 2 gm/day for 10 days).

Steere AC, Hutchinson GJ, Rahn DW, et al: Treatment of the early manifestations of Lyme disease. Ann Intern Med 99:22–26, 1983.

Overall, **tetracycline** (250 mg qid for 10 days) appeared to be the most effective drug for treating patients with early Lyme disease.

In a study of 108 adult patients, erythema chronicum migrans and its associated symptoms resolved faster in patients treated with **phenoxymethyl penicillin** (250 mg qid for 10 days) or tetracycline (250 mg qid for 10 days) than in those given **erythromycin** (250 mg qid for 10 days) (mean duration 5.4 and 5.7 days vs 9.2 days). None of the 39 patients given tetracycline developed major late complications (meningoencephalitis, myocarditis, or recurrent arthritis), compared with 3 of 40 penicillin-treated patients and 4 of 29 patients given erythromycin. However, in all of the antibiotic-treated groups approximately half of the patients had late minor symptoms such as headache, musculoskeletal pain, and lethargy.

Although the dosage used for each drug in the study was 250 mg qid for 10 days, the authors now recommend phenoxymethyl penicillin (500 mg qid) or **benzathine penicillin** (2.4 million U IM).

Dosage for children:

phenoxymethyl penicillin (50 mg/kg/day for 10 to 20 days, giving at least 1 gm daily, but not over 2 gm daily).

erythromycin (30 mg/kg/day for 15 to 20 days)

During the first 24 hours of antibiotic therapy, 14 per cent of patients had intensification of symptoms with higher fever, redder rash, and greater joint pains. This Jarisch-Herxheimer–like reaction probably resulted from rapid killing of spirochetes by tetracycline or penicillin and tended to occur in patients with more severe disease.

Bruhn FW: Lyme disease. Am J Dis Child 138:467–470, 1984.

Anecdotal experience with corticosteroid abounds, but there are no controlled studies of its true effectiveness.

Children over seven years of age should be treated with oral **tetracycline**

(40 mg/kg/day in four divided doses for 10 to 20 days, to a maximum of 250 mg qid).

Younger children should receive **penicillin V** (250 mg qid for 10 to 20 days) *or* **erythromycin** (40 mg/kg/day in four divided doses).

Neurologic manifestations of Lyme disease (such as meningitis), which begin four weeks after the tick bite, should be treated with intravenous **penicillin G sodium** (20 million units/day IV in divided doses for 10 days).

Hurwitz S: Erythema chronicum migrans and Lyme disease. Pediatr Dermatol 2:266–274, 1985.

Review of the literature indicates that relapses of fever, malaise, or arthritis are best treated with nonsteroidal anti-inflammatory agents such as salicylates (80 to 100 mg/kg/day) or tolmetin sodium (Tolectin 10 to 30 mg/kg/day). In some instances corticosteroids (prednisone 2 mg/kg/day) may also be advisable.

It is difficult to make predictions—particularly about the future.
CONFUCIUS

Erythema Multiforme

Acyclovir
Antibiotics
Corticosteroids
Azathioprine

Here is a disease to summon all of your skills: in detecting its cause, treating and eliminating its source, and preventing its recurrence. Erythema multiforme is an immunologically determined reaction pattern with as many causes as a fever of undetermined origin.

The most common cause is herpes simplex infection with subclinical viremia. This leads within a day or two to vasculitic target lesions at points of trauma and loci minora resistentiae. As many as one in six of the erythema multiforme patients can give a history of a preceding herpes lesion, but even more probably have occult attacks of herpes simplex as a trigger for the disease. Oral acyclovir should help these patients if given immediately at the time of the appearance of the herpes lesion (200 mg q4h for 14 days). Acyclovir ointment (Zovirax) applied every three hours to the herpes lesion and any sequential erythema multiforme lesions is also helpful.

We prophylactically completely remove the virus-filled vesicles or bullae of herpes simplex lesions on the initial day of appearance, using surgical subsection with a Gillette Super Blue Blade. This has prevented the appearance of post-herpetic erythema multiforme in some patients. Immediate epidermal excision of the viral lesions of orf should similarly prevent development of erythema multiforme in the sensitized farmer or veterinarian.

The second common cause of erythema multiforme is *Mycoplasma pneumoniae* pneumonitis. A chest roentgenogram should be obtained, and if signs of infection are present a course of erythromycin (250 mg qid for seven days) should be immediately prescribed. Gram-negative infections of the small bowel are also known to trigger erythema multiforme, such as yersiniosis, which is responsive to tetracycline. The patient must also be checked for possible urinary tract infection, sinusitis, and dental abscesses. In severe forms of erythema multiforme such a survey must be exhaustive and requires hospitalization. Intravenous antibiotics may be required for the control of certain gram-negative infections. In any event, antibiotics are a rational, necessary weapon for the control of many examples of erythema multiforme.

The third common family of causes includes drugs of all types, configurations, and dosages. Ideally, every single drug the patient is taking or using should be eliminated, including eye drops. We prefer to widen the net even further by interdicting chemical exposures of all sorts. This includes work-related allergens and such home-related allergens as cosmetics, vitamins, toothpaste, and household sprays. One of the worst examples of bullous erythema multiforme (Stevens-Johnson syndrome) we have ever seen resulted from a single drop of an obscure complex organic acid falling on a chemist's skin. In this regard, 9-bromofluorene consistently sensitizes and produces erythema multiforme in many who work with it.

A host of other causes may have to be considered. Prominent among these in the older age group are malignant tumors. Elimination of the tumor and its antigen is the only cure, and recurrence of the erythema multiforme tells us immediately that the tumor has recurred.

For the seriously afflicted patient with no discernible cause of erythema multiforme, systemic steroids in high dosage are de rigueur. Despite lack of controlled studies, systemic steroids immediately make both the patient and the physician feel better. Since the disease is usually self-limiting, a tapered three-week course is all that is required. We prefer intramuscular Kenalog (40 to 80 mg) to oral steroids, as it gives 21 days of even dosage.

Local treatment can be as varied as the severity of the lesions, ranging from emollient topical steroids (Synalar ointment) to cooling Burow's solution compresses or tap-water tub soaks. In all cases of the major form of erythema multiforme (Stevens-Johnson syndrome), ophthalmologic consultation and specialized care are mandatory, as the eyes may be severely affected. Similarly, good oral hygiene is necessary, with frequent cleansing and oral Mycostatin suspension rinses.

The patient must be instructed that this disease can recur. He should see you promptly as an emergency if any lesions or known antecedents develop. In the totally idiopathic case a short course of erythromycin may abort the lesions of erythema multiforme.

Tonnesen MG, Soter N: Erythema multiforme. J Am Acad Dermatol 1:357–364, 1979.

Comprehensive review. No specific treatment available. Elimination of all suspected etiologic factors is of prime importance.

Huff JC, Weston WL, Tonnesen MG: Erythema multiforme: A critical review of characteristics, diagnostic criteria, and causes. J Am Acad Dermatol 8:763–775, 1983.

Lists 99 causes for this acute self-limited, destructive process: 33 infections, 40 drugs, 26 miscellaneous. Use it as an aide memoire in your sleuthing for a cause. Includes 76 references. Do not forget to look for:

hepatitis B	infectious mononucleosis
dental infections	syphilis
Trichomonas	tinea
inhalants	pollen shots
eye drops	

Brettle RP, Gray JA, Sangster G, Murdoch JM, Dick HM: The mucocutaneous syndromes—erythema multiforme, Stevens-Johnson and ectodermosis erosiva pluriorificialis. J Infection 4:149–160, 1982.

Review of their 78 cases over 30 years in Edinburgh showed 1.2 per cent mortality. All patients need extensive microbiologic screening. Most common complications: nephritis, blindness. Treat for *Mycoplasma pneumoniae* infection if any respiratory signs present.

Edmond BJ, Huff JC, Weston WL: Erythema multiforme. Pediatr Clin North Am 30:631–640, 1983.

Minor form: antihistamines, warm tub-water soaks, oral hygiene with half-strength H_2O_2.

Major form: hospitalize, antibiotics, ophthalmologic consultation, high-dose steroids (1 to 2 mg/kg/day) while lesions are extending, then taper over one to three weeks.

Ting HC, Adam BA: Erythema multiforme: Response to corticosteroids. Dermatologica 169:175–178, 1984.

Prednisone (40 to 60 mg/day for two to four weeks) made no difference in the course of 25 patients with erythema multiforme minor except to shorten the febrile period (from 5.6 to 2.7 days).

Sontheimer RD, Garibaldi RA, Krueger GG: Stevens-Johnson syndrome associated with *Mycoplasma pneumoniae* infections. Arch Dermatol 114:241–244, 1978.

Treat with **erythromycin** if any pulmonary signs. Diagnosis requires cultural isolation of organism or elevation of complement-fixing antibody titer to 1:64 or above (or threefold increase in titer of convalescent over acute sera). Cold hemagglutins alone are not specific for *Mycoplasma pneumoniae* infection.

Jones RR: Azathioprine therapy in the management of persistent erythema multiforme. Br J Dermatol 105:465–467, 1981.

Azathioprine (100 mg/day) for three months and (150 mg/day) for three years, respectively, was necessary to control and cure two cases of persistent erythema multiforme of unknown etiology. Steroids could be stopped in both cases. Azathioprine inhibits both T and B cell function.

Arstikaitis MJ: Ocular aftermath of Stevens-Johnson Syndrome. Arch Opthalmol 90:376–379, 1973.

Among 67 children with Stevens-Johnson syndrome, 33 had eye involvement and 9 had residual ocular defects. Keratitis sicca with corneal pannus developed in five, while single cases had corneal pannus alone, symblepharon, entropion, and stricture of the lacrimal puncta. May require artificial tears, a moisture chamber, or surgical intervention, but always ophthalmologic specialist care during the acute illness.

Brody I: Topical treatment of recurrent herpes simplex and postherpetic erythema multiforme with low concentrations of zinc sulphate solution. Br J Dermatol 104:191–194, 1981.

Aqueous **zinc sulfate** ($ZnSO_4 \cdot 7H_2O$) as a compress or mouthwash was helpful in treating five patients with active herpes simplex lesions and preventing recurrences of both herpes simplex and erythema multiforme (follow-up 16 to 23 months). Zinc ions have been shown experimentally to irreversibly inhibit replication of herpes simplex virus type I.

compress
- active lesions: (0.025 to 0.05 per cent) 10 minutes/day
- maintenance: (0.05 per cent) once weekly for four weeks, then twice a month

mouthwash
- active lesions: (0.01 to 0.025 per cent) one to three minutes/day
- maintenance: (0.025 per cent) once weekly for four weeks, then twice a month

Fawcett HA, Wansbrough-Jones MH, Clark AE, Leigh IM: Prophylactic topical acyclovir for frequent recurrent herpes simplex infection with and without erythema multiforme. Br Med J 287:798–799, 1983.

No help. Double-blind controlled cross-over trial with 16 patients studied 5 per cent **acyclovir** in a modified aqueous cream (with 40 per cent **propylene glycol**).

Shelley WB: Bacterial endotoxin (lipopolysaccharide) as a cause of erythema multiforme. JAMA 243:58–60, 1980.

Treat with appropriate antibiotics. Gram-negative bacterial antigens (no longer commercially available) reproduced erythema multiforme lesions in a 47-year-old woman found to have *Proteus mirabilis* on urine culture. Treatment with **ampicillin** (500 mg qid), Kenalog (40 mg IM), and, later, **dapsone** (100 mg/day) was curative, with maintenance dosage given for five months.

The "fibrin star" test (in vitro fibrin clot formation) also can be used to identify hypersensitivity to the gram-negative bacterial endotoxin, lipopolysaccharide. A positive test should lead to a thorough search for infection in the respiratory, gastrointestinal, and urinary tracts. (Although experimental, this test is easily performed—for details see Br J Dermatol 96:577–586, 1977).

Lonsdorf G, Neubert U: Yersinsiosis. Hautarzt 29:127–129, 1978.

Can be a cause of erythema multiforme. Responds well to **tetracyclines**.

Gottschalk HY, Stone OJ: Stevens-Johnson syndrome from ophthalmic sulfonamide. Arch Dermatol 112:513–514, 1976.

Protect patient from casual drugs in any form. Here, the offender was a commonly prescribed sulfacetamide sodium ophthalmic ointment, used for only one day in a 71-year-old man with a history of bullous drug reaction to a sulfonamide.

Rosato FE, Shelley WB, Fitts WT Jr, Miller LD: Non-metastatic cutaneous manifestations of cancer of the colon. Am J Surg 117:277–281, 1969.

In case of malignancy-induced erythema multiforme, excision is curative. Later recurrence of skin lesions is indicative of recurrence of cancer.

Fitzpatrick JE, Thompson PB, Aeling JL, Huff C: Photosensitive recurrent erythema multiforme. J Am Acad Dermatol 9:419–423, 1983.

In a 31-year-old white man, hydroxychloroquine (200 mg/day) dramatically cleared erythema multiforme, proven by phototesting to be due to UVL. Lesions appeared on sun-exposed areas 24 to 36 hours after a sunburn, apparently unrelated to cold sores on his lip. Sun avoidance and use of sunscreens may help patients with erythema multiforme due to herpes simplex infections.

Bahmer FA, Zaun H, Luszpinski P: Thalidomide treatment of recurrent erythema multiforme. Acta Derm Venereol 62:449–450, 1982.

A treatment of promise is **thalidomide** (experimental study only). A 39-year-old man with virtually continuous attacks that had not responded to steroids, **levamisole**, **gamma globulin**, or vaccinations to polio and herpes virus cleared completely within a few days of taking thalidomide (200 mg/day). Maintenance dose (100 mg/day) kept him free of attacks for more than six months.

Horio T, Danno K, Okamoto H, Miyachi Y, Imamura S: Potassium iodide in erythema nodosum and other erythematous dermatoses. J Am Acad Dermatol 9:77–81, 1983.

Potassium iodide (300 mg tid—in form of 100-mg pill) given for two weeks rapidly cleared 14 of 16 cases of erythema multiforme. Only one patient had recurrence. No side effects except for occasional mild gastric distress.

Huff JC, Weston WL: Isomorphic phenomenon in erythema multiforme. Clin Exp Dermatol 8:409–413, 1983.

Lesions are induced by circulating factors localizing at sites of previous inflammation or trauma, including scars, nail folds, and folliculitis. Avoid stiff toothbrush, dental floss, and intradermal skin tests at time of attack.

Gebel K, Hornstein OP: Drug-induced oral erythema multiforme—Results of a long-term retrospective study. Dermatologica 168:35–40, 1984.

Positive patch tests specifically incriminated offending drug in four cases, while scratch tests were positive in three cases. Worthy of trying to help patients avoid recurrences.

Lewis JE: Surgical treatment of recurrent herpes simplex. Cutis 26:567, 1980.

Epidermal excision of early lesions (less than 36 hours old) of herpes simplex prevented appearance of postherpetic erythema multiforme.

Agger WA, Webster SB: Human orf infection complicated by erythema multiforme. Cutis 31:334–338, 1983.

Erythema multiforme developed in a woman 21 days after she acquired lesions of orf on her fingers. Treatment with **prednisone** (20 mg qid) and **bacitracin** ointment caused improvement of the lesions within three days. (We feel that immediate surgical excision of the primary orf lesions by epidermal subsection could have prevented the erythema multiforme.)

Phoon WH, Chan MOY, Rajan VS, et al: Stevens-Johnson syndrome associated with occupational exposure to trichloroethylene. Contact Dermatitis 10:270–276, 1984.

Trichloroethylene, a solvent used for degreasing parts in an electronics factory, was shown to be the cause of erythema multiforme in five patients who also suffered liver damage.

Nethercott JR, Albers J, Guirgius S, et al: Erythema multiforme exudativum linked to the manufacture of printed circuit boards. Contact Dermatitis 8:314–322, 1982.

Formaldehyde used in the manufacture of circuit boards was the apparent cause of erythema multiforme in four workers after 6 to 12 weeks of exposure. Liver involvement occurred in three of the cases. Because of good ventilation, trichloroethylene was felt not to be the cause.

Green JA, Spruance SL, Wenerstrom G, Piepkorn MW: Post-herpetic erythema multiforme prevented by oral acyclovir. Ann Intern Med 102:622–633, 1985.

Acyclovir (Zovirax, 200 mg five times a day for seven days, then tid for five months) completely prevented attacks of herpes simplex and erythema multiforme in a 26-year-old man. For 12 years he had had three to five episodes of labial herpes virus infection per year. For the past two years each had been invariably followed three to seven days later by severe erythema multiforme.

Record what you see, hear, and do. The patient (and his lawyers) expect no less of you.

Erythema Nodosum

Antibiotics	Colchicine
Iodides	Steroids
Indomethacin	Underlying cause

Erythema nodosum is another example of a monomorphic inflammatory skin reaction with multiple causes. Ideally the cause should be ascertained, and treatment directed toward this. In actual practice this ideal is not commonly achieved, and treatment must center on anti-inflammatory measures of a nonspecific nature.

Sensitization to circulating bacterial antigens is the most common discernible cause. Antigens from streptococcal pharyngitis or yersinial enterocolitis lodge in blood vessels in the lower legs presumably damaged by clinical bruises. There they initiate a progressive inflammatory sequence that involves a complex cascade of inflammatory mediators, from histamine to leukotrienes and prostaglandins. Hence, many types of antibiotics may be helpful in eliminating the primary source of antigen, and both steroidal and nonsteroidal anti-inflammatory agents may interrupt the inflammatory cycle at various points.

Unless the therapeutic response occurs within a few days, any drugs used may receive undeserved accolades, as the average case of erythema nodosum fades spontaneously in about six weeks. Such a course suggests that the responsible primary infection (and antigen source) is self-limiting.

We screen our patients for infections in the pharynx, chest, bowel, and teeth. We rule out sarcoidosis and, if they are from endemic areas, coccidioidomycosis and histoplasmosis. We ascertain whether or not they are taking a contraceptive. If none of these avenues, including a health profile, CRP titer, and ASO titer, suggests a specific therapeutic attack, we favor conservative management with reduction in activity, bedrest as much as possible, and erythromycin (250 mg qid). For control of pain we prescribe aspirin or Indocin, alerting the patient to expect results within 48 hours. If this improvement is not forthcoming, potassium iodide is prescribed on a short-term trial basis. Both the patient and the physician should be impatient for rapid symptomatic and clinical help in this disease.

Soderstrom RM, Krull EA: Erythema nodosum: A review. Cutis 21:806–810, 1978.

Streptococcal infection is the most commonly recognized cause, while sarcoidosis is the disease most commonly associated with erythema nodosum. Thus, all patients deserve a throat culture, ASO titer, chest roentgenogram, and skin testing with PPD.

Fine RM, Meltzer HD: Chronic erythema nodosum. Arch Dermatol 100:33–38, 1969.

Study of nine patients. Although usually short-term and self-limited, erythema nodosum can persist or recur for years, without any identifiable cause. In idiopathic cases, treatment centers on trials of antibiotics, **dapsone**, **chloroquine**, **indomethacin**, iodides, and steroids.

Schulz EJ, Whiting DA: Treatment of erythema nodosum and nodular vasculitis with potassium iodide. Br J Dermatol 94:75–78, 1976.

After taking **potassium iodide** (300 to 900 mg/day), 24 of 28 patients with erythema nodosum had symptomatic relief within 48 hours and clearing within two weeks and had no need for treatment after three weeks. Prior treatments included **aspirin**, **phenylbutazone**, **indomethacin**, **sulfonamides**, and steroids. Seven of these patients had tonsillitis and received concurrent antibiotics. Other causes or associated conditions included influenza (seven), sarcoid (four), contraceptives (two), pregnancy (two), dental sepsis (two), and sinusitis (one).

Horio T, Imamura S, Danno K, Ofuji S: Potassium iodide in the treatment of erythema nodosum and nodular vasculitis. Arch Dermatol 117:29–31, 1981.

Of 15 patients with erythema nodosum, 11 had symptomatic relief in 24 hours and complete disappearance of lesions within 10 to 14 days of starting **potassium iodide** (300 mg orally tid). Patients with positive C-reactive protein tests, joint pains, or fever showed the best response.

Barr WG, Robinson JA: Chronic erythema nodosum treated with indomethacin. Ann Intern Med 95:659, 1981.

Indocin (25 mg tid for one month) led to permanent disappearance of all nodules in a 32-year-old woman with iodiopathic erythema nodosum of three years' duration. **Aspirin** had been without effect, and **prednisone** had provided only temporary remission.

Ubogy Z, Persellin RH: Suppression of erythema nodosum by indomethacin. Acta Derm Venereol 62:265–267, 1982.

Three patients with severe debilitating erythema nodosum secondary to antecedent streptococcal pharyngitis showed no response to **erythromycin**, **penicillin**, or **aspirin**. Dramatic clearing occurred with **indomethacin** (Indocin 50 mg tid for two weeks). There were no recurrences, and relief was noted within 24 hours.

Elizaga FV: Erythema nodosum and indomethacin. Ann Intern Med 96:383, 1982.

Indomethacin (25 mg qid for four months) provided prompt symptomatic relief and complete involution of nodules of arms and legs in a 57-year-old man with successfully treated tuberculosis (liver, spleen) and acute myelogenous leukemia.

Lehman CW: Control of chronic erythema nodosum with Naproxen. Cutis 26:66–67, 1980.

Naprosyn (250 mg bid for one month) gave prompt resolution within 96 hours and clearing in 14 days of erythema nodosum that had been refractory to **phenylbutazone** and **aspirin**. The patient was a 28-year-old woman who had recurrent erythema nodosum for seven years. Several relapses occurred 6 months after stopping therapy, but the condition would promptly respond again to Naprosyn.

De Coninck P, Baclet JL, Di Bernardo C, et al: Traitement de l'érythème noueux par la colchicine. Presse Med 13:680, 1984.

Colchicine (2 mg/day for three days, followed by 1 mg/day for two to four weeks) cleared erythema nodosum lesions in five women. Regression was noted within 72 hours, and there were no recurrences when the drug was stopped.

MacFarlane JT: Recurrent erythema nodosum and pulmonary sarcoidosis. Postgrad Med J 57:525, 1981.

Prednisolone (15 mg/day for four months) induced complete clearing of pulmonary changes and associated erythema nodosum lesions in a 36-year-old woman. Over 20 years she had had three separate episodes, separated by complete remissions.

Debois J, Vandepitte J, Degreef H: *Yersinia enterocolitica* as a cause of erythema nodosum. Dermatologica 156:65–78, 1978.

Tetracycline therapy may be valuable in treating bowel infection due to *Yersinia enterocolitica*, which triggers erythema nodosum. Eight of 54 patients with erythema nodosum had elevated antibody titers to *Y. enterocolitica*. Note that enterocolitis symptoms may precede erythema nodosum lesions by two weeks.

Ellis ME, Pope J, Mokashi A, Dunbar E: Campylobacter colitis associated with erythema nodosum. Br Med J 285:937, 1982.

A 24-year-old woman with a one-week history of frequent watery, bloody diarrhea, ulcer on the lower lip, and concurrent erythema nodosum experienced prompt involution of all problems without therapy. The symptoms mimicked inflammatory bowel disease, which would probably have been diagnosed if stool cultures had not been obtained.

Linaker BD: Erythema nodosum presenting before inflammatory bowel disease. Lancet 2:931, 1977.

Seventeen days after the onset of erythema nodosum, an 18-year-old woman (who also had alopecia totalis) developed signs of inflammatory bowel disease, which required Azulfidine (**sulfasalazine**), intramuscular **corticotropin**, and later a colectomy.

Hicks JH: Erythema nodosum in patients with tinea pedis and onychomycosis. South Med J 70:27–28, 1977.

Among five women with erythema nodosum and onychomycosis, unilateral erythema nodosum occurred in three patients on the same side as unilateral tinea pedis. All cleared with **griseofulvin** therapy (500 mg/day). Lesions could be reproduced with *Trichophyton* antigen (0.1 ml) injected subcutaneously on the legs.

Whitaker DC, Lynch PJ: Erythema nodosum and coccidioidomycosis. Ariz Med 36:887–889, 1979.

Asymptomatic coccidioidomycosis was found in 6 of 22 patients (27 per cent) with erythema nodosum, based on serologies, skin test conversion, and chest roentgenogram. The authors recommend bedrest, elastic wrap compression, and **aspirin**. Four of six patients had spontaneous resolution of nodules.

Ozols II, Wheat LJ: Erythema nodosum in an epidemic of histoplasmosis in Indianapolis. Arch Dermatol 117:709–712, 1981.

None of 11 patients with erythema nodosum as a complication of histoplasmosis infection required antifungal treatment. In most cases the erythema nodosum lasted only two to three weeks and resolved spontaneously, presumably as the result of rapid elimination of the organism. One patient with longer lasting erythema nodosum and arthritis was treated successfully with a saturated solution of **potassium iodide** on two different occasions.

McMillan A: Reiter's disease in a female, presenting as erythema nodosum. Br J Vener Dis 51:345–347, 1975.

Prednisolone for 10 days induced rapid involution of erythema nodosum lesions in a 20-year-old woman who also had recurrent cystitis, sore throat, aching in her joints, and an effusion in one knee. However, recurrence of skin lesions required 1 week of conjoint **tetracycline** (250 mg qid) and **phenylbutazone** (100 mg tid) to achieve a lasting remission.

Jillson OT: Erythema nodosum. Cutis 29:142–146, 1982.

Look for and treat tuberculosis if a child develops erythema nodosum.

Alinovi A, Lui P, Benoldi D: Syphilis—Still a cause of erythema nodosum. Int J Dermatol 22:310–311, 1983.

A 28-year-old man had erythema nodosum of the arms and legs as part of secondary syphilis. Both were cured with **penicillin** therapy.

Chalmers RJG, Proctor SJ, Marks JM: Erythema nodosum and Hodgkin's disease. Br J Dermatol 106:593–595, 1982.

Recurrent erythema nodosum was a presenting sign of Hodgkin's disease in three patients.

Sato A, Mikami M, Konno H, Usuba M: Non-Hodgkin's lymphoma simulating erythema nodosum. J Dermatol 10:167–176, 1983.

Unilateral chronic indurated erythema on the leg resembled erythema nodosum in two patients. A biopsy of the lesions was necessary for directing treatment.

Vesey CMR, Wilkinson DS: Erythema nodosum: A study of seventy cases. Br J Dermatol 71:139–155, 1959.

Seven of these cases (all in middle-aged women) occurred in association with chronic bronchitis. Fever, fatigue, lassitude, and cough accompanied the abrupt onset of erythema nodosum.

The odds on the therapeutic success vary inversely with the number of therapies being touted.

Erythroderma

Homeostatic measures	Erythromycin
Compresses	Etiologic approaches
Steroids	
Topical	
Systemic	

Erythroderma is the ultimate inflammatory response of the skin. Here, one must treat 2 square meters of angry red scaling skin that is out of control. Its massive vasodilation adds a circulatory shunt that strains the heart. Its vascular bed and sweat glands no longer provide thermoregulatory control, leaving the patient truly poikilothermic. Its role as the impermeable membrane interface with the environment is destroyed, allowing critical losses of water, proteins, and electrolytes. Moreover, its pathologic permeability makes normally innocuous topical agents a source of local irritant reactions and toxic systemic effects. Finally, its constant shedding of keratin scales leads to nutritional deficits, especially protein depletion.

The *Sturm und Drang* of this generalized exfoliative dermatitis calls for intense yet gentle therapy. Every effort is made to assist the patient in his homeostatic crisis. The environment must be warm and humid. The patient must be at rest, preferably in the hospital; only the blandest compresses and lubricants are to be used. Nutritional supplements in the form of high protein feedings and multivitamins with minerals are essential.

Since erythroderma is a nonspecific end-stage reaction pattern, all of these patients respond to the same anti-inflammatory regimens. We favor physiologic saline compresses (30 minutes qid) to selected areas to remove scales, serum, bacteria, and debris. Avoid the aluminum of Burow's solution and Bluboro compresses on a skin so permeable. The saline compresses supplement a short, warm daily bath in which no soap or washcloth is used, and the body is rapidly patted dry with the softest of towels. Some therapists favor colloidal baths, but one should be wary of rare sensitivities. We once had a patient with erythroderma of 11 months' duration due solely to oatmeal sensitivity from his daily colloidal baths, started in a hospital elsewhere.

Following each bath and compress, we favor generalized lubrication with Synalar ointment 0.025 per cent (since it is preservative free).

Erythromycin (250 mg qid) has proven to be the best prophylactic and therapeutic agent for secondary bacterial growth in this moist damaged skin. We use it routinely. In the more severe recalcitrant erythrodermas, systemic steroids are necessary. We favor intramuscular Kenalog (40 mg once or twice), since control of the dosage is in the hands of the physician, and it offers 21 days of even, sustained levels of systemic triamcinolone.

Any specific therapy for erythroderma must arise from a knowledge of the cause. Thus, if psoriasis has been the antecedent, we treat with methotrexate (25 mg IM weekly). A prior stasis dermatitis requires specific attention to correction of the vascular problem. Protection from contact sensitizers, sprays, and drugs taken prior to the onset of erythroderma is absolutely essential, and can be curative in selected patients.

All patients deserve a careful hospital search for underlying lymphoma or occult internal cancer. This may include skin and lymph node biopsies, blood studies, computed tomography, and exploratory surgery at times. This need becomes magnified in elderly patients, and in anyone in whom the cause of the erythroderma is not clearly apparent. Appropriate chemotherapy may be the only chance of resolving this type of erythroderma.

Throughout all of this, the patient needs compassionate care and support during the weeks and months of recovery. Fortunately, today we can add to this a sense of optimism, which surely shortens the days and nights until the shedding stops and the patient can rejoice in his newborn skin.

Nicolis GD, Helwig EB: Exfoliative dermatitis: A clinicopathologic study of 135 cases. Arch Dermatol 108:788–797, 1973.

A survey of 135 patients studied at the Armed Forces Institute of Pathology over a 36-year-period revealed the following:

Cause	*Percentage*
Drug reaction	40
Preexisting dermatosis	27
Lymphoma, leukemia	18
Internal cancer	3
Unknown	12

Pneumonia was the most common cause of death. Lymphadenopathy was present in 83 patients, hepatomegaly in 50, and splenomegaly in 31.

Anderson PC, Loeffel ED: Erythrodermatitis: A review of 40 cases. Mo Med 67:252–255, 1970.

Approximately 25 per cent of erythrodermas are due to psoriasis, 25 per cent are due to eczemas (atopic, contact, stasis with autoeczematization) and 15 to 20 per cent are due to leukemia or lymphoma. Advise hospitalization, sedation, analysis, wet dressings, Acid Mantle creme, systemic steroids, and **methotrexate** (if due to psoriasis). The ultimate answer is prevention by good early management of prior lesions. Direct job counseling, visiting the patient's employer, and utilizing rehabilitation experts are helpful for patients with persistent erythroderma.

Abrahams I, McCarthy JT, Sanders SL: 101 cases of exfoliative dermatitis. Arch Dermatol 87:96–101, 1963.

A survey of 101 patients at Columbia Medical Center from 1930 to 1960 revealed that 19 of the 101 died as a result of their erythroderma. Common causes of death: pneumonia, heart failure, or septicemia. Nearly half of the cases could not be classified as to etiology.

Kannangara DW, Smith B, Cohen K: Exfoliative dermatitis during Cefoxitin therapy. Arch Intern Med 142:1031–1032, 1982.

In an 84-year-old man receiving **cefoxitin** (Mefoxin 1 gm IM q6h), an erythematous scaly eruption began around the injection sites on the 17th day of treatment and became generalized by the 25th day. The skin returned to normal eight days after the drug was stopped. Management of erythroderma requires elimination of any and all drugs suspected as being a cause, as well as careful monitoring and control of body temperature, electrolytes, fluid balance, serum albumin, and dependent edema. Sensitivity to antibiotics (penicillin and sulfonamides) accounts for many drug-induced erythrodermas, but each of the following drugs has been responsible for some cases:

Antimicrobial Agents
Sulfonamides
Dapsone
Trimethoprim
Penicillins
Tetracyclines
Streptomycin sulfate
Isoniazid
Para-aminosalicylic acid
Amithiozone
Quinine sulfate
Quinacrine hydrochloride

Anticonvulsants
Barbiturates
Phenytoin sodium
Mephenytoin
Phenacemide
Pheneturide
Trimethadione

Heavy Metals
Arsenicals
Antimonials
Mercurials
Gold salts

Analgesics
Aspirin
Codeine phosphate
Phenylbutazone
Lidocaine hydrochloride

Antiarrhythmic Drugs
Quinidine salts
Practolol

Miscellaneous
Dimercaprol
Iodides
Chlorpropamide
Phenothiazines
Allopurinol
Dactinomycin
Potassium thiocyanate
Diethylstilbestrol
Vitamin A

Solinger AM: Exfoliative dermatitis from captopril. Cutis 29:473–474, 1982.

In a 57-year-old man with refractory congestive heart failure, **captopril** (Capoten 100 mg q8h), an angiotensin–converting enzyme blocker, induced erythroderma within 14 days of starting treatment. It cleared two months after stopping the captopril and introducing **prednisone** (60 mg/day). However, tapered doses of prednisone were required over the following two years.

Yantis PL, Bridges ME, Pittman FE: Cimetidine-induced exfoliative dermatitis. Dig Dis Sci 25:73–74, 1980.

Only 33 tablets of **cimetidine** (300 mg qid) induced erythroderma in a 68-year-old woman, who required hospitalization and subsequent therapy with **prednisone** (60 mg/day tapered to 5 mg/day) over six weeks. A warning signal was pruritus, noted following the second tablet!

Rosin MA, King LE Jr.: Isoniazid-induced exfoliative dermatitis. South Med J 75:81, 1982.

Careful study of a 75-year-old man ruled out the following antecedents of erythroderma:

psoriasis
seborrheic dermatitis
atopic dermatitis
contact dermatitis
pityriasis rubra pilaris
malignant disease

Subsequent oral challenge with **INH** established it as the true cause. The rash initially appeared nine days after INH (300 mg/day) was started, and cleared within one week after INH was stopped. When INH was restarted, pruritus appeared within six hours, and exfoliation developed over two days. Despite the stopping of the drug, the rash took three months to resolve.

Kuhnley EJ, Granoff AL: Exfoliative dermatitis during lithium treatment. Am J Psychiatry 136:1340–1341, 1979.

Lithium carbonate (900 to 1200 mg/day) induced a morbilliform eruption on the ninth day of therapy in a 16-year-old manic-depressive boy. This was followed over two weeks by chills, fever, malaise, and erythroderma, which cleared spontaneously once the lithium was stopped.

Slagel GA, James WD: Plaquenil-induced erythroderma. J Am Acad Dermatol 12:857–862, 1985.

A 31-year-old woman with psoriasis developed erythroderma 11 days after starting **hydroxychloroquine** (Plaquenil 200 mg bid) for treatment of arthritis. **Prednisone** (60 mg/day tapered over three weeks) cleared all of the skin lesions, including the psoriatic plaques, and she remained clear for six months. Relapse occurred after nine months.

Review of 152 patients in the literature revealed that 31 per cent of psoriatic patients treated with antimalarials developed acute generalized eruptions, including 11 cases of exfoliative dermatitis that occurred 10 to 27 days after starting treatment. All of the cases cleared well, but relapsed after several months.

(Could this be a new form of therapy for psoriasis, analogous to the therapeutic exfoliation induced by massive doses of **vitamin A** for pityriasis rubra pilaris?)

Schillinger BM, Berstein M, Goldberg LA, Shalita AR: Boric acid poisoning. J Am Acad Dermatol 7:667–673, 1982.

Self-administered boric acid, 14 gm or less, resulted in generalized "boiled lobster" erythema and massive desquamation in a 44-year-old black woman. Treatment included hemodialysis, **gentian violet** applications to denuded areas, Burow's solution soaks, and daily baths with $KMnO_4$ (1 : 80,000). Alopecia, common in boric acid poisoning, was seen on the thirteenth day after ingestion of boric acid.

Chesney PJ, Jaucian R-M C, McDonald RA, et al: Exfoliative dermatitis in an infant. Association with enterotoxin F–producing staphylococci. Am J Dis Child 137:899–901, 1983.

A fatal example of bullous erythroderma in a two-month-old premature infant girl due to a *Staphylococcus aureus* toxin. The exfoliative dermatitis may have been a form of toxic shock syndrome.

Rosen T, Chappell R, Drucker C: Exfoliative dermatitis: Presenting sign of internal malignancy. South Med J 72:652–653, 1979.

Carcinomas of the colon, prostate, and lung, respectively, accounted for the exfoliative dermatitis in three black men, ages 59 to 69. In the case of prostatic carcinoma, roentgen therapy of the tumor had a dramatically beneficial effect on the erythroderma.

Clues for suspecting malignant disease include:

- insidious development of erythroderma
- progressive debility
- resistance of erythroderma to standard treatment
- absence of prior skin disease

Wishart JM: Generalized exfoliative dermatitis due to contact with an antiperspirant. Br J Clin Pract 28:264, 1974.

Patch test–proven sensitivity to a spray antiperspirant and its perfume used in an 18-year-old man led to axillary dermatitis and then erythroderma. The erythroderma required three weeks of hospitalization (with **prednisolone** 30 mg/day and **betamethasone** ointment) and a further two months of outpatient steroid therapy for complete healing.

Reuler JB, Jones SR, Girard DE: Hypothermia in the erythroderma syndrome. West J Med 127:243–244, 1977.

A remarkable example of severe hypothermia in an 88-year-old man with psoriatic erythroderma. His rectal temperature was 32.2°C (90°F) as the result of increased heat loss by radiation, conduction, and evaporation. Warm peritoneal dialysis temporarily raised his temperature to 36.1°C (97°F), but he died after two days.

Commens CA, Greaves MW: Anhidrosis following exfoliative dermatitis. Clin Exp Dermatol 3:99–101, 1978.

A 32-year-old Iraqi man developed permanent generalized anhidrosis following pruritic erythroderma of unknown cause, which included alopecia, nail loss, and mucosal ulceration. Therapy: air conditioning. (We have personally seen three examples of this following **atabrine** exfoliative dermatitis.)

Cataldo MF, Varni JW, Russo DC, Estes SA: Behavior therapy techniques in treatment of exfoliative dermatitis. Arch Dermatol 116:919–922, 1980.

Prednisone, **erythromycin**, and **dicloxacillin** failed to control the pruritus of exfoliative dermatitis that began in the area of an insect bite 3½ years previously in a 37-year-old man. Excoriations were reduced in number when the patient kept careful count and used pleasurable distractions.

No patient wants a second opinion if the first doctor inspires confidence and radiates friendship and compassion.

Erythromelalgia

Cold
Aspirin
Inderal
NSAID

Here is a disease that is neither easy to spell nor to treat. It is hard to spell because of the polysyllabic alternatives, erythromelalgia or erythermalgia. It is hard to treat, as the literature attests with its polynomial drug list. Since there is no singular drug for this chronically painful affliction, one must acquaint the patient with the need for hunting for the right key.

We are especially alert to the primary need of ruling out underlying causes, such as drugs, chemicals, or disease. We have cured two patients by eliminating the artificial sweetener, cyclamate, from their diet. This avenue of dietary management should be explored in view of the hundreds of esoteric chemicals added to foods. We are eager to eliminate spices, cola drinks, mouthwashes, monosodium glutamate (Accent), coffee, and tartrazine on a trial basis. A careful history will reveal other suspects. In every case the known drug offenders, calcium channel blockers and dopamine agonists, must be discontinued. Smoking, taking snuff, and chewing nicotine gum should also be contraindicated until a positive or negative trial has been achieved. We look for underlying disease, recognizing that erythromelalgia may be one of the early signs of diabetes mellitus, thrombocythemia, or multiple sclerosis.

Aspirin has pride of place in the polypharmacy of this disease. Even in a low dose it will prevent the platelet aggregation that causes the capillary occlusion accounting for the symptoms in some patients. In addition, it inhibits prostaglandin synthesis and thereby reduces inflammation.

By the time patients reach you, they are already aware of the relief obtained from the ice bath or cold compresses. But it is well to reinforce the need for avoiding hot environments. They also need to avoid long periods of standing, as venous stasis adds to the malfunction of their vessels.

Many patients derive major benefits from a beta-blocker, indicating that the complex underlying mix of vasodilation and vasoconstriction may represent an abnormal response to epinephrine or norepinephrine. We prescribe Inderal (20 mg tid initially, with ascending dosage), remembering that there is a real sevenfold variability in the dose requirements for this drug. Patients receiving Inderal should carry a card warning against being given epinephrine, since it may induce a hypertensive response via the nonblocked alpha-adrenergic receptors.

For the aspirin- and Inderal-resistant patient, the field is still open, ranging from nonsteroidal anti-inflammatory drugs to steroids and immunosuppressants. These patients, however, must be protected from narcotics. Rare as they are, these patients must not be orphaned. They deserve your continued study and thought. Surely, in the scores of remedies proposed in the 150 years since this disease was first described, you can find one that is right for your patient.

Ratz JL, Bergfeld WF, Steck WD: Erythermalgia with vasculitis: A review. J Am Acad Dermatol 1:443–450, 1979.

Treatment of this rare painful erythema centers on empiric use of vasoconstrictors, vasodilators, and anti-inflammatory agents. This excellent review reports a 70-year-old man whose problem with swollen, red burning feet was not helped by any of the following commonly recommended remedies:

propranolol hydrochloride	Midrin
acetylsalicyclic acid	indomethacin
hydroxychloroquine	hydrochlorothiazide
dapsone	methysergide maleate
nitroglycerine ointment 2 per cent	prednisone
ergotamine with caffeine	betamethasone
ephedrine sulfate	azathioprine
phenoxybenzamine	IV dextran
phenylbutazone	

Uno H, Parker F: Autonomic innervation of the skin in primary erythermalgia. Arch Dermatol 119:65–71, 1983.

This study of one patient showed a marked reduction in the affected skin of autonomic nerve endings of both the adrenergic and cholinergic type. The vasomotor responses resemble the denervation hypersensitivity state seen after sympathectomy, with stagnation of circulating catecholamines in the receptor site of vascular smooth muscle cells.

Thompson GH, Hahn G, Rang M: Erythromelalgia. Clin Orthop 144:249–254, 1979.

An extremely detailed account of primary familial erythromelalgia in a 14-year-old girl with symmetric involvement of her lower legs and feet since age 3, which led to bilateral knee disarticulations at age 13. She achieved best results through environmental control with a special cooling unit and by avoidance of heat-producing situations. She had no help from the usual approaches, as well as ultrasound, transcutaneous nerve stimulation, **ibuprofen**, and subcutaneous hypertonic saline injections.

Note: Any patient over 40 years old should be screened for an underlying primary problem such as:

diabetes mellitus	gout
polycythemia vera	hypertension
nephritis	multiple sclerosis
systemic lupus erythematosus	syphilis
rheumatoid arthritis	

Such patients usually have asymmetric involvement of both the arms and the legs. Symptoms may be reproduced by the application of local heat between 32° and 36°C.

Fitzgerald G, McCarthy D, O'Connell LG: Burning feet. Br Med J 1:1149, 1976.

Phlebotomy (4 units in 10 days) cured a 74-year-old woman whose only sign of polycythemia vera was a burning erythema of the soles of 18 months' duration.

Michiels J, Lindemans J, Vermeiden I, et al: Erythromelalgia and peripheral gangrene in thrombocythaemia. Br J Dermatol 102:750, 1980.

Often the first sign of thrombocythemia, this type of erythromelalgia was successfully treated in 20 patients with:

low-dose **aspirin** to prevent platelet aggregation
busulfan (Myleran) for the underlying myeloproliferative disease

Redding KG: Thrombocythemia as a cause of erythermalgia. Arch Dermatol 113:468–471, 1977.

Heparin (IV) gave rapid relief in two patients with erythromelalgia whose arterioles were occluded by platelet aggregates. This was followed by appropriate chemotherapy for the underlying myeloproliferative process.

Fisher JR, Padnick MB, Olstein S: Nifedipine and erythromelalgia. Ann Intern Med 98:671–672, 1983.

Nifedipine (Procardia 20 mg tid), a calcium-channel blocker, successfully relieved angina in a 44-year-old woman, but after eight weeks it induced erythromelalgia. Stopping the drug resulted in total clearing in 48 hours. Resumption of the drug later again produced the symptoms of burning pain and redness of her feet.

Eisler T, Hall RP, Kalavar KAR, Calne DB: Erythromelalgia-like eruption in parkinsonian patients treated with bromocriptine. Neurology 31:1368–1370, 1981.

Bromocriptine (Parlodel 100 mg daily for more than one year), an ergot alkaloid derivative with dopamine agonist properties, was proven responsible for erythromelalgia in 9 of 110 patients with Parkinson's disease. The symmetric tender warm areas of pain, erythema, and edema involuted within 10 days of stopping the drug and reappeared on challenge.

Monk BE, Parkes JD, Du Vivier A: Erythromelalgia following pergolide administration. Br J Dermatol 111:97–99, 1984.

Two patients with Parkinson's disease developed erythromelalgia of the shins 6 to 18 months after beginning treatment with **pergolide**, a powerful vasoconstricting ergot derivative. **Bromocriptine**, a similar ergoline, which is likewise a dopamine agonist, can have the same effect. Neither patient would discontinue the drug because of its beneficial effect on their parkinson's disease.

Jørgensen HP, Søndergaard J: Pathogenesis of erythromelalgia. Arch Dermatol 114:112–114, 1978.

In two patients with erythromelalgia, best results were achieved by elevating the legs and cooling the feet. **Aspirin** (3 gm/day) to inhibit prostaglandin synthesis was also of some help.

Hammar H: Plantar lesions of lichen sclerosus et atrophicus accompanied by erythermalgia. Acta Derm Venereol 58:91–92, 1978.

In a 52-year-old man, **aspirin** (3 gm/day, then tapering dose) gave complete relief of erythromelalgia, but had no effect on the lichen sclerosus et atrophicus.

Bada JL: Treatment of erythromelalgia with propranolol. Lancet 2:412, 1977.

Dramatic relief of erythromelalgia was achieved with beta-blockade of the adrenergic receptors using **propranolol** (Inderal 10 mg tid) in a 48-year-old woman who had suffered for 10 years.

Özsoylu S, Coskun T: Sodium nitroprusside treatment in erythromelalgia. Eur J Pediatr 141:185–187, 1984.

Two children with primary erythromelalgia were cured of their symptoms with **sodium nitroprusside** (Nipride IV 1 to 5 μg/kg/min for 48 and 120 hours, respectively). This drug, which has been used in treating ergotism, gave relief within three hours, and there was no recurrence in the following two years.

Putt AM: Erythromelalgia—A case for biofeedback. Nurs Clin North Am 13:625–630, 1978.

Training a female patient to relax promoted blood flow to her toes and aided management of incapacitating erythromelagia. Switching from polyester to cotton sheets also helped relieve symptoms at night.

Mandell F, Folkman J, Matsumoto S: Erythromelalgia. Pediatrics 59:45–48, 1977.

An 11-year-old Japanese girl had incapacitating erythromelalgia resistant to **hydantoin**, **reserpine**, **diazepam**, **chlorpromazine**, **carbamazine** and **phenobarbital**, as well as the commonly used **aspirin**, **methysergide**, and **prednisolone**. Her only relief came from submersion of her feet in ice water, contained in an ice bucket she carried with her.

Cohen IJK, Samorodin CS: Familial erythromelalgia. Arch Dermatol 118:953–954, 1982.

A 20-year-old brother and 14-year-old sister with primary erythromelalgia were not helped by **naproxen** (Naprosyn 250 mg tid), **aspirin** (650 mg q6h), or **dipyridamole** (Persantine 25 mg tid).

Some patients are compulsive gamblers and will continue to bet against incredible odds as long as you keep the betting window open.

Erythropoietic Protoporphyria

Beta-carotene	Transfusion
Canthaxanthin	Vitamin E
Cholestyramine	

Fortunately, patients with this rare error in heme metabolism can be accurately identified by laboratory study and effectively treated with a systemic "sunscreen," beta-carotene. This has consistently proven to be the best single therapy for these patients, but the dose must be adequate, and it must be given every day from April through August every year.

Chronic changes include shallow, waxy, pitted scars, which eventually develop over the nose, cheeks, and dorsal area of the hands, along with thickening and premature aging of the dorsal area of the hands. During sun exposure these patients experience itching and burning of the skin, followed within hours by erythema and edema of exposed skin.

Pathak MA, West JD: Porphyrias: Office procedures and laboratory tests for diagnosis of porphyrin abnormalities. Acta Derm Venerol (Suppl 100):91–105, 1982.

Precise directions for biochemically differentiating the entire set:

- erythropoietic protoporphyria
- erythropoietic porphyria
- porphyria cutanea tarda
- acute intermittent porphyria
- variegate porphyria
- hereditary coproporphyria

For erythropoietic protoporphyria:

Take a detailed family history.

Do a skin biopsy from a light-exposed area and PAS staining to see deposits around blood vessels in papillary dermis.

Obtain quantitative RBC and stool protoporphyrins.

Poh-Fitzpatrick MB: Erythropoietic protoporphyria. Int J Dermatol 17:359–369, 1978.

The specific therapy for this rare disease is beta-carotene (Solatene 30 to 60 mg qid). It must be given for one month before patients note increased light tolerance. Thus the drug should be started in April and stopped in late August. Protection from sunlight persists for a month after the drug is stopped.

For laboratory diagnosis, place 5 to 7 cc of blood in a heparinized tube, wrap the test tube in aluminum foil, and mail immediately for quantitative determination of RBC protoporphyrins. A thin blood smear may also be examined for RBC fluorescence under a fluorescence microscope with appropriate filters (details given).

Fusaro RM, Runge WJ: Erythropoietic protoporphyria. IV. Protection from sunlight. Br Med J 1:730–731, 1970.

Dihydroxyacetone (3 per cent) and **lawsone** (0.13 per cent) in a vanishing-cream base (applied at bedtime starting seven days prior to sun exposure) allowed patients to enjoy an outdoor environment. Presumably the dihydroxyacetone-**naphthoquinone** mixture structurally altered the keratin in the stratum corneum to reduce ultraviolet light penetration. Treated skin had a chemical color simulating a tan.

The same two chemicals in a 50 per cent isopropyl alcohol–water solution did *not* induce adequate light protection.

Eales L: The effects of canthaxanthin on the photocutaneous manifestations of porphyria. S Afr Med J 54:1050–1052, 1978.

Canthaxanthin (4,4-diketo-beta-carotene, 100 mg/day for six weeks) significantly improved sun tolerance in four of five adult patients and in two children with erythropoietic protoporphyria. It is preferred over **beta-carotene** because it gives a suntanned appearance, in contrast to a sickly yellow coloration.

Bloomer JR: Pathogenesis and therapy of liver disease in protoporphyria. Yale J Biol Med 52:39–48, 1979.

Cholestyramine resin (Questran 12 gm/day), to interrupt the enterohepatic circulation of protoporphyrin, and **vitamin E** (Aquasol E 100 U/day for 11 months), to decrease porphyrin production, dramatically reduced the lifelong photosensitivity of a 26-year-old housewife who had protoporphyria. Concomitantly there were a rapid drop in plasma protoporphyrin levels, improvement in liver function tests, and healing of the liver with decreased protoporphyrin deposits noted on liver biopsy after one year of therapy. Long-term therapy was continued.

Bechtel MA, Bertolone SJ, Hodge SJ: Transfusion therapy in a patient with erythropoietic protoporphyria. Arch Dermatol 117:99–101, 1981.

In an eight-year-old boy, transfusions with washed packed RBCs (1 unit, once a month, for five months) markedly decreased the free erythrocyte protoporphyrin levels and gave a 15-month clinical remission of photosensitivity. After exacerbation, three additional transfusions again gave clinical improvement. He had had two years of earlier success with beta-carotene (120 mg/day), but declined to continue it because of intractable diarrhea of uncertain etiology. Long-term use of transfusions is not warranted because of several risk factors, but infrequent, careful use of transfusions in childhood and adolescence may be helpful.

Romslo I, Gadeholt HG, Høvding G: Erythropoietic protoporphyria terminating in liver failure. Arch Dermatol 118:668–671, 1982.

Report of a seventeenth patient in the literature in whom progressive liver failure led to death. A 38-year-old man with erythropoietic protoporphyria developed cholestatic jaundice and rapidly deteriorating liver function. Treatment with **cholestyramine** resin (4 gm tid) and vitamin E (50 mg tid) made him feel better, but he died after two months from massive bleeding from esophageal varices.

Therapeutic serendipity favors the common disease over the rare.

Flushing

Dietary control	Indocin
Inderal	Pyridoxine
Antihistamines	Steroids
Aspirin	

Even as those who blush, patients who flush are at the mercy of their autonomic nervous system. Every emotion and every embarrassing thought can send a stream of impulses to actively dilate the vessels of the face, neck, and upper chest. These patients are not hyperemotional. Rather, their vessels are hypersensitive because of increased catecholamine in the nerve endings or increased beta-type adrenergic receptors in the muscle of the blood vessel walls.

We call this the adrenergic flush. Our therapy for it begins with Inderal (**propranolol** HCl 20 mg tid before meals), a drug tailored to block the beta-receptors. It is this drug that counters the same adrenergic-induced angina pectoris, migraine, and even stage fright. The dose is gradually increased to a therapeutic level, watching always for signs of intolerance. We cannot use it in patients with cardiac insufficiency, asthma, or the suspicion of a pheochromocytoma. If there is associated sweating, an additional or alternate treatment is the anticholinergic Pro-Banthine (**propantheline bromide** 15 mg tid).

If blocking the sympathetic nervous system is of no help, we proceed to blocking the non-neural mediators of vasodilatation, such as histamine and prostaglandin. We use conjoint **chlorpheniramine** (Chlor-Trimeton 4 mg) and **cimetidine** (Tagamet 200 mg) to achieve both H_1 and H_2 receptor blockade. If the antihistaminics prove inadequate, we prescribe **aspirin** coupled with **indomethacin** (Indocin) to block the prostaglandin synthetase. We prescribe Periactin (**cyproheptadine** HCl) for its antiserotoninergic action and **chlorpromazine** for its action against bradykinin. If no response is seen, steroids are ultimately tried in the form of Kenalog (40 mg IM).

Throughout all this, we instruct the patient to look for clues. He must recognize that many drugs can cause a flush. **Nicotinic acid**, sometimes hidden within a vitamin complex, is a prime example. Is the sun a factor? Does he realize that alcohol produces flushing? But more importantly, does he know that drugs, such as those used in treating diabetes, may produce a flush not noted with alcohol alone. Even certain mushrooms and, of course, Antabuse (**disulfiram**) can trigger this idiosyncratic alcohol flush. It apparently results from drugs depressing the acetaldehyde oxidase so that vasoactive levels of acetaldehyde build up when alcohol is consumed. Does he know that sulfites in salads, or nitrites in hot dogs can trigger flushing? And finally we alert him to the hazard of Accent, the monosodium glutamate seasoning so popular in Chinese cooking. Here, the best treatment is avoidance, although prophylactic **pyridoxine** (50 mg/day) can prevent the Chinese restaurant syndrome.

As the doorways close with still no view of the cause, we reach out for the rarities. Even the hyperendorphin syndrome must now come under consideration. We secure a skin biopsy and measure blood histamine and plasma catecholamines. We also test the urine for 5-HIAA and vasoactive intestinal polypeptide (VIP). We have radiographic studies for endocrine secretory tumors, such as bronchogenic carcinoma, pancreatic and carcinoid tumors, and VIPomas.

The search can be long and unrewarding, but serious unremitting episodic flushing demands that we look through the window of their skin at more than their thoughts and emotions.

Wilkin JK: Flushing reactions. *In* Rook AJ, Maibach HI (eds): Recent Advances in Dermatology, Number Six. London, Churchill Livingstone, 1983, pp 157–187.

A master source with everything from the fact that aspirin will block the nicotinic acid flush to the fact that a cold cup of coffee may make a rosacea patient wince but not flush.

Flushing produced by autonomic activity is associated with sweating. Vasoactive agents acting on vascular smooth muscle (without neural mediation) cause dry flushing.

I. *Flushing reactions related to alcohol:*
  - There is increased susceptibility in mongoloid populations.
  - Occupational "degreasers'"flush occurs in workmen drinking beer after exposure to industrial solvents:
    - trichloroethylene vapor
    - N,N-dimethylformamide
    - N-butyraldoxime
  - Fermented alcoholic beverages (beer, sherry) may contain tyramine or histamine, which induce flushing.
  - Drugs
    - disulfiram (Antabuse)
    - **chlorpropamide** (Diabinese)
    - **calcium carbamide** (urea)
    - **phentolamine** (Regitine)
    - **griseofulvin**
    - **metronidazole** (Flagyl)
    - β-lactams with methyltetrazolethiol side chain (cephalosporin antibiotics)
      - **cefamanadole** (Mandol)
      - **cefoperazone** (Cefobid)
      - **moxalactam** (Moxam)
  - Eating mushrooms
  - Carcinoid flushing—Alcohol may release a catecholamine that acts on tumor cells.

II. *Flushing related to food additives:*
  - Monosodium glutamate (MSG) in a large dose may cause Chinese restaurant syndrome.
  - Sodium nitrite in cured meats (frankfurters, bacon, salami, ham) may cause headache and flushing.
  - Sulfites (potassium metabisulfite) may cause wheezing and flushing.

III. *Flushing associated with eating:*
  - Hot beverages cause flushing through countercurrent heat exchange into blood vessels leading to the anterior hypothalamus.
  - Auriculotemporal flushing: unilateral flushing, heat, and sweating following parotid gland injury with misdirected regeneration of parasympathetic nerves.
    - Treatment:
      - Avoid cheese, chocolate, lemon, highly spiced foods.
      - Apply scopolamine or atropine in a cream base.
  - Gustatory flushing: bilateral flushing, salivation, sweating, lacrimation, and

nasal secretion with no history of parotid gland injury. This may be reproduced by chewing a chili pepper (*Capsicum minimum*) and holding it in the mouth for five minutes.

Treatment:

Avoid eating chili peppers and washing red chili peppers (as the active chemical, capsaicin, may be absorbed through abraded fingertips).

Cool the body temperature.

Dumping syndrome: Facial flushing is associated with tachycardia, sweating, dizziness, weakness, and gastrointestinal disturbances. Symptoms begin after gastric surgery and are provoked by a meal or ingestion of hot fluids or hypertonic glucose. The syndrome becomes worse with menopause.

IV. *Neurologic flushing:*

anxiety
simple blushing
brain tumors
spinal cord lesions (autonomic hyperreflexia)
orthostatic hypotension
migraine headaches
Parkinson's disease

V. *Flushing due to drugs:*

all vasodilators (e.g., nitroglycerin)
all calcium channel blockers:
  nifedipine (Procardia)
  verapamil (Calan)
  diltiazem (Cardizem)
nicotinic acid (not nicotinamide)
  may block flush with **aspirin** and **indomethacin**
morphine
amyl nitrite and **butyl nitrite** (recreational drugs)
cholinergic drugs
  e.g., **metrifonate**, an anthelminthic (not available in the United States)
  may block flush with **atropine**
bromocriptine (Parlodel) used in Parkinson's disease
thyrotropin-releasing hormone (TRH)
tamoxifen (Nolvadex)
cyproterone acetate
oral **triamcinolone** used with psoriatic arthritis
cyclosporin A (Sandimmune)

Wilkin JK: Flushing reactions: Consequences and mechanisms. Ann Intern Med 95:468–476, 1981.

The transient vasodilatation of flushing is mediated through nerves or local vasodilators. Inappropriate alcohol flushing suggests that the patient is taking a drug (e.g., **cephalosporins**, **griseofulvin**), working with the solvent trichloroethylene, eating mushrooms, or has a tumor (carcinoid, carcinoma of the thyroid, mastocytosis).

Waldhäusl W: To flush or not to flush? Comments on the chlorpropamide-alcohol flush. Diabetologia 26:12–14, 1984.

The following are the real or putative vasoactive mediators for flushing:

histamine	kallikrein
prostaglandins	lysyl-bradykinin
serotonin	met-enkephalin
acetaldehyde	substance P

Each deserves continuing therapeutic attention.

Mulley GP: Flushing. J R Coll Physicians Lond 12:359–364, 1978.

Look for tumors producing catecholamines, vasoactive hormones, or other mediators, e.g., pheochromocytoma, bronchogenic carcinoma, pancreatic tumor, thyroid medullary carcinoma.

Ginsburg J: Flushes in women—and men. Br Med J 287:242–243, 1983.

The beta-blocker **propranolol** (Inderal) is mentioned as one of a number of empiric remedies to try.

Prichard BNC, McDevitt DG, Shanks RG: Uses of beta-adrenoceptor blocking drugs. J R Coll Physicians Lond 11:35–57, 1976.

Propranolol (Inderal 20 mg tid to 1000 mg qid) also has a dramatic effect on reducing the somatic expressions of anxiety, tachycardia, and tremors. It is not to be used in patients with asthma or cardiac insufficiency.

Groop L, Eriksson CJP, Huupponen R, et al: Roles of chlorpropamide, alcohol and acetaldehyde in determining the chlorpropamide-alcohol flush. Diabetologia 26:34–38, 1984.

In the body, alcohol is metabolized to acetaldehyde, a powerful vasodilator. Drugs such as **chlorpropamide** inhibit the enzymatic oxidase responsible for removal of this acetaldehyde. Thus, reducing either the intake of alcohol or the dosage of drug can provide relief from this type of flushing.

Moral: Drink less or drug less.

Tan OT, Stafford TJ, Sarkany I, et al: Suppression of alcohol-induced flushing by a combination of H_1 and H_2 histamine antagonists. Br J Dermatol 107:647–652, 1982.

The combination of **cimetidine** (200 mg) and **chlorpheniramine** (4 mg), taken 30 minutes prior to drinking alcohol, eliminated the flush of sherry (1 ml/kg), apparently by reducing the rate of absorption of the alcohol. Larger amounts of alcohol overcame the suppressive effect of the medications and induced flushing.

Wilkin JK: Oral thermal-induced flushing in erythematotelangiectatic rosacea. J Invest Dermatol 76:15–18, 1981.

Neither cool coffee (180 ml) nor caffeine (200 mg) at 22°C (72°F) produced flushing, whereas both hot coffee and plain water at 60°C (140°F) induced flushing. A careful study of 24 subjects.

Mulley G, Mitchell JRA: Menopausal flushing: Does oestrogen therapy make sense? Lancet 1:1397–1398, 1976.

A tightly reasoned position paper speaks against the mindless traditional use of estrogens for hot flashes. This problem, hard to grade and occurring in a group richly populated with placebo responders, deserves more than hand-jerk prescription writing for a potentially harmful hormone.

Clayden JR, Bell JW, Pollard P: Menopausal flushing: Double-blind trial of a non-hormonal medication. Br Med J 1:409–412, 1974.

Although a pronounced placebo effect was seen in this series of 100 patients, **clonidine** (25 to 75 μg bid), an alpha-adrenergic agonist, did have a demonstrably significant effect in controlling the number, severity, and duration of flushes.

Sturdee DW, Wilson KA, Pipili E, Crocker AD: Physiological aspects of menopausal hot flush. Br Med J 2:79–80, 1978.

Hot flushes in 11 menopausal women were associated with evidence of sudden transient increases in sympathetic drive, including peripheral vasodilatation, acute rise in skin temperature, increase in heart rate, and decrease in skin resistance. (An ideal area for Inderal therapy!)

Wilkin JK: Climacteric flushing in a patient with carcinoid tumor. Br J Dermatol 112:357–361, 1985.

In a 70-year-old man, orchiectomy for adenocarcinoma of the prostate was followed by frequent flushing attacks. **Diethylstilbestrol** (2 mg/day orally for six weeks) gave rapid complete remission of the flushing attacks. A non-functioning carcinoid tumor found in the midgut proved to be irrelevant to the flushing, showing that carcinoid flushing requires biochemical confirmation, not just tissue identification.

Eaton AC, McGuire N: Cyproterone acetate in treatment of post-orchiectomy hot flushes: Double-blind cross-over trial. Lancet 2:1336–1337, 1983.

Cyproterone acetate (100 mg tid), an androgen receptor blocker (not available in the United States), was of distinct value in 12 men with carcinoma of the prostate and surgically induced climacteric flushing. Orchiectomy in men causes a sudden reduction in sex steroids, with resulting vasomotor dysfunction similar to that of menopausal women.

Folkers K, Shizukuishi S, Willis R, et al: The biochemistry of vitamin B_6 is basic to the cause of the Chinese restaurant syndrome. Hoppe Seylers Z Physiol Chem 365:405–414, 1984.

Pyridoxine (vitamin B_6 50 mg/day for three months) prevented the facial flushing, burning, and pressure of the glutamate-mediated Chinese restaurant syndrome, as proven in 12 volunteers by a double-blind challenge with 6 gm monosodium glutamate. Individuals susceptible to Chinese restaurant syndrome apparently have a subclinical pyridoxine deficiency. Correction of this by supplemental pyridoxine should permit them to enjoy glutamate (Accent)-seasoned Chinese food without discomfort. This includes won ton soup (the main culprit).

Goldstein DJ, Keiser HR: A case of episodic flushing and organic psychosis: Reversal by opiate antagonists. Ann Intern Med 98:30–34, 1983.

In a 29-year-old woman, episodic attacks of flushing associated with psychiatric symptoms and skin, bone, and abdominal pain resolved within 1 minute of **naloxone** (Narcan 0.4 mg IV) or within 20 minutes of **naltrexone** (50 to 200 mg by mouth).

Melmon KL, Sjoerdsma A, Mason DT: Distinctive clinical and therapeutic aspects of the syndrome associated with bronchial carcinoid tumors. Am J Med 39:568–581, 1965.

In two women with carcinoid, flushing was completely controlled with **prednisone** (15 mg daily on a long-term basis).

Rosenstein BJ, Engelman K: Diarrhea in a child with catecholamine-secreting ganglioneuroma: Case report and review of the literature. J Pediatr 63:217–226, 1963.

Marked flushing and diarrhea in a 15-month-old boy was cured by surgical removal of the responsible catecholamine-secreting tumor of sympathetic ganglion cells lying above one adrenal gland.

Bednarek J, Reid W, Matsumoto T: Frey's syndrome. Am J Surg 131:592–594, 1976.

Gustatory sweating and flushing of the right cheek, which started eight months after parotid surgery in a 57-year-old woman, was controlled with **atropine** cream (0.5 per cent applied every morning to the affected area). She had previously been helped by **acetylsalicylic acid** (10 grains daily) and **scopolamine** cream (3 per cent applied every morning), but had developed dizziness, tachycardia, fainting, and contact allergy from the scopolamine.

Mooney E: The flushing patient. Int J Dermatol 24:549–554, 1985.

A comprehensive review (69 references) with further valuable insights:

Xylene or carbon disulfide exposure favors alcohol flushing.

Chloramphenicol and quinacrine are medications associated with the alcohol flush.

Patients with horseshoe kidneys experience flushing, nausea, and pain (Rovsing syndrome), which are relieved by an antiflexed position.

Flushing may signal the presence of rare tumors, such as malignant histiocytoma, neuroblastoma, ganglioneuroma, renal cell carcinoma, or basophilic granulocytic leukemia.

When it comes to appointments, if the patient thinks it's an emergency, it is an emergency.

Once trouble comes, you will find the "informed consent" was signed by a patient who was never fully informed and never fully consented.

Folliculitis

Antimicrobial soaps	Accutane
Xerac AC	Chlor-Trimeton
Antibiotics	Aquasol A
Ketoconazole	

The clinical diagnosis of folliculitis is not a reliable guide to therapy. One needs to study the history, distribution, and prior response to therapy. Furthermore, bacterial cultures and a skin biopsy may be necessary to direct effective treatment.

The banal form on the back or buttocks, induced by *Staphylococcus aureus*, deserves daily cleansing of the body surface with a commercial antibacterial bar soap or prescription antimicrobial liquid soap (pHisoHex, Hibiclens, or Desquam-X 5 Wash). To further reduce the surface bacterial flora and the sweating that favors their growth, we use Xerac AC (6.25 per cent aluminum chloride hexahydrate in anhydrous ethyl alcohol) applied to the area each night. If the skin is dry, a preparation such as Neosporin ointment or Silvadene cream is helpful. We usually also start systemic erythromycin (1 gm daily).

If the culture shows a specific pathogen, sensitivity studies may clearly indicate the appropriate systemic antibiotic. For gram-negative folliculitis, ampicillin has been our general weapon, and now Accutane provides a powerful alternative approach. *Pityrosporum* folliculitis, common on the oily areas of the chest, responds to Selsun shampoo or systemic Nizoral. One of our patients, with folliculitis for six years, experienced dramatic resolution of his problem within a week of starting oral Nizoral (200 mg/day). If the culture shows no growth, a search must be made elsewhere as to the cause and cure. Particularly misleading are cases of folliculitis due to contactants, acting as either primary irritants or sensitizers. Industrial greases and oils are notorious hazards in this respect. We have also seen chemical allergens in powder form specifically localize in the hair follicles, producing a focal contact dermatitis presenting as folliculitis. Oral vitamin A (Aquasol A 50,000 IU tid) or Accutane (20 to 80 mg/day) is valuable for "cleaning-out" these hair follicles and restoring normal keratinization. Dapsone (100 mg/day) may also help to reduce the neutrophil component of the folliculitis.

Systemic causes are rare but significant, including ulcerative colitis and hemodialysis. We also see a folliculitis of pregnancy clearing at the time of delivery.

All in all, a seemingly banal, yet wretchedly chronic, folliculitis can be a tremendous challenge to your therapeutic skills.

Marzulli FN, Bruch M: Antimicrobial soaps: Benefits versus risks. *In* Maibach HI, Aly R (eds): Skin Microbiology Relevance to Clinical Infection. New York, Springer-Verlag, 1981, pp 125–134.

Currently available bar soaps have broad gram-positive and gram-negative antimicrobial action:

Dial (1.5 per cent triclocarban)
Coast (triclocarban)

Irish Spring (0.75 per cent triclocarbon, 0.25 per cent triclosan)
Safeguard (1.5 per cent triclocarban)
Zest (triclocarban)

Taplin D: Antibacterial soaps: Chlorhexidine and skin infections. *In* Maibach HI, Aly R (eds): Skin Microbiology: Relevance to Clinical Infection. New York, Springer-Verlag, 1981, pp 113–124.

pHisoHex (3 per cent **hexachlorophene**) and Hibiclens (4 per cent **chlorhexidine gluconate**) both reduced new skin infections. However, pHisoHex was ineffective against gram-negative organisms.

Lowbury EJL: Topical antimicrobials: Perspectives and issues. *In* Maibach HI, Aly R (eds): Skin Microbiology Relevance to Clinical Infection. New York, Springer-Verlag, 1981, pp 158–168.

Although simple washing with a detergent or applying 70 per cent alcohol greatly reduces the number of bacteria on skin, there is 99 per cent removal after six washings with Betadine (10 per cent **povidone-iodine**), Hibiclens, or pHisoHex. Hibiclens proved to be the most effective.

Shelley WB, Hurley HJ: Anhydrous formulation of aluminum chloride for chronic folliculitis. JAMA 244:1956–1957, 1980.

Single daily application of 6.25 per cent **aluminum chloride hexahydrate** in absolute ethyl alcohol (Xerac AC) cleared all five cases of antibiotic-resistant chronic folliculitis of the buttocks within two weeks. Similar results on the chest, but not on the scalp. Modus operandi: Kills bacteria and inhibits sweating.

Leyden JJ, Marples RR, Mills OH, Kligman AM: Gram-negative folliculitis—A complication of antibiotic therapy in acne vulgaris. Br J Dermatol 88:533–538, 1973.

Fifty cases (out of 1200 acne patients) due to use of antibiotics and hexachlorophene, which allowed overgrowth of gram-negative organisms. **Ampicillin** (1 gm/day for two weeks, then maintenance dose) was the drug of choice.

Plewig G, Nikolowski T, Wolff HH: Action of isotretinoin in acne rosacea and gram-negative folliculitis. J Am Acad Dermatol 6:766–785, 1982.

Gram-negative folliculitis (13 cases): Dramatic, consistent response with disappearance of lesions, as well as organisms, from both skin and reservoir site of nasal mucosa. Bacteria die as mucosa becomes dry. The **isotretinoin** (Accutane 40 to 80 mg/day) was given for three to six months.

Leyden JJ, McGinley KJ, Mills OH: *Pseudomonas aeruginosa* gram-negative folliculitis. Arch Dermatol 115:1203–1204, 1979.

Source: otitis externa
Treatment: Cortisporin otic drops (bid), acetic acid compresses (1 per cent tid), Cortisporin cream (bid)
Cure: three patients

Gustafson TL, Band JD, Hutcheson RH, Schaffner W: *Pseudomonas* folliculitis: An outbreak and review. Rev Infect Dis 5:1–8, 1983.

Alkaline, hypochlorinated whirlpool bath water was the origin of *Pseudomonas aeruginosa*. Folliculitis specifically involved apocrine sweat glands (axillae, glands of Montgomery of breast). Made worse with steroids, but healed spontaneously. Watch for associated green nails, otitis externa, and toe web intertrigo. Lists 39 references.

Potter BS, Burgoon CF, Johnson WC: *Pityrosporum* folliculitis: Report of seven cases and review of the *Pityrosporum* organism relative to cutaneous disease. Arch Dermatol 107:388–391, 1973.

Widespread follicular pustules and papules on back and chest responded to appplication twice a day of: 2 per cent **salicylic acid**, 5 per cent **benzoic acid**, and 20 per cent **isopropyl alcohol** in hydrophilic ointment.

Berretty PJM, Neumann HAM, Hulsebosch JH: Folliculitis door pityrosporum-organism geinduceerd. Ned Tijdschr Geneeskd 124:1818–1821, 1980.

Favors Selsun shampoo, but good results also with MicaTin cream or sodium thiosulfate.

Neumann HAM, Berretty PJM: Treatment of *Pityrosporum* folliculitis with ketoconazole (R41400). Mykosen 24:167–171, 1981.

Eight cases cleared within three weeks of systemic Nizoral therapy.

Ford GP, Ive FA, Midgley G: *Pityrosporum* folliculitis and ketoconazole. Br J Dermatol 107:691–695, 1982.

Twelve patients were given Nizoral (200 mg/day) for three weeks: 10 cases were cleared; 2 were helped. Rapid relapse on stopping: Required maintenance dose of 200 mg twice weekly.

Maibach HI: Scalp pustules due to *Corynebacterium acnes*. Arch Dermatol 96:453–455, 1967.

Six cases responded to **tetracycline** (1 gm/day). One required maintenance dosage (500 mg/day) for four years.

Cutler TP: Eosinophilic pustular folliculitis. Clin Exp Dermatol 6:327–332, 1981.

Case report: Widespread pruritic pustular folliculitis on trunk, buttocks, and proximal limbs of a young Chinese man. Associated with eosinophilia (26 per cent), lesions sterile. Required systemic steroids and maintenance **erythromycin** (500 mg/day).

Anderson KE, Petri M: Occupational irritant contact folliculitis associated with triphenyl tin fluoride (TPTF) exposure. Contact Dermatitis 8:173–177, 1982.

In marine paint plant worker.

Heckman BH: Jeans folliculitis. N Engl J Med 305:525, 1981.

Six cases due to working, dancing, and jogging in ultratight jeans. Cure: Res ipse loquitor.

Rifkin A, Kurtin SB, Quitkin F, Klein DF: Lithium-induced folliculitis. Am J Psychol 130:1018–1019, 1973.

Folliculitis developed in 12 patients after taking lithium for 1 to 12 months. Three cases cleared when lithium was stopped.

Burkhart CH: Perforating folliculitis: A reappraisal of its pathogenesis. Int J Dermatol 20:597–599, 1981.

Case Report: Responded to intralesional steroid.

White CR, Heskel NS, Pokorny DJ: Perforating folliculitis of hemodialysis. Am J Dermatopathol 4:109–116, 1982.

Three patients with perforating folliculitis lesions on legs after beginning hemodialysis for chronic renal failure. All resistant to treatment. One case cleared when hemodialysis was stopped after renal transplant.

Zoberman E, Farmer ER: Pruritic folliculitis of pregnancy. Arch Dermatol 117:20–22, 1981.

Six cases, onset in fourth to ninth month of pregnancy, cleared spontaneously after delivery.

O'Loughlin S, Perry HO: A diffuse pustular eruption associated with ulcerative colitis. Arch Dermatol 114:1061–1064, 1978.

Diffuse sterile pustular eruption in two patients. Biopsy: suppurative folliculitis. Improved with IV systemic steroids and antibiotic therapy of colitis, but cleared only after colectomy.

Jung LKL, Engelhard D, Kapoor N, Pitt K, Good RA: Pyoderma, eczema and folliculitis with defective leukocyte and lymphocyte function: A new familial immunodeficiency disease responsive to a histamine-1 antagonist. Lancet 2:185–187, 1983.

Dramatic response of both father and son with atopic eczema to simple **chlorpheniramine** (Chlor-Trimeton 4 mg q6h). No response to **cimetidine**, the H_2 blocker.

Owen WR, Wood C: Disseminate and recurrent infundibulofolliculitis. Arch Dermatol 115:174–175, 1979.

Vitamin A (50,000 IU bid) greatly helped five of six black patients with diffuse pruritic follicular papules in four to six weeks.

Steffen C: Eosinophilic pustular folliculitis (Ofuji's disease) with response to dapsone therapy. Arch Dermatol 121:921–923, 1985.

Dapsone (100 mg/day for two weeks) completely cleared this sterile pustular rash on the face of a 50-year-old man.

The drug is not the variable; the patient is.

Folliculitis Keloidalis

Selsun	Intralesional steroids
Drysol	Surgery
Vleminckx' solution	Vitamin A
Antibiotics	Accutane

Folliculitis keloidalis is an orphan in the literature of therapy. There are no grand reviews, no controlled studies. We are left with clinical improvisation based on an awareness that this chronic progressive disease of the black male and female occiput is a mixture of bacterial folliculitis, ingrown hairs, and keloids.

We center our attack initially on the folliculitis. Scrupulous cleanliness with daily shampoo is mandatory. Our favorite is Selsun because of its powerful antibacterial action. Each night anhydrous aluminum chloride solution in the form of Drysol is applied to the area. If the area is tender we prescribe Vleminckx' solution compresses (sublimed sulfur) or Vlemasque (6 per cent sulfurated lime topical solution) for 20 minutes each day. Systemic antibacterial therapy (erythromycin or minocycline) is regularly employed on a long-term basis. If tenderness and inflammation are not easily curbed, we extend the antibiotic spectrum to dicloxacillin, metronidazole, and ketoconazole. Alternate topical preparations include benzoyl peroxide (Desquam-X 10 gel), Neosporin cream, and Silvadene cream.

The ingrown hair factor is best controlled by seeing that tne area is never shaved. Curving ingrowing hairs should be mechanically removed, and often the patient's family can be persuaded to do this on a once-a-week basis.

The most formidable feature is the follicular keloid formation that gradually becomes a massive pebbly growth. In the early cases after the bacterial infection has been cleared, the nightly application of a potent fluorinated steroid ointment such as Diprolene (betamethasone dipropionate 0.05 per cent) is advisable to induce atrophy of the follicular scars. If the keloid formation is marked, injections of triamcinolone acetonide suspension (Kenalog 10 mg/ml or 40 mg/ml) has a marked "debulking" effect. Surgical excision remains the treatment of choice for advanced examples. As in all keloids, however, there may be postsurgical recurrence.

Finally, Aquasol A (50,000 IU tid for three months) may help calm the folliculitis. Accutane also holds promise for the early stage in view of its remarkable curative effect of gram-negative folliculitis.

Hollander L: Treatment of folliculitis keloidalis chronica nuchae (acne keloid). Arch Dermatol 64:639-640, 1951.

In the past, cryosurgery, electrolysis, electrocoagulation, intralesional **penicillin**, x-ray, and oral **stilbestrol** were all of little avail. Massive electrodesiccation, described in this report, gave satisfactory results in two patients.

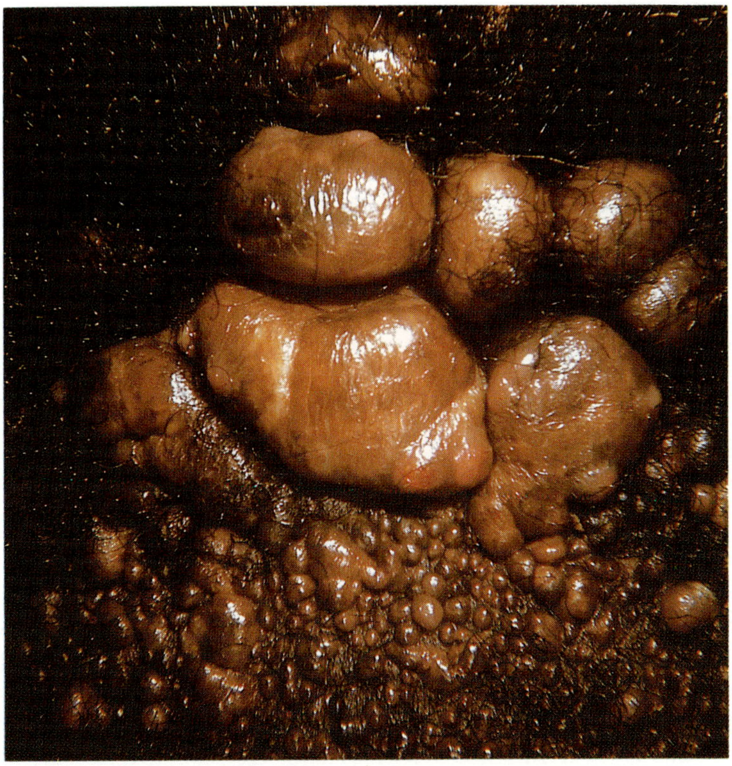

Kenney JA: Management of dermatoses peculiar to Negroes. Arch Dermatol 91:126-129, 1965.

The still modern approach is manual depilation, intralesional steroids, local and systemic antibiotics, and excision of scar tissue down to the skin surface level.

Cosman B, Wolff M: Acne keloidalis. Plast Reconstr Surg 50:25-30, 1972.

Recommends wide excision with skin grafts, but in 50 per cent of 14 cases new keloids developed within an average of eight months.

Malherbe WDF: Sycosis nuchae and its surgical treatment. Plast Reconstr Surg 47:269-271, 1971.

Advises excision with primary closure, although the large size of the defect means that the patient's head must be bent backward for closure, and the neck is very tight at first (one patient requested a good book on astronomy). Excellent results in eight cases over five-year follow-up. Better cosmetic result than skin grafting.

Vasily DB, Breen PC, Miller OF III: Acne keloidalis nuchae: Report and treatment of a severe case. J Dermatol Surg Oncol 5:228-230, 1979.

One case with many sinus tracts was cured by surgical excision down to the erector spinae and trapezius muscles of the neck, followed by a split-thickness skin graft.

Not bathing is the poor man's antipruritic.

Foreign Bodies

Tweezers	Paper clip
Razor blade	String
Face mask	Lidocaine
Suction tube	

Foreign bodies range from the visible to the invisible, from the gross to the microscopic. If the patient has not succeeded in removing the object or in recognizing the source of tenderness and pain, it is your challenge. Often the patient is unaware of a foreign body having entered the skin. As an example, we removed an unsuspected plant stem 7 cm long from the foot of a woman who had been limping for two months following a hike in the Scottish Highlands. Once we also removed a triangular fragment of glass from the sole of a patient in whom the shadow of the glass had been seen on x-ray examination, but disregarded as an emulsion defect. (When we saw him he was on crutches, having had unsuccessful surgery for what was viewed as a glomus tumor.)

The most common problem involves bristles, tiny spines, or splinters embedded in the thick stratum corneum of the sole. Here, we use the Gillette Super Blue Blade to free the object, which is then lifted out by lateral traction or with an ultrafine Swiss jeweler's tweezer (Dumont, pattern 5, 4⅜ inches, stainless, Roboz Surgical Instrument Co., 1000 Connecticut Ave., Washington, DC 20036). The removal of any foreign body brings instant relief of pain to the patient and delight to the physician for an "instant cure."

Putnam MH: Simple cactus spine removal. J Pediatr 98:333, 1981.

Several thousand cactus spines were embedded in the skin of a 22-month-old boy who fell into a household plant. Tweezer and tape techniques were inadequate and painful.

Avon's Aloe Smooth Peel-off facial mask was applied to all areas involved. After 20 minutes in front of a large fan, the mask dried and was peeled off, removing several hundred spines. Eight successive painless peels cleared most areas, and the "game of pat, propeller, and peel" was enjoyed by the child.

Lawton MB: Resourceful women unmask cactus spines. JAMA 253:2830, 1985.

Method of removing fiberglass and multiple tiny redwood slivers in the skin:

Generously apply a peel-off type of facial mask.
Air dry for five minutes.
Peel off mask to extract slivers.

Gelbard MK: Removal of small cactus spines from the skin. JAMA 252:3368, 1984.

Apply a thick layer of woodworking glue (white, water soluble), cover with a piece of linen, and dry for 30 minutes. Then peel off linen and glue layer, extracting the spines.

Deeken JH: Tape treatment for fiberglass splinters. Arch Dermatol 114:623, 1978.

Fiberglass splinters in the hands and forearm from installing home insulation are easily extracted by applying the extremely adhesive plumber's duct tape directly to the affected areas.

Shelley WB, Pillsbury DM: Fingertip hyperesthesia: Solitary sign of new occupational dermatosis due to silica hair curlers. JAMA 170:1779–1781, 1959.

Unexplained fingertip hyperesthesia in a 40-year-old hairdresser was viewed by a succession of physicians as being possibly due to glomangiomas, peripheral neuritis, peripheral vascular disease, acrodynia, cervical rib syndrome, spinal cord lesion, syringomyelia, tumor, malingering, or hysteria. The correct diagnosis proved to be a foreign body reaction: Particles of silica had become embedded in the superficial skin as a result of using sand-coated hair curlers. Cure was achieved by superficial razor blade tangential excision of the subepidermal and epidermal skin of the fingertips.

Shelley WB: Fingertip hyperesthesia due to scouring pad. JAMA 215:1503, 1971.

In a 44-year-old housewife, roentgenogram revealed wire fragments in the tip of the right index finger, which had been tender for four months. Only then could the patient relate the problem to the use of steel wool scouring pads.

Baruch AD, Haas A: Injury to the hand with metallic mercury. J Hand Surg 9A:446–448, 1984.

A suction catheter (fine 10 cm long, curved Baron suction tube) was used during surgical exploration of the hand for immediate removal of mercury in the skin of two patients following broken-thermometer accidents. Check the wound areas with postoperative roentgenograms and also check lung roentgenograms for mercury emboli.

Thompson MP: Removing objects from the external auditory canal. N Engl J Med 311:1635, 1984.

Traditional devices: wire loop curette, alligator forceps, suction
Thompson device: a paper clip. Under otoscope visualization, make contact with the object, using the tip of a straightened wire paper clip that has been moistened with a rapidly drying glue (cyanoacrylate—less than 1 drop). Allow glue to dry for a few seconds and slowly withdraw the attached object. Especially good for small hard objects such as a plastic bead.

Brauer EW, Leider M: How to unhook persons hooked on fishhooks. J Dermatol Surg Oncol 6:668–669, 1980.

Tie a string on the free curve of the fishhook, so that the buried tip and barb are repositioned into the line of entry. Pull the string firmly to extract the barb back through the path it entered into the skin. If the barb has passed out through the skin, simply clip it off and use the same removal technique for the remainder of the hook. Don't forget the need for a tetanus booster and possible antibiotics.

Benforado JM: Removal of ticks. JAMA 252:3368, 1984.

1. Warm the tip of a large eight- to ten-penny size nail in a match flame.
2. Slide a flat knife blade under the tick's abdomen.
3. Place the heated nail tip on the dorsal surface of the tick.
4. When the tick's legs wiggle, turn the knife blade 90 degrees to stand the tick on its head.
5. Keeping the tick between the nail tip and knife blade, lift the blade, tick, and nail away from the skin. The trick is to get the tick to open its mouth in pain and thereby ensure a perfect "lift off." Try to annoy the tick, rather than roast it.

O'Toole K, Paris PM, Stewart RD, Martinez R: Removing cockroaches from the auditory canal: Controlled trial. N Engl J Med 312: 1197, 1985.

Simply spray 2 per cent **lidocaine** solution into the canal and the roach will instantly exit. You don't even need to yell "Fire." (Mineral oil killed the roach in the opposite ear, but subsequent removal of the creature proved difficult.)

Andrus CH: Instrument and technique for removal of subungual foreign bodies. Am J Surg 140:588, 1980.

An 18-gauge needle is an effective instrument for transungual removal of foreign bodies when the nail plate has been separated from the nail bed by fluid or trauma. Cut 2-mm windows with an 18-gauge disposable needle, using the needle as a small scalpel blade. Windowing of the nail plate may be done without anesthesia, and the foreign body may be lifted out with fine forceps.

Needham GR: Evaluation of five popular methods for tick removal. Pediatrics 75:997–1002, 1985.

Recommendations:

Tweezer or shielded fingers.
Grasp entire tick.
Use straight upward, steady, even pull.
Never use bare hands or crush tick, since it may harbor infectious agents.

Needham does not favor the four other methods: hot match, isopropyl alcohol, fingernail polish, or petroleum jelly.

Cantrell H: More on removing cockroaches from the auditory canal. N Engl J Med 314:720, 1986.

Cantrell prefers mineral oil for removal, since lidocaine spray will induce an alarming, although temporary, vertigo should the patient have even a tiny perforation of the eardrum, allowing entrance of the anesthetic into the middle ear cavity.

I always use the newest medicines quickly before their effectiveness runs out.

Sir William Osler

Fox-Fordyce Disease

Retin-A cream	UVL
Accutane	Dermabrasion
Enovid	Electrocoagulation
Corticosteroids	Excision

Shelley WB: Treatment of Fox-Fordyce disease. JAMA 222:1069, 1972.

The cornerstone of therapy has been the systemic contraceptive, such as Enovid (**norethynodrel** + **mestranol**), but isolated cases have been helped or cured by dermabrasion, surgical excision, intralesional **triamcinolone acetonide** (10 mg/ml), and tranquilizers. For many women the cure has to await the arrival of menopause. (Fourteen years later, we can add our new success: **Isotretinoin** [Accutane 40 mg bid for three months] cleared a 29-year-old male patient of Fox-Fordyce disease.)

Giacobetti R, Caro WA, Roenigk HH Jr: Fox-Fordyce disease: Control with tretinoin cream. Arch Dermatol 115:1365–1366, 1979.

Tretinoin cream (Retin-A 0.1 per cent, every other evening for four weeks) was associated with markedly reduced pruritus, mild regression of papules, and considerable regrowth of axillary hair in a 21-year-old woman with Fox-Fordyce disease for three years. The same therapy was required as maintenance to control pruritus.

Helfman RJ: A new treatment of Fox-Fordyce disease. South Med J 55:681–684, 1962.

A 17-year-old black female with Fox-Fordyce disease of the axillae for three years had complete resolution of all lesions following nine injections of **triamcinolone acetonide** to the right axilla given over a three-month period. The control left axilla showed no change. Relief of symptoms immediately followed the first injection of triamcinolone acetonide (Kenalog 10 mg/ml, 0.5 ml diluted with equal volume of 1 per cent lidocaine, given at each of four sites). There was residual hypopigmentation, but no atrophy at the site of lesions.

Pinkus H: Treatment of Fox-Fordyce disease. JAMA 223:924, 1973.

Several patients experienced long-lasting remissions following erythema doses of ultraviolet light therapy (hot quartz given once weekly for four to six weeks). The dosage level to produce exfoliation presumably unplugs the horny material and opens the apocrine ducts. Talc was used for relief of sunburn, with avoidance of ointments, creams, and deodorants.

Kronthal HL, Pomeranz JR, Sitomer G: Fox-Fordyce disease: Treatment with an oral contraceptive. Arch Dermatol 91:243–245, 1965.

Norethynodrel plus **mestranol** (Enovid given on days 5 through 25 of each cycle) was extremely effective in controlling pruritus and inducing the resolution of papules in two women with Fox-Fordyce disease. The therapeutic result is similar to that seen during pregnancy.

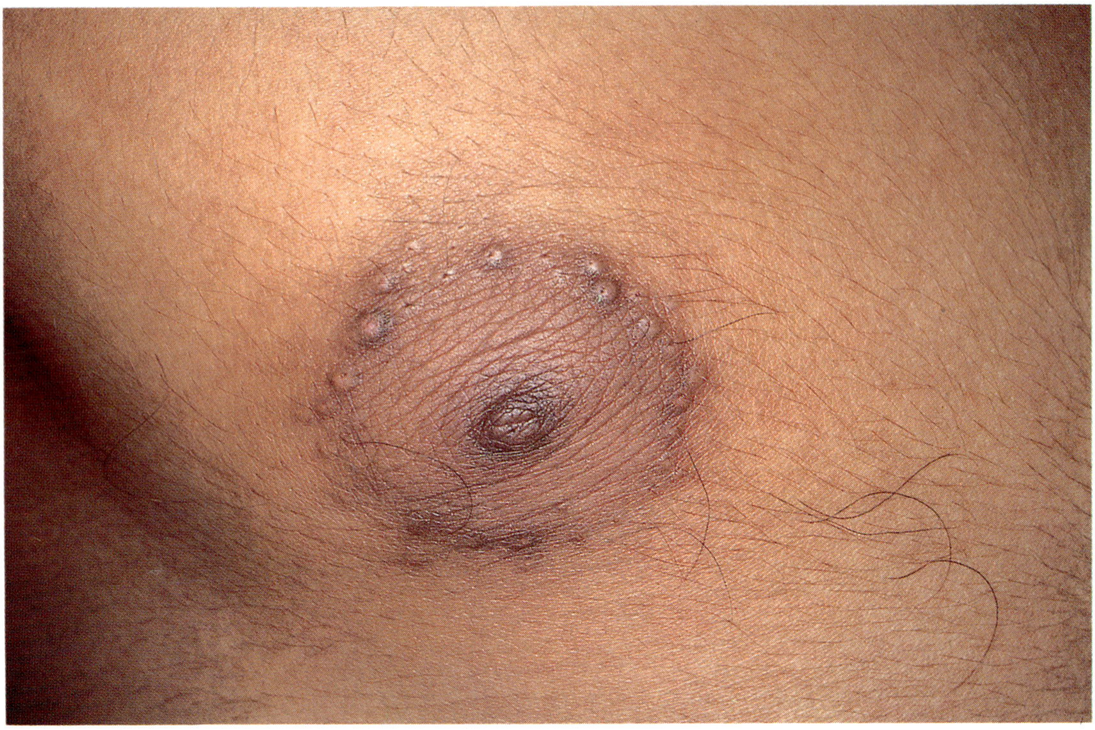

Pasricha JS, Nayyar KC: Fox-Fordyce disease in the post-menopausal period treated successfully with electrocoagulation. Dermatologica 147:271–273, 1973.

A report of two postmenopausal women (ages 50 and 46) with recent onset of extremely pruritic papules, who had complete clearing as a result of electrocoagulation of each lesion to a depth of 3 to 4 mm. Each procedure was done under local anesthesia and consisted of treatment of a 4-sq cm area. Several sittings were necessary for completion. There has been no recurrence in one year.

Storino WD, Engel GH: Office surgical management of recalcitrant axillary lesions. Cutis 21:338–341, 1978.

Fox-Fordyce disease, because of its focal nature, can be eliminated by excision of the affected area and closure with superior and inferior Y advancement flaps.

Getting well means more to a patient than getting a diagnosis.

Furunculosis

Erythromycin
Cephalosporin
Incision
Topical antibiotic

The treatment of the common boil is straightforward: (1) a systemic antibiotic to eliminate the pathogenic *Staphylococcus aureus* and (2) incision and drainage if the lesion is fluctuant. Since many strains of staphylococci are penicillin resistant, we usually prescribe erythromycin, a cephalosporin, or cloxacillin for a 10-day period. Culture and sensitivity tests are valuable, particularly if the patient is immunocompromised or the lesion is large, as in the carbuncle class. Hot compresses with a concentrated solution of Epsom salts ($MgSO_4 \cdot 7H_2O$ 20 minutes tid) are soothing, provide the patient with an active role, and probably hasten the "coming to a head." Carbuncles require higher antibiotic dosage and more active surgical intervention, with debridement of necrotic tissue and sometimes eventual skin grafting.

The approach to the patient with recurring boils is much more complex, as the challenge is prophylaxis and the goal illusory—the elimination of invisible pathogens. Not only the patient but also his infectious contacts must be treated. Even after the furuncles have faded, the pathogenic staphylococci continue to colonize the skin of the patient and his family contacts. Moreover, pets such as a dog with mange are often carriers of the organism. Other possible contributing factors should be sought, such as diabetes mellitus, anemia, or leukemia. Only rarely, usually in children, does a granulocyte or immunologic defect prove responsible. A greatly elevated serum IgE level may point to the "hyper IgE" syndrome in adults.

The patient and his entire family should use a commercial bacteriostatic soap (e.g., Dial or Safeguard), with scrupulous attention paid to cleansing the underarm and genital areas daily. Frequent shampooing of the hair to eliminate scalp bacteria is also vital. Compulsive attempts to sterilize clothing are probably not helpful. If the communal group has used antibacterial soaps regularly and exclusively without success, we prescribe Hibiclens (chlorhexidine gluconate) or pHisoHex (hexachlorophene) as a liquid soap.

The carrier state is best attacked by having the family apply a topical antibiotic ointment such as bacitracin (available without prescription) over the entire skin surface each night for two weeks. This course may have to be repeated, but it offers the best hope of reducing the pathogen load. Nasal carriage of staphylococci can also be reduced with Neosporin ointment applied three times a day to the anterior nares.

Immunity may be enhanced in some individuals by the administration of oral zinc or cimetidine. Finally, all patients should be instructed to avoid excess carbohydrate intake, since elevated skin glucose levels favor bacterial growth. Demonstration of abnormally elevated postprandial blood glucose levels may be of assistance in changing the habits of the "sweets addict" who has boils.

Hedstrom SA: Recurrent staphylococcal furunculosis: Bacteriological findings and epidemiology in 100 cases. Scand J Infect Dis 13:115–119, 1981.

Study of 100 cases in three years showed that in virtually every instance *Staphylococcus aureus* was the pathogen and that in half the cases other members of the family had furuncles. Phage typing of strains from lesions and nares is considered essential for epidemiologic analysis.

Bartzokas CA, Paton JH, Gibson MF, Graham R, McLoughlin GA, Croton RS: Control and eradication of methicillin-resistant *Staphylococcus aureus* on a surgical unit. N Engl J Med 311:1422–1425, 1984.

Frequent and energetic total body washing with **triclosan** (2 per cent antiseptic liquid tid) cleared patients and "staff" carriers within two to three weeks. Weekly cultures of anterior nares, axillae, and perineum monitored progress. Heavy contamination of environment was found in dust of patient and support rooms, toilets, showers, and bathrooms, and daily methodical cleansing was required for one week for clearing.

Effective whole-body antiseptics (with high skin substantiveness and prolonged effect):

chlorhexidine (Hibiclens)
hexachlorophene (pHisoHex)
triclosan (Irish Spring)

Not effective:

—iodophors (Betadine)
—alcohol

Taplin D: Pitfalls in eradicating contagious boil epidemic. JAMA 241:444, 1979.

Pitfalls:

1. Simply incising and draining the boils
2. Treating with **penicillin** or **tetracycline**
3. Failure to treat with **cloxacillin**
4. Failure to treat contacts who have boils

Broughton R: A cure for recurrent furunculosis. Cutis 23:808, 1979.

Apply **bacitracin** ointment to every square inch of body each night for 10 nights. Success in 15 cases. No controls.

Smith IM: A plague of boils. JAMA 251:3010, 1984.

Definition of a plague: 10 or more boils, or boils for six months or longer.

Studied 100 families. Most were treated successfully with one to four courses of total-body **bacitracin** ointment (500 U/gm daily or bid for two weeks) to each family member. Staphylococci are carried in anterior nares (as high as finger can reach), axillae, and perineum, which require fastidious care.

Brody I: Treatment of recurrent furunculosis with oral zinc. Lancet 2:1358, 1977.

Oral **zinc sulfate** (45 mg Zn^2 tid) given to eight patients restored serum zinc levels to normal and prevented further furuncles.

Mattson L, Rombo L, Holmgren B: Vaccination against furunculosis with staphylococcal vaccine. No difference in therapeutic effect can be noted between vaccine and placebo. Lakartidningen 79:743–744, 1982.

An instructive title.

Mattson L, Blomgren H, Holmgren B, Jarstrand C: Bestatin treatment for the correction of granulocyte dysfunction in patients with recurrent furunculosis. Infection 11:205–207, 1983.

Decreased phagocytic activity of granulocytes was found in 19 patients with furunculosis. Oral administration of **bestatin** 40 mg (a metabolite of *Streptomyces olivoreticuli*), given to 10 patients restored the phagocytic activity of granulocytes to normal within three hours. Clinical trials are still in the research and development stage in Sweden.

Bork K, Schram P: Furunkuloide myiasis durch larven von *Dermatobia hominis*. Hautarzt 32:141–144, 1981.

When a larval fly induces the furuncle, simply incise and cover with Vaseline. The larva will crawl out within 48 hours.

Meure-Haik C, Garcia-Valasco J: Carbuncle: Discussion and a report of two cases. Int J Dermatol 13:63–68, 1974.

In addition to control of diabetes and administration of antibiotics such as synthetic **penicillin**, **erythromycin**, or **lincomycin** (Lincocin), these cases required excision of necrotic tissue and skin grafting.

Fontana G, Lorente F, Rodriguez G, Ojeda JA: Defective neutrophil chemotaxis and hyperimmunoglobulinemia E—A reversible defect. Acta Paediatr Scand 65:509–511, 1976.

Rifampicin for two months and control of severe atopic eczema with diet (no eggs, milk, or fish) for four months stopped recurrent *Staphylococcus aureus* subcutaneous abscesses. While the IgE level remained high (3900 IU), eosinophilia and neutrophil chemotaxis returned to normal.

Davis SD, Schaller J, Wedgwood RJ: Job's syndrome—Recurrent, "cold," staphylococcal abscesses. Lancet 1013–1015, 1966.

Two girls with red hair, eczema, recurrent respiratory infections, and cold abscesses required continuous antibiotic prophylaxis for even partial control.

McDaniel DH, Welton WA: Furunculosis and hidradenitis suppurativa response. Arch Dermatol 120:437, 1984.

The nonsteroidal anti-inflammatory agent **tolmetin sodium** (Tolectin, 400 mg tid or 8 to 10 mg/kg/day) induced nearly complete clearing within days to weeks when given to four patients (ages 4 to 30 years) with antibiotic-resistant furunculosis of several years' duration. The furunculosis reappeared when the tolmetin was stopped and remitted on resumption of the drug. Tapering the dose slowly over several months induced lesion-free remissions of up to one year after discontinuing tolmetin.

Most patients long for someone in whom they can confide their troubles.

WANFIELD T. LONGCOPE

Gianotti-Crosti Syndrome

Erythromycin

The treatment here is not for the child, but for the parents. It consists of finding which of the known viruses has triggered the reaction pattern. Knowledge of this and the course of the eruption, lymphadenopathy, and lymphocytosis, which ordinarily fade within three weeks, is the best therapy possible.

The most commonly observed viral antecedent is hepatitis B, but comprehensive serologic testing, blood counts, blood chemistry profile, and liver function studies are indicated. A chest roentgenogram and culture for *Mycoplasma* may indicate the need for a course of erythromycin. Finally, check for hepatosplenomegaly and lymph node enlargement.

Gianotti F: Papular acrodermatitis of childhood and other papulo-vesicular acro-located syndromes. Br J Dermatol 100:49–59, 1979.

In this authoritative account by the eponymic father of this unique reaction pattern, he remains silent regarding therapy. The salient features include:

1. Symmetric erythematous papular rash on face, buttocks, and limbs, which lasts three weeks
2. Paracortical hyperplasia of lymph nodes, mainly inguinal and axillary
3. Acute anicteric hepatitis, lasting two months, which may progress to chronic liver disease
4. Hepatitis B surface antigenemia, subtype ayw (HBsAg)

Eiloart M: The Gianotti-Crosti Syndrome. Report of forty-four cases. Br J Dermatol 78:488–492, 1966.

It is transient, it is benign, and it usually occurs in toddlers whose parents need your hand.

Spear K, Winkelmann RK: Gianotti-Crosti Syndrome: A review of ten cases not associated with hepatitis B. Arch Dermatol 120:891–896, 1984.

An upper respiratory infection in the patient or family is a common antecedent of this 21-day eruption that is apparently a virus-related response. Viruses implicated to date include hepatitis B, Epstein-Barr, Coxsackie, and parainfluenza. If petechiae are noted in the rash, the virus is probably hepatitis B. Acute hepatitis may last up to three months.

Recommended laboratory evaluation:

liver enzymes
serologic test—hepatitis B virus
serologic test—EBV
viral throat culture
CBC

Berant M, Naveh Y, Weissman I: Papular acrodermatitis with cytomegalovirus hepatitis. Arch Dis Child 58:1024–1025, 1983.

Case report: A one-year-old boy in Israel had fever, cough, jaundice, lymphadenopathy, and enlarged liver and spleen. One week later, after other symptoms had abated, a symmetric maculopapular rash appeared on face, limbs, and buttocks. CMV antibodies appeared eight days after onset of the rash, the titer rising to 1 : 160 after three weeks. The eruption slowly faded after 20 days.

Secure serologic tests for:

HBsAg and Ab
hepatitis A
Epstein-Barr virus
cytomegalovirus (CF antibodies)
herpesvirus
toxoplasma
adenovirus

Iosub S, Santos C, Gromisch DS: Papular acrodermatitis with Epstein-Barr virus infection. Clin Pediatr 23:33–34, 1984.

Case report: A nine-month-old black male with fever, paroxysmal cough, papular rash, nasal discharge, pharyngeal exudate, lymphadenopathy, and enlarged liver and spleen. Laboratory values included WBC 39,000 with 60 per cent atypical lymphocytes and elevated sedimentation rate and LDH. The EBV titer rose from 0 to 1 : 160 over a three-week period.

Additional serologic tests that may be helpful include:

parainfluenza viruses
respiratory syncytial virus
Mycoplasma pneumoniae

Fiocchi A, Codara L, Colombini A, Rota M: Epidemiologic significance of infantile papular acrodermatitis. J Pediatr 104:163, 1984.

To detect the source of the infection, specific serologic screening is mandatory, not only for the immediate family, but also of all contact relatives. In this report of two cases, clinically unrecognized HBV infection was demonstrated serologically in several contact relatives, but not the immediate family.

James WD, Odom RB, Hatch MH: Gianotti-Crosti-like eruption associated with coxsackie virus A-16 infection. J Am Acad Dermatol 6:862–866, 1982.

A two-year-old boy had rhinorrhea and typical erythematous papules on the face, arms, legs, and buttocks, along with generalized lymphadenopathy and hepatomegaly.

Viral infection confirmed by:

initial throat culture
repeat stool culture at six weeks
acute and convalescent sera (16-fold increase)

If you can't be the first doctor seen, take time to be the best.

Granuloma Annulare

Steroids	KI
Dapsone	Chlorambucil
Niacinamide	

Here is a hypersensitivity reaction pattern hidden in the dermis. It ranges from the trivial to the disfiguring and disabling. It may result from no more than a rap on the knuckles, a finger prick, or a bruise. Rarely, it may be a generalized disseminated eruption, alarming and without known cause. Accordingly, therapy must be tailored to each patient's needs. We suggest a search for underlying tinea, candidiasis, streptococcal infection, insect bites, and localized trauma and the appropriate therapeutic measures. In one of our cases, Nizoral proved to be curative, while in another, erythromycin stopped both the strep throat and the granuloma annulare.

For the mildest examples, simple reassurance that the lesions are neither cancer nor a sign of cancer is sufficient. When a patient consults you it does not always mean he wants treatment. He may only seek knowledge.

A topical high-potency steroid cream applied at night with or without Saran wrapping has the potential for inducing some involution. However, injection of steroid directly into the lesion is more effective and for small lesions is probably the treatment of choice.

The disseminated form may call for systemic steroids or even an immunosuppressant, such as chlorambucil (Leukeran). The common thread of success for the many varied drugs used seems to be interference with the immune system. Thus, one of our patients with large disseminate lesions responded dramatically to phenytoin (Dilantin), which has mild immunosuppressant activity.

Wells RS, Smith MA: The natural history of granuloma annulare. Br J Dermatol 75:199–205, 1963.

Half of 115 cases cleared spontaneously within two years (thus favoring the "latter-day" therapist). Fifty-two patients had biopsies with no resolution.

Sparrow G, Abell E: Granuloma annulare and necrobiosis lipoidica treated by jet injector. Br J Dermatol 93:85–89, 1975.

Intralesional injection of **triamcinolone acetonide** (5 mg/ml) resulted in clearing in 32 of 45 patients within two to four weeks, but new lesions developed elsewhere. Transient atrophy from injections was disappointing.

Ravits HG: How I treat granuloma annulare. Postgrad Med 48:176–177, 1970.

Cordran tape applied daily.

Moyer DG: Papular granuloma annulare. Arch Dermatol 89:41–45, 1964.

Gnat bites (*Culicoides furans*) in three children were the cause. Systemic steroids helped but relapses occurred until insect exposure was eliminated.

Saied N, Schwartz RA, Estes SA: Treatment of generalized granuloma annulare with dapsone. Arch Dermatol 116:1345–1346, 1980.

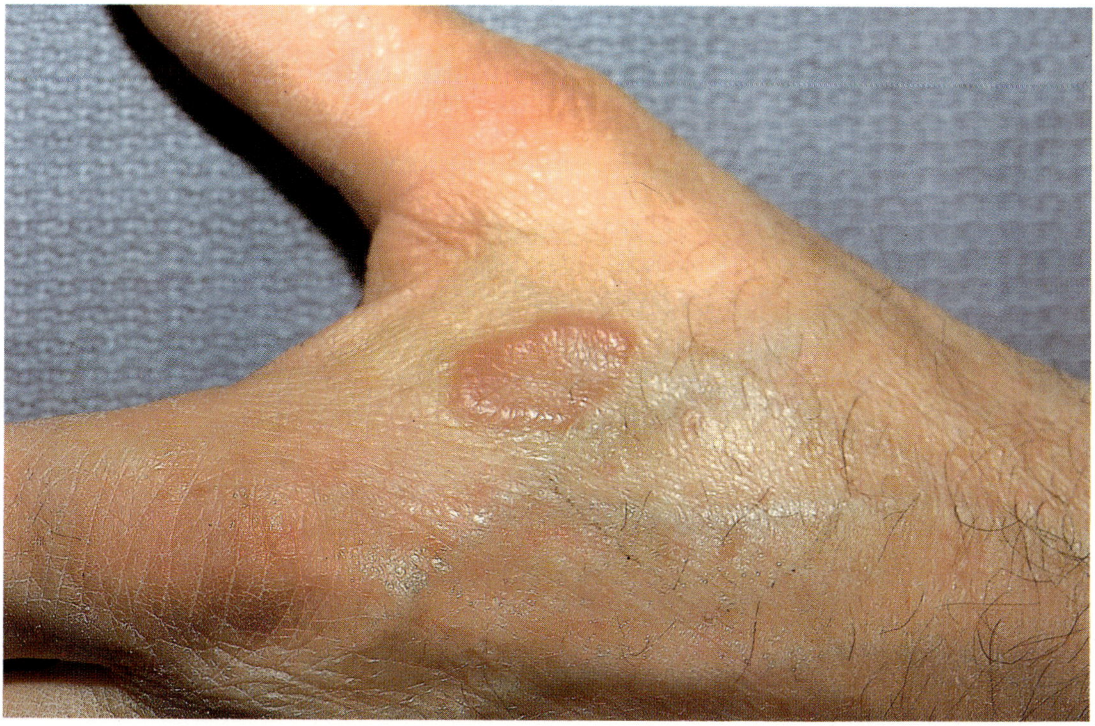

Two cases cleared in two to four weeks with dapsone (100 to 200 mg daily). No relapse when dapsone was discontinued three to six months later.

Ma A, Medenica M: Response of generalized granuloma annulare to high-dose niacinamide. Arch Dermatol 119:836–839, 1983.

One case cleared after six months of **niacinamide** (1.5 gm daily). Relapse on reduced dose, remission on return to 1.5 gm/day.

Giessel M, Graves K, Kolivas J: Treatment of disseminated granuloma annulare with potassium iodide. Arch Dermatol 115:639–640, 1979.

SSKI (1.0 ml daily) for three months helped two of four patients.

Marsch WD, Stuttgen G: Granuloma annulare-eine indication fur der photochemotherapie? Z Hautkr 56:44–49, 1981.

Single case report of success with **8-methoxypsoralen** (0.15 per cent emulsion) and UVA (10.2 J/sq cm, over a six-week course).

Kossard S, Winkelmann RK: Low-dose chlorambucil in the treatment of generalized granuloma annulare. Dermatology 158:443–450, 1979.

Clearing in four of six patients after three to four months. Hazard: thrombocytopenia in one.

Rudolph RI: Disseminated granuloma annulare treated with low-dose chlorambucil. Arch Dermatol 115:1212–1213, 1979.

One case cleared in two months with **chlorambucil** (2 mg tid). No relapse when drug was discontinued after three and one-half months. Warning: Possible irreversible bone marrow suppression.

Charles CR, Johnson BL, Damm SR: Granuloma annulare. Int J Dermatol 15:655–665, 1976.

Fallen warriors in the battle against granuloma annulare:

antihistamines	incision
chloroquine	pantothenic acid
cryotherapy	penicillin
diethylstilbestrol	vitamin E
gold injections	x-ray

73 references.

Steiner A, Pehamberger H, Wolff K: Sulfone treatment of granuloma annulare. J Am Acad Dermatol 13:1004–1008, 1985.

In 14 patients with either localized or generalized granuloma annulare given **dapsone** (100 mg/day for 2 weeks to 4.5 months):

Complete remission occurred in six patients within six weeks, but in adult patients relapses developed within three months of discontinuing therapy.
Partial response in seven patients.
No response in one patient.

The musical score of therapy comes from books, journals, and colleagues. But the performance—ah, that is what you do in your office.

Granuloma Faciale

Dapsone	Cryosurgery
Chloroquine	Dermabrasion
Intralesional steroid	Laser
PUVA	Excision

Guill MA, Aton JK: Facial granuloma responsive to dapsone therapy. Arch Dermatol 118:332-335, 1982.

In a 37-year-old woman, **dapsone** (100 mg/day for six months) resulted in improvement within two weeks in a large, painful erythematous indurated plaque of facial granuloma. This had previously been unresponsive to Grenz ray therapy (2000 rads for 17 days), intralesional **triamcinolone acetonide** (10 mg/ml, 1 ml on four occasions), **liquid nitrogen**, **erythromycin** (250 mg qid for 10 days), **dicloxacillin sodium** (500 mg qid for 14 days), **tetracycline** (500 mg for 10 days), **cephalexin** (500 mg qid for 14 days), **sulfamethoxazole** (2 gm qid), and **potassium iodide** (0.5 ml for 10 days). The pain was so severe as to require **meperidine** (Demerol). Within one month after dapsone was started, the pain was controllable with **ibuprofen** (Motrin 1600 to 2400 mg/day), and after three months all pain medication could be discontinued. The lesions were completely healed after six months, and the tapered dose of dapsone was discontinued. There was no recurrence in the following year.

Milligan MP, Goette DK: Dapsone-responsive granuloma faciale. J Assoc Mil Dermatol 10(1):30–31, 1984.

Another patient showing excellent response to **dapsone** (50 mg/day, later reduced to 25 mg/day) is a 66-year-old man with a 2-cm violaceous plaque on the scalp that cleared within several months. The lesion had not changed following intralesional **triamcinolone acetonide** (10 mg/ml once monthly for three months).

Pedace FJ, Perry HO: Granuloma faciale: A clinical and histopathologic review. Arch Dermatol 94:387–395, 1966.

A review of 21 cases at the Mayo Clinic:

1. It may occur on other areas of the body.
2. The course is chronic (in these patients up to 21 years).
3. There was no consistent response to therapy. In one case intralesional steroid produced clearing, while another case cleared with **chloroquine** (500 mg/day for four years).

Johnson WC, Higdon RS, Helwig EB: Granuloma faciale. Arch Dermatol 79:42–52, 1959.

Analysis of 15 cases at the Armed Forces Institute of Pathology indicated that:

1. Excision or destruction by electrodesiccation or dermabrasion of the lesion gave the greatest promise of cure, but recurrences did arise in some scars.
2. The following systemic treatments were ineffective in one or more patients: bismuth, calciferol, chloroquine, Fowler's solution, INH, iodides, PABA, penicillin, steroids, testosterone.

Graham GF, Stewart R: Cryosurgery for unusual cutaneous neoplasms. J Dermatol Surg Oncol 3:437–442, 1977.

Granuloma faciale plaques of the nose and cheeks, present for 14 years in a 54-year-old man, were successfully eradicated by cryosurgery (double freeze-thaw cycles of 3 minutes, 45 seconds to −40°C, with thermocouple thaw times of 5 minutes and clinical thaw times of 11 minutes). In one plaque in which the granuloma went down to subcutaneous fat, a freeze time of 3½ minutes and a thaw time of 8 minutes were necessary. There was one recurrence that was again treated effectively with cryosurgery. Hypertrophic residual scarring occurred in some areas.

It is important to note that these lesions had for 14 years resisted the following approaches used in a variety of dermatologic and plastic surgery centers:

- excision and grafting
- liquid N_2 by cotton swab
- freezing with solid carbon dioxide
- intralesional steroids
- radiotherapy
- nitrogen mustard topically
- antimalarials
- systemic corticosteroids

Bergfeld WF, Scholes HT, Roenigk HH Jr: Granuloma faciale—Treatment by dermabrasion: Report of a case. Cleve Clin Q 37:215–218, 1970.

Granuloma faciale of four years' duration in a 31-year-old woman was eradicated by dermabrasion, with a good cosmetic result and no recurrence at six months. The lesions had previously not responded to either intralesional injections of **triamcinolone acetonide** (0.5 to 2.0 mg every two to four weeks for six months) or to **hydroxychloroquine sulfate** (200 mg/day for six months).

Hudson LD: Granuloma faciale: Treatment with topical psoralen and UVA. J Am Acad Dermatol 8:559, 1983.

Granuloma faciale on the nose of a 62-year-old man, unresponsive to **dapsone** (50 mg/day for six weeks), completely involuted following 10 weeks of treatment with topical **psoralen** and UVA (total dose 24 joules over 10 weeks: weeks 1 to 6, 0.5 joule three times a week; weeks 7 to 8, 1 joule three times a week; weeks 9 to 10, 1.5 joules three times a week).

No recurrence was noted at six months.

Apfelberg DB, Druker D, Maser MR, et al: Granuloma faciale: Treatment with the argon laser. Arch Dermatol 119:573–576, 1983.

Three patients were cleared completely of their granuloma faciale lesions by use of an argon laser. A single treatment with this intense blue green laser light (480 to 520 nm, 100 to 125 joules/sq cm of treated area, 0.6 to 1.8 W of power, 40 to 108 seconds' duration) gave rapid persistent resolution with no recurrence in up to two years.

Good luck is sometimes better than good medicine.

Granuloma Inguinale

Tetracycline Bactrim DS Minocycline

The causative organism, *Calymmatobacterium granulomatis* (that old Donovan body) is sensitive to a broad spectrum of systemic antibiotics, but tetracycline (2 gm/day) is the treatment of choice.

Rosen T, Tschen JA, Ramsdell W, et al: Granuloma inguinale. J Am Acad Dermatol 11:433–437, 1984.

An excellent survey of current therapeutic options, including some old ones:

chloramphenicol (2 gm/day)

streptomycin (20 to 30 gm IM over 5 to 10 days)

Tetracycline (2 gm/day) is the treatment of choice, whereas ampicillin should not be used because of variable response.

Bactrim DS (1 tablet bid) completely cleared granuloma inguinale in 6 patients who had not responded to **tetracycline** (2 gm/day for two weeks). An additional 14 patients had equally good responses to Bactrim DS (**trimethoprim** 160 mg/**sulfamethoxazole** 800 mg). All 20 patients were healed in two to five weeks and experienced no relapse.

Velasco JE, Miller AE, Zaias N: Minocycline in the treatment of venereal disease. JAMA 220:1323–1325, 1972.

Dose: Minocycline (Minocin 200 mg stat, then 100 mg bid for 15 days).

Disease	***Patients***	***Median healing time***
Granuloma inguinale	6	21 days
Chancroid	6	16 days
Lymphogranuloma venereum	5	15 days

Werman BS, Herskowitz LJ, Olansky S, et al: A clinical variant of chancroid resembling granuloma inguinale. Arch Dermatol 119:890–894, 1983.

Sixteen patients with nonsyphilitic, nonherpetic genital ulcerations had the precise clinical features of granuloma inguinale, but no Donovan bodies were present. *Hemophilus ducreyi* was regularly cultured from these lesions and established the diagnosis of chancroid. Significantly, healing did not occur in three weeks in any of six patients treated with **tetracycline** (500 mg qid), whereas in five of eight patients receiving **minocycline** (Minocin 100 mg bid) healing occurred in two weeks.

Sehgal VN, Prasad ALS: Donovanosis: Current concepts. Int J Dermatol 25:8–16, 1986.

A carefully referenced review of 112 papers on this subject emphasizes the following:

Tetracyclines are drug of first choice, e.g., **oxytetracycline** (2 gm/day for two weeks).

Alternate effective drugs include **trimethoprim-sulfamethoxazole** (2 tablets bid for two weeks) or chloramphenicol (2 gm/day for two weeks).

Other reported successes have been with **erythromycin, triacetyloleandomycin,** and **gentamicin.**

Streptomycin, although effective, is not favored owing to its side effects.

Penicillin is ineffective.

Lucky is the doctor who has a lucky person as his patient.

Hailey-Hailey Disease

Compresses	Dapsone
Antibiotics	Lithium
Ketoconazole	Surgery
Acyclovir	

The treatment of Hailey-Hailey disease is the treatment of infection. Although the primary lesion is a friction-induced acantholysis, it is the secondary infection that brings the patient to you. The complex infection arises and thrives in the unique world of warmth and moisture of the axillae and groin, with numerous and varied organisms whose exact mix changes in response to therapy. The ecologic balance frequently shifts as new pathogens emerge to contribute to the continuing malodorous exudation.

In the initial assessment we are best guided by a Gram stain of the exudate and bacterial and yeast cultures. Initially, we usually prescribe compresses such as acetic acid ($\frac{1}{4}$ per cent 15 minutes bid), Silvadene cream (silver sulfadiazine bid), and erythromycin (250 mg qid). If a quick response is not forthcoming, we move to other topical and systemic antibiotics as indicated by laboratory sensitivity tests. If there is evidence of yeast infection or of a relapse while the patient is receiving antibiotics, we prescribe ketoconazole (Nizoral 200 mg/day). We suspect an occasional recalcitrant patient also may have secondary herpes simplex infection, which can be helped with acyclovir (Zovirax 200 mg, one capsule six times a day).

In resistant cases, dapsone (100 mg/day) is especially valuable. At times it is necessary to give an injection of Kenalog (triamcinolone acetonide 40 mg IM) to reduce the inflammatory element. For continuous, life-spoiling lesions, hospitalization may be necessary to restore the epidermis to a functional state. In two of our patients complete surgical excision of the affected areas was necessary to reach a cure. One of these has remained cured for more than 16 years, with no recurrence in the anhidrotic grafted skin of her axillae.

A serendipitous observation in another of our patients with active long-standing Hailey-Hailey disease is of interest. She experienced rapid, complete disappearance of all lesions once lithium therapy was started. We suspect that the increase in circulating neutrophils induced by lithium may have been critical, although an effect on keratinization may have been responsible.

Once the lesions clear, prophylaxis is most important, since all of these patients have life-long inborn fragility of their epidermis. We alert them to the dangers of tight underclothing, back packs, sunburn, and vigorous exercise such as jogging. But most importantly, we stress the importance of keeping the predisposed areas dry. We prescribe Xerac AC to inhibit sweating and lower the bacterial population. We recommend Dial soap as well. The patients are asked to wear loose, airy clothing and to change clothing if wet (e.g., do not sit around in a wet bathing suit). We urge that they avoid working in hot, humid environments and prescribe air conditioning in the car, work place, and home.

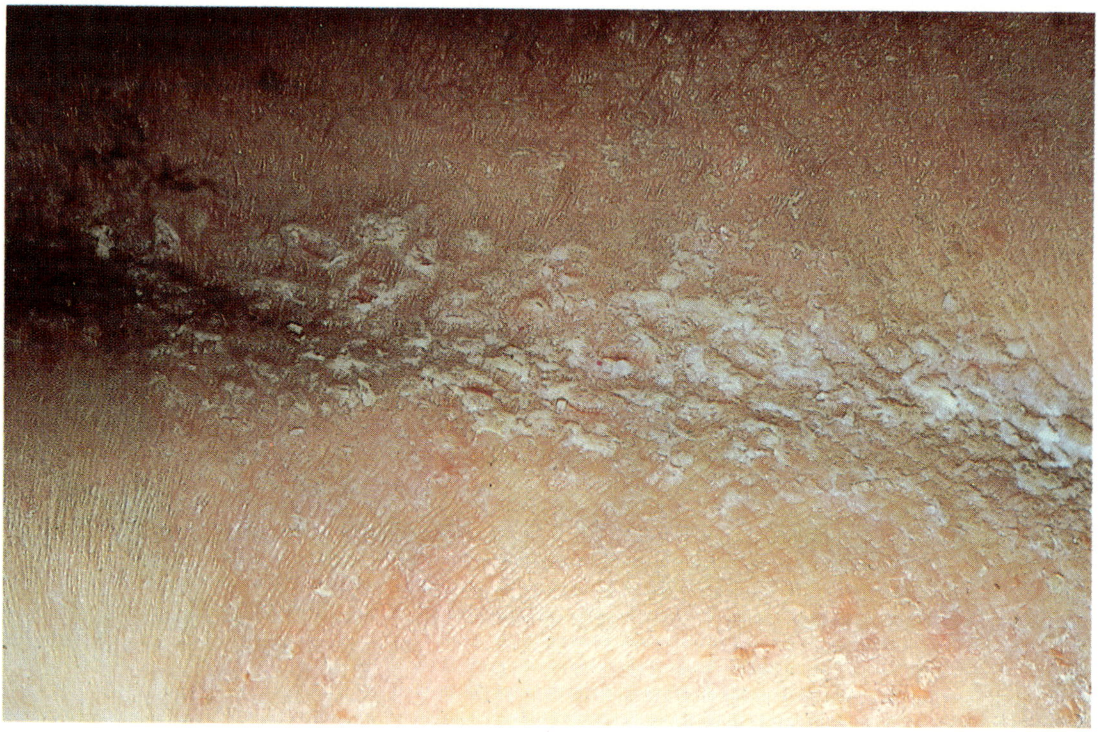

Genetic counseling is advisable since three out of four of these patients give a positive family history of the disease. The bad news is that it is transmitted as an autosomal dominant, but the good news is that it has quite incomplete penetrance.

Our message to all of these patients is that they have a strange familial predilection to infection in areas of friction. Such infection is best prevented by availing themselves of the best of all antibiotics—dryness of the skin surface.

Michel B: Commentary: Hailey-Hailey disease. Familial benign chronic pemphigus. Arch Dermatol 118:781–783, 1982.

Notable improvement can be achieved with oral and topical antibacterial and antiyeast therapy. Topical, intralesional, and systemic steroids are helpful. Dapsone (100 mg/day, then maintenance 50 mg/day or every other day) also deserves a trial. Surgery provides the only cure.

Shelley WB, Pillsbury DM: Specific systemic antibiotic therapy in familial benign chronic pemphigus. Arch Dermatol 80:554–556, 1959.

Both bacteria and friction play significant roles in precipitating acute attacks of this disease. Attacks can best be controlled with specific systemic antibiotics, as determined by antibiotic-sensitivity testing of bacterial isolates from each successive attack.

Palmer DD, Perry HO: Benign familial chronic pemphigus. Arch Dermatol 86:493–502, 1962.

Antibiotics provide the best treatment and air conditioning the best prophylaxis (study of 23 patients at the Mayo Clinic).

Levene GM: The treatment of pemphigus and pemphigoid. Clin Exp Dermatol 7:643–652, 1982.

Grenz ray therapy is also of help in the treatment of familial benign chronic pemphigus.

Sire DJ, Johnson BL: Benign familial chronic pemphigus treated with dapsone. Arch Dermatol 103:262–265, 1971.

Dapsone (100 mg/day) produced a splendid response in three patients within one to two weeks. In one patient maintenance dapsone (50 mg/day) could be stopped after three months, with no return of symptoms after one year.

Burns RA, Reed WB, Swatek FE, Omieczynski DT: Familial benign chronic pemphigus: Induction of lesions by *Candida albicans*. Arch Dermatol 96:254–258, 1967.

Initially, **tetracycline** controlled lesions in three patients, but a sequential *Candida albicans* superinfection required specific candicidal therapy with **nystatin** cream (Mycostatin).

Cram DL, Muller SA, Winkelmann RK: Ultraviolet-induced acantholysis in familial benign chronic pemphigus: Detection of the forme fruste. Arch Dermatol 96:636–641, 1967.

The hazard of sunlight to these patients and their asymptomatic relatives was demonstrated by induction of lesions with UVB phototesting (long-wave UVL due to Corning glass filter, 20-minute exposure on lower back, read and biopsy at 24 hours). Lesions were produced in two patients and in two of their clinically normal siblings.

Peled I, Weinrauch L, Kaplan H, Wexler MR: Surgical management of Hailey-Hailey disease: Report of a case. J Dermatol Surg Oncol 6:662–663, 1980.

Excision of all chronically affected areas, followed by split-thickness grafts, cured a 56-year-old man with disabling Hailey-Hailey disease of the groin and perianal area.

Kauten JR, Zook EG, Kumar AA, Kinkead LR: Surgical management of familial benign chronic pemphigus by excision and primary closure. Ann Plast Surg 9:337–343, 1982.

An impressive cure of long-standing Hailey-Hailey disease of the axillae, groin, and perineum in a 54-year-old man following full-thickness excision without grafting. Primary closure was possible and is recommended, since the skin in these intertriginous areas is lax. The photographs are convincing.

Berger RS, Lynch PJ: Familial benign chronic pemphigus: Surgical treatment and pathogenesis. Arch Dermatol 104:380–384, 1971.

Postoperative immobilization, fever, sweating, and maceration led to a widespread flare of familial benign chronic pemphigus on the back of a 51-year-old man following groin excision and split-thickness skin grafting. Use of a Stryker frame to relieve pressure and maceration and **hydrocortisone** 1 per cent in Schamberg's lotion cleared the lesions.

Decreased sweating in the groin after surgery was felt to be responsible for clinical improvement. (Decreased sweating may also be achieved with topical **aluminum chloride hexahydrate** 6.25 per cent in anhydrous ethyl alcohol [Xerac AC, applied at bedtime] after skin lesions have healed. Use of this product prophylactically on the back also might have prevented maceration and new lesions in this patient.)

A fully informed patient is a fully frightened patient.

Hand Eczema

Protection	Erythromycin
Detection	Phototherapy
Corticosteroids	

Hand eczema provides an intellectual challenge for any practice. The patient literally brings you the whole world of dermatology in the palm of his hand. It is for you to find out which part of the world is causing the trouble and to do something about it.

Nothing is more heterogeneous in its origins—ranging from bare-handed work with "guts" in a slaughterhouse to the wearing of gloves in the operating room. Getting these answers demands the art of detection. Nowhere are good history taking and patient orientation more important. Ultimate cures come only from finding the cause and eliminating it.

But while the analysis proceeds, the patient needs immediate help. We provide this with Synalar ointment 0.025 per cent (preservative-free) applied each night, Nutraderm lotion (lanolin-free) applied frequently during the day, and systemic erythromycin (250 mg qid). The last is invaluable, since so many of these patients come to see you only after nonpurulent secondary infection has made the problem intolerable.

There are nearly as many different answers to hand eczema as one can imagine. Very few patients share anything but the common pathway of a nonspecific eczematous reaction. It takes hard work and time to solve many of these hand eruption puzzles. But always there is the shared delight of patient and physician when the cause is identified, and both come out of the black box of ignorance.

Many times the cause is a silent, innocent-appearing contactant. One of the most common is herbal shampoo, well tolerated by the scalp but not the hands. Anecdotes abound, but here are three of ours:

1. The widower's hand eruption appearing shortly after his wife's death, not due to grief but to sensitization to the oils from the skin of oranges that he was now hand squeezing for the first time
2. The woman with a six-year history of eczema of the palms due to sensitivity to the steering wheel of their six-year-old car
3. The woman with eczema of the right palm of 21 years, proven to be due to sensitivity to the cocobolo wood handle of a carving knife given her as a wedding present those 21 years before

But not all hand eruptions are due to contactants. We recall the dentist who was virtually ready to give up his practice because of a chronic recalcitrant hand eruption. The answer was sensitivity to coffee. And then there are some patients for whom empiric therapy holds the cure, if not the answer. One of our patients had a defiant hand eruption that cleared only after dapsone (100 mg/day) was prescribed.

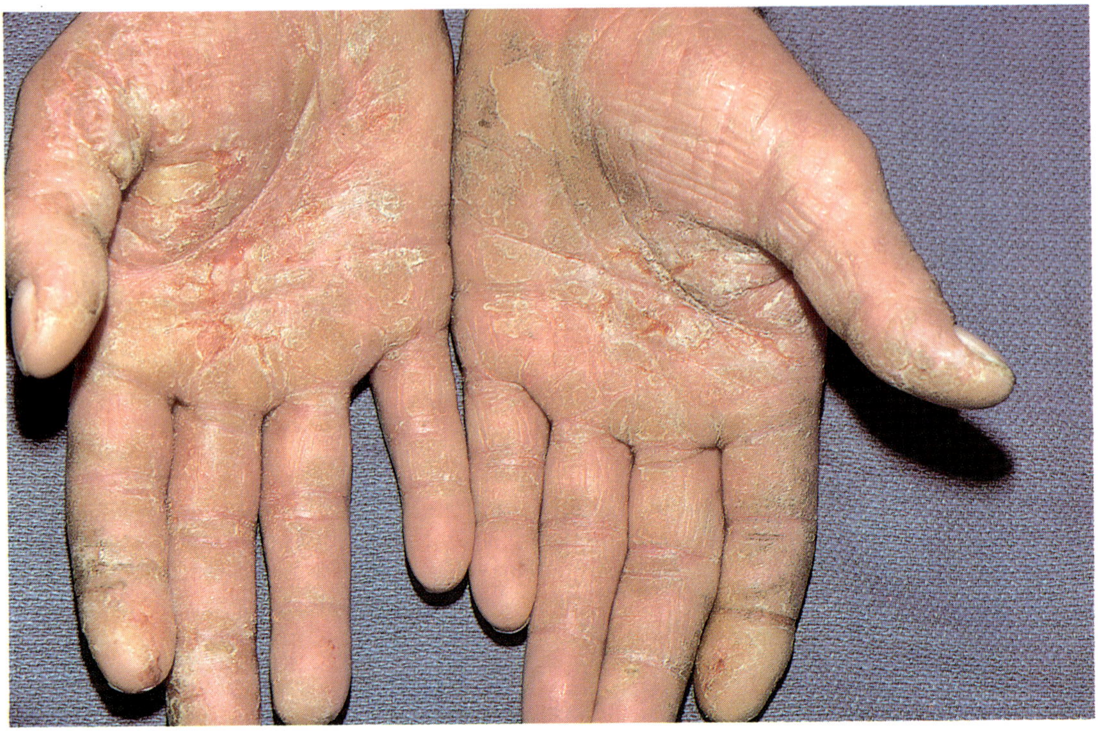

But no matter what the cause may prove to be, once hand eczema has cleared, a period of six months of convalescence is required. During that time the patient must protect the newly healed skin from even minor irritation or potential allergens. It is the most difficult stage for the patient to understand. But unless the hands are treated as "convalescents," relapse is to be expected. In this regard, one of our octagenarian Vermont farmer patients (whom we were proudly discharging from our care because we had cleared his hand dermatitis of 30 years) said with a shrug of gratitude, "Thank you, so far."

Epstein E: Hand dermatitis: Practical management and current concepts. J Am Acad Dermatol 10:395–424, 1984.

Monographic in scope, this 30-page review is a classic. Instructions to the patient stress protection during treatment and four months of convalescence:

1. Wear waterproof heavy-duty vinyl gloves (Cyralon) for wet work or when handling citrus fruits, potatoes, or tomatoes, or when using polishes, paints, or solvents.
2. Wear leather gloves when doing outdoor work, cotton gloves for dry housework.
3. Use a dishwasher, washing machine for laundry, and family help.
4. Wash hands with only a trace of mild soap and lukewarm water and with rings removed. All soaps are irritating.
5. Use nothing on the hands other than that advised by the physician.

Specific therapy:

1. Hand lubricant: white **petrolatum** (15 per cent) incorporated into **hydrocortisone cream** (1 per cent). Dispensed in several jars to keep in the bathroom, kitchen, and work place and apply frequently.

2. **Prednisone** (60 to 80 mg the first day; reduce by 10 to 20 mg each day thereafter for a four- to seven-day course) for severe blistering hand dermatitis
3. **Erythromycin** systemically if secondary infection
4. Treatment of underlying disease, e.g., psoriasis, tinea
5. Patch testing for specific allergens to eliminate.

Shelley WB, Shelley ED: Chronic hand eczema strategies. Cutis 29:569–573, 581–584, 598, 1982.

The LLTT strategy:

*L*isten:

analyze the patient's past therapy, systemic medications, cleansing routine, occupation, and hobbies, as well as a possible atopic or psoriatic background for therapeutic attack areas

*L*ook:

inspect the whole skin from the fossae to the feet for evidence of atopic dermatitis, psoriasis, ichthyosis, scabies, candidiasis, tinea, and mycosis fungoides, and for clues to problems that deserve special treatment.

*T*est:

patch test, photopatch test, scrapings, oral challenge with foods and medications, biopsy.

*T*reat:

protection—two pairs of gloves—light cotton gloves beneath Playtex rubber or plastic covering gloves for all work

topical—**fluocinolone acetonide** ointment (Synalar 0.025 per cent)

systemic—erythromycin (250 mg qid)

Rystedt I: Factors influencing the occurrence of hand eczema in adults with a history of atopic dermatitis in childhood. Contact Dermatitis 12:185–191, 1985.

Patients with a history of atopic dermatitis often have persistent hand eczema as adults or develop it after exposure to irritants or at work.

Livingood CS, Pillsbury DM: Specific sensitivity to foods as a factor in various types of eczematous dermatitis. Arch Dermatol 60:1090–1115, 1949.

Hand eruptions that seem to persist interminably can be due to specific food allergens, detectable only by painstaking dietary control and oral challenge. This paper details data on 26 patients sensitive to one or more of the following:

pork	canned pears	rye
eggs	paprika	sweet potatoes
milk	white potatoes	cheese
seafood	rice	pepper
citrus fruits	cinnamon	cauliflower
wheat	peaches	pimento
nuts	carrots	coffee
chocolate	onions	pineapple
tomatoes	peas	tea
broccoli	Scotch whisky	apricots
chicken	butter	cabbage
sweet corn	veal	string beans
vanilla extract	beef	lima beans

Simons RDG Ph: Eczema of the Hands: Investigations into Dyshidrosiform Eruptions, 2nd ed. New York, S. Karger, 1966, 104 pp.

Genuine pompholyx or "dyshidrosis" remains an idiopathic disease. It is *not*:

a disease of the eccrine glands	a bacterid reaction
industrial dermatitis	allergic contact dermatitis
a dermatophytid reaction	

Adams RM: Occupational Skin Disease. New York, Grune & Stratton, 1983, 477 pp.

This comprehensive, indispensable book includes 77 pages of descriptions of various occupations with their irritants and allergens and precisely how to test with them. Exposure data, ranging from air hammer operators to welders, give all you need to know.

Foussereau J, Benezra C, Maibach HI: Occupational Contact Dermatitis: Clinical and Chemical Aspects. Philadelphia, WB Saunders Co, 1982, 452 pp.

Another superb reference source for the hazards of 50 occupations that people get their hands into.

Calnan CD, Bandmann HJ, Cronin E, et al: Hand dermatitis in housewives. Br J Dermatol 82:543–548, 1970.

A study in six European countries of 281 women with contact dermatitis of the hands revealed an allergic basis in 50 per cent. In order of frequency, the following allergens were identified by patch testing:

balsams	rubber
nickel	chromate
medicaments	benzocaine
cobalt	paraphenylenediamine

Thus, hand dermatitis is as frequently due to specific allergens as to primary irritants.

Sinha SM, Pasricha JS, Sharma RC, Kandhari KC: Vegetables responsible for contact dermatitis of the hands. Arch Dermatol 113:776–779, 1977.

Patch testing (0.05 ml of fresh juice) of 53 patients with hand eczema due to contact with vegetables showed the following sensitivities:

garlic	(44)
onion	(30)
tomatoes	(10)
carrots	(9)
ginger	(6)
radish	(5)
cauliflower	(5)
potato	(4)
gourd	(3)
pea	(2)
cucumber	(1)
bean	(1)
spinach	(1)
turnip	(1)

Feuerman EJ: Housewives' skin and the hazards of detergents. Curr Probl Dermatol 7:187–190, 1978.

In Israel 455 of 500 women with housewives' eczema were patch-test–proven sensitive to chromates (potassium dichromate 0.5 per cent aqueous solution), which were found in all 15 detergents used. The largest amount of chromates was found in detergents used for bleaching. Specific protection was afforded by an anion-exchange ointment reactive with chrome (Ivosin). Positive patch tests to nickel sulfate (1 per cent aqueous solution) were seen in 47 women.

Cronin E, Kullavanijaya P: Hand dermatitis in hairdressers. Acta Derm Venereol 59(Suppl 85):47–50, 1979.

Contact with shampoos was the most common cause of hand dermatitis in hairdressers. Atopy did not appear to be a significant factor. They should be encouraged to wear gloves while shampooing and also to apply emollients.

Fisher AA: Hand dermatitis—A "baker's dozen." Cutis 29:214–221, 1982.

Thirteen causes of bakers' dermatitis:

1. Chromates in flour
2. Cinnamon (vermouth, toothpaste)
3. Irritants (e.g., acids, yeast, iodides, bleaches)
4. Paronychia (candidal, bacterial)
5. Food mites (flour, sugar)
6. Ammonium persulfate (bleach)
7. Benzoyl peroxide
8. Sorbic acid (preservative—rye bread)
9. Karaya gum (meringue)
10. Inhalants (dyshidrotic eczema)
11. Atopic dermatitis allergens (especially flour dust causing asthma)
12. Flour (contact urticaria)
13. Trauma (baker's psoriasis)

Alomar A, Conde-Salazar L, Romaguera C: Occupational dermatoses from cutting oils. Contact Dermatitis 12:129–138, 1985.

Occupational dermatitis constitutes 50 per cent of all occupational illnesses in Spain.

A study of 230 patients with occupational hand dermatitis due to cutting oils proved that the eruption began as an irritant dermatitis that allowed contact allergens to enter and produce an allergic reaction in some. A patch test to the cutting oil (diluted 1 in 10 with water) was positive in 48 per cent, and specific sensitivities to paraphenylenediamine, chromium, and cobalt were most commonly demonstrated.

Rystedt I: Work-related hand eczema in atopics. Contact Dermatitis 12:164–171, 1985.

This study of 827 patients with hand eczema discovered that job exchange was not usually of benefit to the patient.

Advises atopic individuals not to select an occupation in which there is a large degree of exposure to chemicals, water, soil, and wear.

Advises that patients with hand eruption not be involved in providing medical services or in the food trade because of transmission of *Staphylococcus aureus*, which regularly colonizes such dermatitic skin.

Lammintausta K, Kalimo K, Havu VK: Occurrence of contact allergy and hand eczemas in hospital wet work. Contact Dermatitis 8:84–90, 1982.

Nickel, cobalt, and fragrances were the most common allergens in a group of 115 of 536 hospital workers studied, with an incidence of contact allergy of 21 per cent. Present or previous hand dermatitis was detected in 46 per cent.

Cronin E: Contact Dermatitis. London, Churchill Livingstone, 1980, 915 pp.

An encyclopedic view of the world of chemical irritants and contact allergens that is invaluable in assessing and treating hand eczemas.

Furia TE (ed.): Handbook of Food Additives, 2nd ed. Cleveland, CRC Press, 1972, 1980. Vol 1. 998 pp, Vol 2 412 pp.

These two volumes detailing the complexity of what we handle and eat are of help for hand eczema detective work.

Jensen O: Pustulosis palmaris et plantaris: The value of routine radiographic examinations in the detection of an infectious focus. Acta Derm Venereol 59:537–539, 1979.

Elimination of occult infectious foci detected by roentgenography, such as abscessed teeth in 8 of 46 patients and sinusitis in 3 of 52 patients, did not affect the course of the disease.

Stoughton RB: The influence of soap on eczematous dermatitis. Arch Dermatol 92:281–282, 1965.

Routine use for five weeks of Ivory soap for bathing and hand washing had no detectable adverse effect on the course of hand eczema in 57 women.

Christensen OB, Kristensen M: Treatment with disulfiram in chronic nickel hand dermatitis. Contact Dermatitis 8:59–63, 1982.

Disulfiram (Antabuse 200 mg/day for eight weeks) greatly improved pompholyx-type hand dermatitis in 8 of 11 women with nickel sensitivity, and 2 more were completely healed. Mild relapses occurred in all patients 2 to 16 weeks after stopping treatment. Disulfiram chelates metals and presumably acted by sequestering the nickel ion. Liver enzymes should be carefully monitored during disulfiram therapy.

Mørk N-J, Austad J: Short-wave ultraviolet light (UVB) treatment of allergic contact dermatitis of the hands. Acta Derm Venereol 63:87–89, 1983.

UVB (0.2 J/sq cm gradually increased to 1.2 J/sq cm, twice weekly for five to seven months, average total dose 18.4 J/sq cm) was successful treatment for 7 of 10 patients with longstanding contact dermatitis of the hands. Maintenance treatment with UVB (1.2 J/sq cm once weekly or every two weeks) was necessary to maintain clearing.

Murray D, Corbett MF, Warin AP: A controlled trial of photochemotherapy for persistent palmoplantar pustulosis. Br J Dermatol 102:659–663, 1980.

PUVA therapy (8-*MOP* 30 mg followed two hours later by UVA, using Sylvania fluorescent tubes, initially 0.5 to 2.0 J/sq cm, four times a week for a total of 30 treatments) completely cleared pustular eruption of the hands and feet in 12 of 22 patients, almost cleared it in 5, and significantly improved it in 4. No results were obtained with a twice-weekly treatment protocol, and no improvement was seen even with four treatments weekly until after five weeks of therapy. Several patients required weekly maintenance PUVA after clearing.

Fisher AA: Management of dermatitis due to surgical gloves. J Dermatol Surg Oncol 11:628–631, 1985.

Recommends Elastyren glove (styrene-butadiene block copolymer, Hermal Pharmaceutical Laboratories, Inc., Rt 145, Oak Hill, NY 12460, 1-800-HERMAL-1, 518-239-4714) for the surgeon whose chronic hand dermatitis is produced or made worse by use of rubber gloves, which commonly contain the sensitizers mercaptobenzothiazole and tetramethylthiuram. Alternate commercially available hypoallergenic surgeon's gloves include Ultraderm, Eudermic, Dermaprene, and Neolon.

Fisher AA: Contact Dermatitis, 3rd ed. Philadelphia, Lea & Febiger, 1986, 954 pp.

Patch tests with a standard scout tray will reveal contactants to be avoided in one out of ten cases of hand dermatitis. The ultimate reference!

Statistics don't lie; in fact, they don't even speak about your patient.

Herpes Gestationis

Pyridoxine	Plasma exchange
Corticosteroids	
Topical	
Systemic	

Therapy for herpes gestationis has finally come into focus and so has the disease. No longer is it blurred and confused with dermatitis herpetiformis, erythema multiforme, and polymorphic eruption of pregnancy. Immunofluorescent studies have shown it to be a distinctive recognizable entity. It is an immunologically mediated pemphigoid reaction at the basement membrane. With this knowledge has come the focus on corticosteroid therapy, rather than the use of an ill-defined mix of empiric drugs that had varying degrees of hazard for the passive little recipient in utero.

Although the drug of choice for this rare autoimmune disease is a corticosteroid, the therapy of choice is moderation. Never use a systemic steroid when a topical steroid will do, and never use a topical steroid when an emollient will do. Good clinical judgment calls for restraint in treating any pregnant woman, but it is especially necessary in a disease in which premature births and even fetal deaths have been recorded.

The patient, once clearly distinguished, should be given an assessment of her problem:

1. It will probably flare at delivery time and then completely clear within one month.
2. The baby will most likely be healthy, but the possibility of stillbirth or premature birth is present.
3. The disease will usually recur in any subsequent pregnancy.
4. Recurrences may be induced by contraceptives.
5. Relapse can occur later, at the time of menses.

It is wise to allow the patient to look at these somewhat harsh statistical facts through a window curtained with your understanding and empathy. It is comforting for the patient to know that any medical prognosis is an area rich in exceptions. Still, herpes gestationis is not a disease in which one has the optimism associated with its common counterpart, pruritic urticarial papules and plaques of pregnancy.

Holmes RC, Black MM: The specific dermatoses of pregnancy. J Am Acad Dermatol 8:405–412, 1983.

Herpes gestationis, also known as pemphigoid gestationis, has become a distinct disorder, although it has many similarities to bullous pemphigoid. All patients have C3 at the basement membrane zone on direct immunofluorescence, while only about 25 per cent have similar deposition of IgG.

Holmes RC, Black MM, Dann J, et al: A comparative study of toxic erythema of pregnancy and herpes gestationis. Br J Dermatol 106:499–510, 1982.

A study of 24 patients with herpes gestationis showed:

1. There were no fetal abnormalities, although one infant developed large bullae on the scalp.
2. The bullous form clears within one month post partum, while the urticarial form may persist for more than one year.
3. Autoimmune thyrotoxicosis may be associated.
4. There was recurrence in 93 per cent of subsequent pregnancies.
5. Steroids are the best therapy.
6. The incidence is estimated to be 1 in 60,000 pregnancies.

Carruthers JA, Black MM, Ramnarain N: Immunopathological studies in herpes gestationis. Br J Dermatol 96:35–43, 1977.

While two patients had no need for therapy, another required **prednisone** (15 to 30 mg/day) during pregnancy and for more than one year post partum. An additional patient required **prednisolone** (10 to 40 mg/day) during pregnancy and for more than two years after delivery, with no steroid-sparing effect from **azathioprine** (Imuran 150 mg/day for three months).

Lawley TJ, Stingl G, Katz SI: Fetal and maternal risk factors in herpes gestationis. Arch Dermatol 114:552–555, 1978.

A detailed analysis of 41 cases (including 7 of their own) revealed:

23 per cent incidence of prematurity
four causes of fetal death
systemic steroid therapy (**prednisone** 20 to 40 mg/day) frequently necessary

Kolodny RC: Herpes gestationis. A new assessment of incidence, diagnosis and fetal prognosis. Am J Obstet Gynecol 104:39–45, 1969.

Therapy of years past:

ACTH **pyridoxine**
hydrocortisone **sulfapyridine**
progesterone **testosterone**

de Wiel AV, Hart H Ch, Flinterman J, et al: Plasma exchange in herpes gestationis. Br Med J 281:1041–1042, 1980.

A 40-year-old woman in the twenty-sixth week of her fifth pregnancy had hypertension and herpes gestationis. Since antihistaminics and pyridoxine were of no help and systemic steroids were contraindicated, she received three exchanges in which 8 liters of plasma were replaced with an albumin and Haemaccel solution. This gave complete remission, but relapse occurred within 48 hours of parturition, requiring four additional plasma exchanges over one week (12 liters total). Rationale: removal of the pathogenic circulating IgG factor. The authors consider the procedure safe, simple, and effective.

Burkhart CG: Pyridoxine-responsive herpes gestationis. Arch Dermatol 118:535, 1982.

Pyridoxine hydrochloride (vitamin B_6, 400 to 4000 mg/day) induced resolution of lesions in a 26-year-old woman in the third trimester. Skin lesions recurred when she stopped the medication after delivery, but disappeared when she resumed the same high-dose medication for one more month.

Physician confidence inspires patient compliance.

Herpes Simplex

Acyclovir L-Lysine Teldrin Silvadene cream

The introduction of acyclovir promises to convert the therapy of this disease from the complex to the simple. Formerly the therapy of this life-long, insidiously recurring viral infection involved following a labyrinthine trail. The hapless victim received a score of prophylactic exhortations ranging from "Avoid stress, sunlight and sin" to "Take two aspirins." He was given vaccines of all types, as well as supplements of animal, vegetable, and mineral origin. Once the sore appeared it was battered, rammed, and crushed with chloroform, ultrasound, and phototoxic dyes, to mention but a few of the popular punitive measures. This common cold sore got more treatment than any common cold.

But now, all this has been quietly replaced by a prescription for acyclovir (Zovirax 200 mg q4h), to be taken at times of stress or fever and at the moment of the earliest sensory warning that a vesicle is imminent. When used in this anticipatory fashion, acyclovir is remarkably effective in preventing herpes simplex. It is not helpful, however, as a treatment for the established lesion in the non-immunocompromised patient. Nor is its topical form (Zovirax ointment 5 per cent) effective as therapy. It is a drug, so to speak, that prevents the patient from falling down the stairs, not one that heals his fracture. Thus the patient must carry his immediate supply of Zovirax capsules with him 24 hours a day, month in and month out. He cannot wait until he goes to the drugstore or goes home to start taking the pill. Once started, the drug is continued for at least three days past the trigger point. The patient must understand that although the drug does not kill the virus in the neural ganglion, it can prevent its harmful growth in the skin.

With individuals who have frequent attacks of unexplained origin, or individuals immunocompromised by either drug therapy or AIDS, we recommend that Zovirax be given indefinitely in a dose of 400 mg bid.

For the patient who already has the herpetic lesion, we advise any one of a number of local measures to speed drying of the vesicles and prevent the commonly occurring secondary bacterial infection. We like Silvadene cream (silver sulfadiazine), Drysol (aluminum chloride hexahydrate 20 per cent in anhydrous ethyl alcohol), or Neosporin ointment (neomycin, polysporin, bacitracin). We strongly caution against topical corticosteroids in the first few days, but once the vesicles are gone these may aid in reducing inflammation.

We advise that the lesions in the early stage are highly contagious, so for that brief period kissing and sexual contact (if the lesion is genital) must be avoided. The lesion is likewise a source of danger for the patient's own eyes. He must

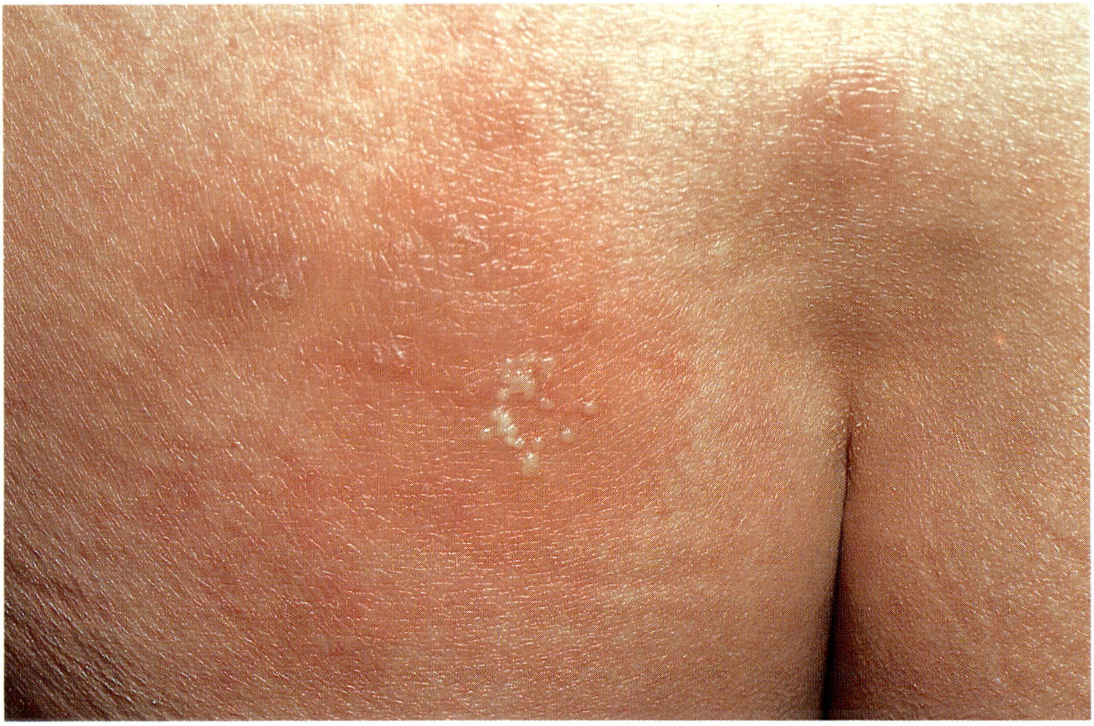

scrupulously wash his hands and avoid as much as possible direct or indirect transfer of the vesicular fluid to the eye region. Any conjunctivitis calls for immediate ophthalmologic consultation, as herpetic keratitis may cause blindness.

We reassure all patients that their virus does not cause cancer, despite newspaper reports to the contrary. However, the presence of herpetic infection in the cervix or vagina of a pregnant woman at term demands intensive acyclovir therapy and often a cesarean delivery to avoid the tragedy of infecting the newborn passing through the birth canal.

Given the patient who declines acyclovir therapy for the prophylaxis of recurrent herpes simplex we recommend:

1. Long-term L-Lysine (Enisyl 500 mg tid)
2. Avoidance of sunburn by use of sun screens (sun protective factor 15)
3. Teldrin or Chlor-Trimeton (chlorpheniramine—12 mg hs for two weeks before each period) if the attacks are premenstrual
4. Inderal (**propranolol** 20 mg tid) before and during times of significant stress
5. Superficial epidermal subsection of the lesion if recurrences are at the same site

It is estimated that Americans suffer at least a hundred million attacks of herpes simplex each year, and it is likely that each has his own treatment. However, the new remedy, acyclovir, is proving to be an ounce of prevention worth more than all these other pounds of cure.

Spoor HJ: The course and management of recurrent herpes. Cutis 24:309–313, 335–336, 1979.

Of 281 patients observed over a 20-year period 18 per cent could relate their attacks of herpes to upper respiratory infection, 10 per cent to sunburn, 9 per cent to emotional stress, and 8 per cent to surgery or trauma.

Strauss SE: Herpes simplex virus infection: Biology, treatment, and prevention. Ann Intern Med 103:404–419, 1985.

This comprehensive NIH conference (with 132 references) stresses the usefulness of **acyclovir** for treating and suppressing HSV infection, but emphasizes the unanswered questions of long-term safety and emergence of drug resistance.

No effective vaccines are yet available for HSV infections.

Anderson H, Scarffe JH, Sutton RNP, et al: Oral acyclovir prophylaxis against herpes simplex virus in non-Hodgkin lymphoma and acute lymphoblastic leukaemia patients receiving remission induction chemotherapy. A randomized double-blind, placebo controlled trial. Br J Cancer 50:45–49, 1984.

Prophylactic oral **acyclovir** (Zovirax 200 mg q6h during six weeks of chemotherapy) reduced the incidence of clinical HSV infection from 60 per cent in the placebo group to 5 per cent in those taking acyclovir. The study involved 41 patients.

Mindel A: Long term oral acyclovir in disseminated mucocutaneous herpes simplex: A case report. Br J Vener Dis 60:125–126, 1984.

Acyclovir (200 mg qid for 12 weeks) continuously suppressed genital herpes infection in a 24-year-old woman with Crohn's disease (controlled with **azothiaprine** 100 mg/day and **prednisolone** 7.5 mg/day). Lesions reappeared promptly once the acyclovir was stopped at the end of three months.

Laskin OL: Acyclovir and suppression of frequently recurring herpetic whitlow. Ann Intern Med 102:494–495, 1985.

Acyclovir (200 mg tid) gave a 30-year-old woman doctor six months of complete freedom from herpetic whitlow, which had been recurring approximately 12 times a year for four years. Three days after stopping the acyclovir she developed a herpes lesion at the same site. Since acyclovir does not eradicate latent herpesvirus infections, long-term continuous use would seem advisable, but at present treatment is recommended for only six months because of lack of data on possible adverse effects from longer administration.

Lagnew DC Jr, Furlow TG, Hager WD, Yarrish RL: Disseminated herpes simplex virus infection in pregnancy. Successful treatment with acyclovir. JAMA 252:2058–2059, 1984.

Acyclovir 7.5 mg/kg (430 mg IV q8h for 20 doses) dramatically improved and cleared disseminated HSV infection in a 26-year-old woman in the third trimester of pregnancy. A normal healthy infant was delivered by cesarean section. This type of infection may be life-threatening because of impaired cell-mediated immunity during the third trimester.

Robinson GE, Underhill GS, Forster GE, et al: Treatment with acyclovir of genital herpes simplex virus infection complicated by eczema herpeticum. Br J Vener Dis 60:241–242, 1984.

Acyclovir (200 mg five times daily for five days) cleared two cases of eczema herpeticum. One patient also needed oral antibiotics for secondary bacterial infection.

Bryson YJ, Dillon M, Lovett M, et al: Treatment of first episodes of genital herpes simplex virus infection with oral acyclovir. A randomized double-blind controlled trial in normal subjects. N Engl J Med 308:916–921, 1983.

Acyclovir (200 mg five times daily for 10 days) proved to be a successful treatment for the primary attack of genital herpes simplex in 48 young adults. However, it did not alter the recurrence rate of 70 per cent in patients observed for four to nine months.

Meyers JD, Wade JC, Mitchell CD, et al: Multicenter collaborative trial of intravenous acyclovir for treatment of mucocutaneous herpes simplex virus infection in the immunocompromised host. Am J Med 73(Suppl 1A):229–235, 1982.

Intravenous **acyclovir** (250 mg/sq m IV over a one-hour period every eight hours for one week) was a safe, effective treatment in 97 immunocompromised patients with mucocutaneous HSV infection. Viral shedding and healing time were both shortened.

Richards DM, Carmine AA, Brogden RN, et al: Acyclovir: A review of its pharmacodynamic properties and therapeutic efficacy. Drugs 26:378–438, 1983.

A splendid comprehensive review.

Acyclovir ointment 3 per cent is helpful for herpes simplex dendritic keratitis, but does not protect from recurrences or the development of deeper herpetic ocular disease.

Herpes simplex virus type 2 calls for a larger dose than type 1, based on inhibitory concentrations.

Alexander S: The prevention of recurrent herpes simplex with aspirin. Br J Dermatol 74:83–85, 1962.

Six of nine patients with recurrent menstrual herpes were able to prevent attacks by charting for three months their daily temperatures upon awakening in relationship to the onset of herpes lesions and the onset of menstruation, and then taking **aspirin** (5 grains qid) to block any evidence of fever. In most patients temperature elevation occurred either 48 hours prior to the onset of menstruation or between days 12 and 16 of their cycles. Patients were instructed to take the aspirin for 24 hours preceding the day of the expected temperature rise. In one case, recurrent erythema multiforme triggered by herpes infection was also prevented.

McCune MA, Perry HO, Muller SA, O'Fallon WM: Treatment of recurrent herpes simplex infections with L-lysine monohydrochloride. Cutis 34:366–373, 1984.

A prospective, randomized, double-blind, placebo-controlled cross-over study of 41 patients showed that oral ingestion of 1248 mg/day of L-lysine decreased the recurrence rate, but not the severity, of herpes simplex attacks. A smaller dosage (624 mg/day) was of no value. Chocolate was considered to be the most common food factor triggering attacks. Other "herpetogenic" foods, which are high in arginine content, were believed to be cola drinks, cashew nuts, and peanuts. Some patients claimed, in decreasing order of frequency, the following food triggers:

chocolate	peanuts
peas	gelatin
cola drinks	cashews
grain cereals	beer

Foods with a high lysine content, which should be encouraged, include:

dairy products	potatoes
milk	brewer's yeast

Shelley WB: Surgical treatment for recurrent herpes simplex. Lancet 2:1021-1022, 1978.

Superficial horizontal epidermal excision of active herpetic lesions during the first 48 hours was effective therapy and prevented recurrence at that exact site in 20 patients. Excision was performed using half of a flexible razor blade (Gillette Super Blue Blade) while the skin was held under firm traction. Presumably, subepidermal fibrosis from the surgery prevented reinnervation of the epidermis and thus stopped further viral shedding and herpetic attacks at the surgical site.

Yeo JM, Fiddian AP: Acyclovir in the management of herpes labialis. J Antimicrob Agents Chemother 12(Suppl B):95–103, 1983.

The failure of topical **acyclovir** (Zovirax ointment 5 per cent) in ordinary practice may be attributed to too low a concentration, poor penetration of the drug, too few applications, and use too late in the course of the disease. Acyclovir cream in a propylene glycol base appeared to be more promising in treating herpes labialis (not available in the United States).

Whitley RJ, Levin M, Barton N, et al: Infections caused by herpes simplex virus in the immunocompromised host: Natural history and topical acyclovir therapy. J Infect Dis 150:323–329, 1984.

But note that the value of topical **acyclovir** ointment could be discerned in treatment of extensive herpetic lesions in immunocompromised hosts. This double-blind, placebo-controlled study of 63 consecutive patients assessed the value of one-inch strips of acyclovir ointment (polyethylene glycol base, applied six times a day for 10 days) to herpetic lesions. There was accelerated clearance of virus and accelerated resolution of pain and healing of lip and skin lesions. The benefit was most marked in patients with lesions more than two inches in diameter.

Brody I: Topical treatment of recurrent herpes simplex and post-herpetic erythema multiforme with low concentrations of zinc sulphate solution. Br J Dermatol 104:191–194, 1981.

In 25 patients, gauze compresses soaked with lukewarm **zinc sulfate** solution (0.025 to 0.05 per cent for cutaneous lesions, 0.01 to 0.025 per cent for mucosal lesions, applied 10 minutes daily for 14 days, tapering to once a week) prevented relapses of herpes simplex lesions that had previously occurred regularly following upper respiratory infections. Zinc ions selectively inhibit replication of herpes virus type I.

Glogau RG: How I treat herpes simplex. Med Times 108(3):66–68, 1980.

For pain:

salicylates, codeine
lidocaine ointment 5 per cent, on fourchette or perirectal skin
Celestone Soluspan (6 mg in 1 ml IM) or **prednisolone** (60 mg/day in divided doses for two to three days) for herpetic whitlow
Stoxil (**idoxuridine** 0.1 per cent solution) or Vira-A ophthalmic ointment (**vidarabine** 3 per cent) for cornea infection

For prevention:

good hygiene
condom
RVPaba sun stick
avoidance of prolonged hot baths or saunas

For secondary infection:

Burow's solution (Domeboro powder packets and tablets)
antibiotic ointment (**polymyxin B-neomycin-gramicidin**)
miconazole cream
erythromycin orally

Jarratt M, Smith R, Knox JM: Therapy of herpes simplex infection. Int J Dermatol 18:357–361, 1979.

Thymol (4 per cent in chloroform applied bid for two to three days), especially for herpetic whitlow and herpes progenitalis
Glutaraldehyde (2 per cent buffered to pH 7.5 with sodium bicarbonate, apply bid)
Corticosteroid creams
Silvadene cream (**silver sulfadiazine**)
Liquid N_2
DNCB
Betadine (**povidone-iodine**)
Intralesional **triamcinolone acetonide**

First law of therapy: Prevent secondary bacterial infection.

Curry SS: Cutaneous herpes simplex infections and their treatment. Cutis 26:41–58, 1980.

Antiviral treatments—usefulness not confirmed in controllable studies:

idoxuridine
cytosine arabinoside
adenine arabinoside
neutral red (aqueous 0.1 per cent) plus fluorescent light for 15 minutes, repeat in six hours

Old treatments of doubtful value:

vaccines (smallpox, BCG, herpes)
chlorpromazine (Thorazine 50 to 100 mg hs)
griseofulvin
Betadine (povidone-iodine) topically
glutaraldehyde topically
ethyl ether topically

Primary herpetic gingivostomatitis:

Benadryl gargle
Xylocaine viscous
Mycostatin suspension
aspirin

Thiers BH: Unusual treatments for herpesvirus infections. I. Herpes simplex. J Am Acad Dermatol 7:811–816, 1982.

Some more recent contenders of doubtful value:

amantadine topical
betadine
boric acid
chloroform
cimetidine
diethylether
epinephrine
ice
levamisole
psychotherapy
thymol
transfer factor
ultrasound
vitamin E
zinc

Two aspirin and a "wake-up-doc" call may have some value, since prostaglandin inhibitors seem to be potent inhibitors of viral replication in vitro.

van de Staak WJBM, Govaert FJ: Treatment of recurrent herpes-simplex infection with liquid nitrogen. Dermatologica 146:373–374, 1973.

In 19 of 25 patients there was no recurrence of herpes at sites treated on one to three occasions with **liquid nitrogen**.

Vonderheid EC, Milstein HJ, Thompson KD, Wu BC: Chronic herpes simplex infection in cutaneous T-cell lymphomas. Arch Dermatol 116:1018–1022, 1980.

Sulfadiazine silver cream 1 per cent (Silvadene) seemed useful in five patients with very extensive herpetic erosions.

Hunter DT: Sodium hypochlorite in the treatment of herpes simplex virus infections. Cutis 31:328–332, 1983.

Sodium hypochlorite (0.5 per cent freshly prepared from 5 per cent stable aqueous stock solution) used locally twice daily seemed beneficial in this uncontrolled study of 36 patients. For mucosal lesions, use 0.1 per cent solution (e.g., mouthwash 30 seconds bid). The action of this chlorine-releasing chemical is presumed to be virucidal.

Takagaki K, Jidoi J: Topical application of ethyl ether to recurrent herpes simplex. J Dermatol (Tokyo) 8:109–111, 1981.

Twenty patients were helped by applying a cotton swab soaked in ethyl ether (10 minutes tid for the first two days of the lesion—must protect nasal and oral mucosa from ether vapor). They found that healing was rapid and remissions were prolonged. Remember, however, that ether is not only inflammable but explosive. No controls.

Lieb J: Remission of recurrent herpes infection during therapy with lithium. N Engl J Med 301:942, 1979.

Two convincing examples:

1. Labial herpes, regularly recurring before each menstrual period, was completely prevented during eight months of **lithium** (900 mg/day) therapy. When the patient stopped taking lithium the herpes recurred at the time of her next period and has recurred every month since then.
2. Herpes progenitalis, attacks one to two times per month for eight years, cleared for three months with lithium carbonate (1200 mg/day) therapy. On stopping, the next attack occurred in three weeks. Resumption of lithium again induced remission.

Kit S, Kit M: Herpes simplex virus vaccines—Where are we? Clin Obstet Gynecol 28:164–177, 1985.

Nothing clinically useful yet. Five types currently under study are:

1. Inactivated herpes virus, e.g., the European Lupidon G.
2. Subunit
3. Biosynthetic vaccine
4. Recombinant hybrid
5. Modified live virus

Laird SM, Roy RB: Treatment of primary attacks of genital herpes with co-trimoxazole. Br J Clin Pract 29:37–42, 1975.

In 46 patients with primary HSV genital infections, **co-trimoxazole** (Septrin—**trimethoprim** 80 mg plus **sulfamethoxazole** 400 mg—two tablets q12h for five days) gave impressive symptomatic relief in 90 per cent within 7 days and complete healing in most patients in 11 to 12 days.

Gosling PH: Treatment of herpes simplex with co-trimoxazole. Br Med J 1:41, 1975.

Approximately 80 per cent of patients with recurrent herpes simplex infections respond favorably to **co-trimoxazole** (two tablets bid for seven days). Children may be treated with lower proportionate doses. Concurrent treatment with **penicillin** nullifies the effect.

Herpes zoster responds favorably to the same treatment continued for 10 to 14 days.

Amantadine (Symmetrel 100 mg bid) may help patients who do not respond to co-trimoxazole.

Being agreeable is the best antidote for the disagreeable patient.

Herpes Zoster

Acyclovir	Chlorprothixene
Steroids	Pimozide
ACTH	Cryotherapy
Cimetidine	

These are exciting times. We are truly in the age of anti-DNA therapy. For years we have had specific compounds that interfere with the DNA machinery of the cell. Witness the remarkable clinical effect of 5-fluorouracil on actinic keratoses. And now we have the laboratory-synthesized nucleosides, which specifically interfere with viral DNA replication but not with the DNA of the host cell. Acyclovir is the only available example that can be given orally, and it or an analogue, such as bromovinyl deoxyuridine (BVDU), should receive wide usage.

Thus, the promises of yesterday have become the treatment of today. Our initial therapy of acute herpes zoster is now high dose **acyclovir** (Zovirax, four 200 mg capsules every four hours five times a day for 10 days). Formerly, we gave **ACTH** (40 U IM daily) for five days, or **triamcinolone acetonide** (Kenalog 40 mg IM, once a week) until healing had occurred. We coupled this with erythromycin (250 mg qid) to prevent secondary bacterial infection. The course of zoster is so capricious as to keep us yet uncertain as to whether the new is better than the old.

Topically we use Burow's compresses (warm, 15 minutes qid) until vesiculation has cleared. Each compress is followed by application of Zovirax (acyclovir) ointment. After this phase we prescribe a steroid cream such as Valisone cream. Analgesics are prescribed as needed, but often a heating pad provides sufficient relief. In cases of zoster of the thorax, a degree of splinting by means of an Ace bandage, a chest binder, or a tight vest gives symptomatic help. We prefer that the patient not work during the acute phase, since he may have a viremia and needs rest. Those with involvement of the face must be seen by an ophthalmologist at once for detection and treatment of any eye lesions.

We alert patients to the fact that this is "second-time" chickenpox. They must refrain from contact with infants and children who have not had varicella. More importantly, they must not be in contact with immunocompromised individuals. This may mean temporary separation from a spouse who is undergoing chemotherapy, has an organ transplant, or has leukemia. We advise that contagiousness is minimal once all of the vesicles have healed.

We instruct patients that although the sensory nerves are almost invariably the target cell, motor neurons may be involved. Thus we see facial motor paralysis in the Ramsay Hunt syndrome and may observe inability to void when a pelvic dermatome is affected.

We do not do exhaustive testing for a systemic disorder or internal malignant disease but do study any symptomatic leads the patient may provide. We also regularly secure a health profile, chest roentgenogram, and usually a CEA de-

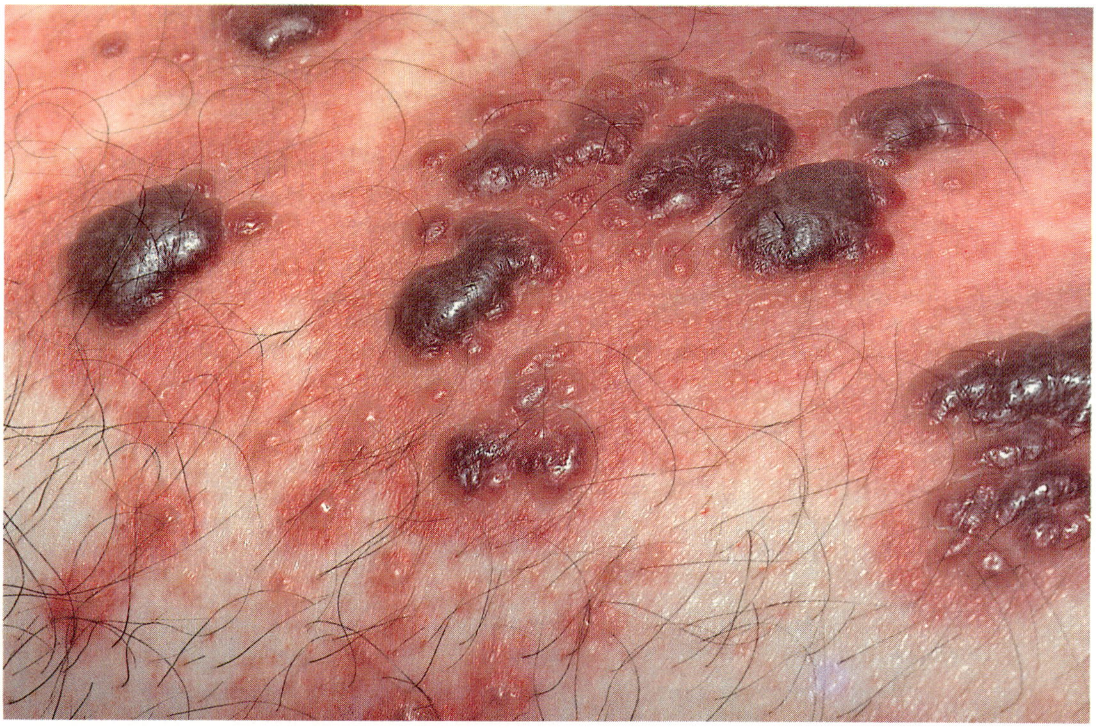

termination in the older group. However, it is rare that we find any underlying cause for this recrudescence of the varicella virus in zoster patients.

The older the patient, the more likely the therapeutic challenge will be not the acute attack but rather the chronic neuralgia that develops. We have little evidence that current treatments of the acute attack, including oral acyclovir, have any influence on the development of postherpetic neuralgia. Major help is provided by codeine and other strong analgesics, but in some the pain is so unremitting and so severe that the patient will embrace treatments ranging from acupuncture to cordotomy. All of these individuals need your close attention and selected trials of drugs such as Tagamet, Taractan, and Orap. These patients need your hand, your encouragement, and your continued help in the months to come. If it is not there, the depression of these elderly people can become so profound as to destroy their will to live. Remember Richard Asher's prescription of "hope not dope."

Burgoon CF Jr, Burgoon JS, Baldridge CD: The natural history of herpes zoster. JAMA 164:265–269, 1957.

Observation of 206 zoster patients revealed:

The disease is acute and self-limiting: More than half of the cases clear within two weeks.

Postherpetic neuralgia occurred in 20 patients. Only four of the group had neuralgia lasting longer than six months.

Zoster is more severe and prolonged in older patients.

Frengley JD: Herpes zoster: A challenge in management. Primary Care 8:715–731, 1981.

Acute phase:

- Burow's compresses
- drying lotions
- analgesics (e.g., **codeine** 60 mg, not prn, but regular doses to prevent pain buildup)
- tricyclic antidepressants—**doxepin** (Sinequan 10 to 25 mg tid)

Postherpetic neuralgia defies all therapeutic attempts.

Finn R, Smith MA: Oral acyclovir for herpes zoster. Lancet 2:575, 1984.

Acyclovir (Zovirax 200 mg five times a day—given q4h when awake for five days) completely aborted zoster in five of five patients treated within 24 hours of onset. The drug had no effect on five other patients with zoster in whom the treatment was not begun until after the second day of the disease.

Novelli VM, Marshall WC, Yeo J, McKendrick GD: Acyclovir administered perorally in immunocompromised children with varicella-zoster infections. J Infect Dis 149:478, 1984.

Acyclovir (400 mg five times daily for 10 days) was helpful in the treatment of herpes zoster in 10 children with leukemia and other malignant diseases.

Esmann V, Ipsen J, Peterslund NA, et al: Therapy of acute herpes zoster with acyclovir in the nonimmunocompromised host. Am J Med 73(1A):320–325, 1982.

Acylovir (5 mg/kg IV bolus tid for five days) was shown to increase the rate of pain disappearance during the first two weeks in this exquisitely detailed double-blind study of 27 patients. There was no difference in the course between the drug and placebo groups at one- and three-month checkpoints. Interestingly, trigeminal lesions healed faster than those elsewhere.

McGill J, Chapman C, Copplestone A, Maharasingam M: A review of acyclovir treatment of ocular herpes zoster and skin infections. J Antimicrob Chemother 12(Suppl B):45–49, 1983.

IV **acyclovir** (five days) helped resolve skin lesions, but did not clear ocular involvement. Topical acyclovir (Zovirax ointment 3.3 per cent five times daily) controlled herpes zoster keratouveitis with no recurrences. It was much superior to topical steroids, which should not be used concomitantly.

Nicholson KG: Antiviral therapy: Varicella-zoster virus infections, herpes labialis and mucocutaneous herpes, and cytomegalovirus infections. Lancet 2:677–681, 1984.

The need for antiviral therapy is enormously magnified in immunocompromised patients. This sound current appraisal with 67 references is a joy to read.

King DH, Galasso G: Proceedings of a symposium on acyclovir. Am J Med 73(1A):1–393, 1982.

Nearly 400 pages of details concerning the only oral antiviral drug currently available for treating zoster.

Öberg B, Johansson N-G: The relative merits and drawbacks of new nucleoside analogues with clinical potential. J Antimicrob Chemother 14(Suppl A):5–26, 1984.

An entrancing molecular biology story of four drugs synthesized to act by specific enzymatic inhibition of viral replication. These are not drugs from the bark of trees or the roots of plants, but from laboratories dedicated to the study of differences in DNA metabolism between man and virus. The four clinically useful drugs are **idoxuridine**, **vidarabine** (ara-A), **acyclovir**, and the newest, **bromovinyl deoxyuridine** (BVDU).

Brigden D, Whiteman P: The mechanism of action, pharmacokinetics and toxicity of acyclovir—a review. J Infect 6(Suppl 1):3–9, 1983.

Acyclovir is a nontoxic, nonmutagenic compound that selectively inhibits specific, critical polymerases found in viruses but not in the host cells.

Clemmensen OH, Anderson KE: ACTH versus prednisone and placebo in herpes zoster treatment. Clin Exp Dermatol 9:557–563, 1984.

ACTH (1 mg IM, three times/week for two weeks) gave more relief from pain during the first four days than **prednisone** (45 mg/day for the first week, 30 mg/day for the second week, and 15 mg/day for the third week). There was no evidence that either reduced the incidence of postherpetic neuralgia. The study was done in a controlled fashion on 60 patients. The authors suggest that ACTH may block pain by attaching to endorphin receptors.

Eaglestein WH, Katz R, Brown JA: The effects of early corticosteroid therapy on the skin eruption and pain of herpes zoster. JAMA 211:1681–1683, 1970.

Although oral **triamcinolone** (48 mg/day for one week, 24 mg/day for a second week, and 16 mg/day for the third week) had no effect on the pain of acute zoster, it did significantly reduce the duration of postherpetic neuralgia. A controlled study of 35 patients. There was no evidence that corticosteroids made the eruption spread.

Keczkes K, Basheer AM: Do corticosteroids prevent post-herpetic neuralgia? Br J Dermatol 102:551–555, 1980.

Yes! Only 15 per cent of patients receiving **prednisone** (40 mg/day for 10 days, then tapered over one month) developed postherpetic neuralgia, whereas the control group receiving **carbamazepine** (Tegretol 100 mg qid) showed a 65 per cent incidence. This study of 40 patients over 50 years of age emphasized the need to treat as soon as possible. (Please alert your office staff to this—the patients need immediate appointments.)

Epstein E: Treatment of herpes zoster and postzoster neuralgia by subcutaneous injection of triamcinolone. Int J Dermatol 20:65–68, 1981.

Describes treatment of 272 patients who had acute herpes zoster and 128 patients who had postzoster neuralgia with sublesional **triamcinolone acetonide** suspension (Kenalog-40, Aristocort Forte, or Aristospan, diluted with normal saline to a final concentration of 2 mg/ml). Every day for 5 to 14 days 30 ml were injected, using a 25-gauge ⅝-inch needle. The striking observation is that 65 per cent of the author's patients with postherpetic neuralgia were helped.

Riopelle JM, Naraghi M, Grush KP: Chronic neuralgia incidence following local anesthetic therapy for herpes zoster. Arch Dermatol 120:747–750, 1984.

Temporary relief from pain in 72 patients referred to a pain clinic with acute herpetic neuralgia was given by:

- Stellate ganglion block (**bupivacaine** 0.25 to 0.5 per cent)
- Epidural block (bupivacaine 0.125 to 0.5 per cent)
- Intralesional infiltration (bupivacaine 0.25 per cent with or without **triamcinolone acetonide** 0.2 per cent)
- Peripheral nerve block (bupivacaine 0.25 to 0.5 per cent)

None of these procedures prevented the development of persistent pain in nine patients.

Whitley RJ, Soong S-J, Dolin R, et al: Early vidarabine therapy to control the complications of herpes zoster in immunosuppressed patients. N Engl J Med 307:971–975, 1982.

Ara-A (**vidarabine** 10 mg/kg/day IV over 12 hours for five days) accelerated the rate of healing, reduced the chance of disseminated lesions, and decreased postherpetic neuralgia in this double-blind study of 121 patients.

Merigan TC, Rand KH, Pollard RB, et al: Human leukocyte interferon for the treatment of herpes zoster in patients with cancer. N Engl J Med 298:981–987, 1978.

High-dosage purified interferon (still experimental) significantly decreased new vesicle formation and the severity of postherpetic neuralgia and reduced visceral complications by sixfold in 90 patients carefully studied under a double-blind, randomized study protocol.

Whitley RJ, Ch'ien LT, Dolin R, et al: Adenine arabinoside therapy of herpes zoster in the immunosuppressed. N Engl J Med 294:1193–1199, 1976.

Adenine arabinoside, a purine nucleoside (**vidarabine** 10 mg/kg/day IV over 12 hours for five days) shortened the disease course in 47 patients. It must be given in the first six days of the disease. This controlled multicenter study used randomized cross-over techniques.

Stevens DA, Merigan TC: Zoster immune globulin prophylaxis of disseminated zoster in compromised hosts: A randomized trial. Arch Intern Med 140:52–54, 1980.

Zoster immune globulin (ZIG 5 ml IM in each buttock) was no better than pooled gammaglobulin (IM) in alleviating either zoster pain or dissemination in a study of 97 patients.

Sulliger JM, Imbach P, Barandun S, et al: Varicella and herpes zoster in immunosuppressed children: Preliminary results of treatment with intravenous immunoglobulin. Helv Paediatr Acta 39:63–70, 1984.

Two immunosuppressed children with herpes zoster benefited from large intravenous doses of polyvalent intact immunoglobulin (IgG 0.4 gm/kg/day, one to seven doses IV). It was more effective if given early. In one patient, uncontrollable pain subsided within a few hours of the first infusion.

The risk for reactivation of herpes zoster in children and adults with cancer is 15 to 52 per cent, being about 33 per cent in children.

Kramer PW: The management of postherpetic neuralgia with chlorprothixene. Surg Neurol 15:102–104, 1981.

Taracten (**chloroprothixene**) gave good to excellent relief of postherpetic pain in 12 of 16 older patients who had suffered for more than two years. This phenothiazine derivative should be given in ascending dosage to the point of relief (10 to 100 add mg qid).

Through the years, this bête noir of neuralgia has been attacked with the following medications and procedures:

autohemotherapy
carbamazepine
diphtheria vaccine
histamine
immune blood
intravenous puncture
iron sulfate
mocassin venom
phenytoin
protamine
quinine
radiation
smallpox vaccination
sodium iodide
vasopressin
vitamin B compounds
alcohol block
cordotomy
cortical extirpation
lobotomy
neurectomy
phenol block
rhizotomy
skin undermining
sympathectomy
thalamotomy

Cordotomy is the ultimate weapon, since the pain is not of peripheral origin.

Duke EE: Clinical experience with pimozide: Emphasis on its use in postherpetic neuralgia. J Am Acad Dermatol 8:845–850, 1983.

Orap (**pimozide** 2 mg tid) gave dramatic complete relief of neuralgic pain in four of eight patients. The medication must be continued for months, since the pain recurs if it is stopped.

Suzuki H, Ogawa S, Nakagawa H, et al: Cryocautery of sensitized skin areas for the relief of pain due to postherpetic neuralgia. Pain 9:355–362, 1980.

Five of 14 patients, refractory to conventional therapy, had relief of pain following cryotherapy of affected skin sites with dry ice (carbon dioxide stick, 1 cm diameter, apply for one minute—induces bullae, pain, and depigmentation). Must preanesthetize area. Each patient had approximately eight treatments, two to three weeks apart.

Toyama N: Sympathetic ganglion block therapy for herpes zoster. J Dermatol (Tokyo) 9:59–62, 1982.

Anesthetic block of local sympathetic ganglia with **lidocaine** 1 per cent (8 to 10 ml) was effective in 38 of 43 patients. The pain disappeared within five minutes and did not return for one to two hours, after which it was much attenuated. Injections should be given as early as possible for full effectiveness, especially on the head and face.

Thiers BH: Unusual treatments for herpesvirus infections. II. Herpes zoster. J Am Acad Dermatol 8:433–436, 1983.

A valuable reference source of diverse remedies ranging from **emetine** to **levodopa**.

Burton WJ, Gould PW, Hursthouse MW, et al: A multicentre trial of Zostrum (5% idoxuridine in dimethyl sulphoxide) in herpes zoster. N Z Med J 94:384–386, 1981.

Idoxuridine (5 per cent in DMSO applied bid) relieved pain and reduced vesiculation in 46 patients in a multicenter randomized controlled study. (Adherence to the caveat that treatment must be started within 48 hours of the onset reduces its usefulness in clinical practice.)

Hayne ST, Mercer JB: Herpes zoster: Treatment with cimetidine. Can Med Assoc J 129:1284–1285, 1983.

In a 61-year-old man, **cimetidine** (600 mg q8h) and zinc sulfate (200 mg tid) appeared to markedly decrease pain and accelerate healing.

Shandera R: Treatment of herpes zoster with cimetidine. Can Med Assoc J 131:279, 1984.

Cimetidine (600 mg q8h) plus **zinc sulfate** (200 mg tid with food) gave dramatic relief of pain within 36 hours to 14 of 15 patients with herpes zoster.

Gordon HH: Glutaraldehyde in treating herpes simplex and herpes zoster. Arch Dermatol 112:1178, 1976.

Glutaraldehyde (2 per cent, alkaline-buffered to pH 7.5 with soda bicarbonate, applied bid for two weeks) helped four patients with zoster. The lesions dried quickly, and symptoms were reduced.

Krulig L, Jacobs PH: Flexible collodion. Arch Dermatol 110:466–467, 1974.

Painting herpes zoster lesions and the immediately surrounding area with flexible collodion every 12 hours provides real relief from pain. After the ether evaporates, a transparent tenacious film forms that helps to prevent irritation.

Boundy CAP, Bamford JAC: Treatment of herpes zoster with "protamide." Med J Aust 1:528–531, 1968.

Protamide (colloidal suspension of denatured proteolytic enzyme from pig stomach mucosa) was advertised and used for more than 20 years in treating herpetic neuralgia. This four-year multicenter double-blind controlled study of 138 patients was the first to critically assess its worth. Conclusion: Protamide is of no help. Moral: Avoid "blind" acceptance of drugs that come without "double-blind" credentials.

Lawrence RM: Autoimmune therapy for herpes zoster. West J Med 130:271, 1979.

Draw 20 ml of the patient's blood and immediately inject 10 ml IM into each buttock (daily for four days). The author claims good results in treating several hundred patients.

(Comment: Is this the poor man's **ACTH** or the poor man's placebo? Autohemotherapy is another approach that has never been subjected to rigorous clinical evaluation. It was popular in a period when any attempt to compare it with saline injections was viewed as a violation of both the patient's trust in the doctor and the doctor's trust in the treatment. The inquiring, doubting mind has only slowly gained access to the bedside.)

Weidmann MJ: Surgical relief of post-herpetic pain by excision of scarred skin. Med J Aust 1:472–473, 1976.

Surgical excision (with primary closure) of the scarred skin site of zoster pain cured three patients and gave appreciable relief to three others in this study of ten patients.

Gershon AA: Prevention and treatment of varicella-zoster virus infection. Pediatr Infect Dis 3(Suppl 3):S34–S36, 1984.

Varicella-zoster immune globulin (VZIG) injections provide no prophylaxis for zoster. However, if given within three days of household exposure to a person at high risk for developing severe varicella, it will modify the disease (dosage: 1.25 ml/10 kg body weight IM).

Wildiers J, De Clercq E: Oral (E)-5-(2-bromovinyl)-2′-deoxyuridine treatment of severe herpes zoster in cancer patients. Eur J Cancer Clin Oncol 20:471–476, 1984.

Bromovinyl deoxyuridine (BVDU 7.5 mg/kg/day PO = 125 mg tid to qid for five days) stopped progression of zoster within 24 hours in 12 of 20 patients and within one to five days in 6 additional patients. This new experimental nucleoside drug offers the greatest promise, since its 50 per cent inhibitory dose for 10 strains of varicella-zoster virus in cell culture is only 0.0024 μg/ml, whereas that of **acyclovir** is 4.64 μg/ml.

Sklar SH, Blue WT, Alexander EJ, Bodian CA: Herpes zoster: The treatment and prevention of neuralgia with adenosine monophosphate. JAMA 253:1427–1430, 1985.

Adenosine monophosphate (AMP, 100 mg in aqueous gel IM three times weekly for one month) provided relief from pain and postherpetic neuralgia in this randomized, placebo controlled, double-blind study of 32 adults with herpes zoster. After four weeks, 88 per cent of AMP-treated patients were pain free, in contrast to only 43 per cent in the placebo group.

Balfour HH: Acyclovir therapy for herpes zoster: Advantages and adverse effects. JAMA 255:387–388, 1986.

The treatment of acute herpes zoster with large dose oral **acyclovir** (Zovirax, 4 grams daily for 10 days) is currently being evaluated in a multicenter US trial, since earlier studies with lower doses produced inconclusive results.

It's better to know the best treatment than all the rest.

Hidradenitis Suppurativa

Accutane	Antibiotics
Surgery	Dapsone
Drysol	

Surgery is the treatment of choice for hidradenitis. It is indeed the only treatment that promises a real cure. But patients resist it. As with breaking a leg, there is no convenient time for such surgery. The patient prefers to procrastinate, pleading for physician prescriptions. Witness the 8 to 10 years of suffering the average patient accepts before coming for surgery.

We carefully explain to all our patients the need for early surgery. We completely excise early localized apocrine abscesses of the axilla, as incision and drainage are simply inadequate. And we urge patients with advanced chronic lesions to have an experienced plastic surgeon remove the entire apocrine-sweat-gland-bearing panniculus, not only the infected lesions. We emphasize that a few months of convalescence is far less disabling than decades of tenderness, pain, suppuration, drainage, and the possibility of cancer in the area.

But for the patient who will not submit to surgery, our first prescription is Accutane (40 mg bid). We couple this with dapsone (100 mg/day). The area is regularly washed with Desquam-X 10 Wash (benzoyl peroxide), and Drysol (aluminum chloride hexahydrate 20 per cent in absolute ethyl alcohol) is applied locally each night to reduce eccrine sweating.

If improvement is not prompt we initiate supplemental therapy with clindamycin (Cleocin 150 mg qid) and pack any sinuses with 10 per cent benzoyl peroxide gel. We often prescribe zinc in the form of zinc sulfate (220 mg tid) with food.

Further steps into antibiotic therapy are guided by culture and sensitivity tests using needle aspirates of pus. The laboratory must be specially directed to look for anaerobes.

Although patients may persuade us to temporize with ameliorative antibiotics for years, we recognize that definitive surgery provides the one bright shining hope for cure. It is our treatment of choice. It should be theirs.

Dvorak VC, Root RK, MacGregor RR: Host-defense mechanisms in hidradenitis suppurativa. Arch Dermatol 113:450–453, 1977.

A careful study of seven patients who had suffered hidradenitis for 5 to 17 years revealed the following parameters of host defenses to be normal:

- immunoglobulins
- cell-mediated immune function
- granulocyte phagocytic activity
- granulocyte intracellular bactericidal activity
- granulocyte adherence
- granulocyte chemotaxis

Morgan WP, Leicester G: The role of depilation and deodorants in hidradenitis suppurativa. Arch Dermatol 118:101–102, 1982.

Shaving and the use of chemical depilatories and deodorants had no role in the pathogenesis of this disease.

Brenner DE, Lookingbill DP: Anaerobic microorganisms in chronic suppurative hidradenitis. Lancet 2:921–922, 1980.

Bacteroides fragilis and **B. melaninogenicus** were isolated from draining hidradenitis lesions in five patients. Treatment for severe cases: hospitalization with **clindamycin** (300 to 600 mg IV q6h for two to three weeks), local soaks, and whirlpool cleansing.

Highet AS, Warren RE, Staughton RCD, Roberts SOB: *Streptococcus milleri* causing treatable infection in perineal hidradenitis suppurativa. Br J Dermatol 103:375–382, 1980.

In three cases of severe anogenital hidradenitis suppurativa, *Streptococcus milleri* was isolated as the only or predominant bacterium. This common commensal in the gastrointestinal and female genital tracts is not an obligate anaerobe and is **metronidazole** resistant.

All patients improved with antibiotics, some of which were aimed at eliminating *S. milleri* from the gut. However, it was difficult to eliminate the pathogenic bacteria from the deep-seated dermal sinuses.

In one patient the treatment sequence of daily therapy was:

nystatin (4 million units PO)	**gentamicin** (240 mg IV)
vancomycin (2 gm PO)	**benzylpenicillin G** (16 million U IV)
neomycin (2 gm PO)	**doxycycline** (100 mg IV)

A second patient received oral nystatin, vancomycin, neomycin, and doxycycline, while a third patient had substantial improvement with **erythromycin** (2 gm daily PO).

Ginder PA, Ousley M, Hinthorn D, et al: Hidradenitis suppurativa: Evidence for a bactericidal defect correctable by cholinergic agonist *in vitro* and *in vivo*. J Clin Immunol 2:237–241, 1982.

A 70-year-old man with hidradenitis suppurativa of 10 years in the axillae and groin had striking improvement in one month and healing in 14 months with **bethanechol chloride** (Urecholine 50 mg tid). Laboratory studies revealed a defective bactericidal function in his polymorphonuclear leukocytes. Cultures showed both aerobic and anaerobic flora (staphylococci, streptococci, *Escherichia coli, Klebsiella, Enterobacter, Corynebacterium* spp., *Bacteroides melaninogenicus*). Multiple drainage procedures, marsupialization twice, and multiple courses of antimicrobial drugs (**cephalexin** six weeks, **gentamicin** four weeks, **moxalactam** two weeks, **cefoxanide** three weeks) had had only limited short-term benefit. Healing occurred only after the cholinergic agonist corrected the neutrophil-killing defect.

Kress DW, Graham WP III, Davis TS, Miller SH: A preliminary report on the use of Staphage Lysate for treatment of hidradenitis suppurativa. Ann Plast Surg 6:393–395, 1981.

Six of seven patients with hidradenitis unresponsive to antibiotics and local surgery had noticeable improvement when given Staphage Lysate (0.1 ml subcutaneously and 0.3 ml intranasally once weekly for three months, then biweekly for six months, then monthly indefinitely). No controls. (This bacterial antigen is made from two lysed strains of *Staphylococcus aureus*.)

Clemmensen OJ: Topical treatment of hidradenitis suppurativa with clindamycin. Int J Dermatol 22:325–328, 1983.

A double-blind study of 27 patients with hidradenitis of the axillae, groin, or both showed **clindamycin** solution (Cleocin T 1 per cent in isopropyl alcohol and propylene glycol) to be superior to placebo over a three-month period.

Dicken CH, Powell ST, Spear KL: Evaluation of isotretinoin treatment of hidradenitis suppurativa. J Am Acad Dermatol 11:500–502, 1984.

Isotretinoin (Accutane 1 mg/kg/day for four months) was used to treat eight patients with long-standing hidradenitis suppurativa. Only one case truly cleared, but three others almost healed. One other showed some improvement, whereas two were unchanged and one continued to worsen. Final evaluation was two months after stopping treatment.

McDaniel DH, Welton WA: Furunculosis and hidradenitis suppurativa response. Arch Dermatol 120:437, 1984.

Two patients with long-standing hidradenitis showed notable improvement when given **tolmetin sodium** (Tolectin 10 mg/kg/day in divided dosage). This improvement persisted after the drug was tapered and stopped, presumably because of increased suppressor T cell activity. This and other nonsteroidal anti-inflammatory agents deserve further trial.

Storino WD, Engel GH: Office surgical management of recalcitrant axillary lesions. Cutis 21:338–341, 1978.

Excellent results were seen in 20 patients following direct excision of localized infected areas. Although primary closure was usually possible, in six patients advancement flaps or bipedicle flaps were necessary.

Duncan WC: Surgical treatment of hidradenitis suppurativa. J Dermatol Surg 2:153–157, 1976.

Successful surgical treatment in two patients consisted of unroofing all sinus tracts with a cutting diathermy current, removal of tract linings with the cutting loop, and final desiccation. Surgery is followed by dry dressings and daily cleansing with shower sprays and sitz baths. This may require general anesthesia and hospitalization. Re-epithelialization occurred in three to six weeks.

Ariyan S, Krizek TJ: Hidradenitis suppurativa of the groin, treated by excision and spontaneous healing. Plast Reconst Surg 58:44–47, 1976.

Direct excision of all affected tissue down to fascia was successful in three patients. This required general anesthesia, electrocoagulation control of bleeding, 10 to 21 days in the hospital, and whirlpool baths four times a day. Patients were able to walk from the first day on. No skin grafts were used. Healing by wound contraction was complete in two months.

Morgan WP, Harding KG, Hughes LE: A comparison of skin grafting and healing by granulation, following axillary excision for hidradenitis suppurativa. Ann R Coll Surg Engl 65:235–236, 1983.

A paired comparison study of 20 axillae in 10 patients showed greater patient acceptance of excision of a 10- by 8-cm area of axillary skin followed by use of Silastic foam dressings (Dow) for three months, than of similar excision with skin grafting.

Hermanson A: Surgical treatment of axillary hidradenitis suppurativa. Scand J Plast Reconstr Surg 16:163–165, 1982.

A study of eight patients revealed:

Incision and drainage gave temporary relief only.

Excision and suture led to recurrence.

Radical excision with flap closure resulted in cure with only one month of disability.

Broadwater JR, Bryant RL, Petrino RA, et al: Advanced hidradenitis suppurativa: Review of surgical treatment in 23 patients. Am J Surg 144:668–670, 1982.

Multiple organisms were cultured from sinus tracts in 11 of 23 patients. Even after wide and deep excision, 9 of 41 areas (22 per cent) showed some recurrence. In these sites cure was achieved only after the remaining apocrine glands were excised.

Billet A, Stueber K, Vaughan L: Hidradenitis suppurativa of unusual severity. Ann Plast Surg 10:231–234, 1983.

A 52-year-old man totally confined to his home because of severe pain and foul odor of hidradenitis of the buttocks was cured by total excision of the skin of both buttocks down to fascia. This tour de force required split-thickness grafts, a colostomy, and six months' convalesence, after which the colostomy was closed.

Humphrey LJ, Playforth H, Leavell UW Jr: Squamous cell carcinoma arising in hidradenitis suppurativum. Arch Dermatol 100:59–62, 1969.

This was the sixth example in the literature of a squamous cell carcinoma arising within an area of hidradenitis suppurativa. In this 48-year-old man widespread hidradenitis had been present for eight years, and the tumor developed between the coccyx and the sacrum. Treatment required a permanent sigmoid colostomy followed by radical perineal resection closed by a pedicle flap and skin graft.

Our main business is not to see what lies dimly at a distance, but to do what lies closely at hand.

THOMAS CARLYLE

Hidrocystoma

Atropine ointment
Excision

We have been very pleased with the results of simply removing each one of these cosmetically annoying sweat traps. For the multiple eccrine type around the eyelid, we excise them using curved iris scissors and no sutures. On the cheek, we remove them with a trephine (punch) of appropriate size (1 to 3 mm) and close with a single 6-0 suture.

Sperling LC, Sakas EL: Eccrine hidrocystomas. J Am Acad Dermatol 7:763–770, 1982.

Isolated lesions are best excised, but the multiple sweat-filled cysts under the eyes of a 66-year-old woman remained invisible after applications of **atropine sulfate** (1 per cent in Aquaphor applied once weekly). Untreated lesions were not affected.

Hagan WE, Riveras E, Duplechin JK: Hidrocystoma of apocrine derivation. Arch Otolaryngol 111:772–775, 1985.

Surgical excision is the preferred treatment of an apocrine hidrocystoma, which usually appears as a solitary nodule. It is also preferred for isolated eccrine hidrocystomas, since simple incision or puncture produces only temporary remissions.

The Index Medicus *is your passport to an international conference at your medical school library. Any day, any subject, any expert you want!*

Hirsutism

Contraceptive	Bleach
Corticosteroid	Pluck
Cimetidine	Epilate
Clomiphene	Shave
Cyproterone acetate	Electrolysis
Spironolactone	Depilatory

All women with true hirsutism deserve more than cosmetic advice. They deserve careful endocrinologic studies. In most instances the abnormal hair signals only a mild, almost physiologic, elevation in androgen production by the adrenal or the ovary. However, to simply dismiss the next patient with hirsutism is to deny the possibility (admittedly rare) that she could have a curable endocrine tumor.

The least that should be done is examination for clinical evidence of more than a subtle increase in androgens, namely, virilization: breast atrophy, muscle hypertrophy, deepened voice, clitoral enlargement, and male hair patterning other than on the face. Then ask: Is hirsutism common in her family or genetic background? Are her periods irregular? Is she taking a drug such as the antihypertensive minoxidil (Loniten)?

From the laboratory, secure the levels of free testosterone, prolactin, LSH, and FSH. The testosterone level should be secured several times during a one-month period, since it fluctuates. If abnormalities are found, further endocrinologic review is mandatory, including the dexamethasone suppression test, computed tomography for adrenal tumor, ultrasound studies for ovarian tumors, and careful evaluation of possible therapy.

It is important for the patient to understand that mild annoying hirsutism of nontumor origin should not be treated by internal medical measures, since these are, at best, helpful only while being taken. Furthermore, they are, at times, hazardous, expensive, and only partially effective. The patient should explore the safe, although tedious avenues of plucking, wax epilation, depilatories (Surgex), and electrolysis (never on the upper lip, a frequent site of scarring).

For the woman with truly heavy male pattern hair growth, there is a need for endocrinologic guidance through the somewhat empiric choices of contraceptives, corticosteroids, and antiandrogens. The best and most effective antiandrogen, cyproterone acetate, used widely in Europe, is still awaited in the United States. Unfortunately the local use of these antiandrogens, although widely studied, has not proven helpful. The systemic use of any agent to block androgen production, transport, or local follicle stimulation calls for much patience on the part of both patient and doctor. Results are never seen in less than four months.

In summary, when we see a patient with hirsutism we say, "What this patient needs is a good endocrinologist."

Biffignandi P, Massucchetti C, Molinatti GM: Female hirsutism: Pathophysiological considerations and therapeutic implications. Endocr Rev 5:498–513, 1984.

Nearly all hirsute women have demonstrable increases in production rates and plasma levels of androgens (testosterone or its precursor, androstenedione) of either ovarian or adrenal origin. Other determinants are (1) serum levels of carrier proteins (albumin and globulin), which bind circulating androgens; (2) androgen metabolism in the perifollicular area; (3) binding capacity and sensitivity to androgen of the hair follicle itself.

Hatch R, Rosenfield RL, Kim MH, Tredway D: Hirsutism: Implications, etiology and management. Am J Obstet Gynecol 140:815–830, 1981.

An elevation of the plasma free (unbound) testosterone is the single most consistent finding in hirsutism. This may be elevated when the total plasma testosterone is normal. Dexamethasone suppression testing often aids in detecting the source of hyperandrogenemia:

If free androgen level stays high, suspect ovary (polycystic ovary syndrome variants).
If free androgen level stays very high, suspect tumor or Cushing's syndrome.
If free androgen is suppressed, suspect adrenogenital syndrome, prolactinoma, idiopathic hyperandrogenemia, or obesity.

Dewis P, Anderson DC: A practical approach to the hirsute patient. Practitioner 226:223–233, 1982.

The speed of onset of hirsutism is important for detecting women with androgen-secreting tumors.

A vaginal examination should be performed on all hirsute patients to search for ovarian tumors.

Additional help may be gained from ordering:

- sex hormone binding globulin level
- gonadotropin level
- prolactin level
- CT (adrenal tumor)
- ultrasound (ovarian tumor)

Recommended treatment:

For patients desiring to get pregnant
prednisolone (7.5 mg) or **dexamethasone** (Decadron 0.5 to 0.75 mg) daily, in divided doses with twice as much given in the evening as in the morning
For patients not desiring pregnancy
oral contraceptive with **ethinylestradiol** (50 μg) + **ethinodiol** (500 μg) (Demulen is the closest equivalent in the United States)
For postmenopausal women or those intolerant of the pill
spironolactone (Aldactone 100 mg/day)

Recommended cosmetic measures:

electrolysis
shaving with an electric razor (as often as necessary)—may combine with bleaching
depilatory creams
avoid plucking and depilatory waxes if undergoing electrolysis (because of scarring at base of hair follicles)

Rentoul JR: Management of the hirsute woman. Int J Dermatol 22:265–272, 1983.

Hirsutism is not curable unless it is due to rare Cushing's disease, prolactinoma, or androgen-secreting tumor of the adrenal or ovary.

Ferriman D, Gallwey JD: Clinical assessment of body hair growth in women. J Clin Endocrinol 21:1440–1447, 1961.

Based on an analysis of 430 women, the classic grading system for evaluating the response of hair growth to treatment includes a score of 1 to 4 at 11 anatomic locations. Sites of hair growth related to hormonal sensitivity include the upper lip, chin, chest, upper and lower back, upper and lower abdomen, arm, and thigh. Hair on the forearm and leg is thought to be protective in nature and "sexually indifferent."

Elias AN, Gwinup G: Hirsutism. New York, Praeger Publishers, 1983, pp 89–104.

The definitive monograph:

The average woman with idiopathic hirsutism is most likely to be helped by an oral contraceptive, which may act by increasing synthesis of sex hormone–binding globulin and thereby reduce the amount of free active androgen responsible for hirsutism.

Other approaches:

dexamethasone (0.5 mg hs) to reduce adrenal androgen output

clomiphene citrate (50 to 100 mg/day for five days each month for three months), an antiestrogen

cimetidine (300 mg five times a day for three months), an H_2 receptor antagonist, which also binds to dihydrotestosterone receptors

spironolactone (100 mg bid), an androgen antagonist

Do not look for results before four months!

Rentoul JR, Aitken AA: The cosmetic treatment of hirsutism. Practitioner 224:1171–1175, 1980.

Drug therapy

Requires long-term treatment to control androgen-dependent hair and may cause serious side effects. This prospect is daunting, particularly in women of child-bearing age. Even while taking these drugs, patients still have to remove hairs cosmetically.

Shaving

The easiest, cleanest, cheapest way of removing hair. May have to do it twice a day.

Waxing

Probably the best home method for hair removal. May space up to six-week intervals, as must wait until the hairs are long enough to be gripped by the wax. The wax is applied in several layers in different directions, with a spatula, and then stripped off rapidly (against the direction of hair growth) before the wax hardens. May be painful, especially on the upper lip. May need bleach between times.

Depilatory creams

Usually **calcium thioglycolate**, which reduces disulfide binding of molecules in the hair keratin. Must apply it in a thick layer, but do not rub in. After a given time, lift off the cream with a spatula, then use moist cotton to rub the hairs away.

Electrolysis

Expensive, painful, time-consuming, and requires numerous treatments to each follicle to stop hair growth. Scarring can occur.

Hair-removing glove

Made of fine sandpaper in the shape of a mitten. Used with a circular motion, it will remove fine stubble. May be used several times daily.

Plucking

Safe and simple. May cause pustules.

Bergfeld WF: Hirsutism. *In* Provost TT, Farmer ER (eds): Current Therapy in Dermatology, 1985 · 1986. St. Louis, C. V. Mosby Co., 1985, pp 119–123.

The most common disorder is the acquired adult-onset type of hirsutism due to minor adrenal hyperplasia with resulting hyperandrogenemia. Check for elevated dihydroepiandrosterone sulfate (DHEA-S), a specific marker for this condition.

The following drugs can induce excessive hair growth:

testosterone
danazol (Danocrine)
ACTH
metyrapone (Metopirone)
phenothiazines
anabolic steroids (e.g., Maxibolin, Dianabol, Winstrol)
acetazolamide (Diamox)
progesterone
Dilantin
Dyazide (hydrochlorothiazide-triamterene)
minoxidil
glucocorticoids
chlorobenzene
penicillamine (Cuprimine)
psoralens

The basic laboratory work-up for hirsutism should include these determinations:

1. Ovarian androgen excess
   free testosterone
   androstenedione
2. Adrenal androgen excess
   DHEA-S
   androstenedione
   17-hydroxyprogesterone
   compound S (serum 11-deoxycortisol)
   cortisol
3. Pituitary
   prolactin

Burton JL, Marshall A: Hypertrichosis due to minoxidil. Br J Dermatol 101:593–595, 1979.

A 50-year-old man with severe essential hypertension developed moderate hypertrichosis after treatment with **minoxidil** (Loniten 15 mg bid for five months). Increased hair growth occurs in nearly all patients treated with this drug. It is not due to androgen production, but is related to cutaneous blood flow, since minoxidil is a strong vasodilator.

Earhart RN, Ball J, Nuss DD, Aeling JL: Minoxidil-induced hypertrichosis: Treatment with calcium thioglycolate depilatory. South Med J 70:442–443, 1977.

Five female patients with serious hypertension and hypertrichosis (thin, non-terminal hair) due to **minoxidil** successfully used Surgex hair removal cream (**calcium thioglycolate** + **calcium hydroxide** + **strontium hydroxide**, two- to five-minute application, wash off with soap and water). **Hydrocortisone** cream (1 per cent) was used to counter any irritation. Treatment was necessary every two to four weeks. Better than **barium sulfide**!

Heise VH, Geidel H, Valerius B: Hirsutismus als seltene Komplikation der PUVA-Therapie. Dermatol Monatsschr 166:611–615, 1980.

A 31-year-old woman with psoriasis noted increased hair growth on her face after receiving PUVA therapy for two months. This was not associated with changes in hormonal blood levels. The photosensitizing psoralen was thought to change the metabolism of androgens in the skin.

Vigersky RA, Mehlman I, Glass AR, Smith CE: Treatment of hirsute women with cimetidine. N Engl J Med 303:1042, 1980.

In four of five severely hirsute women, **cimetidine** (300 mg five times a day for three months) induced an average decrease of 64 per cent in the rate of hair growth. Four of the patients had polycystic ovary syndrome. No changes were found in hormonal levels, suggesting that the antiandrogen effect of cimetidine occurs through inhibition of dihydrotestosterone binding to androgen receptors on hair follicles.

Hammerstein J, Moltz L, Schwartz U: Antiandrogens in the treatment of acne and hirsutism. J Steroid Biochem 19:591–597, 1983.

Cyproterone acetate is the only pure antiandrogen drug currently available in several countries (not available in the United States). **Spironolactone** also has antiandrogen activity.

Severe hirsutism
Cyproterone acetate (100 mg/day until satisfactory response, then decrease to 50, 25, or 10 mg daily)

Mild hirsutism
Cyproterone acetate (2 mg) + **ethinyl estradiol** (50 μg) (Diane—a low-dose oral contraceptive) daily

General rules for treatment:

1. Antiandrogen treatment should not be instituted unless androgen-producing tumors have been excluded with certainty. Otherwise, one could lose valuable time for tumor therapy that requires surgical intervention, not medication.
2. Antiandrogens must not be given unless a woman is shown not to be pregnant and is taking contraceptives, since they can induce intersexual malformations of the male fetus.
3. Do not expect results before the third month and do not expect more results than seen at the ninth month.
4. Reduce the dose once an acceptable result is obtained to minimize risk. Explain to the patient that hirsutism will return if the drug is stopped.
5. Use these drugs only with severe hirsutism.

Messina M, Manieri C, Biffignandi P, et al: Antiandrogenic properties of spironolactone. Clinical trial in the management of female hirsutism. J Endocrinol Invest 6:23–27, 1983.

There was a significant decrease in hair growth and shaft diameter in 11 of 18 women treated with **spironolactone** (Aldactone 200 to 400 mg/day for 250 days). Beneficial effects were noted only after 100 days of treatment. Menstrual irregularities were the major side effect.

Cumming DC, Yang JC, Rebar RW, Yen SSC: Treatment of hirsutism with spironolactone. JAMA 247:1295–1298, 1982.

Spironolactone (Aldactone 200 mg/day) had a clear beneficial effect on the quantity and quality of facial hair growth in 19 of 20 patients with moderate to severe hirsutism. The effect was seen within two months and was maximal at six months. The drug reduces androgens of ovarian, but not adrenal, origin and also interferes with peripheral androgen action.

Nielsen PG: Treatment of idiopathic hirsutism with spironolactone. Dermatologica 165:194–196, 1982.

After low-dose **spironolactone** (50 mg/day for seven months) 15 of 21 women noted that their hair was softer and lighter in color. The average frequency of hair removal was reduced by half.

Jones KR, Katz M, Keyzer C, Gordon W: Effect of cyproterone acetate on rate of hair growth in hirsute females. Br J Dermatol 105:685–692, 1981.

Nine of ten patients receiving the antiandrogen **cyproterone acetate** (50 mg/day for days 5 to 14 of their cycle) then Diane (cyproterone acetate 2 mg + **ethinyl estradiol** 0.05 mg for days 5 to 25, followed by a seven-day break) for one year found an overall reduction in hair growth, with hairs being softer, thinner, and brighter in color. Measurements were made with an ingenious trichometer. (Drugs not available in the United States.)

Garner PR, Poznanski N: Treatment of severe hirsutism resulting from hyperandrogenism with the reverse sequential cyproterone acetate regimen. J Reprod Med 29:232–236, 1984.

Seven severely hirsute hyperandrogenic women had reductions in both plasma testosterone and sex hormone–binding globulin levels within two months of starting **cyproterone acetate** (100 mg daily for days 5 to 14 of their menstrual cycle) and **ethinyl estradiol** (50 μg for days 5 to 25 of each cycle). Hair growth was not clinically reduced until after four months. The main side effects included fatigue and loss of libido. (Drug available in Canada and Europe but not in the United States.)

Rigaud C, Couzinet B, Schaison G: Treatment of hyperandrogenic states in women. Horm Res 18:135–142, 1983.

Remember that although the majority of cases of hirsutism are of idiopathic origin and their treatment is only palliative, all patients with significant hirsutism should be studied for the presence of a tumor or congenital adrenal hyperplasia.

The most effective antiandrogen for idiopathic hirsutism is combined estrogen and cyproterone acetate. Because of its antiestrogen effects, cyproterone acetate must be combined with estrogen to permit regular menstrual bleeding (**cyproterone acetate** 50 mg + **ethinyl estradiol** 50 μg for 21 days/month). Improvement in hirsutism is noted after 6 to 9 months and becomes marked after 12 to 18 months. Hair growth reappears one month after discontinuation of therapy.

Wagner RF, Tomich JM, Grande DJ: Electrolysis and thermolysis for permanent hair removal. J Am Acad Dermatol 12:441–449, 1985.

Electronic or high-frequency tweezers (Depilatron, Depillex, Permatron, Removatron, Bioepilator) have been declared by the Food and Drug Administration to be no better than household tweezers.

Even with electrolysis or diathermy, epilation regrowth occurs in 15 to 50 per cent of the treated hair follicles.

Case reports are the catalysts for the clinical mind.

Hyperhidrosis

Drysol	Drionic device
Anticholinergics	Surgery
Glutaraldehyde	

The pied piper of advertising for the billion-dollar-a-year antiperspirant-deodorant industry keeps most patients with axillary hyperhidrosis out of your office. But those who come in despair over the results of using "soft-touch" antiperspirants (effective only in the normhidrotic axilla) will be pleased with what can be achieved.

We prescribe Drysol (aluminum chloride hexahydrate 20 per cent in anhydrous ethyl alcohol). Its successful use requires patient instruction, follow-up, and even auxiliary measures at times. We give the following instructions:

1. Accept no substitutes. The preparation must be water-free to minimize irritation and must be free of all other chemicals, such as buffers, to maintain its potency. Extemporaneous preparations made by pharmacists "the same day" are not acceptable, since rapid formulation can be achieved only by adding water. Solubilization of the hexahydrate aluminum chloride crystals in anhydrous alcohol requires three weeks.
2. Apply the Drysol sparingly *only* to the center of the axilla and only at bedtime. It is at this time that sympathetic impulses to the gland are minimal, and the Drysol can remain in place without being flushed out by an egress of sweat.
3. Do not apply the Drysol to moist or wet skin. This means the patient must not wash the area before application or have been sweating recently. Use of a hair dryer to blow dry the skin before application is a valuable aid. If sympathetic calm and hence temporary sweat cessation cannot be achieved by relaxation in the evening, we prescribe the anticholinergic, Pro-Banthine (propantheline bromide 15 mg two hours before bedtime) for initial treatments. We repeat, the skin must be *dry* and not sweating at the time of application. To ignore this is to invite irritation and hence patient noncompliance.
4. Do not use Drysol on recently shaved or irritated skin. Do not rub in. If Drysol produces irritation, treat the area with 1 per cent hydrocortisone cream the morning after application.
5. Wash Drysol off upon arising. It is strongly acidic and can be destructive to certain clothing.
6. If the sweating is not eliminated after a week of applications nightly or every other night, we advise the patient to apply Saran wrap over the Drysol-treated skin area. This can be wadded into the armpit and kept in place overnight by wearing a T-shirt. It appreciably enhances penetration of Drysol into sweat pores, producing greater keratin blockage of sweat.
7. Once control is achieved, the Drysol is applied as needed, usually one night a week.

8. If the Drysol is irritating despite its proper careful use, we prescribe the milder form, Xerac AC (6.75 per cent aluminum chloride hexahydrate in anhydrous ethyl alcohol). The same instructions must be followed, and for many this gives the same excellent help as Drysol, but not as rapidly.

We explain to the patient that reduction in axillary sweating is safe and sensible. Axillary sweating serves no thermoregulatory or excretory function. Furthermore, Drysol and Xerac AC are nonallergenic, have no systemic effects, and can be used indefinitely.

For the patients who do not wish to persist with a topical approach or in whom Drysol and Xerac AC are regularly irritating, we give relief surgically by excising the central portion of each axilla that bears most of the hyperhidrotic eccrine glands.

Drysol also controls hyperhidrosis of the palms and the soles, but here longer periods of treatment are needed, as well as more frequent application for maintenance.

For all three areas, alternate treatment is now available in the form of iontophoresis. The patient can purchase a Drionic unit, and with simple tap water iontophoresis produce poral closure and control of hyperhidrosis.

In the rare patient with socially or occupationally devastating hyperhidrosis of the palms who fails to respond to local measures, recourse to sympathectomy is recommended. A neurosurgeon *experienced* in this area can provide lifelong cure for these unfortunate individuals. We do not recommend sympathectomy for the axilla, since direct excision of the gland-bearing skin has been so successful.

The patient with local hyperhidrosis in focal or segmental distribution deserves study as to the nature of the problem. Only then can appropriate measures be taken, if at all. Even more meaningful can be the uncovering of the cause for generalized hyperhidrosis, such as diabetes, thyrotoxicosis, or acromegaly.

It is important to know that sweating a little over your patient's problem can mean your patient will sweat a lot less.

Grice K: Treatment of hyperhidrosis. Clin Exp Dermatol 7:183–188, 1982.

Aluminum chloride hexahydrate (20 per cent in absolute ethyl alcohol) has pride of place in the treatment of localized hyperhidrosis. In patients with generalized hyperhidrosis look for an underlying cause such as:

pyrexia	hyperpituitarism
hypoglycemia	pheochromocytoma
hyperthyroidism	familial dysautonomia

A splendid comprehensive review!

Hölzle E: Therapie der hyperhidrosis. Hautarzt 35:7–15, 1984.

Detailed review of the topical, systemic, and surgical approaches to the problem of localized hyperhidrosis. The author points out that tap water iontophoresis is a safe, simple technique that is gaining in popularity. Some patients benefit from one of the following:

psychotherapy	biofeedback
tranquilizers	hypnosis
sedatives	

Quinton PM: Sweating and its disorders. Annu Rev Med 34:429–452, 1983.

An exquisite look at what goes on inside this little gland that, knowing its thermoregulatory role, never aspired to be an organ. As a result, it and its two million unincorporated colleagues can deliver as much as a gallon of hypotonic fluid every hour for evaporative cooling. Receiving its central direction from the primitive hypothalamus, where afferent impulses are integrated, the gland is innervated by the sympathetic nerves whose terminal neurotransmitters are paradoxically parasympathetic agonists. Thus, all sweat gland activity can be blocked by oral or topical anticholinergic drugs. 209 references.

Episodic systemic hyperhidrosis is usually due to:

1. Autonomic nervous system disturbance, e.g.:
   - pheochromocytoma
   - thyrotoxicosis
   - hypotension
   - hypoglycemia
2. Thermoregulation disorder, e.g.:
   - postmenopausal hot flashes
   - nightsweats
   - diabetes mellitus neuropathy
   - diabetes insipidus
3. Hypersensitivity to stimulation, e.g.:
   - allergic disease
   - anxiety nervosa
   - familial dysautonomia
   - cold exposure

Raff SB, Gershberg H: Nightsweats: A dominant symptom in diabetes insipidus. JAMA 234:1252–1253, 1975.

A 10-year-old boy developed night sweats following diffuse cerebritis, not associated with polydipsia or nocturia. Eventually a diagnosis of diabetes insipidus was made, and treatment with **vasopressin tannate** (Pitressin 0.5 ml in oil IM every three days) promptly terminated the night sweats.

Sohar E, Shoenfeld Y, Udassin R, et al: Cold-induced profuse sweating on back and chest: A new genetic entity? Lancet 2:1073–1074, 1978.

In two sisters (ages 20 and 21) whose parents shared a common grandfather, **atropine sulfate** (0.5 to 1 mg PO one hour before cold exposure) completely blocked profuse sweating of the chest and back that was usually precipitated by exposure to cold. Other abnormalities included a high, arched palate and inability to fully extend the elbow.

Scholes KT, Crow KD, Ellis JP, et al: Axillary hyperhidrosis treated with alcoholic solution of aluminum chloride hexahydrate. Br Med J 2:84–85, 1978.

Excellent control of axillary hyperhidrosis was achieved in 64 of 65 patients who applied $AlCl_3 \cdot 6H_2O$ (in absolute alcohol at bedtime for one week, then as needed every 7 to 21 days). Irritation in 29 patients was easily controlled with **hydrocortisone** cream (1 per cent applied the following morning).

Yarrow H: Treatment of axillary hyperhidrosis. Br Med J 282:150, 1981.

The **aluminum chloride hexahydrate** must be used only in anhydrous alcohol and must not be applied to a moist or wet axilla to minimize irritation.

Jensen O, Karlsmark T: Palmoplantar hyperhidrosis: Treatment with alcoholic solution of aluminum chloride hexahydrate: A simple method of transpiration measurement. Dermatologica 161:133–135, 1980.

Aluminum chloride hexahydrate (25 per cent in absolute alcohol applied nightly without occlusion) controlled palmar hyperhidrosis in 12 of 13 patients after a month of usage. It achieved similar control of plantar hyperhidrosis in 10 of 11 patients after six weeks of daily usage. Thereafter, maintenance control required application every four to seven nights.

Control of axillary hyperhidrosis was achieved more rapidly and with fewer applications for maintenance.

MacFarlane IA, Knass D, Beardwell CG, Shalet SM: Hyperhidrosis in acromegaly: Effectiveness of topical aluminum chloride hexahydrate solution. Br Med J 2:901–902, 1979.

Aluminum chloride hexahydrate (20 per cent in anhydrous alcohol) was also effective in treating hyperhidrosis of the forehead, limbs, and axillae in three patients with acromegaly. In a two-month double-blind study, excessive sweating returned when treatment was stopped for two weeks.

Sato K: Frey's syndrome. JAMA 253:2735, 1985.

Advises daily application of Drysol (**aluminum chloride hexahydrate** 20 per cent in anhydrous ethyl alcohol) for treatment of gustatory sweating following facial trauma or surgery around the parotid gland. Apply to the affected facial area immediately after sweating has subsided and dry quickly with a hair dryer to minimize irritation.

Tap water iontophoresis on the face would be an alternative method of treatment.

Juhlin L, Hansson H: Topical glutaraldehyde for plantar hyperhidrosis. Arch Dermatol 97:327–330, 1968.

Excellent control of plantar hyperhidrosis and odor was achieved in 25 patients by applying **glutaraldehyde** solution (10 per cent aqueous solution, buffered to pH 7.5 by adding 16.5 gm sodium bicarbonate to each 100 ml, applied to one foot three times per week for four weeks). This preparation had no effect on axillary hyperhidrosis. After treatment was stopped, sweating reappeared in five to seven days. Because of brown discoloration of the skin, this treatment was not cosmetically acceptable for the palms.

Cullen SI: Topical methenamine therapy for hyperhidrosis. Arch Dermatol 111:1158–1160, 1975.

Methenamine, a condensation product of formaldehyde and ammonia (Mandelamine 5 per cent in a solid gel stick, applied twice a day for three weeks to one hand or one foot), effectively decreased palmar and plantar sweating in 24 of 26 individuals. The study was double blind in a placebo-controlled fashion, and sweating was recorded with starch-iodine tests.* Continuing relief persisted one to three weeks after stopping treatment.

Frankland JC, Seville RH: The treatment of hyperhidrosis with topical propantheline—A new technique. Br J Dermatol 85:577–581, 1971.

Sweating and macerative keratolysis were reduced in 38 institutionalized mentally retarded patients with plantar hyperhidrosis by spraying the soles with the anticholinergic drug **propantheline** (Pro-Banthine 1.85 or 3.60 mg/dose in ethanol, delivered by metered aerosol twice a day). Each treatment consisted of three metered doses, with one each to the dorsum of the foot, plantar surface, and toe clefts from below.

Bednarek J, Reid W, Matsumoto T: Frey's syndrome. Am J Surg 131:592–594, 1976.

Atropine sulfate (dl-hyoscyamine cream 0.5 per cent once daily) was effective in eliminating both sweating and flushing in a 57-year-old woman

---

* Directions for starch-iodine test:

Dry palms or soles with a facial tissue.

Paint with a mixture of 3 per cent iodine + 3 per cent potassium iodide in 95 per cent ethanol, then fan dry.

Place a hand or foot on a sheet of bond paper (with a starch-surface sizing) for one minute.

who had had partial resection of her right parotid gland. **Acetaminophen** (Tylenol 10 grains PO before meals) gave relief of the burning pain that was precipitated by mastication. (In the United States, use Atropine Sulfate 0.5 per cent or 1 per cent S.O.P. ophthalmic ointment.)

Juhlin L, Evers H, Broberg F: Inhibition of hyperhidrosis by topical application of a local anesthetic composition. Acta Derm Venereol 59:556–559, 1979.

A cream containing a eutectic mixture of 5 per cent **lidocaine** and 5 per cent **prilocaine** (EMLA—not available in the United States) inhibited palmar and axillary hyperhidrosis for one to six hours after application in 15 of 17 patients. The efficacy of the preparation usually disappeared after continued daily use for three to four weeks. (In the United States parenteral prilocaine hydrochloride is available as Citanest hydrochloride 1 to 4 per cent.)

Tkach JR: Indomethacin treatment of generalized hyperhidrosis. J Am Acad Dermatol 6:545, 1982.

Indomethacin (Indocin 25 mg tid) completely abolished lifelong idiopathic generalized hyperhidrosis within four days in a 61-year-old woman. Hyperhidrosis returned when the drug (prescribed for arthritis) was stopped and remitted upon its resumption. Careful study had ruled out the following known causes of hyperhidrosis:

diabetes	neurologic disease
hypoglycemia	dumping syndrome
thyroid disease	lymphoma
acromegaly	carcinoid syndrome
tuberculosis	drug or alcohol withdrawal
brucellosis	

Kuritsky A, Hering R, Goldhammer G, Bechar M: Clonidine treatment in paroxysmal localized hyperhidrosis. Arch Neurol 41:1210–1211, 1984.

Two women with paroxysmal localized hyperhidrosis were given **clonidine hydrochloride** (Catapres 0.25 mg three to five times a day) with rapid total long-term relief. In one patient paroxysmal sweating of the upper trunk had been associated with flushing 15 to 20 times daily. During the 12 months of clonidine therapy she did not have a single attack.

Chan P, Kao GF, Pierson DL, Rodman OG: Episodic hyperhidrosis on the dorsum of hands. J Am Acad Dermatol 12:937–942, 1985.

In a 21-year-old man with intermittent heat-induced attacks of hyperhidrosis on the dorsum of one or both hands, spontaneous improvement occurred after Drysol (applied once every other day) proved to be too irritating to use. Localized hyperplasia of the eccrine glands and ducts was found.

Causes of hyperhidrosis limited to one segment of the skin surface include:

cerebrovascular accident	syringomyelia
brain tumor	lung carcinoma
brain abscess	spinal cord injury
subclavian aneurysm	osteoma of vertebra

Alexander WD: Systemic side effects with eye drops. Br Med J 282:1359, 1981.

A puzzling case of idiopathic generalized hyperhidrosis for two years occurred in a 59-year-old man completely blind from glaucoma and also suffering from fatigue, muscle weakness, and diarrhea. All symptoms cleared after discontinuation of his eye drops, which contained the powerful anticholinestase **echothiophate iodide** (Phospholine iodide 0.25 per cent). This emphasizes the importance of a full drug history, including topical medications.

Peterson JL, Read SI, Rodman OG: A new device in the treatment of hyperhidrosis by iontophoresis. Cutis 29:82–89, 1982.

Includes details on the new Drionic device (battery operated, 7 to 20 ma) now available to the public for home tap water iontophoretic treatment of hyperhidrosis of the palms, soles, or axillae. In 10 patients (treated 20 minutes three times a week for two weeks) sweating was reduced for up to six weeks. Sweat prints were recorded on Persprint paper.

Hölzle E, Pauli M, Braun-Falco O: Leitungswasser-iontophorese zur behandlung von hyperhidrosis manuum et pedum. Hautarzt 35:142–147, 1984.

Ten treatments with tap water iontophoresis gave 80 per cent suppression of hyperhidrosis of the palms and soles in seven patients resistant to aluminum chloride treatment. The anhidrotic effect lasts for two weeks.

Ashby EC: Treatment of hyperhidrosis. Br Med J 2:503–504, 1978.

Cryotherapy is advocated for axillary hyperhidrosis, using three or four 40-second applications per axilla. An 18-mm diameter discoid nitrous oxide cryoprobe is surrounded by bunched-up anesthetized axillary skin. Blistering and post-treatment pain may be severe enough to require **pentazocine** (Talwin 30 mg IM) and postoperative observation for two hours. Depilation and depigmentation are permanent side effects. The technique was successful in 40 patients for up to three years.

Thorner MO, Chait A, Aitken M, et al: Bromocriptine treatment of acromegaly. Br Med J 1:299–303, 1975.

Bromocriptine (Parlodel 5.0 mg qid) stopped hyperhidrosis within a few days in each of 21 acromegalic patients studied. A slowly increasing dose regimen over approximately three months, starting with bromocriptine (2.5 mg at bedtime), is recommended to avoid side effects of nausea, vomiting, constipation, and postural hypotension.

Lerer B, Jacobowitz J: Treatment of essential hyperhidrosis by psychotherapy. Psychosomatics 22:536–538, 1981.

A 19-year-old woman who had suffered from emotional hyperhidrosis of the palms, soles, and axillae since age five had greatly diminished sweating after a few one-hour weekly sessions with the psychotherapist. After 14 months of weekly therapy her self-confidence had increased, aspirations were more realistic, and sweating remained decreased. The long-term result was equally good. The sweating seemed to act as a signal of anxiety, which forced the patient to withdraw from stress-provoking situations.

Duller P, Gentry WD: Use of biofeedback in treating chronic hyperhidrosis: A preliminary report. Br J Dermatol 103:143–146, 1980.

Biofeedback training sessions (30 minutes twice a week until improvement or for a maximum of 10 sessions if no improvement) enabled 8 of 14 patients to relax to the point of "no sweat," which persisted for six weeks after the training was over. An additional three patients also had decreased sweating. The poorest response occurred in patients with generalized hyperhidrosis.

Stenquist B: Axillary hyperhidrosis: A simple surgical procedure. J Dermatol Surg Oncol 11:388–391, 1985.

Excellent results were achieved in 14 consecutive patients (refractory to topical **aluminum chloride** therapy) following excision of a bat-shaped area of hyperhidrosis. No undermining was required, and primary closure was achieved. Prior to surgery, the hyperhidrotic area was mapped, using crepe paper pressed against the vault of the axilla. The edges of the wet spot on the paper were pierced with a pointed wooden skewer loaded with waterproof ink, thus marking the skin.

Also reviews several prior versions of direct excision of the site of hyperhidrosis.

Harahap M: Management of hyperhidrosis axillaris. J Dermatol Surg Oncol 5:223–225, 1979.

Tabulation and drawings of surgical variants of the Hurley-Shelley operation for axillary hyperhidrosis. Another technique is described, with removal of subcutaneous tissue through two parallel 5- to 6-cm transverse incisions in the axilla, located 4 to 5 cm apart, followed by primary closure and use of a bulky dressing for one week.

Bass A, Inovrotzlavski S, Adar R: Upper dorsal sympathectomy for palmar hyperhidrosis. Isr J Med Sci 19:112–115, 1983.

This operation done bilaterally in 133 patients gave immediate success in 98 per cent, but one third of the patients had troublesome compensatory hyperhidrosis of the trunk and legs. Although 26 per cent had return of moisture in the palms within 3 to 12 months, only 5 per cent had true recurrence of hyperhidrosis.

Kenawi MM, El Mofty M, Wishahy AH: The surgical treatment of associated axillary and palmar hyperhidrosis. J R Coll Surg Edinb 28:116–120, 1983.

To avoid postsurgical compensatory hyperhidrosis of the trunk due to major sympathectomy, these surgeons combined the Hurley-Shelley procedure of axillary skin excision with upper thoracic sympathectomy at the same time. Using the same incision in the axilla, they divided the sympathetic chain just below the third ganglion to achieve anhidrosis of the palms. Good results were seen in three patients.

McCoy BP: Apical pulmonary adenocarcinoma with contralateral hyperhidrosis. Arch Dermatol 117:659–661, 1981.

Hyperhidrosis of the right side of the head and trunk in a 58-year-old man was traced to stimulation of the contralateral cervicothoracic sympathetic chain by a metastatic adenocarcinoma of the lung. Usually the tumor is on the same side as the hyperhidrosis.

Pleet DL, Mandel S, Neilan B: Paroxysmal unilateral hyperhidrosis and malignant mesothelioma. Arch Neurol 40:256, 1983.

Roentgen therapy (5000 rad) to the mesothelioma that invaded the sympathetic fibers of the right side of the chest in a 35-year-old man did not relieve the profuse sweating of the right side of his face, right side of the upper trunk, and right arm.

Ottomo M, Heimburger RF: Alternating Horner's syndrome and hyperhidrosis due to dural adhesions following cervical spinal cord injury: Case report. J Neurosurg 53:97–100, 1980.

In a 30-year-old man with quadriplegia, cure of facial hyperhidrosis was achieved by freeing dense adhesions between the spinal cord and the dura mater.

Disease thrives on pessimism.

Hypertrichosis Lanuginosa

Cancer work-up
CEA

Find and treat the underlying internal malignant tumor!

Sindhuphak W, Vibhagool A: Acquired hypertrichosis lanuginosa. Int J Dermatol 21:599–601, 1982.

Of the 24 cases of hypertrichosis lanuginosa reported in the world's literature, 22 were due to proven malignant tumors in the following sites:

- breast
- lung
- mediastinum
- liver
- pancreas
- gallbladder
- ovary
- urinary bladder
- colon
- rectum

Price ML, Hall-Smith SP: Hypertrichosis lanuginosa acquisita. Clin Exp Dermatol 10:255–257, 1985.

A 63-year-old woman developed long fine hairs on the face, ears, arms, and trunk, along with liver metastases from a carcinoma of the colon removed two years previously. The tumor had not recurred locally, but her carcinoembryonic antigen (CEA) was greatly increased (found in tumors of the gastrointestinal tract, lung, and breast).

Doctors and lawyers are among the most difficult patients. The former want risk-free overnight cures prescribed in the hallway. The latter want risk specified, and guaranteed cures in a contractually specified time.

Ichthyosis

Hydration	Retin-A
Emollients	Propylene glycol
Ultra Mide	Accutane
Lacticare	Tigason
Keralyt	Aquasol A

The doctrine of signatures surely applies to the therapy of ichthyosis. Here is a disease named for its distinctive fishlike scaling. It is this name that bespeaks the therapy, i.e., water. It is a skin made not for land or air, but for the sea, and all of these patients benefit from seeking out the natural milieu of the fish. Since this is an impractical therapeutic maneuver for other than short periods, attention must be paid to maintaining an aqueous microenvironment for the skin.

Most patients derive real help from applying a water-barrier ointment immediately after showering or bathing. Classically this is petrolatum (Vaseline), but many moisturizing derivations are available over the counter, such as:

Complex 15	Mi Fine Skin Cream
Curél	Moisturel
Eucerin	Nivea cream
Formula 405	Purpose cream
Lubriderm	Sween cream

For bathing we caution the patient against using an alkaline soap such as Ivory. We prefer an antibacterial bar such as Dial.

Further help can be given by prescribing creams that contain urea (Ultra Mide has 25 per cent) or lactic acid (LactiCare lotion). These agents are well tolerated and give some symptomatic relief. We tend to use neither the salicylic acid formulations (Keralyt) nor the vitamin A acid preparations (Retin-A) because of irritation and expense. Much is a matter of trial and observation.

For the individual with severe disabling ichthyosis we regularly prescribe Aquasol A (50,000 IU tid). A distinct improvement should be noted within six weeks; if not, we discontinue the drug. (We do not use the generic form of this drug because of uncertainties regarding capsule composition and hence absorption.)

The ultimate treatment of ichthyosis centers on the new retinoids that profoundly alter the keratinization sequence. Accutane has given some of our patients enormous relief from a lifetime of dreadful scaling, cosmetic disfigurement, and social isolation. Even more dramatic in its action is Tigason. One of our patients is taking this on an experimental basis for the treatment of her epidermolytic hyperkeratosis. It has transformed her life, removed the daily onus of two hours of skin care, and accordingly made her a "retinoid addict." Every effort is being made to find the minimal maintenance by alternate-day dosage.

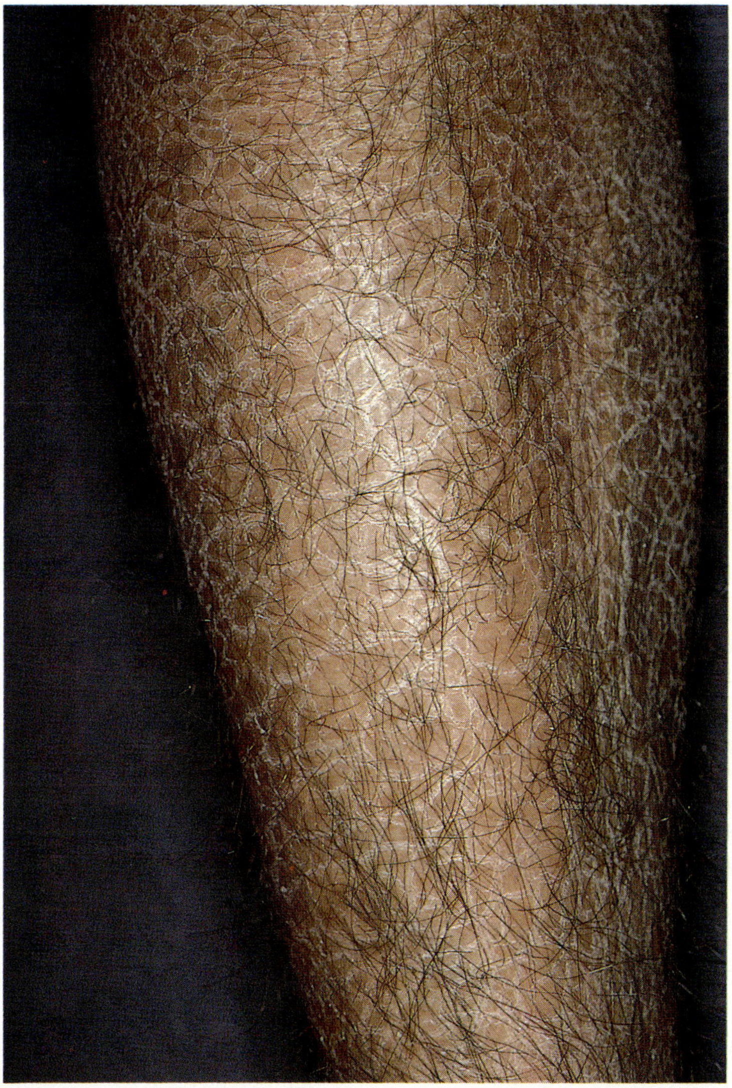

It is important to note that Aquasol A, Accutane, and Tigason do not cure ichthyosis, but act only on a temporary basis. Once these drugs are stopped the ichthyotic skin invariably returns. Furthermore, they have to be used in doses much larger than for the treatment of acne. Already we are seeing the skeletal hyperostosis resulting from Accutane (3 to 4 mg/kg/day for two years). Other toxic effects that will evolve on a long-term basis could be equally serious. The rapidly reversible effects of the retinoids make for the development of addiction. Once severely afflicted ichthyotic patients have known the joy of "newborn" skin, it is almost impossible to return them to the miseries of their former lives. They are already victims who have decided, "Give me liberty from my ichthyosis or give me death."

With all the attention being given to the local and systemic care of this disease, one must not forget that patients who develop ichthyosis later in life deserve careful study for the presence of underlying disease, especially lymphomas, sarcoidosis, malignant tumors, and leprosy. Malnutrition in the alcoholic may likewise be responsible for acquired ichthyosis. In these patients a true cure may be achieved, since they do not suffer from an irreversible inborn error of metabolism.

Rand RE, Baden HP: The ichthyoses—A review. J Am Acad Dermatol 8:285–305, 1983.

The definitive source of information on every aspect of this disease group. It details the "big four" (ichthyosis vulgaris, X-linked ichthyosis, lamellar ichthyosis, and epidermolytic hyperkeratosis) as well as the rarities (e.g., KID syndrome, Rud's syndrome, Refsum's disease). All patients derive benefit from hydration via water in the air, bathtub, or emollient.

Griffiths WAD: Ichthyosis and dry skin. Clin Exp Dermatol 7:551–556, 1982.

The best treatment for ichthyosis is a daily bath followed by use of a topical emollient. Temporary improvement is easy to achieve with a variety of chemicals, but treatments are so messy and unappealing that patients abandon them.

Swanbeck G: The ichthyosis. Acta Derm Venereol Suppl 95:88–90, 1981.

Genetic counseling:

Prenatal diagnosis a possibility
Ichthyosis vulgaris—incidence 1:300, autosomal dominant
X-linked ichthyosis—transmitted only to sons by unaffected mother—recessive
Ichthyosiform erythroderma—autosomal recessive
Mutations possible

Parental counseling:

Before the child enters school, inform parents of other children in the class of the serious, but noncontagious, nature of the skin disease.

Marks R, Dykes PJ (eds): The Ichthyoses: Proceedings of the 2nd Annual Clinically Oriented Symposium of the European Society for Dermatologic Research. New York, SP Medical and Scientific Books, 1978, 205 pp.

The monograph on this subject!

Van Scott EJ, Yu RJ: Commentary: Ichthyosis and keratinization. Arch Dermatol 118:860–861, 1982.

All ichthyosis scales show:

- thickened stratum corneum
- enhanced corneocyte adhesion
- low water-binding capacity

Grekin JL, Basler RSW: New treatments for ichthyosis. Cutis 25:432–434, 1980.

Advises:

frequent bathing with tar soap
vigorous scrubbing off of scales with a firm-bristled brush
then application of topical medication:

- **petrolatum**
- **urea** cream
- **salicylic acid** in propylene glycol (Keralyt)
- **lactic acid**
- Retin-A cream (for lamellar ichthyosis)

Pope FM, Rees JK, Wells RS, Lewis KGS: Out-patient treatment of ichthyosis: A double-blind trial of ointments. Br J Dermatol 86:291–296, 1972.

In 84 patients with ichthyosis vulgaris or X-linked ichthyosis, **urea** cream 10 per cent was superior to **salicylic acid** ointment 2 per cent, **lanolin** moisturizing cream, and an oily cream. Note that ichthyosis vulgaris, but not X-linked ichthyosis, clears with age.

Baden HP, Alper JC: A keratolytic gel containing salicylic acid in propylene glycol. J Invest Dermatol 61:330–333, 1973.

Keralyt gel (6 per cent **salicylic acid** in 60 per cent **propylene glycol** gel) applied under plastic dressing occlusion after five minutes of hydration of the skin cleared 21 of 29 cases of ichthyosis vulgaris and 6 of 6 with sex-linked ichthyosis, but none of 6 cases of lamellar ichthyosis. The treatment also helped plantar hyperkeratosis.

Swanbeck G: A new treatment of ichthyosis and other hyperkeratotic conditions. Acta Derm Venereol 48:123–127, 1968.

The skin of seven patients with ichthyosis became soft and pliable following the use of a 10 per cent **urea** cream.

Van Scott EJ, Yu RJ: Control of keratinization with α-hydroxy acids and related compounds. Arch Dermatol 110:586–590, 1974.

Lactic acid and its congeners (5 per cent in hydrophilic ointment bid) were the most effective of 60 compounds studied in the treatment of six patients with lamellar ichthyosis, three with X-linked ichthyosis, two with ichthyosis vulgaris, and one with epidermolytic hyperkeratosis.

Frost P, Weinstein GD: Topical administration of vitamin A acid for ichthyosiform dermatoses and psoriasis. JAMA 207:1863–1868, 1969.

Impressive improvement followed use of **vitamin A acid** (0.1 to 0.3 per cent in petrolatum or cold cream) in 17 patients with lamellar ichthyosis and 10 patients with epidermolytic hyperkeratosis. It was not helpful in 8 patients with ichthyosis vulgaris and 8 patients with X-linked ichthyosis.

Mirrer E, McGuire J: Lamellar ichthyosis-responsive to retinoic acid (tretinoin): A case report. Arch Dermatol 102:548–551, 1970.

Tretinoin (0.05 per cent in 70 per cent **isopropyl alcohol** applied tid) caused marked improvement in a 12-year-old boy. However, resultant irritation necessitated decreasing the applications to once daily or once every other day using topical steroids (**triamcinolone acetonide** cream 0.025 per cent).

Günther S: Topical treatment with retinoic acid in various dyskeratoses of childhood: Keratosis plantaris, verrucous naevus, and autosomal dominant ichthyosis. Dermatol Monatsschr 159:721–732, 1973.

Eight patients with ichthyosis vulgaris responded well within three to eight weeks when **retinoic acid** (0.1 per cent in Vaseline) was applied every second day. Results were seen in two weeks, and maintenance applications were needed once a week. Relapse began in all patients four weeks after withdrawal of therapy. Do not use in atopic patients.

Goldsmith LA, Baden HP: Propylene glycol with occlusion for treatment of ichthyosis. JAMA 220:579–580, 1972.

Propylene glycol (40 to 60 per cent aqueous, under tubular plastic or polyethylene film occlusion) induced complete clearing in 18 patients with ichthyosis vulgaris and 10 patients with X-linked ichthyosis. The scales came off in the bath after three applications. It had no effect if used without occlusion. Propylene glycol was also very helpful in keratosis palmaris et plantaris and gave partial improvement in lamellar ichthyosis and epidermolytic hyperkeratosis.

Audebert C: Un traitement simple des ichtyoses: Le propylene-glycol sous occlusion. Ann Dermatol Venereol 104:423–424, 1977.

Another endorsement of 40 to 60 per cent **propylene glycol** in water applied at night under occlusion. This study included nine patients with ichthyosis vulgaris.

Lykkesfeldt G, Høyer H: Topical cholesterol treatment of recessive X-linked ichthyosis. Lancet 2:1337–1338, 1983.

Cholesterol cream (10 per cent bid for six weeks) was more effective than urea cream (10 per cent bid for six weeks) in 13 of 20 males with steroid-sulfatase deficiency and recessive X-linked ichthyosis; 18 patients were significantly benefited by the cholesterol cream, including 8 patients who showed complete remission.

Ibsen HH, Brandrup F, Secher B: Topical cholesterol treatment of recessive X-linked ichthyosis. Lancet 2:645, 1984.

Another Danish team, in follow-up of the previous study, demonstrated in a paired comparison double-blind trial that the base used in the **cholesterol** cream was just as effective as the cholesterol cream itself in 9 of 11 patients studied. One case, in a five-year old boy, cleared completely.

Cooke JP, Winkelmann RK: Response of bullous congenital erythroderma to high-dose vitamin A. Cutis 29:44–46, 1982.

Short-term benefit in a 27-year-old black man following 740,000 U Aquasol A/day for two weeks. Desquamation began on the fourth day and became generalized on the fifth day. This treatment was well tolerated by the patient. Skin biopsy showed epidermolytic hyperkeratosis.

Baden HP, Buxman MM, Weinstein GD, Yoder FW: Treatment of ichthyosis with isotretinoin. J Am Acad Dermatol 6:716–720, 1982.

Accutane (2 mg/kg/day) in a multicenter study gave these results:

Lamellar ichthyosis: All 59 patients improved. Many noted increased heat tolerance, the ability to sweat, and improvement in ectropion.
Epidermolytic hyperkeratosis: Improvement occurred in 20 of 22 patients.
Ichthyosis vulgaris: There was improvement in 4 of 9 patients.
X-linked ichthyosis: Improvement occurred in 4 of 5 patients.
Congenital ichthyosiform erythroderma (unclassified): There was improvement in 3 of 4 patients.

The clearing effect was generally less noticeable on the lower half of the body, and in patients with very thick scales clearing was less complete.

Pehamberger H, Neumann H, Holubar K: Oral treatment of ichthyosis with an aromatic retinoid. Br J Dermatol 99:319–324, 1978.

Tigason (1 mg/kg/day) completely cleared three cases of lamellar ichthyosis and two cases of X-linked ichthyosis in three weeks. When Tigason was stopped, the ichthyosis reappeared within six weeks.

Mashkilleysson AL, Mashkilleysson NA: Treatment of congenital ichthyosiform erythroderma in mother and son with oral aromatic retinoid Ro 10-9359. Z Hautkr 58:1127–1129, 1983.

Tigason (25 to 50 mg/day) given to a mother and son suffering from nonbullous ichthyosiform erythroderma resulted in complete disappearance of all clinical signs of disease in two weeks. Relapse in one patient occurred six weeks after the drug was stopped. Reinstitution of treatment caused clearing in 10 days. Apparently patients need small daily maintenance doses for long periods.

Jagell S, Liden S: Treatment of the ichthyosis of the Sjögren-Larsson syndrome with etretinate (Tigason). Acta Derm Venereol 63:89–91, 1983.

Tigason (50 mg/day for two weeks, then 10 to 25 mg/day maintenance) in conjunction with **urea** cream (10 per cent) cleared within one month six of seven cases of this autosomal recessive subset of ichthyosis (lamellar form associated with mental retardation and spastic diplegia or quadriplegia). Treatment was continued for six months. Patients particularly appreciated being able to cut down on the time-consuming application of creams.

Tamayo L, Ruiz-Maldonado R: Oral retinoid (Ro 10-9359) in children with lamellar ichthyosis, epidermolytic hyperkeratosis, and symmetrical erythrokeratoderma. Dermatologica 161:305–314, 1980.

Another Tigason triumph in 10 children: 8 with lamellar ichthyosis, 5 with erythrokeratoderma variabilis, and 1 with epidermolytic hyperkeratosis. All showed dramatic improvement when given Tigason (2 mg/kg/day). Some were treated for two years, since relapse occurred whenever the drug was stopped.

Hazell M, Marks R: Follicular ichthyosis. Br J Dermatol 111:101–109, 1984.

Describes four cases of a new distinctive form of congenital ichthyosis expressed only at the follicular orifices as horny follicular projections. Three of the patients also had pseudoacanthosis nigricans, and two of them had facial abnormalities. Treatment with Tigason gave good results, but relapse occurred when the drug was withdrawn.

Pittsley RA, Yoder FW: Retinoid hyperostosis: Skeletal toxicity associated with long-term administration of 13-cis-retinoic acid for refractory ichthyosis. N Engl J Med 308:1012–1014, 1983.

Four patients with severe ichthyosis (lamellar) developed arthralgias and related skeletal hyperostosis after two years of high-dose treatment with **13-*cis*-retinoic acid** (Accutane 3 to 4 mg/kg/day). Retinoid hyperostosis may be a distinct rheumatic disorder.

Sillevis Smitt JH, de Mari FR: A serious side-effect of etretinate (Tigason). Clin Exp Dermatol 9:554–556, 1984.

Long-term high-dose **vitamin A** therapy can induce cortical hyperostosis, premature closure of the epiphyses of the long bones, periosteal calcification, and demineralization of the long bones and spine. Accutane similarly can induce skeletal and fascial hyperostosis and calcification. This report documents similar events following five years of Tigason (60 mg/day) therapy for lamellar ichthyosis in a 19-year-old woman. She was found to have bone spicule formation as well as hyperostosis and periosteal calcification, resulting in painful and limited rotation of both forearms. Thus, vitamin A and the related retinoids have profound effects on skin and bones.

Caver CV: Clofazimine-induced ichthyosis and its treatment. Cutis 29:341–343, 1982.

Ultra Mide lotion (25 per cent **urea** applied bid) controlled serious ichthyosis induced by **clofazimine** (100 mg/day) in eight leprosy patients. Improvement was clearly seen within two weeks and was complete in three to four weeks.

Flint GL, Flam M, Soter NA: Acquired ichthyosis: A sign of nonlymphoproliferative malignant disorders. Arch Dermatol 111:1446–1447, 1975.

Ichthyosis not present since infancy can result from drugs (nicotinic acid), hypothyroidism, severe xerosis, or internal malignant disease. This report cites four examples associated with carcinomas of the lung, breast, colon, and cervix. In one patient the ichthyosis improved when cytotoxic drugs temporarily controlled the adenocarcinoma of the breast.

Majekodunmi AE, Femi-Pearse D: Ichthyosis: Early manifestation of intestinal leiomyosarcoma. Br Med J 3:724, 1974.

Excision of a leiomyosarcoma of the small bowel in a 49-year-old man was followed two weeks later by the disappearance of acquired ichthyosis on his legs that had been present for two months. When the tumor recurred, so did the ichthyosis, with spread to the lower abdomen.

Dykes PJ, Marks R: Acquired ichthyosis: Multiple causes for an acquired generalized disturbance in desquamation. Br J Dermatol 97:327–334, 1977.

Varied examples of ichthyosis (generalized dryness and roughness in which large clumps of corneocytes are shed in the absence of signs of inflammation).

1. Malnutrition in a 60-year-old alcoholic man. The ichthyosis cleared with a regular diet and vitamin and folic acid supplements.
2. Reticulum cell sarcoma in a 57-year-old man. Chemotherapy was followed by remission of the ichthyosis.
3. Panhypopituitarism in a 61-year-old man. The ichthyosis involuted following endocrine therapy, but his skin remained dry.

English RS, Hurley HJ, Witkowski JA, Sanders J: Generalized anhidrosis associated with Hodgkin's disease and acquired ichthyosis. Ann Intern Med 58:676–681, 1963.

Hydrophilic ointments relieved the acquired ichthyosis but not the anhidrosis in a 51-year-old man with Hodgkin's disease. The anhidrosis was apparently secondary to vacuolar degeneration of the eccrine secretory cells induced by the lymphoma.

Nagata T: Netherton's syndrome which responded to photochemotherapy. Dermatologica 161:51–56, 1980.

A 22-year-old Japanese woman with ichthyosis linearis circumflexa and hair shaft abnormalities (trichorrhexis invaginata) showed a good response to UVA following 8-MOP topically for two to three weeks. Relapse occurred as soon as therapy was stopped.

Manabe M, Yoshiike T, Negi M, Ogawa H: Successful therapy of ichthyosis linearis circumflexa with PUVA. J Am Acad Dermatol 8:905–906, 1983.

Lesions completely involuted after two weeks of phototherapy (UVA 2 J/sq cm daily after application of 8-methoxypsoralen ointment 0.3 per cent) in an 18-year-old man with serpiginous lesions since birth. Therapy was stopped after one month, and lesions recurred. A second course of PUVA was equally successful.

Klein E, Hahn GM, Solomon JA, et al: Explorations of antimitotic agents in the treatment of a congenital disease, ichthyosis linearis circumflexa. J Surg Oncol 11:85–88, 1979.

Low-dose **cyclophosphamide** (Cytoxan 50 mg every three days) was extremely effective in a 19-year-old man with ichthyosis linearis circumflexa. When it was stopped after nine months, he remained clear of the disease for three months before a milder form returned that was controllable with LCD in Aquaphor. This disabling form of ichthyosis, which exacerbates in three- to five-week cycles, is considered to be a form of Netherton's syndrome.

Peled I, Bar-Lev A, Wexler MR: Surgical correction of ectropion in lamellar ichthyosis. Ann Plast Surg 8:429–431, 1982.

Surgical success is described in treating bilateral ectropion that had led to photophobia, chronic conjunctivitis, keratitis, and corneal erosions in a 25-year-old woman with lamellar ichthyosis. Surgery involved blepharoplasty incisions, temporary tarsorrhaphy to close the eyelids, and skin grafts on both the upper and lower eyelids.

How do you get new ideas? Read! Read! Read!

Impetigo

Erythromycin
Cephalosporins
Clindamycin

Nonbullous impetigo, usually caused by beta-hemolytic streptococci, can be erased like chalk from a blackboard by giving erythromycin orally. A 10-day course is usually adequate for complete re-epithelialization and bacteriologic cure. Bullous impetigo is due to *Staphylococcus aureus,* often a penicillin-resistant strain. We treat these patients also with systemic erythromycin. Bockhart's impetigo, a superficial folliculitis caused by *S. aureus,* is amenable to erythromycin and numerous other antistaphylococcal antibiotics.

It is no longer necessary to scrub the area with antimicrobial soaps or use tedious wet dressings to remove crusts. Simple gentle washing of the area is sufficient. We feel that topical antibiotics used alone are *not sufficient treatment* for impetigo, as healing is slow and only mild cases respond. The more rapid healing produced by systemic antibiotics helps prevent spread and probably reduces the chance and severity of subsequent nephritis, although this remains to be proven. Impetigo is highly contagious, so that any playmates or contacts exhibiting impetigo should be treated. Parents of children with atopic dermatitis should be particularly watchful for early impetigo, which disseminates rapidly in eczematous skin. In the hospital, the possibility of an epidemic of impetigo in the newborn nursery calls for scrupulous cleanliness and keeping the area off limits to any person with even a minor skin infection, including paronychia.

Prophylaxis centers on improved washing hygiene, using antibacterial soaps such as Dial or Safeguard or bactericidal soaps such as Hibiclens (chlorhexidine gluconate) or pHisoHex (hexachlorophene). Likewise, attention should be paid to correcting underlying disease and poor nutrition.

Becker LE, Tschen E: Common bacterial infections of the skin. Primary Care 10:397–409, 1983.

Comprehensive scholarly review with 83 references.

Dillon HC Jr: Topical and systemic therapy for pyodermas. Int J Dermatol 19:443–451, 1980.

Summary of years of data in children favors systemic over topical antibiotic therapy. **Erythromycin** is the drug of choice for bullous impetigo, while oral penicillin is best initially for purulent streptococcal infection. Avoid IM benzathine penicillin G because of pain and discomfort and risk of sensitization. Hold **clindamycin**, cephalosporins, and **dicloxacillin** in reserve.

Dillon HC: Impetigo contagiosa: Suppurative and non-suppurative complications: 1. Clinical, bacteriologic, and epidemiologic characteristics of impetigo. Am J Dis Child 115:530–541, 1968.

Streptococcal impetigo (427 cases) had an average duration of 18 days, whereas staphylococcal bullous impetigo (31 cases) averaged 7 days. Sib-

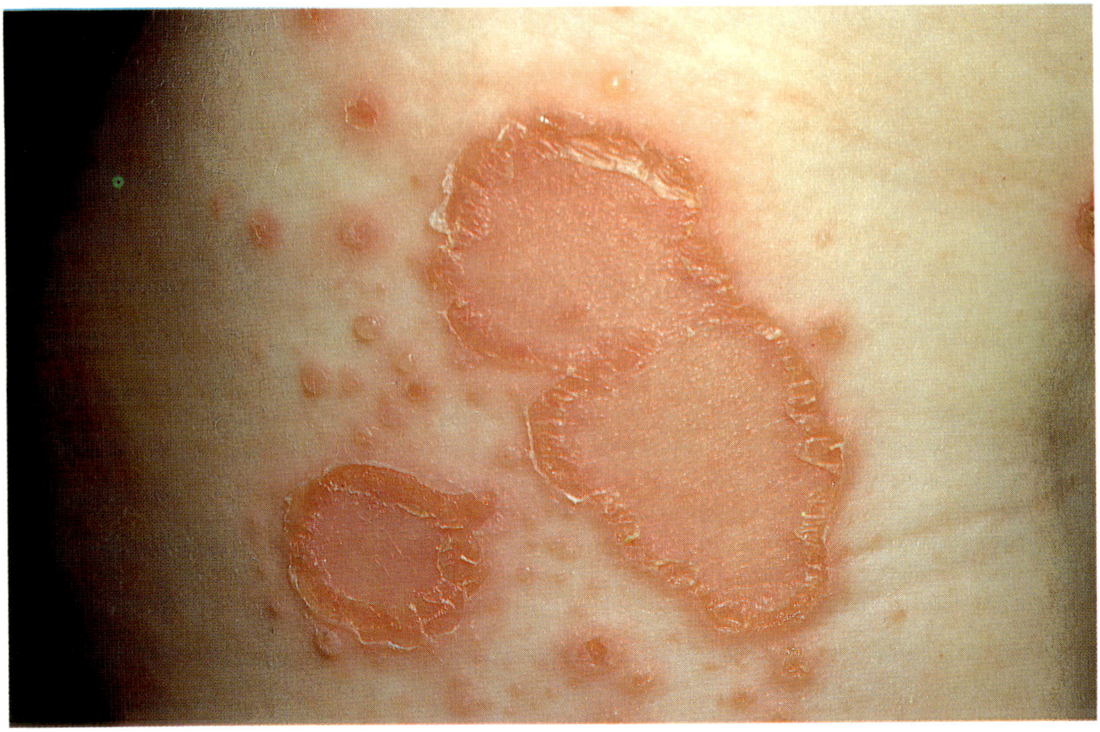

lings are commonly affected. Mosquito bites and minor skin trauma predispose. Nasal carriage of staphylococci may predispose to secondary contamination of lesions initiated by streptococci.

Hall WD, Blumberg RW, Moody MD: Studies in children with impetigo: Bacteriology, serology, and incidence of glomerulonephritis. Am J Dis Child 125:800–806, 1973.

Impetigo contagiosa in 150 children studied over a two-year period was associated with glomerulonephritis (hematuria) in only one instance. Most cases were treated with mechanical cleansing followed by application twice a day of Mycitracin (**bacitracin-neomycin-polymyxin**) ointment.

Hughes WT, Wan RT: Impetigo contagiosa: Etiology, complications and comparison of therapeutic effectiveness of erythromycin and antibiotic ointment. Am J Dis Child 113:449–453, 1967.

Oral **erythromycin** (40 mg/kg/day for five days) was more effective in healing and preventing recurrence than **polymyxin B-bacitracin-neomycin** ointment (applied four times a day). Controlled study of 62 children.

Esterly NB, Markowitz M: The treatment of pyoderma in children. JAMA 212:1667–1670, 1970.

In 209 children, one IM injection of **benzathine penicillin G** (600,000 U) with **procaine penicillin G** (600,000 U) was superior to Neosporin ointment and **gentamicin sulfate** (Garamycin) ointment. **Tetracycline** was not adequate. Favor systemic treatment to, it is hoped, decrease the incidence of nephritis.

Schachner L, Taplin D, Scott GB, Morrison M: A therapeutic update of superficial skin infections. Pediatr Clin North Am 30:397–404, 1983.

Current "batting averages" for impetigo treatments reflect changing strains of streptococci:

cloxacillin (Tegopen)	1000
penicillin V potassium (Pen·Vee K)	470

With **erythromycin**-resistant strains emerging, the authors prefer cloxacillin or **cephalexin** (Keflex).

Dillon HC Jr, Gray BM, Ware JC: Clinical and laboratory studies with cefaclor: Efficacy in skin and soft tissue infections. Postgrad Med J 55(Suppl 4):77–81, 1979.

Cefaclor (Ceclor 30 mg/kg/day in two to four doses) cleared 93 per cent of 67 cases of bullous impetigo in one week.

Dillon HC Jr, Derrick CS: Clinical experience with clindamycin hydrochloride. 1. Treatment of streptococcal and mixed streptococcal-staphylococcal skin infections. Pediatrics 55:205–212, 1975.

Impetigo cure rates in 244 children at one week after oral antibiotics:

erythromycin (Pediamycin 40 mg/kg/day)	99 per cent
clindamycin (HFC capsules 15 mg/kg/day)	97 per cent
phenoxymethyl penicillin (Pen·Vee K 200,000 to 400,000 U tid)	91 per cent

Garcia RL, Bishop ME: Telephoners' impetigo. Arch Dermatol 112:1178, 1976.

Impetigo of the ear in four women required elimination of the phone, as well as the bacteria, for successful treatment.

Ruby RJ, Nelson JD: The influence of hexachlorophene scrubs on the response to placebo or penicillin therapy in impetigo. Pediatrics 52:854–859, 1973.

Daily baths were a unique experience to many of the children studied and thus must be considered a significant form of local therapy.

Stringer HCW: Treatment of impetigo. Drugs 6:413–416, 1973.

Patient should not return to work until clear of pathogens if handling meat, food, or patients. The nares, perineum, and scalp are the most common carrier sites.

Hartman LA, Miller HN, Zack A: Orthotic collar in the treatment of intertriginous impetigo. Phys Ther 56:928–929, 1976.

Cervical four-poster collar permitted critical aeration and drying in antibiotic-resistant impetigo of the neck.

Albert S, Baldwin R, Czekajewski S, Van Soestbergen A, Nachman R, Robertson A: Bullous impetigo due to group II *Staphylococcus aureus*. An epidemic in a normal newborn nursery. Am J Dis Child 120:10–13, 1970.

Crowding of infants plus a change in infant bathing technique (from using 3 per cent **hexachlorophene** liquid to 0.75 per cent hexachlorophene bar soap) was followed by 34 cases of bullous impetigo. In addition to resuming use of 3 per cent hexachlorophene liquid for bathing, therapeutic measures included limitation of staff, strict individual gown technique, limited admissions, earlier discharge, no circumcisions, nasopharyngeal cultures of personnel, antibiotics, and institution of 502 A *Staphylococcus* colonization. Routine bacterial cultures of umbilical cord stumps monitored the *S. aureus* colonization rate in the nursery.

Ferrieri P, Dajani AS, Wannamaker LW: A controlled study of penicillin prophylaxis against streptococcal impetigo. J Infect Dis 129:429–438, 1974.

Evidence that a single IM injection of long-acting **benzathine penicillin** (Bicillin 600,000 U or 1.2 million U) protects children from recurrence of impetigo for four to six weeks and significantly reduces incidence and prevalence of skin lesions for a six-week period.

Beware of patients who call you Doc. They rarely pay their bills.
WILLIAM OSLER

The patient who has TTLT: hard to see, hard to treat.*

* Tiny troublesome little things.

Impetigo Herpetiformis

Prednisone
Calcium-vitamin D
Photochemotherapy
Contraceptives

We view this rare disease as a subset of generalized pustular psoriasis triggered by pregnancy. Rarely do we see it, and rarely do we see it go away until the end of the pregnancy. In our limited experience, systemic steroid therapy has been the best, with the dose kept at levels that suppress rather than eliminate the lesions. Since the unborn child shares in the mother's treatment, the disease cannot be approached as aggressively as its analogue, pustular psoriasis.

The patient should be told of the likelihood of a stillbirth. She should also be advised that subsequent pregnancies, as well as contraceptives, may induce further attacks.

Oumeish OY, Farraj SE, Bataineh AS: Some aspects of impetigo herpetiformis. Arch Dermatol 118:103–105, 1982.

A patient developed the disease in each of nine pregnancies, with fetal or infant death in eight of them. Oral contraceptives produced the same lesions. **Prednisolone** (60 to 120 mg/day) offered the best help.

Oosterling RJ, Nobrega RE, DuBoeuff JA, Der Meer JB: Impetigo herpetiformis or generalized pustular psoriasis? Arch Dermatol 114:1527–1529, 1978.

Prednisone (60 mg/day) was found to be rapidly effective in clearing lesions during the 34th week of pregnancy. Tapering to 17.5 mg/day resulted in slight exacerbation in the 36th week. Spontaneous delivery produced a healthy daughter.

Bajaj AK, Swarup V, Gupta OP, Gupta SC: Impetigo herpetiformis. Dermatologica 155:292–295, 1977.

Dramatic response after two weeks of parenteral **calcium levulinate** (100 mg/day) and **vitamin D** (10,000 U/day) in a 7-months-pregnant woman with a low serum calcium level. Previous antibiotics and steroids had not been helpful. A healthy girl was born 1½ months later.

Ott F, Krakowski A, Tur E, Lipitz R, Weisman Y, Brenner S: Impetigo herpetiformis with lowered serum level of vitamin D and its diminished intestinal absorption. Dermatologica 164:360–365, 1982.

A patient with Crohn's disease who was three months pregnant received no help from steroids, antibiotics, **dapsone**, **calcium**, **vitamin D**, or plasma. A macerated dead male fetus was delivered at 31 weeks, and several days later the patient's skin cleared completely.

Ei-Din Selim MM, Rehak A, Abdel-Hafez K, Al-Saleh K: Impetigo herpetiformis: Report of a case treated with photochemotherapy (PUVA). Dermatol Monatsschr 168:44–48, 1982.

Dramatic clearing of lesions in a 32-weeks-pregnant patient with topical **8-methoxypsoralen** (8-MOP cream 0.1 per cent) applied one hour before exposure to UVA therapy (2J/sq m, four times a week for four weeks). No maintenance required. Steroids (**prednisone** 40 mg/day) had previously caused a flare. One month later a healthy baby was delivered.

Gligora M, Kolacio Z: Hormonal treatment of impetigo herpetiformis. Br J Dermatol 107:253, 1982.

Abortion was performed in the second month of pregnancy, but eruption did not abate. No help from steroids, cytostatic drugs, PUVA, and **dihydrotachysterol** (a blood calcium regulator) in various combinations. Marked improvement occurred within 10 days of starting **mestranol** and an estrogen-progestogen as follows:

Ovaras (Serono, Rome)
- Week 1: 15 μg mestranol
- Week 2: 50 μg mestranol
- Week 3: 50 μg mestranol + 1 μg ethynodiol
- Week 4: 75 μg mestranol + 2 μg ethynodiol

(Ovulen is the analogous compound in the United States, containing 0.1 mg mestranol and 1.0 mg ethynodiol diacetate.)

Count that day lost that does not see a new avenue of therapy explored.

Intestinal Bypass Dermatitis

Metronidazole
Tetracycline
Dapsone
Clindamycin

This mélange of macular, vesicular, pustular, nodular, ecchymotic, urticarial, and erythema nodosum lesions results from absorption and sensitization to bacterial antigens present in a stagnant bypassed loop of bowel or diverticulum. Antibiotics or surgical revision is the answer.

Stein HB, Schlappner OLA, Boyko W, et al: The intestinal bypass arthritis-dermatitis syndrome. Arthritis Rheum 24:684–690, 1981.

The syndrome includes polyarthralgias, nondeforming polyarthritis, pustular cutaneous vasculitis, Raynaud's phenomenon, and paresthesias. Five of ten patients were definitely helped by **tetracycline** (2 gm/day) or **clindamycin** (600 mg/day) for a minimum of five days, but often on a continuous basis. Neither **metronidazole** (Flagyl) nor sulfasalazine (Azulfidine) was effective. Six of nine patients were helped by a sphincteroplasty performed at the anastomosis of the blind loop and transverse colon to prevent bacterial reflux into the blind loop.

Ely PH: The bowel bypass syndrome: A response to bacterial peptidoglycans. J Am Acad Dermatol 2:473–487, 1980.

A comprehensive review with data on 10 more patients. **Prednisone** (10 mg/day) suppressed most symptoms. **Sulfapyridine** (500 mg qid) was effective therapy in two patients. **Metronidazole** (500 mg qid) was of no help for four patients, nor was zinc sulfate (220 mg tid) in two patients. Skin testing with *Streptococcus pyogenes* caused exacerbation of symptoms in all seven patients tested and in three patients provoked the entire clinical syndrome. In two of the above patients, repeat skin tests with *S. pyogenes* five days following reanastomosis of the bypass were negative and did not provoke arthritis.

Drenick EJ, Ahmed AR, Greenway F, Olerud JE: Cutaneous lesions after intestinal bypass. Ann Intern Med 93:557–559, 1980.

Of 81 intestinal bypass patients with episodes of bypass enteropathy 23 had papulopustular or nodular skin lesions. These resolved with spontaneous improvement of the bypass enteropathy or in response to **metronidazole** therapy (Flagyl 750 to 2000 mg/day). After the bypass was dismantled the eruptions disappeared permanently. The problem is a bacterial immune-complex vasculitis resulting from overgrowth of bacteria in the bypassed bowel.

Kennedy C: The spectrum of inflammatory skin disease following jejuno-ileal bypass for marked obesity. Br J Dermatol 105:425–435, 1981.

Dapsone (100 mg/day) abolished or reduced vesicular, pustular, and nodular lesions in two patients. **Metronidazole** (600 mg/day) or **tetracycline** (1 gm/day) or both were given to seven patients for several weeks. Tetracycline helped clear lesions in one patient, but did not prevent new lesions. Metronidazole was of doubtful prophylactic value in two patients. In four other patients no effect was seen.

Fairris GM, Ashworth J, Cotterill JA: A dermatosis associated with bacterial overgrowth in jejunal diverticula. Br J Dermatol 112:709–713, 1985.

A 64-year-old man simultaneously developed diarrhea and target-like vasculitic skin lesions. Multiple diverticula were found in the upper jejunum, along with excess numbers of bacteria in the small bowel (confirmed by hydrogen breath test using glucose). Circulating immune complexes and heavy dermal deposits of IgG, IgM, and fibrin were also present.

Similar to the intestinal bypass syndrome, it also responded to antibiotic therapy (**tetracycline** 500 mg qid and **metronidazole** 400 mg tid for four months).

There will be days when all of the patients are getting better; there will be days when none of the patients is getting better; but most of the days most of the patients will be getting better.

Just Think

Patients invariably underestimate the duration and cost of therapy.

Avoid prescriptions you can't defend in court—when the patient avers, "It was only for a pimple."

Lesions have lives. Therapy works best on the senescent ones.

The best memory is a record made at the time.

WILLIAM GULL

If you treat relatives, charge them and give the money to their *favorite charity. Free advice is freely ignored.*

Don't lose patients—by losing your patience.

A generic drug is about as good as a generic doctor.

Every doctor should have a pet placebo, i.e., a drug he knows works despite what others think.

The secret of being a lucky doctor is to have lucky patients.

Disease favors the chance of a second disease.

Some dermatoses are to be diagnosed, yet never treated. Others are to be treated, yet never diagnosed.

Illegible prescriptions make for an imaginative pharmacist.

There is more than knowing what to do: The patient must know how to do it.

If you see your patient's tears, you know some of her problems are being washed away.

Some patients have symptoms that scatter like leaves in the wind. You will never catch up with every one.

Your prescription may not have helped because it was never taken—to the pharmacist or by the patient.

The number of side effects of a drug is directly proportional to the number known to the patient.

If you have trouble finding the patient's problem, you'll have trouble finding a cure.

When once the itch of literature comes over a man nothing can cure it but the scratching of a pen.

SAMUEL LOVER

The last prescription written for a self-limiting disease always proves to be a wonder drug.

What is so rare as a day in the office when everyone is getting better?

Therapeutic nihilism may be the correct way to approach the facts, but not the patient.

Some patients feel abandoned if not seen often, others abandon doctors who have to be seen often.

A committee is a device for spreading the responsibility for doing nothing.

Anxiety is contagious. Watch out you don't catch it from your patient.

Keratosis Pilaris

Retin-A	Buf-Puf
Aquasol A	Erythromycin
Carmol 20	Bactrim DS

Common, but not common in the dermatologist's office, is keratosis pilaris. It can easily vary all the way from a trivial cosmetic annoyance present in four out of five teenagers, to an inflammatory follicular keratotic process deserving medical attention. For the latter we prescribe erythromycin (250 mg qid) or Bactrim DS (1 tablet at bedtime for several weeks), thus treating it as a folliculitis. To reduce the keratinous plugging of the follicles we prescribe **vitamin A** (Aquasol A 50,000 U tid for two to three months), which may be repeated in the event of relapse.

Topically, we recommend an emollient cream such as Carmol 20. If this gives no relief we use paired comparison trials of LacHydrin lotion versus Retin-A cream (0.05%). We advise use of Neutrogena dry skin soap or Cetaphil lotion for cleansing the area.

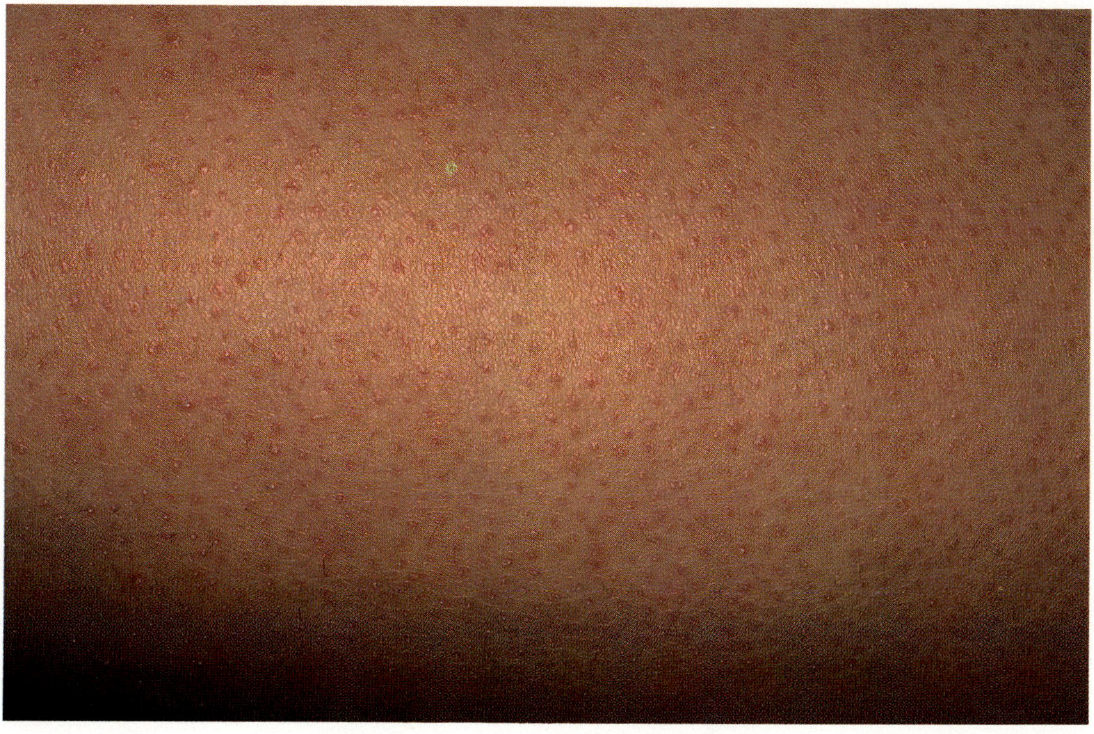

It is important for patients to know that new smooth skin will not be theirs until several months elapse. Follicular renovation cannot be achieved in a few days, but it can be achieved.

Orentreich N, Durr NP, Trancik RJ: Physical methods for altering surface texture of the skin. *In* Frost P, Horwitz SN (eds): Principles of Cosmetics for the Dermatologist. St. Louis, CV Mosby Co, 1982, pp 75–80.

Buf-Puf, a nonwoven polyester web gently rubbed across areas of keratosis pilaris (once daily for 14 days) results in almost complete resolution. This technique specifically concentrates the epidermabrasion on the elevated follicular keratoses of this disease, i.e., it is a folliculoabrasion.

Novick NL: Practical management of widespread, atypical keratosis pilaris. J Am Acad Dermatol 11:305–306, 1984.

The following routine completely cleared or greatly relieved widespread psychologically disabling keratosis pilaris within two to three weeks in 30 patients:

1. Reduce bathing.
2. Use superfatted soap.
3. Keep humidity high in home environment.
4. Apply a medium-potency topical steroid once a day for one week if lesions are inflammatory.
5. Apply 2 per cent **salicyclic acid** in 20 per cent **urea** cream (Carmol 20) using a 5- to 20-second gentle massage with a Buf-Puf after a daily shower.
6. For maintenance, use plain 20 per cent urea cream (Carmol 20) applied with Buf-Puf once or twice a week.

Read widely to avoid being narrow-minded.

Kyrle's Disease

Accutane	Cryotherapy
Aquasol A	Surgery
Retin-A cream	

This strange focal derangement of orientation of keratinization is one that should respond to the new retinoids. Our initial approach today would center on the use of Accutane (40 mg bid). Prior to Accutane we had limited success with Aquasol A (50,000 IU tid) and the conjoint spot use of a topical keratolytic containing salicyclic acid, such as Keralyt (6 per cent salicylic acid gel with alcohol, cellulose, and propylene glycol). Others have reported excellent results with topical retinoic acid. Efudex also deserves consideration.

In the case of recalcitrant lesions, cryotherapy with liquid nitrogen, similar to the treatment of warts, can be an effective method of eradication. Bulla formation is followed by elimination of the keratinous mass and the aberrant clone of keratinocytes responsible for its presence. Finally, excision or destruction by electrodesiccation may also be of benefit.

Tappeiner J, Wolff K, Schreiner E: Morbus Kyrle. Hautarzt 20:296–310, 1969.

The definitive paper on all aspects of this disease. Stresses its resistance to therapy. **Vitamin A** and ultraviolet light give only temporary relief.

Carter VH, Constantine VS: Kyrle's disease. I. Clinical findings in five cases and review of the literature. Arch Dermatol 97:624–632, 1968.

Vitamin A (100,000 U/day) coupled with topical keratolytics produced improvement in two patients, but relapse occurred when treatment was stopped. A third patient showed no response to topical keratolytics, **fluorouracil**, systemic steroids, or **methotrexate**, but improved moderately with vitamin A (100,000 U/day for three months).

Günther S: Morbus Kyrle (Hyperkeratosis follicularis et parafollicularis): lokale und systemische Therapie mit Vitamin-A-Säure (retinoic acid). Z Hautkr 50:507–511, 1975.

Oral **retinoic acid** (20 to 50 mg/day) was helpful in controlling the disease in 10 women over a period of one year. In one case, serum levels of retinol and carotene increased as the patient improved.

Petrozzi JW, Warthan TL: Kyrle disease: Treatment with topically applied tretinoin. Arch Dermatol 110:762–765, 1974.

Retin-A cream (0.1 per cent tid) induced virtual clearing of all lesions within 12 days in a 43-year-old man.

Brand A, Brody N: Keratotic papules in chronic renal disease. Cutis 28:637–639, 1981.

Tretinoin (Retin-A 0.05 per cent cream bid for two months) greatly improved the hyperkeratotic follicular lesions on the legs of three patients undergoing hemodialysis.

Aram H, Even-Paz Z, Livshin R: Kyrle's disease: Response to high-dose vitamin A. Cutis 30:753–759, 1982.

In a 60-year-old man with follicular papules and erythematous verrucous plaques over the extensor surfaces of arms and legs, **vitamin A** (500,000 U/day) therapy resulted in demonstrable improvement in 2 weeks and remarkable improvement in 14 weeks. At that time the dosage was gradually tapered as **vitamin E** (400 IU/day) was added to take advantage of the synergism between vitamin A and vitamin E. All treatment was stopped at 35 weeks without recurrence.

It's preferable to look for a new drug rather than to have your patient look for a new doctor.

Leg Ulcers

Zinc SO_4	Cholestyramine
Antibiotics	Pressure dressing
Benzoyl peroxide	Pinch grafts
DuoDerm	Varicose vein surgery
Debrisan	Arterial graft

About 400 years before Christ, Hippocrates wrote, "In case of an ulcer, it is not expedient to stand, especially if the ulcer be situated on the leg." This was no casual observation, for Hippocrates himself had a leg ulcer. And his advice rings true to this day. Dependency edema has never favored wound healing.

Support hose, Ace bandages, the Unna boot, and casts all serve the same purpose of improving the venous circulation. They provide relief from pain, protection from trauma, and reduction of venous incompetence. They are a keystone in the treatment of nearly all leg ulcers, since nearly all are due to chronic venous insufficiency.

One should first ascertain, however, the underlying cause of any leg ulcer. Such knowledge provides additional help in directing therapy. Thus, one should assess the patient for arterial disease. What is the arterial blood flow? In a few instances, arteriosclerosis of the vessels restricts blood flow to the point of anoxemic pain, as well as ulceration at the site of any physical trauma. Here the prognosis is guarded, as the ulcer may be but a prelude to gangrene. We always try vasodilators such as prazosin HCl (Minipress 2 mg tid), but often the vessel is already unresponsive. It is important to have early review by a vascular surgeon with respect to the need for an arterial graft.

For arterial ulcers we recommend maneuvers that reduce the painful cry of the skin for oxygen: avoidance of cold and avoidance of smoking. We stress the need to keep the extremities warm, the judicious use of alcoholic beverages for vasodilatation, and the value of some dependency of the limbs at night, which can be achieved with 6-inch blocks under the head of the bed. Tight constricting socks are to be avoided, and local heat is distinctly contraindicated, since a burn blister may evolve directly into an ulcer. Always, lights must be kept on at night to avoid inadvertent trauma from bumping into furniture in the dark.

At least 20 times more common is the ulcer of venous disease. While the proximate cause of the ulcer is still trauma, the pathogenesis involves a skin denied its normal venous return. Very often the underlying perforator veins have become incompetent as a result of smoldering or acute phlebitis or simply a varicose vein with valve failure. It is here that physical support by external dressing is so helpful (Unna boot, Primer + Tensoplast changed weekly). For the ulcer itself we use a packing with benzoyl peroxide (10 per cent gel) or a fixed dressing with DuoDerm that we change weekly. We have also used Debrisan, as well as

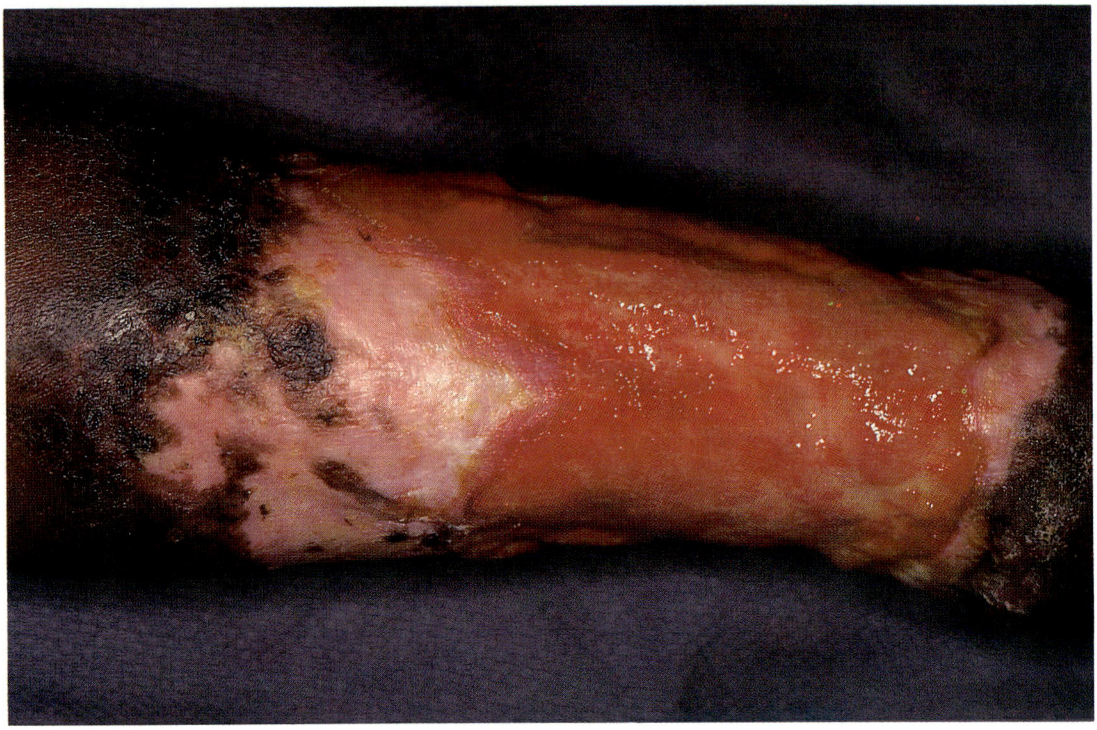

cholestyramine powder (Questran), in the ulcer site with success. No matter what the local regimen, it takes six to eight weeks for the average stasis leg ulcer to heal.

For those that fail to heal in this time frame, pinch grafts may be necessary, but such ulcers must first be reevaluated: x-ray examination for evidence of underlying osteomyelitis; culture for specific pathogens and use of systemic antibiotic therapy; biopsy for underlying disease or vasculitis; check for gamma globulins, cryoglobulins, sickle cell disease, and diabetes. And never forget the possibility of a factitial factor. We had experience with one ulcer that failed to heal even under a cast because of the patient inserting a wire coat hanger under the cast to keep the lesion viable.

We generally prescribe zinc (zinc sulfate 220 mg tid with food) as a nonspecific aid to healing. We stress the importance of not taking long cramped auto or bus rides and of not standing erect and immobile for any period. Finally, all such patients benefit from review by a specialist in peripheral vascular disease to determine the need and value of varicose vein surgery.

Given a cooperative patient, the treatment of leg ulcers can be a gratifying experience. As the door to the ulcer finally closes, you and the patient can look down at the leg and say, "We did that!" Even as Hippocrates knew, medicine has its moments of triumph, always best shared with the patient.

Young JR: Differential diagnosis of leg ulcers. Cardiovasc Clin 13(2):171–193, 1983.

Although there are 57 varieties listed here, 90 per cent of all leg ulcers are due to simple chronic venous insufficiency, 5 per cent are due to arteriosclerosis obliterans, and diabetic neuropathy is involved in most of the remainder.

If the ulcer is atypical in appearance or location or does not respond to treatment, the following laboratory tests may be helpful:

CBC
blood glucose
VDRL
bacterial culture of ulcer
ANA
rheumatoid factor
ESR
serum protein electrophoresis
biopsy of ulcer
chest roentgenogram
gastrointestinal roentgenograms (rule out causes of pyoderma gangrenosum)
bone marrow
arteriography (only if vascular surgery is being considered)

Dodd H, Cockett FB: The Pathology and Surgery of the Veins of the Lower Limb. New York, Churchill Livingstone, 1976, pp 297–314.

Includes detailed differential diagnosis of ulcers of the leg.

The "ankle flare" is the most constant sign of venous pathology associated with ulcers and occurs before ulceration takes place. It consists of a flare of small subcutaneous dilated venules immediately below and behind the internal malleolus, seen best with the patient standing. It may also occur below and behind the external malleolus.

Kitahama A, Elliott LF, Kerstein MD, Menendez CV: Leg ulcer: Conservative management or surgical treatment. JAMA 247:197–199, 1982.

Nonsurgical management cured 59 of 65 indigent patients with chronic venous stasis leg ulcers resulting mainly (67 per cent) from prior phlebitis; 86 per cent needed only pressure dressings changed once weekly in the clinic (coat ulcer with 10 per cent boric acid in petrolatum, cover with gauze and cast padding, wrap with wide elastic bandages 10 to 15 cm).

For large ulcers associated with extreme edema, the patient was hospitalized overnight with the leg elevated. When the edema disappeared, the leg was wrapped with two rolls of gauze saturated with **calamine, glycerin**, and **zinc oxide** (Gelocast boot). A skin-tight plaster of Paris cast was then applied from the toes to below the knee, which remained in place for up to three months.

Lofgren EP: Chronic venous insufficiency. Cardiovasc Clin 13(2):133–154, 1983.

Half a million Americans suffer from leg ulcers associated with incompetent varicose veins. In some, venous surgery can be curative. Removal of varicose veins will not jeopardize venous blood return to the heart and should not be postponed until after childbearing age. Varicose veins are not suitable for grafting in arterial bypass surgery.

Leg cramps due to venous insufficiency occur at the end of the day or shortly after retiring. Relief comes from massaging, walking, or a warm bath. Wearing elastic stockings during the day may help prevent nocturnal leg cramps.

Chronic deep venous insufficiency, with cyanosis, daytime edema from ankles to knees, secondary superficial varicosities, and stasis changes, is best treated nonsurgically. Stasis cellulitis, induration, fibrosis, retraction of subcutaneous tissue, and subcutaneous ossifications are long-term consequences.

Recommendations for treatment:

1. Elastic support: a lifelong necessity. Support is inadequate and must be increased if dermatitis develops.
   - Bandages (10 to 15 cm wide):
     - Apply upon arising and remove at bedtime
     - Begin above the ankle and work toward the base of the toes, then return to the beginning (seven turns of the roll should cover the foot and heel)
     - Apply spiral bandage around the lower leg (with overlap of half the width), above the belly of the calf muscles, and to the popliteal skin fold.
   - Stockings:
     - Knee length is satisfactory in most cases and is tolerated best.
     - Leotards and pantyhose provide excellent support in the thigh, groin, and perineum (especially in pregnancy)
     - The strength of the stocking often must be compromised so the patient will wear it.
     - The severity of the venous insufficiency and the type of occupational life style ultimately determine the type of stocking.
2. Elevation:
   - Assume the supine position (30 minutes one or two times a day) with the ankle 12 inches above the heart—"Toes above the nose."
   - Elevate the legs whenever possible.
3. Exercise:
   - Strengthen the calf muscles with exercise—walking, bicycle riding, and swimming.
   - Avoid prolonged sitting (car or airplane) or standing (walk around).

Husni EA: Skin ulcers secondary to arterial and venous disease. *In* Lee BY (ed): Chronic Ulcers of the Skin. New York, McGraw-Hill, 1985, pp 93–99.

Mechanical, thermal, chemical, or surgical trauma is the immediate cause of all leg ulcers in patients with arterial or venous disease.

Principles of management of venous disease
- good foot hygiene
- elevation
- elastic compression
- venous reconstruction on the basis of phlebography and pressure studies:
  - removal of incompetent saphenous vein as well as all incompetent communicators
  - ligation of all perforators
- postphlebitic disease: fibrinolytic agents, anticoagulants, antibiotics, and diuretics
- no surgery for one year
- evaluation for the presence of tumor, aneurysm, fistula, or scar

Principles of management of arterial insufficiency
- protection 4+
- arterial reconstruction on the basis of arteriography, Doppler studies, and ankle and arm blood pressure indices
- lumbar sympathectomy

Seville RH, Martin E: Dermatological Nursing and Therapy. London, Blackwell Scientific Publications, 1981, p 153.

Good advice to patients:

Never stand still.
Don't be afraid of exercise.
Avoid any obstruction to the veins.
Keep feet up whenever possible.
Keep weight down.
Bandage legs correctly.
Do not let legs get cold.

Alper JC, Welch EA, Maguire P: Use of the vapor permeable membrane for cutaneous ulcers: Details of application and side effects. J Am Acad Dermatol 11:858–866, 1984.

Op-site dressing (a thin transparent synthetic polyurethane semipermeable membrane, applied once or twice weekly) aids healing of nonexudative venous ulcers. If necrotic debris and bacterial contamination lead to rapid accumulation of fluid beneath the membrane, the dressing should be changed two or three times daily.

The dressing may be loosened by wiping it with isopropyl alcohol or isopropyl alcohol and acetone (50:50 mixture) or by soaking the area with soapy water for 30 minutes. Careful peeling off of the dressing is necessary to avoid damaging the underlying epithelium.

Friedman SJ, Su WPD: Management of leg ulcers with hydrocolloid occlusive dressing. Arch Dermatol 120:1329–1336, 1984.

DuoDerm (Squibb, a synthetic absorbent colloidal dressing containing gelatin, pectin, carboxymethylcellulose sodium, and polyisobutylene) proved to be an efficient occlusive dressing for 31 leg ulcers in 22 patients. Changed every five days, it relieved pain and was convenient. However, the healing time of six weeks was the same as for control ulcers treated with wet dressings.

Roenigk HH Jr: Dermabrasion: State of the art. J Dermatol Surg Oncol 11:306–314, 1985.

Reviews the new synthetic wound dressings for postoperative care. Recommends **Vigilon** (Bard-4 per cent polyethylene oxide, in a colloidal suspension in water on polyethylene mesh), which is nonadherent, oxygen permeable, and has a removable exterior polyethylene layer to permit passage of water vapor. It affords a moist environment, absorption of its own weight in exudate, and the possibility of using absorbent dressings over it. It should be changed daily.

Skog E, Arnesjö B, Troëng T, et al: A randomized trial comparing cadexomer iodine and standard treatment in the out-patient management of chronic venous ulcers. Br J Dermatol 109:77–83, 1983.

Cadexomer iodine, 0.9 per cent iodine physically immobilized within biodegradable spherical microbeads (**Iodosorb powder** applied once daily, 3 mm depth for six weeks under compression bandages) was more effective than standard treatment (paraffin-impregnated gauze under compression bandage) for reduction of pain, removal of pus and debris, removal of exudate, stimulation of granulation, and reduction of surrounding erythema. The study was conducted at 10 centers in Norway and Sweden and involved 93 patients who had leg ulcers of at least 2 cm in diameter that had failed to heal during a two-year period despite use of topical enzyme preparations, dextranomer, polymyxin, and silver nitrate. Half of the patients receiving standard treatment showed 5 per cent increase in mean ulcer size at the end of six weeks, whereas the group treated with iodine microbeads showed a 34 per cent decrease in mean ulcer size.

Ramelet A-A, van Melle G: Le benzoyl peroxyde dans le traitement des ulcéres de jambe. Dermatologica 161:315–326, 1980.

Forty leg ulcers were treated with **benzoyl peroxide** (20 per cent lotion bid for six weeks) with very satisfactory results. After six weeks there was a 76.5 per cent reduction in wound area. The bacterial flora of the wounds also changed, with disappearance of streptococci and staphylococci, while *Pseudomonas aeruginosa* became abundant.

Strömberg H-E, Agren MS: Topical zinc oxide treatment improves arterial and venous leg ulcers. Br J Dermatol 111:461–468, 1984.

In 37 geriatric patients with leg ulcers, dry gauze dressings impregnated with **zinc oxide** powder (400 μg/sq cm changed daily for 60 days) healed 83 per cent of ulcers, as opposed to a control rate of 42 per cent.

Söderberg T, Hallmans G, Stenström S, et al: Treatment of leprosy wounds with adhesive zinc tape. Lepr Rev 53:271–276, 1982.

Nonporous waterproof adhesive tape containing zinc oxide (30 per cent) was applied once daily directly to plantar ulcers of hospitalized leprosy patients. Wounds treated with the zinc tape healed significantly faster than those treated with gauze soaked in Eusol. Zinc from the tape is absorbed into granulation tissue and stimulates wound healing.

Hallböök T, Lanner E: Serum-zinc and healing of venous leg ulcers. Lancet 2:780–782, 1982.

Ulcers in patients with a serum zinc level greater than 110 μg/100 ml initially, or after **zinc sulfate** therapy (effervescent tablets 200 mg tid for 18 weeks), healed significantly faster than ulcers in patients with a low serum zinc level. During treatment with zinc, the serum zinc levels remained at about 150 μg/100 ml. This was a double-blind study of 50 patients with chronic venous leg ulcers.

Mathur NK, Bumb RA: Oral zinc in the trophic ulcers of leprosy. Int J Lepr 51:410–411, 1983.

Zinc sulfate (220 mg daily for 3 to 18 months) plus antileprosy drugs and **co-trimoxazole** for secondary infection of ulcers resulted in complete healing of trophic ulcers in 6 to 12 weeks. Skin biopsies after zinc therapy showed neovascularization and endothelial cell proliferation in the dermis. Zinc was also being given for immunostimulation.

Serjeant GR, Galloway RE, Gueri MC: Oral zinc sulphate in sickle-cell ulcers. Lancet 2:891–892, 1970.

Leg ulcers occur in 75 per cent of adults with sickle cell anemia, causing great morbidity. A double-blind study of 34 such patients showed that **zinc sulfate** (220 mg tid for three months) caused the healing rate of ulcers to be three times faster than in the placebo group. In the zinc-treated group 13 of 17 improved, with complete healing in six patients.

Hendricks WM: Pressure ulcers. Ann Intern Med 95:239, 1981.

Ulcerations of the lower legs or the feet, especially in a patient with diabetes or arteriosclerosis obliterans, will heal more rapidly if the head of the bed is elevated 4 to 6 inches and 1 per cent **gentian violet** is applied to the wound surface.

Avoid aggressive surgical debridement, wet to dry dressings, and whirlpool baths, but debride conservatively with **collagenase** ointment and **benzoyl peroxide** lotion (10 per cent Benoxyl) once each week.

Baker PG, Haig G: Metronidazole in the treatment of chronic pressure sores and ulcers: A comparison with standard treatments in general practice. Practitioner 225:569–573, 1981.

Metronidazole (400 mg tid for one week) was more effective in the treatment of foul smelling decubitus ulcers (30 cases) than in venous stasis ulcers (23 cases) but appeared to increase the rate of healing in both types of ulcers. It acts by eliminating anaerobic organisms.

Lishner M, Lang R, Kedar I, Ravid M: Treatment of diabetic perforating ulcers (mal perforant) with local dimethylsulfoxide. J Am Geriatr Soc 33:41–43, 1985.

Dimethylsulfoxide (DMSO) (25 per cent in normal saline, soak 20 minutes tid in 500 ml, for 20 weeks) provided prompt lasting analgesia in painful ulcers of peripheral vascular disease. Of 20 patients with diabetic neuropathy and ulcers of the sole or heel (unresponsive to at least four months of conventional therapy) 14 showed complete healing in one to four months. The DMSO solution was freshly mixed every three days. If ulcers were infected, Garamycin (80 mg) was added to the DMSO solution. DMSO probably increases tissue oxygenation through vasodilatation and decreased platelet aggregation.

Rubinstein A, Pierce CE Jr II, Bloomgarden Z: Rapid healing of diabetic foot ulcers with continuous subcutaneous insulin infusion. Am J Med 75:161–165, 1983.

Report of two cases of intractable foot ulcers in diabetic men which healed completely after six to eight weeks of pump-driven subcutaneous **insulin** therapy (27 units basal dose, 38 units in divided doses in one case; 12 units basal dose and 16 units in divided doses in the other case) that stabilized their blood sugar levels. Good control of blood sugar is probably important for improving wound healing in diabetics.

Helm PA, Walker SC, Pullium G: Total contact casting in diabetic patients with neuropathic foot ulcerations. Arch Phys Med Rehabil 65:691–693, 1984.

Neuropathic ulcers of the foot are both limb threatening and life threatening. In this study of 22 diabetics, 73 per cent of the ulcers healed in an average of 38 days following application of total contact plaster short-leg walking casts, which were changed weekly.

Berginer V, Baruchin A, Ben-Yakar Y, Mahler D: Plantar ulcers in hereditary sensory neuropathy: A plea for conservative treatment. Int J Dermatol 23:664–668, 1984.

The neruopathic ulcer (heredity, diabetes, syphilis, leprosy) may require a cast for six months. Prevention centers on wearing orthopedic shoes, inspecting the feet several times daily, and resting if redness or swelling appears.

Coleman WC, Brand PW, Birke JA: The total contact cast: A therapy for plantar ulceration on insensitive feet. J Am Podiatry Assoc 74:548–552, 1984.

Plantar ulcers present as long as 15 years on a foot without sensation can be healed in six to eight weeks with casting (details of application given, with photographs). Do not use if patient is febrile or there is cellulitis, lymphadenopathy, or a sinus tract or drainage from the ulcer.

Millard LG, Roberts MM, Gatecliffe M: Chronic leg ulcers treated by the pinch graft method. Br J Dermatol 97:289–295, 1977.

Inexpensive, simple, partial-thickness pinch grafting is effective therapy in patients with chronic leg ulcers. But in this study of 49 patients, none of the grafts lasted even six months in the vasculitic ulcer group. In stasis ulcers nearly 50 per cent had broken down within two years, but in arteriosclerotic ulcers 70 per cent remained intact after two years.

Hinz J, Kuhne FW, Stahl KW: Local tetrachlorodecaoxide treatment to improve oxygen supply to non-healing wounds. Lancet 2:630, 1984.

An ingenious water-soluble complex that releases oxygen when applied to the ulcer base. When applied once daily it proved helpful in a double-blind study of 38 patients.

Fischer BH: Treatment of ulcers on the legs with hyperbaric oxygen. J Dermatol Surg 1(3):55–58, 1975.

Topical hyperbaric oxygen chambers (Topox Corporation, 2627 Kennedy Blvd, Jersey City, NJ 07306), which provided an oxygen bath (4 liters/minute flow, under 22 mm Hg pressure, through a hermetic chamber surrounding the ulcer, 2 to 3 hours bid for two weeks to two months), induced healing of previously recalcitrant leg ulcers in 28 of 30 patients. The ulcers were due to burns, pressure, venous stasis, surgical wounding, rheumatoid arthritis, and hypergammaglobulinemia.

Heng MCY: Hyperbaric oxygen therapy for a foot ulcer in a patient with polyarteritis nodosa. Australas J Dermatol 24:105–108, 1983.

Problem:

A large area of necrosis with bare bone exposed on the plantar aspect of the left foot of a 62-year-old man with polyarteritis who was being treated with **prednisone** (20 mg/day) and Cytoxan (50 mg/day). How to avoid amputation?

Answer:

Plastic bag (heavy-gauge polyethylene) filled with O_2 (flow 15 liters/minute, 30 mm Hg pressure, 6 hours/day, 4 days/week for 10 weeks)

Then a walking cast for six months, at which time the ulcer was healed. The only topical therapy: hydrogen peroxide wet-to-dry dressings

Heng MCY, Pilgrim JP, Beck FWJ: A simplified hyperbaric oxygen technique for leg ulcers. Arch Dermatol 120:640–645, 1984.

Hyperbaric oxygen is of no value in treating venous stasis ulcers or ulcers due to incompetent perforators. However, 18 of 27 arterial disease ulcers healed in 6 to 21 days in five of six patients. The affected leg was covered by a disposable polyethylene bag through which oxygen flowed (15 liters/minute, 6 hours/day, 4 days/week). Pressure was monitored and kept at 25 to 30 mm Hg, using a Y tube connected to a sphygmomanometer. Interspersed periods of tissue hypoxia help to stimulate formation of granulation tissue, so that continuous oxygen therapy is not desirable.

Thwaites M, Dean S: Chronic leg ulcers: Ozone and other factors affecting healing. Aust Fam Physician 14:292–298, 1985.

Recommendation

- Weight control
- Edema control
- Ambulation
- **Ascorbic acid** (250 mg/day)
- **Zinc sulfate** (200 mg/day)
- Thiamine HCl (300 mg/day) if diet is inadequate
- Stop adrenoreceptor-blocking agents, since these reduce blood flow to the skin. Cites two patients whose chronic leg ulcers healed by simply withdrawing these beta-blockers.
- Avoid topical antibiotics because of risks of developing sensitization and producing resistant strains of bacteria. Use systemic antibiotics instead.
- Avoid topical steroids because of vasoconstriction and impairment of circulation. However, they may be used in any surrounding dermatitis.

Wounds containing more than 10^5 bacteria per gram of tissue are less likely to heal satisfactorily.

A study of leg ulcer therapy with **ozone** (an allotropic form of oxygen) showed complete healing in 29 of 33 ischemic ulcers and 17 of 21 venous ulcers. Ozone stimulates formation of granulation tissue and has bactericidal, virucidal, and fungicidal properties. The ozone was produced in an ozonator through a high-voltage electrical discharge that ruptures the oxygen molecule and allows recombination of three atoms of oxygen. The ulcers were exposed to the ozonator unit (producing ozone 80 mg/hour) under a bed cradle covered with a sheet (20 minutes q12h for six weeks or more).

Reynolds JEF (ed): Martindale: The Extra Pharmacopoeia, 28th ed. London, Pharmaceutical Press, 1982, p 1834.

Compounds indicated for use in treating ulcers (note that the list does not include new synthetic membranes)

honey	**salicylic acid**
sucrose	**alum**

aluminum sulfate
chromium trioxide
balsams and resins
dextranomer
nitrofurazone
disinfectants and antiseptics
magnesium chloride
chymotrypsin
streptokinase-streptodornase
trypsin
metacresolsulfonic acid-formaldehyde
povidone-iodine
aluminum powder
copper sulfate
gold
silver salts
zinc salts
carmellose sodium
clioquinol
penicillins and other antibiotics
peroxides
adenosine phosphate
cod liver oil
collagenase
porcine skin

Villavicencio JL, Collins GJ Jr, Youkey JR, et al: Nonsurgical management of lower extremity venous problems. *In* Bergan JJ, Yao JST (eds): Surgery of the Veins. Orlando, Grune & Stratton, 1985, pp 323–345.

This extremely valuable and up-to-date book is filled with good advice for the rare physician interested in the neglected field of venous diseases.

Treatment of venous leg ulcers should be preceded by answering these three questions:

1. How is the arterial circulation?
2. Is the ulcer infected?
3. Is the patient diabetic?

Night cramps due to venous insufficiency are best treated with **diphenhydramine** (Benadryl 50 mg hs). Alternative treatments include **quinine sulfate** (200 mg tid) or **potassium** (tablets or syrup).

External elastic support is the single most important therapeutic measure in the management of venous disorders of the extremities:

Apply elastic bandage before getting out of bed.
Wrap bandage from base of toes to just below the knee.
Wear bandage the entire day.
Take two 30-minute rest periods:
  Unwrap and elevate the legs above the heart.
  Best times are 11 to 12 AM and 3 to 4 PM

Episodes of erysipelas-like inflammation with induration and nodular phlebitis are usually due to *Streptococcus.* Healing takes four to eight weeks. Treatment should include:

bedrest—Trendelenburg position
antibiotics
anti-inflammatory agents: **phenylbutazone** (Butazolidin 1 ampule IM every 12 hours for two or three days, then 100 to 200 mg PO tid)
local heat (warm wet towels) for pain control
firm elastic bandages as tolerated

Concerning infected leg ulcers (which are dirty and smelly). There are two types:

type 1: very painful with necrotic tissue, crusts, and infected fascia
type 2: infection of subcutaneous tissue and skin margins
bacteria in exudate (in order of frequency): *Staphylococcus, Streptococcus, Klebsiella, Pseudomonas*
treatment
  hospitalize patient
  antibiotics
  absolute bedrest (Trendelenburg position)
  phenylbutazone (100 to 200 mg bid or tid)
  analgesics
  surgical debridement of type 1 ulcers
  wash leg daily with soap and water
  apply fibrinolytic ointment (e.g., trypsin + streptokinase-streptodornase) to the ulcer once daily

cover the ulcer with thick gauze wet with isotonic saline solution
wrap entire leg with a double-thickness gauze bandage, then cover with a thin plastic sheet to keep ulcer moist. Continue for four or five days, then discharge of patient from hospital
ambulatory treatment:
fibrinolytic ointment and dry dressing
firm compression with rubber cushion and elastic bandage
scheduling for venous surgery when ulcer is clean and granulating

Options for treatment of superficial venous dilatations:

1. Cosmetic coverage or camouflage
2. Electrocoagulation (superfine needle, setting 1.5 bipolar mode, insert needle first and then depress foot pedal, destroy little veins in segments, no anesthesia)
3. Argon laser therapy
4. Sclerotherapy (training required. Not without hazards—often results in hyperpigmentation)

Sclerosing agents:

1. **Dextrose** 65 per cent (use in patients with asthma or allergies)
2. **Hydroxypolyethoxidodecaine** (Aethoxysklerol 0.5 per cent and 1.0 per cent, manufactured in Germany), preferred for telangiectasia
3. **Sodium tetradecyl sulfate** (Sotradecol 1 per cent and 3 per cent)—no longer preferred because of allergic reactions and skin necrosis

(Note: **Morrhuate sodium** (50 mg/ml) is another sclerosing agent available in the United States, although not mentioned in this article. It also causes allergic reactions [from cod liver oil] and skin necrosis.)

Bergan JJ: Conrad Jobst and the development of pressure gradient therapy for venous disease. *In* Bergan JJ, Yao JST (eds): Surgery of the Veins. Orlando, Grune & Stratton, 1985, pp 529–540.

Conrad Jobst, an engineer, was the inventor of gradient compression therapy, which has had the most impact on the treatment of venous stasis disease. He recognized that venous insufficiency was simply a hydrostatic problem that required balancing with correct circumferential pressure. He searched for a proper fabric and came up with a bobbinet weave of closely spaced, prestressed rubber cords. Form fitting was achieved through use of a paper template consisting of a vertical strip of paper with multiple horizontal strips attached that could be wrapped around the foot, ankle, leg, and calf.

Johnson G Jr: The role of elastic support in venous problems. *In* Bergan JJ, Yao JST (eds): Surgery of the Veins. Orlando, Grune & Stratton, 1985, pp 541–550.

There is still variability in the manufacture of elastic stockings, and there is no single best stocking. This chapter includes details of manufacturing and types of knit fabrics.

Elastic stockings compress the superficial venous system, forcing blood into the deep venous system where velocity of flow is increased. Sometimes this allows the superficial veins to regain their tone and valvular competency. Compression of the subcutaneous tissues forces fluid into the vascular system and helps control edema.

Hefton JM, Caldwell D, Biozes DG, et al: Grafting of skin ulcers with cultured autologous epidermal cells. J Am Acad Dermatol 14:399–405, 1986.

Sheets of autologous epidermal cells, grown in culture, were applied to chronic ulcers in five patients. Four of the six ulcers healed completely in three to five weeks.

Patients hear better when you write it down.

Leiomyoma

Nifedipine
Nitroglycerin
Phenoxybenzamine

The old nitroglycerin and the new calcium channel blocker nifedipine offer these patients relief from the pain of the contracting smooth muscle. The nitroglycerin patches may provide an easy method of control.

Abraham Z, Cohen A, Haim S: Muscle relaxing agent in cutaneous leiomyoma. Dermatologica 166:255–256, 1983.

Nifedipine (Procardia 30 mg tid) acting as a calcium channel blocker, smooth muscle relaxant gave a 21-year-old man complete relief from the painful burning sensations of confluent plaque-like lesions of leiomyomas on the right side of the chest.

Engelke H, Christophers E: Leiomyomatosis cutis et uteri. Acta Derm Venereol 59(Suppl 85):51–54, 1979.

The extreme pain experienced by a 32-year-old woman with a massive number of leiomyomas of the skin and uterus was assuaged instantly by **nitroglycerin** (0.8 to 1.6 mg). Longer-lasting relief came from taking **nifedipine** (20 mg/day) and the alpha-adrenergic blocking agent **phenoxybenzamine** (Dibenzyline 20 mg tid) over a two-year period. The fact that 10 other drugs had failed to help had led to earlier suicide attempts.

Thompson JA Jr.: Therapy for painful cutaneous leiomyomas. J Am Acad Dermatol 13:865–867, 1985.

A 24-year-old man with a painful erythematous nodular eruption on the left side of the chest, proven to be leiomyomas, had relief of pain from **nifedipine** (Procardia 10 mg tid). During cold weather the dose was increased to 10 mg qid.

(Other calcium channel blockers that might prove useful include **diltiazem** [Cardizem] and **verapamil HCl** [Calan, Isoptin]).

Drug testing is easy: Control the source and the quantity. If patients don't ask you for more, it's a drug you can ignore.

Leprosy

Dapsone Rifampin Clofazimine Ethionamide

Arnold HL Jr, Fasal P: Leprosy: Diagnosis and Management, 2nd ed. Springfield, Ill., Charles C Thomas, 1973, 93 pp.

A concise and essential reference for details on clinical manifestations and treatment.

Pettit JHS, Parish LC: Manual of Tropical Dermatology. New York, Springer-Verlag, 1984, pp 69–73.

The treatment of choice is **dapsone** (100 mg/day). In the case of tuberculoid leprosy, daily dapsone therapy must be continued for two years after total disappearance of skin lesions. In contrast, lepromatous patients should be treated for life.

Alternate treatments for sulfone-resistant or sulfone-sensitive patients:
- **clofazimine** (100 mg tid)
  - turns the skin red
  - after three months reduce the dose to (100 mg/day) to avoid lymph node necrosis.
- **rifampin** (Rifadin 600 mg/day)

Lepromatous leprosy may require:
- rifampin (1300 mg once a month for one year)
- clofazimine (100 mg tid for three months)
- **Dapsone** (100 mg/day for life)

Erythema nodosum leprosum:
- **chloroquine** (1 tablet tid)
- or
- **prednisone** (20 mg/day)
- or
- **thalidomide** (100 to 500 mg/day)—treatment of choice

Do not interrupt dapsone therapy.

Orthopedic and plastic surgery should wait until the disease is inactive.

Chemotherapy of leprosy. Lancet 2:77–78, 1982.

In 1976 the WHO Expert Committee on Leprosy noted a rising incidence of **dapsone** resistance and recommended that multibacillary cases be treated with at least two effective antileprosy drugs.

In 1982 the same group published new guidelines for therapy (study group: Chemotherapy of leprosy for control programmes. WHO Tech Rep Ser No. 675, 1982):

1. *Multibacillary* (lepromatous + borderline cases)
   - three drugs (standard regimen for two years' minimum)
     - **rifampin** (600 mg once a month supervised)
     - **dapsone** (100 mg/day unsupervised)
     - **clofazimine** (300 mg/month supervised + 50 mg/day unsupervised)
   - supplemental drug—**ethionamide** (Trecator) or **protionamide** (500 mg/month supervised, 250 to 375 mg/day unsupervised)
   - minimum follow-up eight years

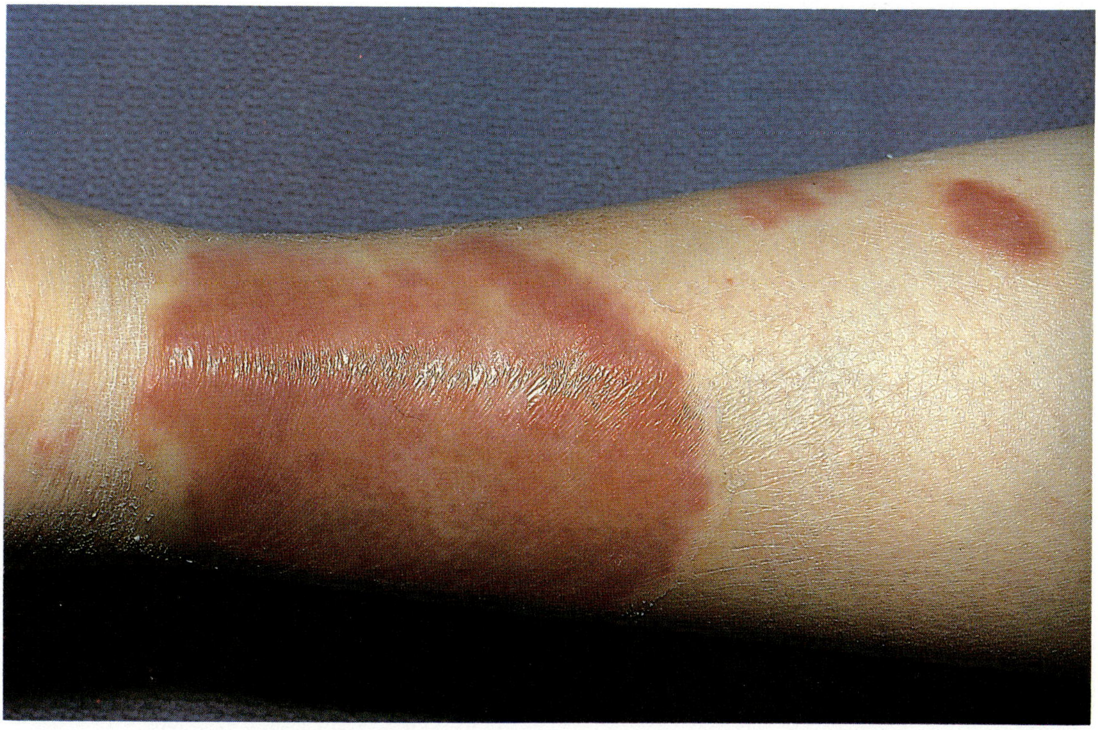

These cases are mainly responsible for the spread of leprosy through discharge of bacilli in nasal and upper respiratory tract mucus.

2. *Paucibacillary* (indeterminate + tuberculoid cases)
   two drugs (take for six months, then stop):
      rifampin (600 mg once/month supervised)
      dapsone (100 mg/day unsupervised)
   minimum follow-up four years

Price EW: The care of the feet. *In* Cochrane RG, Davey TF (eds): Leprosy in Theory and Practice, 2nd ed. Bristol, John Wright & Sons, 1964, pp 510–536.

Feet at risk (having loss of localization to light pressure) should be regularly inspected every 10 days to reduce the incidence of neuropathic ulcers in leprosy.

Practical footwear and footdrop splints are illustrated.

Pursley TV, Jacobson RR, Apisarnthanarax P: Lucio's phenomenon. Arch Dermatol 116:201–204, 1980.

An eight-year delay in making the correct diagnosis of diffuse, non-nodular lepromatous leprosy with widespread vasculitis-like ulcerations (Lucio's phenomenon) in a 38-year-old Mexican woman probably caused her general debility (fever, lymphadenopathy, anemia, splenomegaly). She died after seven months despite treatment with **clofazimine** (100 mg tid), **thalidomide** (100 mg bid), and **prednisone** (80 mg/day).

Treatment recommendations for Lucio's phenomenon:

prevention of secondary infection
prevention of loss of fluid, protein, and blood from the skin
continuation of sulfone therapy
thalidomide (400 mg/day or 6 mg/kg/day in divided doses initially, then maintenance 100 to 200 mg/day)

prednisone (20 to 60 mg/day for months/years)
clofazimine (300 mg/day)

Wallach D, Cottenot F, Bussel A, et al: Plasma exchange therapy in Lucio's phenomenon. Arch Dermatol 116:1101, 1980.

A 76-year-old man with nodular lepromatous leprosy developed widespread ulcerated lesions with evidence of circulating immune complexes. He had been taking **rifampin** (600 mg/day) and **dapsone** (100 mg/day). Despite antireactional treatment with **clofazimine** (100 mg/day) and **thalidomide** (300 mg/day), his condition deteriorated. He was then treated with four plasma exchanges (5 liters/exchange replaced by fresh-frozen plasma) over a 20-day period with remarkable improvement and no relapse after nine months.

Distraction is the art of medicine. If you are having trouble examining a little tot's feet, try taking off your *shoes and stockings first.*

Leukoplakia

Dental care	Excision
Stop smoking	Cryotherapy
Electrodesiccation	Laser
Subsection	

Inducing no symptoms and hiding within the mouth as it does, leukoplakia is easily overlooked or ignored by the patient and, at times, by the doctor. Yet, this white spot, so unremarkable in its presentation, is a lesion to command respect, attention, and treatment. Within it are cells that can become cancerous. They are new cells that have 100 times more potential for malignant change than normal mucosal cells have. Furthermore, one out of every six persistent leukoplakic lesions eventually becomes malignant.

Management thus centers on (1) patient education, (2) elimination of the cause when possible, (3) excision or destruction of localized plaques, and (4) long-term follow-up.

We clearly explain to the patient that he is at risk for cancer if the lesion persists. If he is a smoker or chews tobacco, he must be strongly encouraged to stop. More than half of all cases of leukoplakia disappear after abstinence from tobacco for one year. We also recommend that dental review be undertaken to eradicate any source of chronic irritation, such as denture plaques or cracks, carious teeth, or a malaligned filling.

A blood test for syphilis rules out the need for penicillin therapy, as does a scraping for *Candida* eliminate the need for clotrimazole troches. Ideally, a biopsy is secured to assess the possibility of dysplastic change or clinically occult squamous cell carcinoma. If the plaque is either erosive or painful a biopsy is no longer optional, but usually is necessary.

We instruct the patient to avoid allowing Life Savers, lozenges, aspirin tablets, cough drops, or the like to remain and dissolve in the mouth. The significance of unconscious cheek biting should be emphasized, and in some instances a mild tranquilizer at bedtime may aid. Finally, inquiry should be made into any unusual habits of chewing or sucking on irritating materials.

If a plaque of leukoplakia remains recalcitrant, excision is always desirable. A variety of other methods is also in use today for destruction or removal of leukoplakic sites. These include electrodesiccation, cryotherapy, and now laser therapy.

In the event that removal is not undertaken (and at times the leukoplakia is so widespread or ill defined as to make excision impractical), the patient must return at intervals of six months or less to have careful unbiased inspection and palpation for significant change. The patient must understand the gravity of his condition and the need for definitive help before his lesion develops the very real potential for metastatic growth.

Pindborg JJ: Oral Cancer and Precancer. Bristol, John Wright & Sons, 1980, 177 pp.

A superb reference source for all aspects of this disease in which tobacco smoking and chewing are the principal etiologic factors.

Silverman S Jr, Gorsky M, Lozada F: Oral leukoplakia and malignant transformation: A follow-up study of 257 patients. Cancer 53:563–568, 1984.

On biopsy, 22 of these 257 patients had dysplastic change, whereas in 235 only benign hyperkeratosis was present. Surgical excision was followed by recurrence in one out of three patients. In 17.5 per cent of all patients, squamous cell carcinoma developed within the leukoplakic sites, on an average within eight years. In half of these, pain was a significant symptom. Nonsmokers (27 per cent of the study group) were at high risk for malignant transformation, as were patients with erythroleukoplakia or a verrucous-papillary hyperkeratotic pattern.

Kramer IRH: Oral leukoplakia. J R Soc Med 73:765–767, 1980.

If erosive or speckled, assume that malignant change is present unless proven otherwise. The highest risk of cancer is associated with leukoplakia of the floor of the mouth and the ventral surface of the tongue.

Dorey JL, Blasberg B, Conklin RJ, Carmichael RP: Oral leukoplakia: Current concepts in diagnosis, management, and malignant potential. Int J Dermatol 23:638–642, 1984.

A complete review with 42 references. Approximately 10 per cent of lesions are malignant when the patient is initially examined, and another 6 per cent will become malignant. Lesions larger than 5.5 mm in diameter are more likely to be malignant than smaller ones. The patient should not smoke and should avoid excessive alcohol intake, mouthwashes, and local trauma. If the leukoplakia has a speckled pattern, use **nystatin** to eliminate the associated candidal infection.

Roed-Petersen B: Effect on oral leukoplakia of reducing or ceasing tobacco smoking. Acta Derm Venereol 62:164–167, 1982.

Very helpful. In a study of 138 patients with leukoplakia who either reduced or quit smoking, 56 per cent of lesions disappeared or regressed over a three-month period. After one year, 78 per cent of lesions in those who quit smoking had either regressed or disappeared.

Shah JP, Strong EW, DeCosse JJ, et al: Effect of retinoids on oral leukoplakia. Am J Surg 146:466–470, 1983.

Lozenges of **13-*cis*-retinoic acid** (1 mg/lozenge—10 mg/day for six months) dissolved in the mouth cleared two of five cases, but lesions returned within five weeks of stopping therapy.

Yarington CT Jr, Larrabee WF Jr: Reconstruction following lip resection. Otolaryngol Clin North Am 16:407–421, 1983.

Leukoplakia or carcinoma in situ can be adequately removed by lip peel or vermilionectomy procedure.

Sako K, Marchetta FC, Hayes RL: Cryotherapy of intraoral leukoplakia. Am J Surg 124:482–484, 1972.

Cryotherapy (lidocaine 1 per cent anesthesia, **liquid N_2** for 30 seconds to several minutes, one to five treatments) was successful in treating 60 patients, but 12 of these had recurrence within two to four years, including 4 with squamous cell carcinoma.

Al-Drouby HAL: Oral leukoplakia and cryotherapy. Br Dent J 155:124–125, 1983.

Short-term (two to five years) success in 27 of 30 patients with white lesions of the oral mucosa treated with cryotherapy.

Horch HH, Gerlach KL: CO_2 laser treatment of oral dysplastic precancerous lesions: A preliminary report. Lasers Surg Med 2:179–185, 1982.

Fifteen patients with leukoplakia were treated successfully with the CO_2 laser beam, but four had recurrences within one year.

Greenspan D, Greenspan JS, Conant M, et al: Oral "hairy" leucoplakia in male homosexuals: Evidence of association with both papilloma virus and a herpes-group virus. Lancet 2:831–834, 1984.

Systemic **ketoconazole**, **clotrimazole** troches, and **nystatin** troches eliminated secondary candidal overgrowth but not the primary lesions in this new form of leukoplakia. Seen on the lateral area of the tongue in 37 male homosexuals, it may presage AIDS. The characteristic histology resembled a flat wart of the skin.

You can always make your patient feel better even if you can't make him look better.

Lichen Nitidus

Fluocinonide cream

This is a disease better known than treated. We suspect that the eruption of hundreds of tiny skin-colored papules often represents a reaction pattern to underlying infection such as tinea pedis, cystitis, or pharyngitis. A search for infection with appropriate treatment may be rewarding in rapidly clearing the lichen nitidus.

Wright S: Successful treatment of lichen nitidus. Arch Dermatol 120:155–156, 1984.

Fluocinonide cream (Lidex 0.05 per cent bid for one month) completely cleared lichen nitidus lesions present for 12 years in a 24-year-old woman. Significantly, the control lesions not treated remained unchanged. Subsequently all areas of the body were treated with the same success and there was no recurrence at one-year follow-up.

Lapins NA, Willoughby C, Helwig EB: Lichen nitidus: A study of forty-three cases. Cutis 21:634–637, 1978.

Only 5 of 43 patients had pruritus. The clinical course is unpredictable, but spontaneous resolution without sequelae usually occurs. Most patients had the disease 1 year or less, although one patient had had it for eight years.

Weiss RM, Cohen AD: Lichen nitidus of the palms and soles. Arch Dermatol 104:538–540, 1971.

A five-year series of therapeutic trials in a 37-year-old woman who had lichen nitidus for 20 years demonstrated that the lesions could be flattened, but not obliterated, by using either **fluocinolone acetonide** cream (Synalar 0.025 per cent) or **betamethasone valerate** cream and ointment (Valisone 0.1 per cent) under polyethylene occlusion. Ineffective were **urea** cream (30 per cent), **liquor carbonis detergens** (LCD), and **vitamin A** (50,000 U bid for one month).

Miracle worker: A doctor who cures patients after first convincing them that only a miracle can cure them.

Lichen Planus

Flagyl	Accutane
Bactrim	Steroids
Griseofulvin	

No dermatosis seems easier to recognize and harder to cure than lichen planus. Although steroid responsive, this reaction pattern may reappear even after megadose steroid therapy. The only direct attack is to seek out and eliminate the specific cause in your patient. Search for triggering drugs and underlying infection (especially urinary tract). Failing that, topical, intralesional, and systemic steroids are the main weapons in your armamentarium.

Altman J, Perry HO: The variations and course of lichen planus. Arch Dermatol 84:179–191, 1961.

Average duration is 15 months.

Fellner MJ: Lichen planus. Int J Dermatol 19:71–75, 1980.

List of 19 drugs and chemicals causing lichen planus, gold being the most common:

- amiphenazole
- antimony
- arsenic
- chloroquine
- chlorothiazide
- demeclocycline
- gold
- hydrochlorothiazide
- iodides
- mercury
- para-aminosalicylic acid
- paraphenylenediamine
- phenothiazine
- quinacrine
- quinine
- quinidine
- streptomycin
- tetracycline
- 2-amino-5-diethylamino toluene monochloride (CD2) color film developer

Powell FC, Rogers RS III, Dickson ER: Primary biliary cirrhosis and lichen planus. J Am Acad Dermatol 9:540–545, 1983.

Seventeen cases of lichen planus were induced by D-penicillamine in the treatment of primary biliary cirrhosis.

Shelley WB, Shelley ED: Urinary tract infection as a cause of lichen planus: Metronidazole therapy. J Am Acad Dermatol 10:905–907, 1984.

Two weeks of **metronidazole** (Flagyl 250 mg tid) cleared the disease in a patient with chronic widespread lichen planus. Recurrence three months later cleared with a second course of Flagyl. No further attacks occurred while she was taking a maintenance dose of **nitrofurantoin** (Macrodantin 100 mg/day) during a two-year follow-up.

Abdel-Aal H, Abdel-Aal MA: Treatment of lichen planus with Bactrim. J Egypt Med Assoc 59:547–549, 1976.

Trimethoprim-sulfamethoxazole (Bactrim, 4 tablets daily for five days) cleared acute lichen planus in 8 of 10 patients within two weeks. Relapse occurred two months later, with remission on retreatment.

Sehgal VN, Bikhchandani R, Koranne RV, et al: Histopathological evaluation of griseofulvin therapy in lichen planus: A double-blind controlled study. Dermatologica 161:22–27, 1980.

In India, **griseofulvin** (500 mg/day for two months) cleared 18 of 22 cases.

Massa MC, Rogers RS III: Griseofulvin therapy of lichen planus. Acta Derm Venereol 61:547–550, 1981.

Only 3 of 15 cases cleared with **griseofulvin** in the United States. (Could underlying fungal infection be more common in India? See preceding reference.)

Sloberg K, Hersle K, Mobacken H, Thilander H: Topical tretinoin therapy and oral lichen planus. Arch Dermatol 115:716–718, 1979.

In Sweden, two months of daily application of 0.1 per cent **tretinoin** (retinoic acid) in adhesive base (Orabase) cleared 16 of 23 cases of painful lichen planus of the oral mucosa—erosive, atrophic, and plaque types. (This favors a trial of Retin-A gel or cream.)

We watch for squamous cell carcinoma on a long-term basis in any case of refractory mucous membrane lichen planus.

Handler HL: Isotretinoin for oral lichen planus. J Am Acad Dermatol 10:674, 1984.

In modest dosage **13-*cis*-retinoic acid** (Accutane 10 mg bid for two months) cleared seven cases of lichen planus of both the generalized and oral types.

Ferguson MM: Treatment of erosive lichen planus of the oral mucosa with depot steroids. Lancet 2:771–772, 1977.

Intralesional steroid (40 mg/ml **prednisolone acetate**, 0.5 to 1.0 ml) cleared four of five cases of severe erosive lichen planus in one week. Note the large dose.

Izumi AK: Allergic contact gingivostomatitis due to gold. Arch Dermatol Res 272:387–391, 1982.

Looking for gold allergy in suspected cases of erosive lichen planus may be golden! A 40-year-old Japanese man developed stomatitis and wedding ring dermatitis three years after gold crowns were inserted. Removal of gold crowns cured his mouth. Tests were positive to a patch of **gold chloride** 0.5 per cent and an intradermal injection of **gold sodium thiomalate** 0.05 cc (Myochrysine 50 mg/cc).

Kristjansen A, Reymann F: On the treatment of lichen planus. Acta Derm Venereol 35:143–150, 1955.

Daily **ACTH** therapy cleared 21 of 25 cases within two weeks. Relapses occurred.

Snyder RA, Schwartz RA, Schneider JS, Elias PM: Intermittent mega-dose corticosteroid therapy for generalized lichen planus. J Am Acad Dermatol 6:1089–1090, 1982.

Methylprednisolone (1 gm IV as a single pulse daily for three days) gave dramatic clearing on the third day in a 70-year-old man with generalized lichen planus. Previous treatment failures included conventional steroid therapy, **griseofulvin**, **methotrexate**, and PUVA. This was repeated each month for three times. At six months the lichen planus was still present, but asymptomatic.

Ortonne JP, Thivolet J, Sannwald C: Oral photochemotherapy in the treatment of lichen planus (LP): Clinical results, histological and ultrastructural observations. Br J Dermatol 99:77–88, 1978.

Remission in six of seven patients with PUVA (3 times a week, 17 to 48 treatments, total 58 to 230 J/sq cm).

Väätäinen N, Hannuksela M, Karvonen J: Trioxsalen baths plus UV-A in the treatment of lichen planus and urticaria pigmentosa. Clin Exp Dermatol 6:133–138, 1981.

A modern version of the Finnish bath (50 mg of **trioxsalen** in 20 ml of ethanol added to 150 liters of warm bath water) followed 10 minutes later by UVA (average: 6 J/sq cm, 17 consecutive daily treatments) cleared widespread lichen planus in 16 of 19 patients.

Do something, or else the patient will get credit for the cure.

Lichen Sclerosus et Atrophicus

Corticosteroids
Testosterone ointment

Wallace HJ: Lichen sclerosus et atrophicus. Trans St Johns Hosp Dermatol Soc 57:9–30, 1971.

A splendid source of knowledge from a lifetime of detailed study of 395 patients with lichen sclerosus et atrophicus.

Summary of treatment of anogenital lichen sclerosus et atrophicus in females:

1. Topical or intralesional corticosteroids for control of itching may require fluorinated preparations; discontinue or taper the concentration when practicable, using protective emollients.
2. Treat any vaginal infection or diabetes mellitus. Eliminate irritant antiseptics, douches, and topical medications.
3. Liquid N_2 cryotherapy.
4. Local excision.
5. Regular follow-up every 6 to 12 months and whenever change is noted for detection of sequential leukoplakia or malignancy. Biopsy of every ulcer of more than three weeks' duration.
6. Reassure, reduce anxiety.
7. Avoid vulvectomy.

Friedrich EG Jr: Lichen sclerosus. J Reprod Med 17:147–154, 1976.

Ecchymosis of the vulva is a pathognomonic sign of lichen sclerosus.

Testosterone (2 per cent in petrolatum or a steroid ointment) is the most commonly used therapy for this problem in adult women.

The patient with vulvar dystrophy should have a solution of **toluidine blue dye** (1 per cent) applied to the vulva, which is then washed off after a few minutes with **acetic acid** solution (1 per cent). Any nonulcerated areas that retain blue dye should undergo biopsy.

Siar CH, Ng KH: Oral lichen sclerosus et atrophicus (report of a case). J Oral Med 40:148–150, 1985.

Triamcinolone acetonide 0.1 per cent (Kenalog in Orabase applied four times a day) was effective treatment and relieved the pain of oral lesions in a 25-year-old Indian man with a small, pale, bald, indurated, immobilized tongue and atrophic pearly white patches and fibrosed bands of the buccal mucosa.

Török E, Orley J, Goracz G, Daroczy J: Lichen sclerosus et atrophicus in children. Mod Probl Paediatr 17:262–271, 1975.

An analysis of 33 cases of lichen sclerosus et atrophicus in girls ages 3 to 12 years:

Itching, soreness, and constipation were the presenting complaints.

One fourth had disappearance of symptoms and no significant atrophy within six months to one year.

One half showed improvement in 18 months.

One fourth had persistence of symptoms.

Treatment was limited to relief of symptoms using bland emollients, estrogen ointment, and topical steroids.

Avoiding trauma prevents extension (wear light clothing, avoid bicycling). The authors feel that lichen sclerosus et atrophicus may be a degenerative reaction pattern induced by different inflammatory agents. In two cases lesions appeared soon after streptococcal vulvitis during the time of medical treatment.

Flynt J, Gallup DG: Childhood lichen sclerosus. Obstet Gynecol 53(Suppl 3):79S–81S, 1979.

Hydrocortisone cream (1 per cent) provided total symptomatic relief for a six-year-old girl with anogenital lesions, vulvar pruritus, and burning on urination, but the white plaques remained. The hydrocortisone should be stopped when symptoms disappear to avoid long-term use and epidermal thinning.

Lichen sclerosus will resolve completely in two thirds of premenarchal girls around the menarche, but may recur in three to five years. After the menarche, **testosterone propionate** (2 per cent) may be used as treatment.

Clark JA, Muller SA: Lichen sclerosus et atrophicus in children: A report of 24 cases. Arch Dermatol 95:476–482, 1967.

The complete resolution of lesions in 11 of 24 children (all girls) contrasts with that in adults in whom atrophic parchment-like skin remains. Improvement in children usually occurs during maturation. In this series 25 per cent of patients had only extragenital lesions.

Woodruff JD, Babaknia A: Local alcohol injection of the vulva: Discussion of 35 cases. Obstet Gynecol 54:512–514, 1979.

Alcohol (0.2 ml of absolute ethyl alcohol) injected sublesionally in a 1-cm grid pattern to the anesthetized patient gave long-lasting relief of pruritus in eight patients with lichen sclerosus et atrophicus. All patients were also being treated with **testosterone** (2 per cent in petrolatum).

Yates VM, King CM, Dave VK: Lichen sclerosus et atrophicus following radiation therapy. Arch Dermatol 121:1044–1047, 1985.

Several years after postmastectomy radiation therapy, lichen sclerosus et atrophicus developed within the radiation fields in two women. This parallels the appearance of lichen sclerosus et atrophicus as a Koebner phenomenon in other sites of trauma such as vaccination and excision scars, bruises, and scratch marks.

Rare diseases rarely respond to routine care.

Linear IgA Dermatosis

Dapsone
Prednisone
Azathioprine

Linear IgA dermatoses can be erased line by line with dapsone.

Mobacken H, Kastrup W, Ljunghall K, et al: Linear IgA dermatosis: A study of ten adult patients. Acta Derm Venereol 63:123–128, 1983.

Immunofluorescence has spotlighted this distinctive blistering disease as one with linear deposits of IgA in the basement membrane zone. Like its clinical bedfellow, dermatitis herpetiformis, it usually responds to **dapsone**. In the three of ten patients studied who did not respond to dapsone, the addition of **prednisolone** or **azathioprine** was helpful.

Leonard JN, Haffenden GP, Ring NP, et al: Linear IgA disease in adults. Br J Dermatol 107:301–316, 1982.

This adult version of chronic bullous disease of childhood also responds to **dapsone**. The majority of the 42 patients treated in this multicenter study showed clearing during dapsone treatment, but several required high doses (300 mg/day).

Jones RR, Goolamali SK: IgA bullous pemphigoid: A distinct blistering disorder. Br J Dermatol 102:719–725, 1980.

Another example of linear IgA dermatosis in which **dapsone** (100 mg/day) gave prompt relief. A 76-year-old woman had a large ulcerating eccrine carcinoma of the abdomen surrounded by pruritic bullae on a slightly erythematous background. After the carcinoma was excised, the localized blistering continued, requiring continuation of dapsone.

If you practice half as well as your patients expect you to, a fourth as well as your mother knows you do, and twice as well as your colleagues think you do, you're doing great.

Linear Scleroderma

Lidex cream
Phenytoin
Physical therapy
Zyderm collagen implant

Neldner KH: Treatment of localized linear scleroderma with phenytoin. Cutis 22:569–572, 1978.

Phenytoin sodium (Dilantin 100 mg bid or tid) produced significant reversal of lesions in five patients with linear scleroderma, including one with en coup de sabre. Softening was noted in two to four months and as much as 90 per cent improvement after one to two years.

Since phenytoin impairs vitamin D metabolism in the liver and may lead to osteomalacia after long-term therapy, **vitamin D** (400 U/day) should be given as a supplement. Must also watch for drug interactions with **phenobarbital**, **coumarin** anticoagulants, and **phenylbutazone** (which are other protein-bound drugs).

Rudolph RI, Leyden JJ: Physiatrics for deforming linear scleroderma. Arch Dermatol 112:995–997, 1976.

In a 14-year-old girl with a six-year history of linear scleroderma of the left arm and hand, physical therapy with hot paraffin baths and twice-daily programmed active and passive stretching exercises converted a useless sclerodermatous clawhand into a useful hand.

Bart RS, Kopf AW: Hemifacial atrophy. J Dermatol Surg 4:908–909, 1978.

An 11-year-old girl with hemifacial atrophy (Romberg's disease) received excellent cosmetic correction with injection of **liquid silicone** (six sessions over three years). Shifting of the silicone does not seem to be a problem when it is injected in small amounts.

Stoner JG, Swanson NA, Siegle RJ: Treatment of localized morphea with zyderm collagen implant. J Dermatol Surg 10:626–627, 1984.

In a 25-year-old woman with a four-year history of sclerotic atrophic lesions on the left side of the face, intralesional ZCI (**Zyderm collagen** implants 0.5 ml/month for three months) corrected the contour defect. Her anti-ZCI antibody tests were negative.

Serologic testing for anti-ZCI antibodies is a highly specific test for detecting people at risk for adverse reactions to Zyderm. A positive test occurs in 7 per cent of the control population and 100 per cent of patients with a positive ZCI skin test or ZCI treatment reaction.

Unbelievable cures are usually just that.

Loiasis

Extraction
Hetrazan

Marriott WRV: Loiasis. Int J Dermatol 24:329–332, 1985.

Caused by *Loa loa* and transmitted by *Chrysops* flies is this disease, common to a few tourists and a vast pool of 20 million natives of the rain forests of West Africa. It calls for the following treatment:

1. **Diethylcarbamazine** (DEC) (Hetrazan 0.7 mg/kg tid for two weeks, then three weeks later 2 mg/kg tid for two weeks). Acute symptoms requiring antihistamines or systemic steroids may develop during treatment because of dead parasites. Blood smears should become clear of microfilariae and massive eosinophilia.
2. Extraction via a small incision of all adult nematodes located in the skin or conjunctivae. These worms, having spent a youth of four to five years, may reach a length of 7 cm as adults and can race at a speed of over 1 cm/minute in subcutaneous tissue, where they cause transient nonpitting erythema and itching.

Vermeer BJ, van der Kaay HJ: Loiasis: A case report. Acta Derm Venereol 62:78–79, 1982.

Allergic reactions to migrating adult worms, particularly around joints and eyelids (Calabar swellings, fever) may require systemic steroids for control. Eradication of microfilariae may call for an increasing daily dosage of **diethylcarbamazine** (Hetrazan 50 mg tid, increasing by 50 mg daily up to 6 mg/kg/day for three weeks) and for multiple courses. Corticosteroids (20 mg/day for six days) should be started two days before Hetrazan to counteract allergic reactions. All adult worms should be removed surgically, with use of local anesthesia, whenever they can be clearly located.

Marriott WRV: Loiasis in a young child in Oregon. Int J Dermatol 25:252–254, 1986.

Recurrent nonspecific swelling of the eyelid, eyebrow, and antecubital fossa of 8 to 24 hours duration in a four-year-old girl proved to be the Calabar swellings of loiasis. Cure was achieved by giving **diethylcarbamazine** (12.5 mg (1/4 tablet) tid for 14 days, followed three weeks later by 25 mg tid for another 14 days).

"No shows" are patients who got better or who are looking for a better doctor.

Lymphangioma Circumscriptum

Surgery
Hypertonic saline
X-ray

Kinmonth JB: The Lymphatics: Surgery, Lymphography and Diseases of the Chyle and Lymph Systems, 2nd ed. London, Edward Arnold, 1982, pp 307–315.

The ultimate reference source—clear, comprehensive, and compelling.

Lymphangioma circumscriptum lesions are not connected to main lymphatic channels. They are best removed surgically; procedures may be staged three to four months apart in extensive cases. Preliminary lymphography should always be done. Radiation therapy is not useful. Sometimes useful is the deep injection of hypertonic saline solution in the lymphangioma to induce shrinkage through scar formation.

Bauer BS, Kernahan DA, Hugo NE: Lymphangioma circumscriptum—A clinicopathological review. Ann Plast Surg 7:318–326, 1981.

In three patients with extensive lymphangioma circumscriptum lesions (axilla, arm, and abdomen and groin respectively), in whom prior surgery had failed, success was achieved by thorough complete excision, including all subcutaneous tissue down to fascia. The use of frozen sections may be helpful during surgery.

Whimster IW: The pathology of lymphangioma circumscriptum. Br J Dermatol 94:473–486, 1976.

Nine patients were successfully treated by excision of the deep subcutaneous lymphatic cisterns, leaving the skin and upper subcutaneous layers intact. After surgery, no new vesicles formed and the old vesicles disappeared.

It is futile to remove the superficial skin containing the vesicles while leaving the deep component of the lymphangioma intact, as new vessels will soon "sprout" from the deep cisterns and form new vesicles.

Silverman PM, Korobkin M, Moore AV: CT diagnosis of cystic hygroma of the neck. J Comput Assist Tomogr 7:519–520, 1983.

Computed tomography confirmed the diagnosis of cystic lymphangioma in a five-year-old girl who for eight weeks had a rapidly enlarging soft tissue mass of the neck.

The best theory suggests that these lesions, which usually occur on the neck or lower part of the face, are sequestrations of primitive lymphatic sacs that fail to establish normal communication to the lymphatic system. (Computed tomography also should aid in showing the depth of the lymphangioma circumscriptum.)

Blair WF, Buckwalter JA, Mickelson MR, Omer GE: Lymphangioma of the forearm and hand. J Hand Surg 8:399–405, 1983.

A sober appraisal of results in nine patients with cavernous lymphangioma of the forearm and hand, pointing out that attempted excision will be followed by tumor recurrence, hypertrophic scars, and persistent pain. The best to be expected at excisional biopsy is the debulking and histologic typing of the tumor.

Pang P, Jakobiec FA, Iwamoto T, Hornblass A: Small lymphangiomas of the eyelids. Ophthalmology 91:1278–1284, 1984.

Simple excision of eyelid lesions in three patients was very successful and not followed by recurrence.

O'Cathail S, Rostom AY, Johnson ML: Successful control of lymphangioma circumscriptum by superficial x-rays. Br J Dermatol 113:611–615, 1985.

A large lymphangioma of the chest wall which had recurred despite repeated surgical excisions and therapy with a cautery showed a slow, yet virtually complete, resolution after radiotherapy (single dose 800 cGy, 100 KV, 0.4-mm copper filter).

The number of symptoms the patient has is often inversely proportional to your level of therapeutic success.

Lymphedema

Penicillin	Pressure
Griseofulvin	Surgery
Ketoconazole	

Schirger A: Lymphedema. Cardiovasc Clin 13:293–305, 1983.

An exquisite review:

Treatment involves five desiderata:
1. Fluid mobilization
2. Maintenance of edema-free state
3. Control of recurrent infection
4. General supportive measures
5. Surgical intervention and observation for possibility of malignancy

Fluid mobilization:
1. Hospitalize for three to five days
2. Elevate extremity at a 45-degree angle in a special lymphedema sling
3. **Furosemide** (Lasix 40 to 80 mg/day)—must watch serum potassium
4. Prophylactic **heparin** (subcutaneous low dose—5000 U every eight hours)

Maintenance of the edema-free state:
1. Made-to-measure elastic support Jobst knee or hip length stocking—should be applied while patient is still in the hospital to avoid reaccumulation of fluid
2. Diuretic therapy intermittently: **hydrochlorothiazide** (Hydrodiuril 25 mg) plus **triamterene** (Dyrenium 50 mg) every other day

Control infection:
1. Intermittent antibiotic prophylaxis
   Phenoxymethyl penicillin (250 mg qid for 10 days each month)
   Erythromycin (250 mg qid for 10 days each month)
2. Local antifungal therapy
   Clotrimazole cream 1 per cent (Lotrimin, Mycelex)
   Miconazole cream 2 per cent (Monistat-Derm, MicaTin)
3. Systemic antifungal therapy
   Griseofulvin (125 mg bid) if indicated

General support:
1. Emotional for the patient and family
2. Engage in selected sports (swimming, walking)—avoiding contact sports that might injure the extremity

Surgery:
1. Consultation, if failing to control the lymphedema
2. Alerting of the patient, family, and doctors to the possibility of lymphangiosarcoma, which starts as a nonhealing bruise. Immediate biopsy, then amputation.
3. Do not operate for cosmetic reasons, but to reduce the overall limb size and enhance mobility. The Kondoleon and modified Charles operations are used at the Mayo Clinic.

Kinmonth JB: The Lymphatics: Surgery, Lymphography and Diseases of the Chyle and Lymph Systems, 2nd ed. London, Edward Arnold, 1982, pp 321–325.

Conservative treatment of lymphedema:

skin care—antiseptic soap
treat tinea pedis, if present
avoid trauma
elevate affected part
centripetal massage
massage machines
walk—don't stand
external support—elastic stocking (ankle and lower leg)
diuretics
analgesic for pain

Zanolla R, Monzeglio C, Balzarini A, Martino G: Evaluation of the results of three different methods of postmastectomy lymphedema treatment. J Surg Oncol 26:210–213, 1984.

Each of three groups of 20 mastectomized patients with secondary arm lymphedema was treated with one of the following:

1. Manual **lymphatic massage** (one hour, three times a week for one month, Vodder massage technique). All wore an elastic sleeve during the day and received benzopyrone (60 mg/day).
2. Uniform-pressure **pneumatic compression** (elongated cuff, 90 mm Hg, six hours/day for one week)
3. Differentiated pneumatic massage (using a ratio of 1 : 3 for compression and decompression)

A statistically significant permanent reduction in edema was observed with both the manual massage and the uniform pressure pneumatic massage, but not with the differentiated pressure therapy. The patient satisfaction index correlated with the objective findings.

Alexander MA, Wright ES, Wright JB, Bikowski JB: Lymphedema treated with a linear pump: Pediatric case report. Arch Phys Med Rehabil 64:132–133, 1983.

Programmable intermittent pressure: The **Wright linear pump** was used 8 hours each night in a seven-year-old girl with lymphedema of the right arm and right leg due to Parkes-Weber syndrome (hemihypertrophy of soft tissue with vascular and lymphatic overgrowth). After two years of treatment a difference of $3\frac{1}{2}$ shoe sizes had been eliminated, and both feet were the same shoe size.

Jørgensen J, Gammeltoft M, Schmidt H: Factitious lymphoedema, Secretan's syndrome. Acta Derm Venereol 63:271–273, 1983.

A good review of a condition described in 1901 by Secretan, a Swiss insurance physician. Application of a tourniquet to a limb and physical trauma to the dorsal hand are common methods used. Not easy to diagnose and not easy to treat, with prolonged disability the rule. Protective splints and casts give immediate improvement, but recurrences can be expected.

Savage RC: The surgical management of lymphedema. Surg Gynecol Obstet 160:283–290, 1985.

A magnificent review of surgical treatments available for the unusual, severe instances refractory to nonoperative therapy (strict elevation, custom-fit graded pressure garments [Jobst], and intermittent pneumatic compression).

None of the myriad of operative procedures offers a cure for lymphedema. The two approaches are excisional and physiologic. In the excisional technique, all involved skin and subcutaneous tissue are removed and coverage achieved by grafting. Less drastic is the staged excision of subcutaneous tissue and skin, which in one study of 14 patients achieved a 50 per cent reduction in limb size that was maintained for over one year. The physiologic approaches of lymphangioplasty (Teflon wicks), lymphatic anastomoses, and flaps (omental, pedicle, myocutaneous, and intestinal) have not been as successful or popular.

(For reasons best known to the publisher, this same article appears in the same journal the year before—Surg Gynecol Obstet 159:501–508, 1984. What's good is worth reprinting!)

Hetter GP (ed): Lipoplasty: The Theory and Practice of Blunt Suction Lipectomy. Boston, Little, Brown and Co., 1984, 340 pp.

Useful for congenital lymphedema.

Certainty is a compound, commonly contaminated with doubt.

Patients don't expect you to have supernatural powers. They only hope you do.

Lymphocytoma Cutis

Penicillin	Excision
Demethylchlortetracycline	Radiotherapy
Intralesional steroids	

All of these patients need a careful history as to possible antecedent causes such as insect bites, trauma, scabies, or drugs. Before excision or radiotherapy is undertaken, we usually prescribe a trial 10-day course of demethylchlortetracycline (Declomycin 300 mg/day) or penicillin G (2 million U/day), since in four cases in our practice this has been curative.

None of these lesions should be ignored since they can be premalignant.

Burg G, Braun-Falco O: Cutaneous Lymphomas, Pseudolymphomas and Related Disorders. New York, Springer-Verlag, 1983, pp 415–463.

Lymphocytoma cutis, one of the pseudolymphomas, most often develops after tick bites. Other precipitating factors include scabies, tattoos, herpes simplex, herpes zoster, repeated antigen injections for hyposensitization, and drug reactions. Drug compounds incriminated include anticonvulsants, hydantoin, salicylates, phenylbutazone, phenacetin, menthol, and aromatic plant oils.

Lymphocytoma cutis may involute spontaneously or as a result of treatment with systemic antibiotics, systemic corticosteroids, or small doses of x-rays.

Caro WA, Helwig EB: Cutaneous lymphoid hyperplasia. Cancer 24:487–502, 1969.

Rare examples have been recorded of an association of malignant lymphoma with benign lymphocytoma, but the malignant potential of cutaneous lymphoid hyperplasia is low, as based on this study of 225 lesions in 193 patients.

Andersen BL, Brandrup F, Petri J: Lymphocytoma cutis: A pseudomalignancy treated with penicillin. Acta Derm Venereol 62:83–85, 1982.

Two elderly patients who developed large histologically malignant lesions of lymphoid hyperplasia following the prick of a rose thorn were completely cured by oral **phenoxymethyl penicillin** (penicillin V, Pen-Vee K 500,000 U tid or qid). The first patient had a dramatic reduction in size of the lesion in two days and was clear of it in two weeks. The second patient required seven weeks of penicillin therapy for his cure.

Shelley WB, Wood MG: Observations on occult malignant lymphomas in the skin. Cancer 38:1757–1770, 1976.

Biopsy-proven benign lymphocytoma cutis lesions in a 36-year-old man kept appearing over an eight-year period. While some involuted spontaneously, others cleared following intralesional injections of **triamcinolone acetonide** (Kenalog). A lymph node biopsy showed only benign hyperplasia. After eight years, new lesions that appeared were histologically malignant, and a diagnosis of malignant lymphoma was made by lymph node biopsy as well. The skin lesions and lymphadenopathy disappeared after treatment with **cyclophosphamide** (Cytoxan IV for five days).

Shelley WB, Wood MG, Wilson JF, Goodman R: Premalignant lymphoid hyperplasia: Preceding and coexisting with malignant lymphoma in the skin. Arch Dermatol 117:500–503, 1981.

A 63-year-old woman with firm purplish papules on the back had six biopsy-proven lymphocytoma cutis nodules excised over a four-year period. However, a seventh noduloulcerative plaque that developed proved to be a malignant lymphoma. Four coexisting nodules were benign lymphocytomas. The malignant lymphoma plaque was treated successfully with radiotherapy (2725 rads, 100 kV peak over 17 days), and three weeks later the lesion was flat. There was no recurrence during a two-year follow-up. The four nodules of lymphocytoma were not treated, but involuted appreciably following the radiotherapy of the large plaque and remained small and inactive.

Some patients are medical orphans, without a diagnosis, without a drug, and without a doctor. Adopt one!

Lymphogranuloma Venereum

Tetracycline
Sulfisoxazole
Minocycline

Lynch PJ: Therapy of sexually transmitted diseases. Med Clin North Am 66:915–925, 1982.

Lymphogranuloma venereum:

—due to *Chlamydia trachomatis*
—less than 500 cases reported annually in the United States
—clinical diagnosis best confirmed by complement fixation serologic tests (titers of 1:64 diagnostic; titers between 1:16 and 1:64 suggestive, but could come from infections with non-LGV serotypes of *Chlamydia*)
—responds well to **tetracycline** (500 mg qid for at least three weeks or until all signs and symptoms have abated)
—alternate treatments: **sulfisoxazole** (**Gantrisin** 1 gm qid for three weeks) or **minocycline** (Minocin 200 mg qid)
—aspirate fluctuant lymph nodes to prevent chronic draining sinuses
—perform periodic dilatation if a stricture of the vagina or rectum develops
—search out and treat sexual contacts with CF titers of 1:16 or greater

Thorsteinsson SB: Lymphogranuloma venereum: Review of clinical manifestations, epidemiology, diagnosis and treatment. Scand J Infect Dis Suppl 32:127–131, 1982.

The prognosis is excellent with **tetracycline** therapy (500 mg qid for more than three weeks). It may take several months for a fistula to heal and for enlarged lymph nodes to involute. Relapses after treatment are rare.

Note that some *Chlamydia trachomatis* types are resistant to sulfonamides (**sulfamethoxazole** or triple sulfa 2 to 4 gm daily) and to **rifampicin**, used previously with good results. The efficacy of **erythromycin** is not known. Do not resect inflamed lymph nodes, but aspirate fluctuant buboes to prevent spontaneous rupture and fistula formation.

Felman YM, Phil M, Nikitas JA: Lymphogranuloma venereum. Cutis 25:264–272, 280, 288, 310, 1980.

Sometimes two or more courses of **tetracycline** (500 mg qid for three weeks) therapy are required to produce a clinical response.

Alternate treatments include:

sulfisoxazole (Gantrisin 4 gm initially, then 1 gm qid for three weeks)
sulfamethoxazole (Gantanol 2 gm initially, then 1 gm bid for three weeks)

Rectal strictures require frequent dilatation and may necessitate surgical removal of polypoid masses.

In some patients, drugs produce only side effects.

Lymphomatoid Papulosis

PUVA Methotrexate BCNU Chlorambucil

Here is a disease that remits and relapses with no concern for what the therapist is prescribing. And here is a disease that humbles the histopathologist by looking so very malignant while remaining clinically benign.

We think it is a malignant disease in which the patient's immune forces repeatedly succeed in destroying the malignant cells, leaving a scarred focal battleground. As new clones of malignant cells arise in the skin, new battles ensue, accounting for the strange rhythmic cycles the disease exhibits. The battle is usually won by the patient's forces, but not always, as 10 per cent of these patients eventually develop a true malignant lymphoma that takes the upper hand.

We feel we can help these patients in their battle by using either photochemotherapy or cytotoxic drugs to reduce the "malignant cell" population. In one patient we have had an excellent response to chlorambucil (4 mg/day). Methotrexate is an alternate treatment of proven worth. The newer retinoids, as well as cyclosporine, all deserve attention in trying to master this Jekyll and Hyde disease.

Macaulay WL: Lymphomatoid papulosis. Int J Dermatol 17:204–212, 1978.

An update from the father of this disease:

This disorder has a rhythmic cycle of remission and relapse indifferent to even major chemotherapeutic intervention.

Eventually 10 per cent of these patients do develop real lymphomas.

Lange Wantzin G, Thomsen K: PUVA-treatment in lymphomatoid papulosis. Br J Dermatol 107:687–690, 1982.

In five patients with lymphomatoid papulosis of 1 to 13 years' duration PUVA treatment (total dose 51 to 481 J/sq cm) induced complete remission in one patient (with a one-year history) and partial remission in the other four. In the latter four patients after treatment, lesions were fewer in number, and the life cycle of individual lesions was reduced from three to six weeks to one week.

Everett MA: Treatment of lymphomatoid papulosis with methotrexate. Br J Dermatol 111:631, 1984.

Low-dose oral **methotrexate** (from 2.5 to 5.0 mg every two to six weeks to 15 mg every 7 to 10 days for 6 to 12 months) cleared the lesions in four of eight patients, and no further methotrexate was needed. The other four patients required intermittent methotrexate for control.

Zackheim HS, Epstein EH Jr, Crain WR: Topical carmustine therapy for lymphomatoid papulosis. Arch Dermatol 121:1410–1414, 1985.

By using carmustine topically (10 mg/60 ml, 8 per cent ethanol daily for one to four months) each of seven patients with lymphomatoid papulosis experienced substantial reduction in the number and size of lesions. Maintenance therapy consisted of local application of carmustine (4 mg/ml, 95 per cent ethanol) to individual new papules. Long-term remissions were not seen, and the treatment remained suppressive in nature.

One of the serious side effects of drugs is lawsuits.

As you leave the consultation room, ask yourself, "Is there something more I should be doing for this patient?"

Molluscum Contagiosum

Expression	Cantharidin
Curettage	Retinoic acid
Liquid N_2	Accutane

Easy to diagnose and usually easy to treat, this little lesion usually appears in little patients. A stroke of the curette followed by Monsel's solution, although seemingly barbaric, is still the most effective measure. In bigger patients with bigger lesions, we prefer a "microepisiotomy" with a no. 11 Bard-Parker scalpel blade, followed by expression of the viral bead with a Schamberg comedone extractor. Other methods of picking on this little fellow include pinpoint applications of liquid nitrogen, tincture of iodine, podophyllin, trichloroacetic acid, benzoyl peroxide, retinoic acid, silver nitrate, and light electrodesiccation (can lasers be far behind?). All techniques must avoid scarring, as these lesions often immunologically self-destruct, leaving no trace.

Future hope for the immunocompromised or atopic patient with hundreds of lesions centers on alteration of the host keratinocyte by means of the retinoids topically or systemically.

Brown ST, Nalley JF, Kraus SJ: Molluscum contagiosum. Sex Transm Dis 8:227–234, 1981.

Splendid review with everything you could want to know. Without treatment an individual lesion persists about two months, and the disease persists for six months to three years. Treatment decreases autoinoculation and transmission of the disease. 96 references.

Steffen C, Markman J-A: Spontaneous disappearance of molluscum contagiosum: Report of a case. Arch Dermatol 116:923–924, 1980.

Infected by his son, a dermatologist developed 50 molluscum contagiosum lesions on his chest. Intrigued, he withheld all treatment and watched each of his own lesions become inflamed and completely disappear within three months.

Sturt RJ, Muller HK, Francis GD: Molluscum contagiosum in villages of the West Sepik district of New Guinea. Med J Aust 2:751–754, 1971.

Spontaneous clearing was noted in most of the 401 cases within 18 months. Children under 10 years comprised 93 per cent of the infected group.

Rosenberg EW, Yusk JW: Molluscum contagiosum: Eruption following treatment with prednisone and methotrexate. Arch Dermatol 101:439–441, 1970.

Immunosuppression favors molluscum contagiosum by the hundreds. No treatment for molluscum was given.

Hellier FF: Profuse mollusca contagiosa of the face induced by corticosteroids. Br J Dermatol 85:398, 1971.

Avoid topical steroids, since they depress local immune defenses.

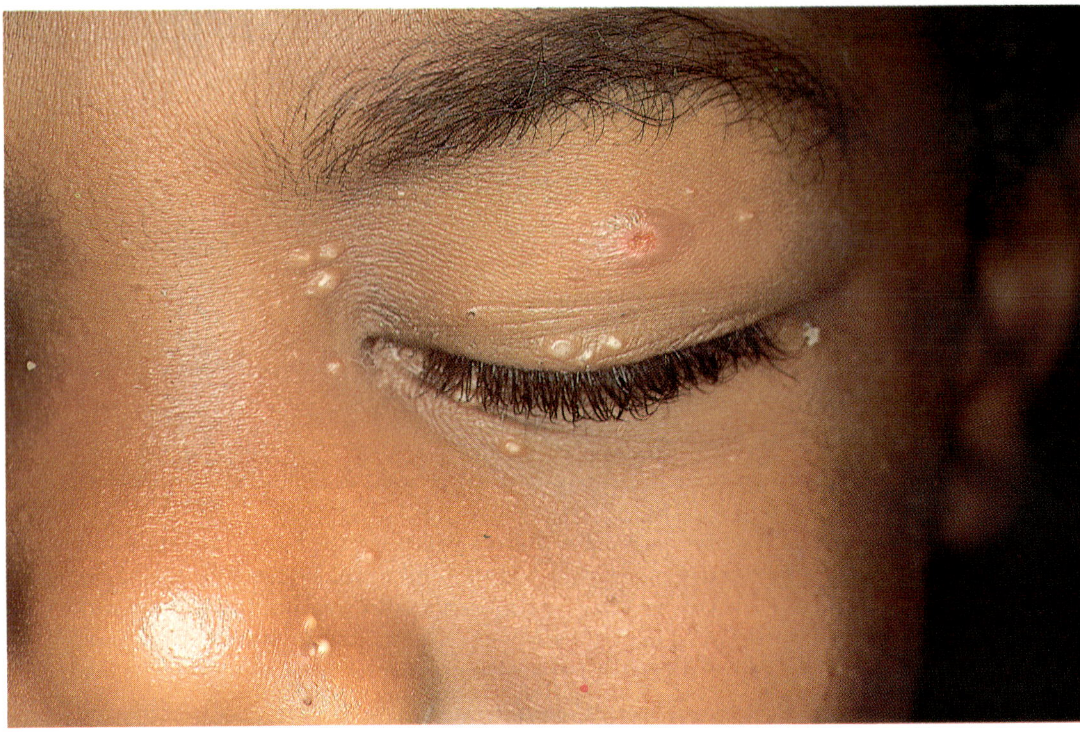

Weston WL, Lane AT: Should molluscum be treated? Pediatrics 65:865, 1980.

The authors say no, since treatment of this self-limited disease is painful and frightening to the child.

Arone di Bertolino R: Psicoterapia del mollusco contagioso nei bambini. Minerva Med 73:1849–1851, 1982.

Eight children under four years of age were successfully treated by hypnotherapy. (Only bambinos can be bamboozled out of their warts and mollusca.)

Resnik SS: A simplified surgical management of lesions of molluscum contagiosum. J Dermatol Surg Oncol 6:982–983, 1980.

Microincision with a no. 11 scalpel blade tip, followed by expression of the white core with a Schamberg comedone extractor.

Nasemann T, Schaeg G: Einfaches Behandlungsuerfahren für Mollusca contagiosa. Hautarzt 24:402–403, 1973.

Lateral pressure with tweezer tip: Pop goes the weasel.

Stanka P: Bemerkungen zur Behandlung des Molluscum contagiosum. Hautarzt 28:208–209, 1977.

Recommends puncturing lesion with a finely pointed toothpick dipped in liquid **phenol**.

Funt TR, Mehr KA: Cantharidin: A valuable office treatment of molluscum contagiosum. South Med J 72:1019, 1979.

Dip the tip of an orange stick or applicator stick into **cantharidin** (0.9 per cent in equal parts of acetone and flexible colloidion USP) or Cantharone

(0.7 per cent of same preparation). Carefully apply only to top of lesion. Lesion blisters, crusts, and exfoliates within four days.

Marchildon A: Le traitement du molluscum contagiosum par cryotherapie. Can J Ophthalmol 9:260–261, 1974.

Punctate cryosurgery.

Kaye JW: Problems in therapy of molluscum contagiosum: Case report. Arch Dermatol 94:454–455, 1966.

Cure in a six-year-old boy only after 607 lesions were removed by curettage (five sessions over four months, general anesthesia).

Fanta D, Kokoschka E-M: Mollusca contagiosa: Übersicht und kritische Betrachtung einer neuen Behandlungsmethode. Wien Klin Wochenschr 87:154–158, 1975.

Common treatment in Europe: Punctate application of **retinoic acid** (0.1 per cent alcoholic tincture tid) cleared 15 cases in 5 to 18 days. (Available in the United States as Retin-A 0.05 per cent solution.)

Vilmer C, de Prost Y, Ricour C, Ferchal F: Molluscum contagiosum profus chez un enfant immuno-déprimé. Essai de traitment par l'acide retinoïque per os. Ann Dermatol Venereol 110:781–782, 1983.

In an immunosuppressed child, oral Accutane cleared multiple molluscum lesions.

Niizeki K, Kano O, Kondo Y: An epidemic study of molluscum contagiosum: Relationship to swimming. Dermatologica 169:197–198, 1984.

The incidence of molluscum contagiosum was 7.5 per cent in the swimming group of 6406 elementary and kindergarten school children, but only 3.6 per cent in the 1066 nonswimmers. The authors recommend that infected children not be permitted to swim in public swimming pools.

It's a given that if you are given a fee, the patient is given a prescription.

Morphea

Diprolene ointment Lidocaine Dilantin Azulfidine

The prognosis here is better than the therapy. Fortunately, most examples of morphea are small in area, cosmetically inoffensive, and self limiting. In such instances, we temporize by prescribing Diprolene ointment to be applied sparingly each night, and we inject the entire site at the time of each visit with 2 per cent lidocaine (without epinephrine, up to 10 cc depending on the lesion size).

In more extensive cases either sulfasalazine (Azulfidine 1 gm bid) or phenytoin (Dilantin 100 mg tid) may be tried. In all instances the patient is heartened by an awareness that the process is not progressive, does not herald internal disease, and will disappear as mysteriously as it arose. Patients should understand, however, that some atrophic scarring is a common keepsake of their disease.

As the patient adapts to his morphea or as it involutes, the intervals between visits should be appropriately lengthened. This remains true for all diseases in which the treatment is not as good as the prognosis.

Czarnecki DB, Taft EH: Generalized morphoea successfully treated with salazopyrine. Acta Derm Venereol 62:81–82, 1982.

In a 60-year-old woman with morphea that had involved the lower half of the trunk, salazopyrine (**sulfasalazine**, Azulfidine 1 gm bid for 10 months) induced complete remission. Softening of the plaques was noticeable within one month of starting therapy. However, the patient's acrosclerosis remained completely unaffected. The drug was stopped, and one year later the morphea recurred on both thighs. It then completely involuted following a subsequent three-month course of Azulfidine.

Stava Z, Kobikova M: Salazopyrin in the treatment of scleroderma. Br J Dermatol 96:541–544, 1977.

Sulfasalazine (Azulfidine 2 to 4 gm/day for five to nine months) aborted acute generalized morphea in two adults. In one patient the disease returned 13 months after the sulfasalazine was discontinued, but was again checked by an additional $4\frac{1}{2}$ months of sulfasalazine treatment.

No effect was seen in eight patients with diffuse scleroderma.

Morgan RJ: Scleroderma: Treatment with diphenylhydantoin. Cutis 8:278–282, 1971.

Phenytoin (Dilantin 100 mg one to four times a day) significantly improved the lesions in 11 of 20 patients with circumscribed morphea. Only 4 of 24 in the control group showed similar resolution.

Person JR, Su WPD: Subcutaneous morphoea: A clinical study of sixteen cases. Br J Dermatol 100:371–380, 1979.

Four of eight patients with this more serious and more inflammatory type of sclerosis of the panniculus or fascia responded well to antimalarial drugs. Three patients responded to **cyclophosphamide**, one to **penicillamine**, and one to **prednisone**. None had complete regression of the sclerosis during a follow-up period of as long as 12 years.

A drug may be neatly placed into a "class," but it often doesn't stay there. Thus, hydroxyzine is not only an antihistaminic, but an anticatecholaminic, an anticholinergic, an antispasmodic, and an anxiolytic agent as well as a CNS depressant. Use any or all of these "six classrooms" to the patient's advantage.

Mucha-Habermann Disease

Sunlight	UVB
Tetracycline	PUVA
Erythromycin	Methotrexate
Dapsone	Ridaura

This is a very serious, necrotizing, scarring process that calls for screening for focal infection. Teeth, sinuses, tonsils, gallbladder, gastrointestinal tract, urinary bladder, vagina, and prostate are areas in which to look for patent or occult infection. Even if no infection is sighted, we still treat empirically with antibiotics, having had more success with tetracycline (2 gm/day) than any other antibiotic. We use erythromycin, ampicillin, metronidazole, or dapsone as alternates until we find a winner.

We consider that Mucha-Habermann disease is another of the skin's many recognizable reaction patterns. As such it can be suppressed either by removing an underlying infection or by modulating the skin's response. For the latter, the use of phototherapy and methotrexate has been successful. With the new availability of oral gold, auranofin (Ridaura), another possible avenue of therapy has been opened.

Takada Y, Irisawa K, Kawada A: Heliotherapy of pityriasis lichenoides chronica. Jap J Dermatol 4:91–94, 1977.

Sunbathing at a resort produced pronounced improvement in 13 of 15 patients with the chronic form of pityriasis lichenoides.

Piamphongsant T: Tetracycline for the treatment of pityriasis lichenoides. Br J Dermatol 91:319–322, 1974.

In 5 of 13 patients with pityriasis lichenoides there was complete disappearance of lesions in two to four weeks when given **tetracycline** (2 gm daily). Seven patients had to continue taking tetracycline (1 gm/day) to keep lesions under control. These findings favor the view that this disease is a hypersensitivity reaction to infectious agents, and indeed four patients had throat cultures yielding coagulase-positive staphylococci.

Shavin JS, Jones TM, Aton JK, et al: Mucha-Habermann's disease in children: Treatment with erythromycin. Arch Dermatol 114:1679–1680, 1978.

Erythromycin (250 mg qid for two to four weeks) completely cleared three children of their lesions within one month. Only one had a recurrence (10 months after the antibiotic was discontinued), and this responded rapidly to a second course of erythromycin.

Powell FC, Muller SA: Psoralens and ultraviolet A therapy of pityriasis lichenoides. J Am Acad Dermatol 10:59–64, 1984.

The distinction between acute (Mucha-Habermann) and chronic (Juliusberg) pityriasis lichenoides is not always clear, since transitional forms occur. On the basis of good results in three patients with PUVA (**methoxsalen** + UVA three times a week for 3 to 12 months), the authors prefer this to previous

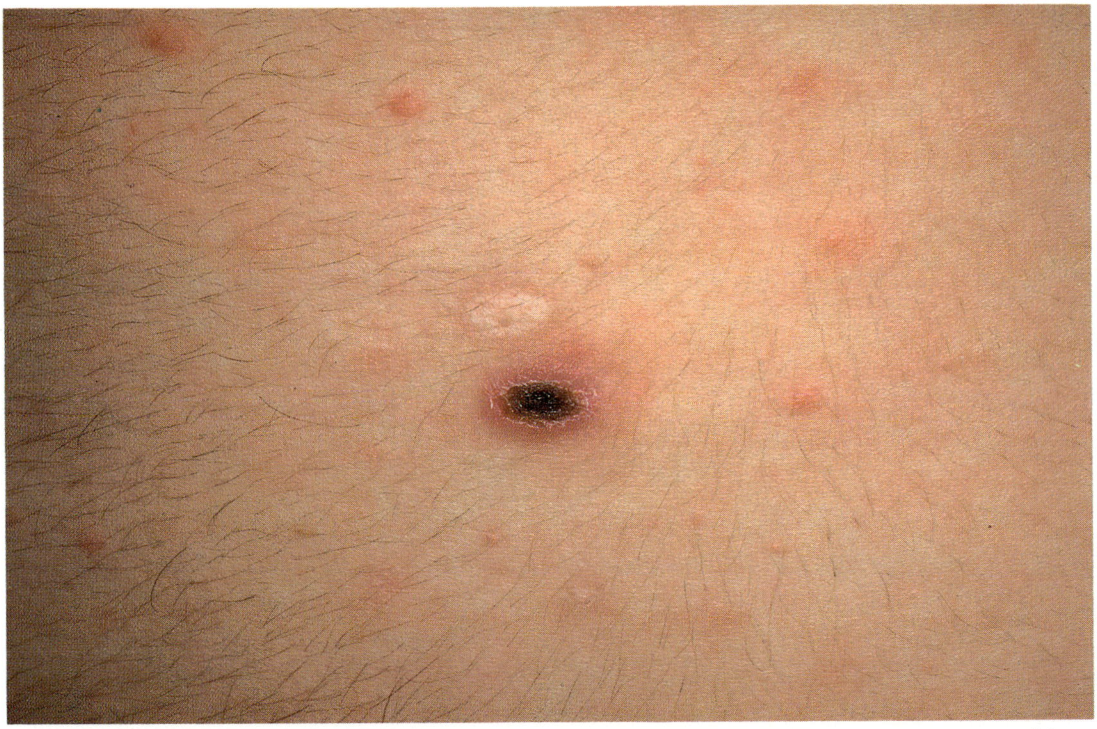

therapies with gold, steroids, **oxyphenbutazone**, **vitamin A**, **vitamin D_2**, antibiotics, **dapsone**, **methotrexate**, and sunlight.

LeVine MJ: Phototherapy of pityriasis lichenoides. Arch Dermatol 119:378–380, 1983.

In each of 11 patients with pityriasis lichenoides chronica, doses of UVB (five times a week) calculated to produce a faint erythema cleared all lesions. This was achieved with an average of 29 treatments (range 10 to 59) and an average UVB dose of 388 millijoules/sq cm.

Cornelison RL Jr, Knox JM, Everett MA: Methotrexate for the treatment of Mucha-Habermann disease. Arch Dermatol 106:507–508, 1972.

Six patients with pityriasis lichenoides et varioliformis acuta (Mucha-Habermann) were treated with low doses of oral **methotrexate** (7.5 to 20 mg weekly); all showed rapid clearing, but lesions usually recurred within one month after treatment was stopped.

There is always another treatment. Find it.

Mycosis Fungoides

Sunlight	Retinoids
Topical corticosteroids	Acyclovir
Nitrogen mustard	Cimetidine
PUVA	Cyclosporine
Declomycin	X-ray
Griseofulvin	Electron beam
Tetracycline	Chemotherapy

Few diseases admit of a wider spectrum of therapy. It extends from a trivial steroid cream in the earliest stages to full combinational chemotherapy for its systemic tumor stage. Therapy may vary from advice to secure a suntan to referral to the radiologist and oncologist for conjoint therapy.

Some feel that since mycosis fungoides is ultimately a fatal T cell lymphoma, therapy should be as early and as fully aggressive as possible. However, it is difficult to persuade most physicians or their patients that a disease that proceeds at a snail's pace needs a lion's attack. To us the rate of change is the key determinant to the specific type of therapy. If the patient has only pruritic, scaly, erythematous macules we prefer to minimize bathing and use a mild emollient or low-potency steroid cream to relieve the itch. We have seen a half dozen such cases in which the disease, although histologically confirmed, never progressed beyond this stage, and in two instances outlived the patients.

Initially, all cases should be completely evaluated and staged as to the extent of the mycosis fungoides. Although staging indices vary, we simply label the macular lesions stage I, the infiltrative plaques stage II, the presence of nodules or tumors stage III, and any lymph node or organ involvement other than the skin stage IV.

It is stage I that may persist for decades and seemingly live in pleasant symbiosis. If new macular lesions are arising or if infiltrative plaques develop, we immediately prescribe topical nitrogen mustard therapy (10 mg powder [1 vial] dissolved in 50 ml tap water, rapidly applied to the entire skin within seconds of preparation). Our sensitization rate is less than 5 per cent, in contrast to many reported series with 40 to 50 per cent sensitization. We attribute this low rate to the absence of sensitizing amines that develop in aqueous solutions upon standing. The fresh solution is applied daily until the lesions have become brownish macules and itching has ceased. Treatment is then stopped.

An excellent alternative therapy for stages I and II is PUVA, but we have not had to employ this.

Stage III usually calls for electron beam therapy, and these patients are referred to the appropriate radiation facility. Once the lymphoma has spread to the lymph nodes or is evident internally (stage IV) the patient should be under the care of an oncologist who can administer one of the multifaceted acronymic chemotherapeutic protocols such as CVP.

It is well to give the full story of this disease to the patient and, at times, the family. Instruct them that the rate of change of the skin lesions is the best index of the course, prognosis, and therapy. It is a disease that can act benign for a lifetime, but can just as easily be fatal within a few months, as in the d'emblée type. No patient to date can be said to be "cured," no matter what the treatment. Indeed, one of our patients, completely cleared of her skin lesions with nitrogen mustard therapy for two years, later died of systemic mycosis fungoides with her skin still totally clear. Once the disease has begun a progressive course, only remissions are achievable.

Nonetheless, radiation and chemotherapy are not the only methods of treatment that can now be proffered to these patients. We have one patient who has had a prolonged remission of his stage III mycosis fungoides following Declomycin therapy. Another case that was in stage I showed involution of lesions following griseofulvin therapy. Although these examples are unusual, duplicate examples are found in the literature with tetracycline and griseofulvin therapy. Equally dramatic have been the responses of a few patients to Tagamet, Accutane, and Zovirax. These new avenues, sketched below, need further study. They certainly add new hope to both patients and physicians much in need of it.

Epstein EH Jr, Levin DL, Croft JD, Lutzner MA: Mycosis fungoides: Survival, prognostic features, response to therapy, and autopsy findings. Medicine 51:61–72, 1972.

This NIH study of 144 patients showed:

All treatments are palliative with no effect on survival time.

Although survival ranged from less than 1 year to 52 years, 50 per cent of patients died within $3\frac{1}{2}$ years of initial histologic diagnosis.

Response rates (percentage of patients improved) for the seven most popular treatment modes of that time were:

Treatment	**Per cent**
Topical nitrogen mustard	75
Orthovoltage radiation	89
Electron beam	88
Systemic methotrexate	82
Systemic cyclophosphamide	62
Systemic nitrogen mustard	59
Systemic steroids	59

Lamberg SI, Bunn PA Jr (eds): Proceedings of the workshop on cutaneous T-cell lymphomas (mycosis fungoides and Sézary syndrome). Cancer Treat Rep 63:561–736, 1979.

Thirty papers covering every aspect of treatment, including the failure of 15 chemotherapeutic agents other than **nitrogen mustard** to be beneficial when applied topically.

Bunn PA Jr, Lamberg SI: Report of the committee on staging and classification of cutaneous T-cell lymphomas. Cancer Treat Rep 63:725–728, 1979.

Staging procedures required for all patients:

1. Complete history and physical examination
2. Whole-body mapping of lesions
3. CBC, platelet count, absolute lymphocyte count, and record of atypical convoluted lymphocytes

4. Serum chemistry studies
5. Chest roentgenogram
6. Skin biopsy, lymph node biopsy
7. Liver and bone marrow biopsies if stage II, III, or IV
8. Evaluation of other organs when indicated by history or examination

Thiers BH: Controversies in mycosis fungoides. J Am Acad Dermatol 7:1–16, 1982.

Two schools of thought regarding ℞:

If MF begins as a benign reactive process, it is inappropriate to begin vigorous toxic antineoplastic treatment early.

If MF begins as a malignant neoplasm early, aggressive therapy seems indicated.

Farber EM, Cox AJ, Steinberg J, McClintock RP: Therapy of mycosis fungoides with topically applied fluocinolone acetonide under occlusive dressing. Cancer 19:237–245, 1966.

Six patients who applied **fluocinolone** cream (0.01 to 0.2 per cent under occlusion for 12 to 24 hours/day) had improvement for the nine-month period of study. This is an early example of one of the most commonly used approaches to MF in its earliest manifestation.

Vonderheid EC: Topical mechlorethamine chemotherapy. Considerations on its use in mycosis fungoides. Int J Dermatol 23:180–186, 1984.

Mechlorethamine (nitrogen mustard, Mustargen 10 mg of powder in vial, dissolved in 50 ml tap water, applied once or twice a day to entire skin except genitalia, after bath, using nylon paint brush) will usually induce regression of lesions in a few weeks, with complete clearing in six months. Continue daily applications for six months past clinical "cure," then alternate days for three years. Occasional monitoring of blood count is advisable. Assistant should wear plastic, not rubber, gloves. Ten-minute daily compresses on thick plaques are helpful.

It is still not known whether such prolonged nitrogen mustard therapy is curative or merely palliative.

Thestrup-Pedersen K, Christiansen JV, Zachariae H: Precautions for personnel applying topical nitrogen mustard to patients with mycosis fungoides. Dermatologica 165:108–113, 1982.

This is an irritant as well as a contact sensitizer and potential carcinogen. Avoid inhalation of dust in preparation of solution and contact with skin or eyes of personnel applying it. Nurses applying the drug should wear protective clothing to cover hair and skin, rubber gloves and boots, and a mask with a special filter that covers the face and eyes.

Volden G, Molin L, Thomsen K: Topical mechlorethamine therapy for mycosis fungoides: Proposed schedule to overcome drug resistance. Arch Dermatol 118:138–139, 1982.

To reduce the chance of carcinogenesis, as well as resistance to treatment, this group advises stopping **nitrogen mustard** applications as soon as complete clinical and histologic remission is achieved. Resume treatment if histologically verified relapse occurs.

Price NM, Hoppe RT, Deneau DG: Ointment-based mechlorethamine treatment for mycosis fungoides. Cancer 52:2214–2219, 1983.

To avoid development of allergic contact sensitivity to **nitrogen mustard**, use anhydrous ointment instead of water as a vehicle. Formula:

nitrogen mustard 90 mg
absolute ethyl alcohol 10 ml
Aquaphor 900 mg

Sig: Apply 15 gm in thin film to entire skin surface once daily. Do not bathe before application.

Since the preparation is stable and only nine vials are used in two months, it is much less costly than one vial (10 mg) a day. Only 1 in 31 patients developed contact allergy to it, and 9 of 12 patients previously sensitized to nitrogen mustard tolerated it. Complete clearing occurred in 26 of 43 patients with stages I to III MF during the 42-month evaluation period.

Constantine VS, Fuks ZY, Farber EM: Mechlorethamine densensitization in therapy for mycosis fungoides: Topical desensitization to mechlorethamine (nitrogen mustard) contact hypersensitivity. Arch Dermatol 111:484–488, 1975.

The patient sensitized to **nitrogen mustard** can be desensitized with intravenous doses given over a one-month period or by this outpatient technique of inducing tolerance: daily total body application of an extremely dilute solution of nitrogen mustard (0.01 to 0.1 mg/100 ml, i.e., 2000 times as dilute as the therapeutic concentration). The concentration is increased (double or more) each week as tolerance permits. It may take nearly a year, but successful desensitization was achieved in four of five of their patients.

Zackheim HS, Epstein EH Jr, McNutt NS, et al: Topical carmustine (BCNU) for mycosis fungoides and related disorders: A 10-year experience. J Am Acad Dermatol 9:363–374, 1983.

This nitrosourea compound provides a topical alternative to nitrogen mustard. It comes in powder form (BiCNU 100-mg vials). It is used topically in 95 per cent or absolute ethanol (200 mg/100 ml), ointments (400 mg/100 gm white petrolatum) or intralesionally in saline solution (1 mg/ml). The preparation of choice is applied to the entire skin surface every day for two months. In this study of 86 patients, clearing was seen within 12 months in 84 per cent of those with less than 10 per cent of the skin surface involved. However, in those with larger areas of involvement, clearing was seen in only 52 per cent after two years. Like nitrogen mustard it is not useful for treating tumors.

Lee LA, Fritz KA, Golitz L, et al: Second cutaneous malignancies in patients with mycosis fungoides treated with topical nitrogen mustard. J Am Acad Dermatol 7:590–598, 1982.

The carcinogenic potential of **nitrogen mustard** is demonstrated by the fact that 4 of 29 patients under treatment for one to three years developed squamous cell and basal cell carcinomas in areas not exposed to the sun. Long-term surveillance is strongly advised.

Powell FC, Spiegel GT, Muller SA: Treatment of parapsoriasis and mycosis fungoides: The role of psoralen and long-wave ultraviolet light A (PUVA). Mayo Clin Proc 59:538–546, 1984.

PUVA therapy with **methoxsalen** (30 to 50 mg orally) two hours before UVA light treatment with an upright Sylvania unit (GTE Sylvania Lighting Products, Danvers, Mass.) three times a week (total dosage 31 to 1433 joules/sq cm) resulted in clearing in ten patients with stage I or II (seven had complete clearing and three had 80 per cent improvement). Nine patients with more advanced MF did not do well, although one of five cases of stage IV cleared. A complete summary of the world's literature on this significant form of treatment shows that although 80 per cent clearing was achieved in stages I and II, less than 40 per cent of patients in stage III showed improvement.

Fischer T, Skogh M: Treatment of parapsoriasis en plaques, mycosis fungoides, and Sézary's syndrome with trioxsalen baths followed by ultraviolet light. Acta Derm Venereol 59:171–173, 1979.

This is PUVA without the pill, given five days per week for two months, then twice weekly for two months, then once weekly indefinitely. Simply soak for 15 minutes in a **trioxsalen** bath (50 mg/150 liter tub) before UVA (given immediately after the bath). Clearing occurred in all seven of their patients with MF stage II with two to six months of treatment and four of five patients with stage III. No value for erythrodermic forms.

Mork BE, Vollum DI, DuVivier AWP: Combination topical nitrogen mustard and photochemotherapy for mycosis fungoides. Clin Exp Dermatol 9:243–247, 1984.

An additive effect of two good treatment regimens was obtained in 29 patients. Note that conjoint phototherapy did not prevent development of sensitivity to **nitrogen mustard**.

Shelley WB: Demethylchlortetracycline and griseofulvin as examples of specific treatment for mycosis fungoides. Br J Dermatol 104:477–480, 1981.

Declomycin (**demethylchlortetracycline** 300 mg bid) resulted in total disappearance of multiple histologically proven MF tumors within one month. Maintenance dosage was stopped after eight years. Tumors reappeared two years later, but completely disappeared again within one month of resumption of Declomycin. The remission continued for more than one year with Declomycin therapy. The response was specific for this patient and was not seen in four other patients with MF.

Thomsen K: Mycosis fungoides responding to tetracycline and griseofulvin. Br J Dermatol 105:483–484, 1981.

Another example of antibiotic-responsive–tumor-stage MF. **Tetracycline** (1 gm/day) was associated with tumors disappearing completely in three weeks. They recurred two months later despite continued tetracycline therapy. Tetracycline was discontinued, but its resumption six months later induced tumors to regress again. The response was unique to this patient and not observed in five other MF patients. One other patient, however, showed tumor regression following griseofulvin (500 mg/day) therapy.

Kessler JF, Meyskens FL Jr, Levine N, et al: Treatment of cutaneous T-cell lymphoma (mycosis fungoides) with 13-cis-retinoic acid. Lancet 1:1345–1347, 1983.

Accutane (2 to 3 mg/kg/daily) induced dramatic improvement in four patients with MF. One patient had nearly complete clearing of extensive plaques and tumors after ten months. Two others had 50 per cent reduction in plaques after six weeks, and a fourth patient had improvement in four weeks, but had to stop because of intense dryness.

Warrell RP Jr, Coonley CJ, Kempin SJ, et al: Isotretinoin in cutaneous T-cell lymphoma. Lancet 2:629, 1983.

Three of seven patients showed excellent response to Accutane (100 mg/sq m, single oral daily dose for one month or more). Most impressive was the total clearing of erythroderma and enlarged lymph nodes in one patient. This remission lasted nine months. Four patients with tumor-stage disease did not improve.

Claudy AL, Delomier Y, Hermier C: Treatment of cutaneous T-cell lymphoma with a new aromatic retinoid (Ro 10-9359). Arch Dermatol Res 273:37–42, 1982.

Nodular MF in a 77-year-old woman flattened completely after one month of Tigason (1 mg/kg/day PO). When the drug was discontinued after four months of therapy, nodules reappeared within three weeks.

Mamus SW, Mladenovic J, Hordinsky MK, et al: Cimetidine-induced remission of mycosis fungoides. Lancet 2:409, 1984.

Case 1: **Cimetidine** (Tagamet 300 mg qid) was associated with total clearing of tumor-stage MF within ten weeks. The remission, which persisted for over three months, is impressive since the tumors had been indifferent to a chemotherapeutic regimen of **chlorambucil**, **cyclophosphamide**, **vincristine**, and **prednisone**. Lesions recurred on stopping the drug after the initial ten weeks of therapy, but cleared again when the drug was restarted.

Case 2: **Cimetidine** (300 mg qid) induced complete remission of plaque-stage MF within seven weeks. Lesions recurred on stopping the drug.

Resnick L, Schleider-Kushner N, Horwitz SN, Frost P: Remission of tumor-stage mycosis fungoides following intravenously administered acyclovir. JAMA 251:1571–1573, 1984.

Acyclovir (Zovirax 5 mg/kg IV q8h—1.2 gm/day for 12 days) induced complete healing within one month of ulcerative tumors in a 58-year-old woman with tumor-stage MF for two years. The tumors reappeared in three months, and a second course of acyclovir was equally effective within one month. The second remission lasted more than three months without further therapy.

Mahrle G, Thiele B, Steigleder GK: Acyclovir in mycosis fungoides. Z Hautkr 59:855–856, 1984.

Two patients with tumor-stage MF treated with IV **acyclovir** (same dosage as above) failed to show any response.

Maddox A-M, Kahan BD, Tucker S, et al: Remission in skin infiltrate of a patient with mycosis fungoides treated with cyclosporine. J Am Acad Dermatol 12:952–956, 1985.

Cyclosporine, a fungal polypeptide popular in preventing graft rejection, since it preferentially inhibits T helper lymphocytes, was temporarily beneficial in controlling symptoms and infiltrates in a 57-year-old woman with MF. The disease had proven refractory to **prednisone** and **nitrogen mustard**, as well as courses of MOPP, CHOP, and MIME. Continuous IV infusion of cyclosporine (5 mg/kg for seven days, then 4 mg/kg for seven days) caused cessation of pruritus within a few days. Oral cyclosporine (7 mg/kg bid) in a dose to keep her serum level at 200 ng/ml, gave a remission of 3½ months. Subsequent recurrence was controlled by 10 weeks of electron beam therapy. Death occurred in an automobile accident.

Kufe DW, Wick MM, Moschella S, Major P: Effect of high-dose thymidine infusions in patients with mycosis fungoides. Cancer 48:1513–1516, 1981.

The response in three patients to **thymidine** (75 gm/sq m/day, continuous IV infusion for four to seven days, four courses) varied from a temporary one-month remission of diffuse erythematous plaques to no response. This was another experimental attempt to inhibit DNA synthesis in a T cell lymphoma.

Gaeke ME, Variakojis D, Sweet DL: Mycosis fungoides. Curr Probl Cancer 6:1–39 (Sept) 1981.

Radiation has been a principal form of therapy since 1902. This may be given locally to tumors or as total body radiation (teleroentgen therapy). Since 1953, megavolt electron irradiation often has been used, since it selectively bathes the skin (but not the rest of the body) in electrons; 2000 to 3500 rads of such electrons induce complete remission in 85 per cent of patients with limited disease.

Borok TL, Farina AT, Leider M: Mycosis fungoides: Retrospect, current understanding, and prospect. J Dermatol Surg Oncol 6:637–645, 1980.

Options for radiation therapy include 120 kVp or 250 kVp orthovoltage and telecobalt-60 (megavoltage). If the patient has systemic MF the authors recommend low-dose megavolt whole-body irradiation (5 to 10 rads/session) coupled with chemotherapy. Whole-body irradiation penetrates the entire body mass (including bone marrow and lymphatics) and partially spares the skin, in contrast to irradiation of the entire skin surface by electron beam, which affects only the skin with an "electron bath."

Hamminga B, Noordijk EM, van Vloten WA: Treatment of mycosis fungoides: Total-skin electron-beam irradiation vs topical mechlorethamine therapy. Arch Dermatol 118:150–153, 1982.

In the early stages of MF this study of 42 patients showed electron beam therapy to be as effective as topical **nitrogen mustard**. In later stages of infiltrative plaques and tumors, however, electron beam therapy is superior in producing complete (although temporary) remissions. Neither is effective in patients with lymph node or systemic spread or both. The authors advise nitrogen mustard treatment after electron beam therapy to prolong remission time. Every one of 21 patients in the "electron skin bath" lost all of his or her hair and nails, and 8 developed marked edema and bullae. Of the 21 receiving nitrogen mustard treatments 18 showed hyperpigmentation, and 11 had an irritant dermatitis. Only one patient became sensitized to nitrogen mustard.

Lo TCM, Salzman FA, Costey GE, Wright KA: Megavolt electron irradiation for localized mycosis fungoides. Acta Radiol Oncol 20:71–74, 1981.

Small, local field, megavolt electron beam irradiation was used to treat 14 patients with localized cutaneous tumors who showed no internal spread; ten (71 per cent) were cured, two still had disease, and two had died over a five-year study period. In contrast, only 16 of 200 patients (8 per cent) with generalized cutaneous MF and treated with total skin electron irradiation had a five-year cure.

Longo DL, DeVita VT Jr: Lymphomas. *In* Pinedo HM, Chabner BA (eds): Cancer Chemotherapy, 1983. New York, Elsevier, 1983, pp 248–281.

The therapeutic efficacy of combination chemotherapy in MF has been examined suboptimally to date, since there was not randomization of most patients, prognostic factors were not stratified, and treatments were heterogeneous.

Tirelli U, Carbone A, Veronesi A, et al: Combination chemotherapy with cyclophosphamide, vincristine, and prednisone (CVP) in TNM-classified stage IV mycosis fungoides. Cancer Treat Rep 66:167–169, 1982.

CVP Protocol, repeated every three weeks for six times.

cyclophosphamide (oral 400 mg/sq m/day on days 1 to 5)
vincristine (1.4 mg/sq m IV on day 1)
prednisone (oral 100 mg/sq m/day, days 1 to 5).

This induced a complete remission of advanced (stage IV) MF in four of nine patients (44 per cent), with a median duration of 7 months (3- to 19-months' range). This is the best record to date for chemotherapy.

Molin L, Thomsen K, Volden G, et al: Combination chemotherapy in the tumour stage of mycosis fungoides with cyclophosphamide, vincristine, VP-16, adriamycin and prednisolone (COP, CHOP, CAVOP): A report from the Scandinavian mycosis fungoides study group. Acta Derm Venereol 60:542–544, 1980.

These drugs (so helpful in Hodgkin's lymphoma) gave no long-term help. Of nine patients, one had complete remission and five had partial remissions, but all were of short term.

Groth O, Molin L, Thomsen K: Tumour stage of mycosis fungoides treated with bleomycin and methotrexate: Report from the Scandinavian mycosis fungoides study group. Acta Derm Venereol 59:59–63, 1979.

Short remissions occurred with **bleomycin** (15 mg IM twice weekly for seven weeks) or bleomycin (same dose) in combination with **methotrexate** (15 mg/sq m IM once weekly for seven weeks). However, 6 of the authors' 19 patients died of complications due to chemotherapy.

Lawrence WT, Robson MC: The treatment of ulcers in patients with mycosis fungoides with split-thickness skin grafts. Ann Plast Surg 13:20–23, 1984.

Surgical grafting of skin ulcers associated with MF and electron beam therapy was generally successful in five patients. Healing of both donor and graft sites was slower than usual.

Fischmann AB, Bunn PA Jr, Guccion JG, et al: Exposure to chemicals, physical agents, and biologic agents in mycosis fungoides and the Sézary syndrome. Cancer Treat Rep 63:591–596, 1979.

Some observations suggesting that long-term antigen persistence in skin may account for induction of hyperplasia and subsequent malignant change in the T cell. Cites example of a worker who after one year of focal contact with creosote developed MF at this exact site.

Rosenthal CJ, Noguera CA, Coppola A, Kapelner SN: Pseudolymphoma with mycosis fungoides manifestations, hyperresponsiveness to diphenylhydantoin, and lymphocyte disregulation. Cancer 49:2305–2314, 1982.

Three patients are described with pruritic exfoliative erythroderma, eosinophilia, lymphadenopathy, hepatosplenomegaly, and Sézary cells, clinically and histologically resembling MF. All signs, symptoms, and immunologic abnormalities (proliferation of T lymphocytes and inhibiton of T_γ-suppressor lymphocytes) totally involuted within one month of stopping Dilantin. To date, there are more than 200 other cases of pseudolymphoma syndrome from Dilantin.

Fischer T, van Vloten WA, Volden G: Internal dissemination of mycosis fungoides despite successful local therapy. Acta Derm Venereol 58:88–89, 1978.

All cases initially staged as skin involvement only need lifelong surveillance. Witness:

Case 1: A 45-year-old man was completely cleared of skin plaques following electron beam therapy (3800 rads, 4 MeV), local x-ray, and topical **nitrogen mustard**. Two months later lymph node involvement became evident, followed by paresis due to an extradural tumor and by death.

Case 2: A 71-year-old man with skin tumors for 10 years was cured of skin lesions with x-ray, ^{32}P, topical **nitrogen mustard**, **bleomycin** and ultraviolet light. He died nine months later of systemic MF.

Case 3: A 69-year-old man was cleared of skin plaques and tumors with 2½ months of topical **nitrogen mustard** therapy. Nine months later he developed inguinal nodes. He was undergoing systemic treatment at the time of the report.

Enter the examining room fast, but leave slowly.

Myiasis

Alexander JO: Cutaneous myiasis. *In* Alexander JO (ed): Arthropods and Human Skin. New York, Springer-Verlag, 1984, pp 87–113.

A classic authoritative review. The aim of treatment is to remove all larvae.

1. Wound myiasis (eggs are laid on wounds)
   - Debridement with irrigation
   - If larvae have burrowed into the tissue and live in sinuses, daily irrigation with ether or chloroform under local or general anesthesia
   - Sterile dressings
   - Heals in one week after larvae have been removed
   - **Lindane** dressings effective, but risky in the very young
   - Prophylaxis
     - cover all wounds
     - eradicate flies
     - sleep indoors
     - good animal husbandry
     - inspect livestock for wounds
     - avoid surgery during "fly season"
     - use repellent creams around wounds
     - destroy breeding grounds of flies (decaying animal and vegetable refuse)
2. Furuncular myiasis (newly hatched larvae are deposited on and penetrate skin)
   - Attempts to express the larva by pressure are fruitless and painful.
   - Bind a piece of pork fat over the lesion for 24 hours and the larva will emerge.
   - (or) Anesthetize the area, incise, and pick out the anesthetized larva.
3. Creeping eruption
   - Place a drop of machine oil on the skin to make the epidermis translucent.
   - Using a lens, locate the larva by spotting black transverse rows of segmental spines (the larva head is approximately 1 cm in front of the visible red linear lesion in the skin).
   - Pick out the larva with a sterile needle.

Kenney RL, Baker FJ: Botfly (*Dermatobia hominis*) myiasis. Int J Dermatol 23:676–677, 1984.

A 43-year-old man who had worked in Panama (where he was frequently bitten by insects) had three erythematous nodules (1.5 to 3.0 cm in diameter), each with a central orifice that drained yellow fluid. Filling the opening of one lesion was a tan blunt object that would retract with pressure.

Protocol for surgical removal:

- local anesthesia
- small incision
- grasp larva with small hemostat
- remove larva
- open packing of wound
- antibiotics as needed

Native remedies include application of pork fat, beeswax, chewing gum, or a drop of nicotine to the larval opening in the skin to interfere with larval respiration and thus prompt migration externally.

Necrobiosis Lipoidica

Aspirin	Benzoyl peroxide
Persantine	Excision and grafting
Triamcinolone, intralesional	

Don't promise too much. This is a disease whose insidious course is measured in years, and it has already scarred by the time you are consulted. Nonetheless, there are things to be done.

Teach the patient to avoid bumps and bruises to the shin, an invariable site of trauma, which accentuate if not initiate the problem. Explain the hazards of physical activities to this area of predilection, ranging from hockey or sailing to simply being clumsy while getting up at night without turning on the lights. Having the patients make a list of hazards increases their self-awareness of this common yet critical self-care factor. One of our patients benefited from lightweight plastic shin guards.

Since two out of three of these patients have diabetes and the others are at risk, careful control and monitoring of the diabetic state are prudent. However, the underlying microangiopathy of these patients does not correlate directly with their diabetic status.

Current management focuses on control of circulating platelet aggregates that localize in areas of trauma, with resulting microvascular occlusion and vasculitis. To prevent heightened platelet aggregability and hypercoagulable blood, long-term aspirin therapy with or without Persantine (dipyridamole) is used to reduce platelet aggregation. Minidose heparin, although not reported, could have the same prophylactic effect as it does in atrophie blanche.

The inflammatory element is most commonly treated with topical or intralesional steroids. In the latter instance, we prefer dilute Kenalog suspension (10 mg/ml diluted 1:10 with 2 per cent Xylocaine) to avoid further atrophy.

Ulcerations, which develop from infarcts in this disease, often respond dramatically to 10 to 20 per cent benzoyl peroxide preparations topically. Some severe ulcerations, however, may necessitate total excision of the lesion and underlying subcutaneous tissue down to fascia, followed by skin grafting to achieve a cure.

Miller SA, Winkelmann RK: Necrobiosis lipoidica diabeticorum: A clinical and pathological investigation of 171 cases. Arch Dermatol 93:272–281, 1966.

Detailed analysis of disorder seen in only 1 of 300 diabetics. Spontaneous resolution occurred in 17 per cent (making anecdotal reports suspect), but one case of involution followed cessation of smoking. The authors favor intralesional steroids.

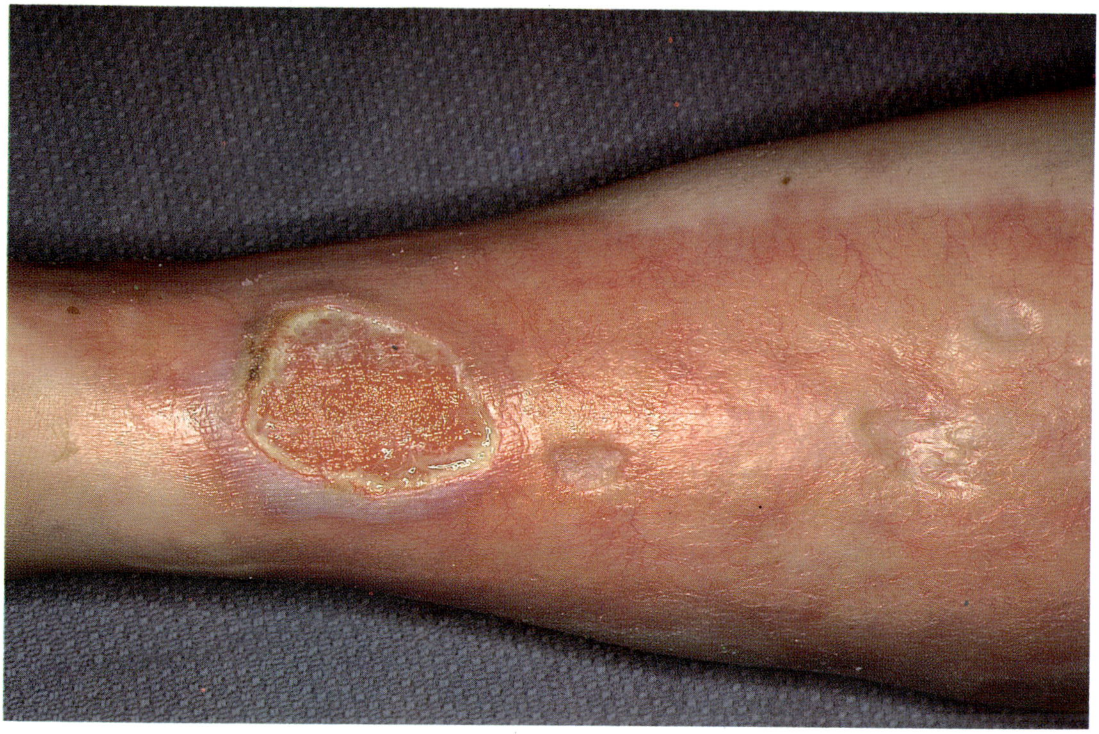

Huntley AC: The cutaneous manifestations of diabetes mellitus. J Am Acad Dermatol 7:427–455, 1982.

Reviews sequence of necrobiosis lipoidica change: occult endothelial cell proliferation, PAS-positive deposits, and basement membrane thickening precede neutrophilic necrotizing vasculitis, collagen destruction, fatty deposits, atrophy, and neovascularization.

Unge G, Tornling G: Treatment of diabetic necrobiosis with aspirin or dipyridamole. N Engl J Med 299:1366, 1978.

Complete healing within five weeks of starting **dipyridamole** (225 mg/day). Case report.

Fjellner B: Treatment of diabetic necrosis with aspirin or dipyridamole. N Engl J Med 299:1366, 1978.

Complete healing with **aspirin** (1.5 to 4.5 gm/day) in two of three patients, after 4 and 12 weeks respectively.

Statham B, Finlay AY, Marks R: A randomized double-blind comparison of an aspirin-dipyridamole combination versus a placebo in the treatment of necrobiosis lipoidica. Acta Derm Venereol 61:270–271, 1981.

When neither patient nor doctor knew what was being given, **aspirin** and **dipyridamole** antiplatelet therapy did nothing in 14 patients.

Karkavitsas K, Miller JA, Dowd PM, Kirby JD: Aspirin in the management of necrobiosis lipoidica. Acta Derm Venereol 62:183, 1982.

A rebuttal, favoring low-dose **aspirin** (3.5 mg/kg every 48 hours) to prevent platelet aggregation without inhibiting elaboration of prostacyclin (a vasodilator, and the natural biologic inhibitor of platelet aggregation). Six of seven patients were helped.

Sahl WT: Necrobiosis lipoidica diabeticorum: Localization in surgical scars. J Cutan Pathol 5:249–253, 1978.

A specific example of localization in traumatized areas.

Ostman J: Can adequate control of diabetes prevent the development of vascular complications? A mini review. Acta Med Scand Suppl 67:5–10, 1983.

Uncertain, despite 58 references.

Hughes A, McVerry BA, Wilkinson L, Goldstone AH, Lewis D, Bloom A: Diabetes, a hypercoagulable state? Hemostatic variables in newly diagnosed type 2 diabetic patients. Acta Haematol 69:254–259, 1983.

More than half the patients have platelet coagulation abnormalities, including platelet aggregates.

Prentice CRM, Lowe GDO: Blood viscosity and the complications of diabetes. Adv Exp Med Biol 164:99–103, 1984.

Blood viscosity is increased, favoring sludging.

Eldor A, Diaz EG, Naparstek E: Treatment of diabetic necrobiosis with aspirin and dipyridamole. N Engl J Med 298:1033, 1978.

Complete healing within six weeks of starting **aspirin** (1 gm/day) and **dipyridamole** (225 mg/day). Case report.

Sidelnikova MV, Zlatkina AR: Lechenie lipoidnogo nekrobioza kozhi geparinom. Vestn Dermatol Venerol 9:64–67, 1977.

Refractory ulcerative lesions of necrobiosis in an 18-year-old girl healed following intralesional injection of **heparin** (2500 U in 5 cc 0.5 per cent Novocain solution) three times a week for three weeks.

Rhodes EL: Fibrinolytic agents in the treatment of necrobiosis lipoidica. Angiology 29:60–64, 1978.

Fibrinolytic agents (**nicotinic acid** derivatives) were helpful in 26 of 30 patients, but only after six months.

Abell E, Sparrow G: Granuloma annulare and necrobiosis lipoidica treated by jet injector. Br J Dermatol 93:85–89, 1975.

Three of five patients injected with **triamcinolone acetonide** (5 mg/ml) showed complete resolution. Do not inject in atrophic sites.

Hanke CW, Bergfeld WF: Treatment with benzoyl peroxide of ulcers on legs within lesion of necrobiosis lipoidica diabeticorum. J Dermatol Surg Oncol 4:701–704, 1978.

Superb result in one patient, using terry cloth dressing impregnated with 20 per cent **benzoyl peroxide** lotion. Apply three times a day, protect normal skin with Vaseline, and cover entire area with Saran wrap. Putrid odor gone in 48 hours, complete healing to firm yellow scars in six weeks. No systemic antibiotics necessary despite aerobic and anaerobic cultures showing *Staphylococcus aureus, Serratia, Pseudomonas aeruginosa*, enterococcus, beta-streptococcus (non group A), *Bacteroides fragilis*, and *Clostridium perfringens*.

Nylen BO, Skoog T: Surgical treatment of necrobiosis lipoidica. Acta Derm Venereol 38:366–371, 1958.

Excellent long-term result in five patients when excision was carried to the level of deep fascia, followed by grafting. There was recurrence in one case in which the subcutaneous fat was left in place.

Marr JJ, Traisman HS, Griffith BH, Schafer MA: Necrobiosis lipoidica diabeticorum in a juvenile diabetic. Treatment by excision and skin grafting. Cutis 19:348–350, 1977.

Single case success, but required subsequent Kenalog 10 injections (1.5 ml) intralesionally for three focal recurrences.

Dubin BJ, Kaplan EN: The surgical treatment of necrobiosis lipoidica diabeticorum. Plast Reconstr Surg 60:421–428, 1977.

Seven cures. Demonstrated deep perforator vessels under center of each lesion. These must be ligated.

Clegg DO, Zone JJ, Piepkorn MW: Necrobiosis lipoidica associated with jejunoileal bypass surgery. Arch Dermatol 118:135–136, 1982.

Developed four years after bypass surgery. Resistant to topical, intralesional, and oral corticosteroids, **aspirin**, and **dipyridamole**. Complete healing within two months after jejunoileal reanastomosis. Convincing photos.

The genius of therapy is blending science, serendipity, and sympathy into your prescription.

Odor

Pimozide
Diet
Metronidazole

Most patients who consult us concerning an offensive body odor have none. What they have is a monosymptomatic hypochondriacal psychosis that manifests itself as a specific delusion of odor. What they need is the new drug, pimozide (Orap 2 to 12 mg in a single dose each day). The delusion is a serious one, leading them into a lonely isolated world. They seek social isolation to avoid the silent rejection they sense in anyone who comes within olfactory range of them.

Most of the patients who have an odor when they consult us are unaware of it, as they have adapted to its presence. The same adaptation accounts for the fact that one is overwhelmed by the aroma of chocolate only on first arriving in Hershey, Pennsylvania. It is these patients who have odor from bacteria acting on their apocrine sweat (bromhidrosis), a *Gardnerella vaginalis* vaginal discharge, a diet of garlic, curry, and beer, incontinence of feces and urine, infected tumors, or even a topical medicament.

Very rarely, the mother's description of a baby's unusual odor will lead to treatment of an underlying metabolic problem. Thus there is an awareness among pediatricians of the mousy, musty odor of babies with phenylketonuria.

Among the rarities of real body odor, which we have seen on eight occasions, is the syndrome of trimethylaminuria. It arises from a failure of liver enzymes to oxidize the trimethylamine absorbed from the gut to a nonodorous form. As a result, the patient smells like rotten fish. Variations in the diet, as well as bacterial flora of the intestine, may account for periods of absence of the odor, so it is well to have the patient seen at a time he and others sense the odor. Gas chromatography of the urine of that day will prove the correctness of the diagnosis, and dietary changes, including elimination of choline, may minimize or eliminate the problem. Avoidance of constipation also helps prevent excessive breakdown of choline and thus decreases odor.

Every patient with odor deserves assessment of its cause and specific treatment. Every patient with the complaint, but not the presence of odor, deserves assessment of the suitability of pimozide therapy.

Riding J, Munro A: Pimozide in the treatment of monosymptomatic hypochondriacal psychosis. Acta Psychiatr Scand 52:23–30, 1975.

Within 3 days, **pimozide** (Orap 2 mg/day) completely cleared the delusion of a 42-year-old man that he was emitting an unpleasant odor due to flatus. Present for six months, the delusional state had led to social isolation and had been unresponsive to phenothiazine drugs (**trifluoperazine, thioridazine,** and **chlorpromazine**). The delusion promptly returned five months later when he stopped the pimozide. Resumption of the drug was soon followed by remission, and he has been free of delusions during two years of continuous pimozide therapy.

Smith M, Smith LG, Levinson B: The use of smell in differential diagnosis. Lancet 2:1452–1453, 1982.

Physicians need to improve their olfactory skills in diagnosis, despite personal distaste for unpleasant odors.

A list of 45 odors and possible explanations includes:

mousy—*Proteus* infection
grapelike—*Pseudomonas*
sweet—marijuana
ammonia—bladder infection
acetone—diabetes mellitus
almond—cyanide poisoning

Lu DP: Halitosis: An etiologic classification, a treatment approach, and prevention. Oral Surg 54:521–526, 1982.

A detailed survey of all aspects, with 46 references. Most cases are caused by bacteria producing hydrogen sulfide, dimethyl sulfide, or methylmercaptan, so that therapy centers on reducing bacteria and these substances. Specifically:

eradication of periodontal pockets
improvement of oral hygiene (brush tongue, teeth, and dentures)
dental care (restore carious teeth, extract unrestorable teeth, regular prophylaxis)
correction of systemic disease
elimination of drugs
protection against xerostomia (stimulate saliva with gum chewing and mint sucking; use **sodium carboxymethyl cellulose** to moisten oral cavity)

Some diseases associated with halitosis:

bronchiectasis
sinusitis
tonsillitis
liver failure
gallbladder dysfunction
kidney failure
scurvy
diabetes mellitus
gastrointestinal disorders
gastrointestinal hemorrhage

Drugs associated with halitosis:

Isordil
ethyl alcohol
iodides
amyl nitrite
chloral hydrate
phenothiazines
dimethyl sulfoxide
antihistamines
antineoplastics
diuretics
tranquilizers
amphetamines

Lists causes of xerostomia:

mouth breathing
heavy smoking
excessive use of mouthwash
aging
diabetes
Sjögren's syndrome
salivary gland aplasia
Mikulicz's disease
macroglobulinemia
radiation therapy
poor oral hygiene
condiments
emotional stress
dehydration
fever
menopause

Eun HC, Kim KH, Lee YS: Unusual body odours due to a nasal foreign body in a child. J Dermatol (Tokyo) 11:501–503, 1984.

Removal of a sponge from the right nostril of a two-year-old gave prompt cure of generalized foul odor. Complete review of the literature.

Molberg P: Body odor from topical benzoyl peroxide. N Engl J Med 304:1366, 1981.

Parents, but not their 15-year-old daughter, noted odor in her clothing and bedding due to the use of **benzoyl peroxide** (10 per cent) topically for acne. To the physician the odor resembled that present in the urine of a patient taking **cloxacillin**, and structural similarities between benzoyl peroxide and cloxacillin were noted, suggesting a common metabolic by-product. Stopping the benzoyl peroxide cleared the odor.

Ashford RFU, Plant GT, Maher J, et al: Metronidazole in smelly tumors. Lancet 1:874–875, 1980.

The putrid odor from anaerobic infection of a fungating metastatic breast tumor of the chest wall was eliminated in a 48-year-old woman by administration of **metronidazole** (Flagyl 200 mg tid). The therapy has allowed the patient to continue working as a teacher.

Shelley ED, Shelley WB: The fish odor syndrome: Trimethylaminuria. JAMA 251:253–255, 1984.

Elimination of fish, eggs, liver, and kidney from the diet immediately lessened the rotten fish odor emanating from a 31-year-old profoundly retarded man with trimethylaminuria. Complete control required a two-week course of **metronidazole** (250 mg tid) and further restriction of soybeans, peas, and mayonnaise from his diet.

Fenwick GR, Butler EJ, Brewster MA: Are Brassica vegetables aggravating factors in trimethylaminuria (fish odour syndrome)? Lancet 2:916, 1983.

Studies with the problem of fishy taint in hens' eggs revealed that cabbage, cauliflower, Brussels sprouts, swede (rutabaga), and kohlrabi contain a chemical that inhibits the liver oxidase responsible for converting the malodorous trimethylamine into its nonvolatile N-oxide. This report suggests that patients with fish odor syndrome should avoid these vegetables, as well as choline (a precursor of trimethylamine), eggs, fish, and legumes.

Rothschild JG, Hausen RC: Fish odor syndrome: Trimethylaminuria with milk as chief dietary factor. Pediatr Dermatol 3:38–39, 1985.

A 10-year-old boy, who consumed two to three liters of milk daily, had been noted to smell like rotten fish for two years, with the odor most noticeable in the summer after exercise. Elimination of milk remarkably decreased the odor, and rechallenge with milk doubled the trimethylamine (TMA) urinary excretion and resulted in recurrence of odor. It is likely that he was drinking milk from cows fed from a wheat pasture, as such milk may contain large amounts of TMA N-oxide. Avoidance of milk and dietary choline (also found in wheat germ, yeast, and lecithin) greatly helped this patient.

Koblenzer CS: The dysmorphic syndrome. Arch Dermatol 121:780–784, 1985.

Haloperidol in low dose (Haldol, 1 to 2 mg/day) is invaluable therapy for patients who have the dysmorphic syndrome, i.e., patients with serious delusions concerning their body structure or function. Eleven such patients treated with this low dose of haloperidol were all symptom-free while taking the drug over a period of 3 months to 3½ years.

Their dysmorphic delusions included body odors causing social ostracism, water-soluble skin (never to be washed), and intense burning of lips, tongue, scalp, or vulva. But most dramatic was the "Haldol help" given a woman who had previously spent $12,000 over a 4½-year period seeing 60 physicians for relief of fancied yet painful distortion of her facial contour.

Chance favors those who take chances.

Onychomycosis

Griseofulvin
Ketoconazole
Loprox cream
Urea ointment

No area of the skin provides a safer haven for invading pathogens than the nail plate. Dermatophytes and yeasts, easily erased from the general skin surface by topical treatment, burrow into hard keratin of the nail plate and live there with impunity. Their eradication calls for prolonged systemic therapy.

If success is to be achieved in fungal infection of the fingernails, the patient should be treated with a daily dose of 1 or 2 gm of griseofulvin for five months. If headaches develop, a lower dose may be tried. In every instance the effectiveness of the drug must be monitored by four- to six-week checkups. At least 2 mm of new healthy nail plate should appear proximally every month. A small file or razor blade mark on the nail plate aids in this evaluation. If no progress is being made with griseofulvin, the dose should be increased or ketoconazole (200 mg or 400 mg/day) should be substituted. If nail growth is slow as a result of age or trauma, zinc supplementation (220 mg tid) or vitamin A (water solubilized, 50,000 U tid) may prove valuable. In a few instances thyroid supplement has been critical. Through all this, regular monitoring of the CBC and blood chemistry profile is appropriate. To eliminate such a prolonged course in the patient with only one or two involved nails, the nail may be surgically avulsed and the bed curetted. Afterward, a short one- to two-month course of griseofulvin or ketoconazole should be prescribed during the early nail replacement growth period.

The treatment of infected toenails is even more arduous, since the growth rate is usually less than one-half that of the fingernails, and the patient may have to take griseofulvin or ketoconazole for as long as two years. The therapy never converts the dystrophic nail plate back to normal, but only allows new healthy nail to form, with resultant slow extrusion of the dystrophic infected nail plate. In an older patient who claims he never has to cut his toenails, it seems futile to start therapy. Furthermore, in view of the high recurrence rate, we usually do not treat asymptomatic onychomycosis of the toes. However, we do treat onychomycosis of the toenails in individuals with ingrown nails, trichophytids, urticaria, or vasculitis of the lower legs.

We generally use Loprox cream topically after the bath or hand wash, as it appears to have the greatest penetrant capability. As a powerful fungicide, it reduces the opportunity for spread to the surrounding skin or other uninfected nails.

Although we have not used keratolytics and occlusion for the chemical removal of nails, a number of therapists employ 40 per cent urea ointment for nail plate dissolution and removal. This is followed by long-term topical imidazole antifungal therapy.

Zaias N, Drachman D: A method for the determination of drug effectiveness in onychomycosis: Trials with ketoconazole and griseofulvin ultramicrosize. J Am Acad Dermatol 9:912–919, 1983.

Rule:

Do not continue treatment if you fail to see 2 mm of new healthy nail plate in great toenails each month. For accurate measure, mark nail plate adjacent to onychomycotic border with a transverse cut and fill with ink.

Rule:

After clinical cure use topical antifungal cream for one year to prevent reinfection.

Results:

Griseofulvin (7 cases)
- 0 cleared with 500 mg/day
- 4 cleared with 1000 mg/day, but all relapsed within six months after stopping medication
- 3 failures with 1000 mg/day

Ketoconazole (9 cases)
- 4 cleared with 200 mg/day
- 3 cleared with 400 mg/day
- 1 improved 80 per cent
- 1 failure with 400 mg/day

Anderson DW: Griseofulvin: Biology and clinical usefulness. Ann Allergy 23:103–110, 1965.

Literature cure rates: fingernails 57 per cent
toenails 17 per cent

Minimal treatment times: fingernails 4 months
toenails 6 months

With aging, as nail growth slows, longer treatment times are required.

Hägermark Ö, Berlin A, Wallin I, Boréus LD: Plasma concentrations of griseofulvin in healthy volunteers and outpatients treated for onychomycosis. Acta Derm Venereol 56:289–296, 1976.

Griseofulvin (500 mg/day for 6 to 24 months) cleared the condition in 11 of 27 patients, with partial improvement also seen in 15 patients. In patients with partial healing there was stagnation of improvement 5 to 20 months into therapy for reasons unknown. Increasing the dose of griseofulvin to 1 gm/day cleared two and improved three additional cases.

Galimberti R, Negroni R, Iglesia de Elias Costa MR, Casala AM: The activity of ketoconazole in the treatment of onychomycosis. Rev Infect Dis 2:596–598, 1980.

Ketoconazole (200 mg daily for seven months) cleared more than 66 per cent of 70 cases of onychomycosis due to either *Trichophyton rubrum* or candidiasis.

Botter AA, Nuijten STM: Further experiences with ketoconazole in the treatment of onychomycosis. Mykosen 24:156–166, 1981.

With ketoconazole (200 or 400 mg/day) the cure rate was 96 per cent for 161 mycotic nails. In 10 of the 41 patients studied a daily dose of 400 mg was required for success. Median treatment time for success was 39 weeks. New healthy nail growth appeared at 2 to 22 weeks (median 8 weeks). Most patients had *Trichophyton rubrum* infections, including four patients not cured after two years of treatment with doses up to 400 mg/day. No side effects were seen.

Candida species caused 40 per cent of onychomycosis of fingernails, but only 10 per cent of toenail infections. Treatment time needed for cure was no different from that for *Trichophyton* infections.

Török I, Simon G, Pap M: An evaluation of two years clinical experience with ketoconazole. Mykosen 25:136–142, 1982.

Twenty-six patients with onychomycosis due to yeasts received ketoconazole (200 mg/day) for 4 to 11 months (mean 7 months): 18 cured, 6 improved, 2 no change.

Farber EM, South DA: Urea ointment in the nonsurgical avulsion of nail dystrophies. Cutis 22:689–692, 1978.

Formulation:

urea	40 per cent
anhydrous lanolin	20 per cent
white wax	5 per cent
white petrolatum	35 per cent

Technique:

1. Protect skin around nail with adhesive tape (over tincture of benzoin).
2. Generously apply thick **urea** paste to nail and cover with plastic wrap under adhesive tape (must be kept dry).
3. After 7 to 10 days lift off nail plate and curette base.
4. Follow with antifungal cream or 3 per cent **thymol** in chloroform twice a day.

Rollman O: Treatment of onychomycosis by partial nail avulsion and topical miconazole. Dermatologica 165:54–61, 1982.

Partially avulse nails, using bone and chalazion ophthalmic curettes, after occlusion with **urea** ointment for three to four days. Use Blenderm no. 1525 plastic tape 25 mm wide for occlusion. Repeat procedure three times, including lateral sulci. Then apply **miconazole** solution 2 per cent (Monistat-Derm) twice a day for eight weeks. Cure rate six months later: 60 per cent of 45 nails in 12 patients. Best for nails with less than 50 per cent involvement of nail bed surface. Very time consuming if several nails involved.

Ishii M, Hamada T, Asai Y: Treatment of onychomycosis by ODT therapy with 20% urea ointment and 2% tolnaftate ointment. Dermatologica 167:273–279, 1983.

Occlusive dressing therapy (ODT) to fingers and toes once daily for 12 to 24 hours cleared onychomycosis in 14 of 20 patients. Maceration without pain appeared in one week, and onycholysis followed in about 33 per cent. Treatment time 1 to 12 months, until newly developed nail appeared normal.

Nolting S: Non-traumatic removal of the nail and simultaneous treatment of onychomycosis. Dermatologica 169(Suppl 1):117–120, 1984.

Principles of treatment:

Identify causative fungi with KOH preparation and culture (to avoid using antifungals unnecessarily).

Remove as much fungus-infected nail as possible (to increase drug bioavailability).

Both doctor and patient must "show a sufficient degree of willingness, consistent action, and perseverance."

Food for thought: Is it necessary to expose 50 to 70 kg of body tissue to an antimycotic drug to reach only 5 to 7 gm of mycotic tissue?

Outlines use of ointment containing **urea** 40 per cent and **bifonazole** 1 per cent for 4 to 14 days to chemically remove nail, followed by bifonazole cream or gel (1 per cent bid). (Bifonazole is a new broad-spectrum antimycotic imidazole derivative [Mycospor—Bayer, Germany—not available in the United States]). Cure rate: "about 50 per cent."

Dorn M, Kienitz T, Ryckmanns F: Onychomykose: Erfahrungen mit atraumatischer Nagelentfernung. Hautarzt 31:30–34, 1980.

Potassium iodide ointment (KI 50 per cent) under adhesive was used by 250 patients to remove 1500 nails chemomechanically. This treatment was combined with **griseofulvin** and topical antifungal preparations. After six months, 101 patients were cured, but the relapse rate was 50 per cent. The authors favor atraumatic nail avulsion as a painless effective alternative to surgical excision in treating onychomycosis.

Kavli G, Midelfart K, Moseng D, et al: *Trichophyton rubrum*–infected toenails treated with ketoconazole and partial nail avulsion. Dermatologica 169:191–193, 1984.

Ketoconazole (Nizoral 200 mg daily) alone for four months gave a cure rate of only 28 per cent, but when combined with **urea** cream (40 per cent) occlusion for one week to give nail debridement (done two weeks after starting ketoconazole), the cure rate was 53 per cent. Final examination was six months after completion of therapy.

Brem J: Effective topical method of therapy for onychomycosis. Cutis 27:69–76, 1981.

How to reach fungi located deep within keratin:

1. Cleanse nail with soap, water, and alcohol.
2. Drill multiple wells in nail plate 2 to 3 mm apart in form of crescent 2 mm distal to cuticle (use sterile 18-gauge needle or power drill with dental burr).
3. Apply **dichloroacetic acid** to wells with a round toothpick.
4. Repeat weekly until nail is covered with a network of holes.
5. Apply keratolytic and fungicidal ointment twice a day to nail plate (**salicylic acid** 6 per cent and **sulfur** 6 per cent in petrolatum).
6. To remove loose nail plate, apply 5 per cent **papain** solution at bedtime for two weeks (as wet dressing under plastic bag).

The above method may also be used to remove large plantar calluses that may also contain fungal hyphae in patients with onychomycosis (or tinea pedis).

Vanderdonckt J, Lauwers W, Bockaert J: Miconazole alcoholic solution in the treatment of mycotic nail infections. Mykosen 19:251–256, 1976.

Miconazole (2 per cent alcoholic solution) applied twice a day for eight months cleared 15 of 20 mycotic nails in 19 male long-term patients. Nurses applied the medication carefully under the front edge and along lateral edges and cuticles of affected nails.

Battistini F, Zaias N, Sierra R, Rebell G: Clinical antifungal activity of thiabendazole. Arch Dermatol 109:695–699, 1974.

Thiabendazole (10 per cent in vanishing cream) applied twice a day under occlusion for four months cleared one of four cases of *Trichophyton rubrum* onychomycosis.

Suringa DWR: Treatment of superficial onychomycosis with topically applied glutaraldehyde. Arch Dermatol 102:163–167, 1970.

Twenty-one toenails on four patients were cleared after application twice a day of 10 per cent aqueous **glutaraldehyde** solution (sodium bicarbonate buffer to pH 7.8, Tween 80 0.1 per cent). Treatment time four weeks to four months, depending on depth of infection in nail plate.

Baran R, Hay RJ: Partial surgical avulsion of the nail in onychomycosis. Clin Exp Dermatol 10:413–418, 1985.

Twenty cases of onychomycosis were successfully treated by combining systemic or topical antifungal agents with surgical removal of only the segment of the nail plate harboring the disease. Parsimony in practice!

It's not how much you read, but what you read that counts.

Orf

Subsection
Idoxuridine

We feel strongly that superficial subsection of this localized bullous viral infection provides immediate relief and cure. The diagnosis is confirmed with electron microscopy by finding typical parapox virions in the skin specimen.

Leavell UM Jr, McNamara MJ, Muelling R, et al: Orf: Report of 19 human cases with clinical and pathological observations. JAMA 204:657–664, 1968.

Nineteen cases of orf healed spontaneously with no scar in an average of 36 days. The natural clinical progression of lesions involves:

Clinical stages	***Duration, days***
Maculopapular	1–7
Target	7–14
Acute	14–21
Regenerative	21–28
Papillomatous	28–35
Regressive	35 to cure

Shelley WB, Shelley ED: Surgical treatment of farmyard pox: Orf, milker's nodules, bovine papular stomatitis pox. Cutis 31:191–192, 1983.

Immediate superficial epidermal removal of the localized bullous lesions of orf by razor blade transection reduces the healing time to one week and eliminates the potential for lymphangitis, lymphadenopathy, secondary bacterial infection, dissemination of lesions, and erythema multiforme. Just because a lesion is viral and self-limited, there is no need to let it run its disagreeable course for more than one month.

Falk ES: Parapoxvirus infections of reindeer and musk ox associated with unusual human infections. Br J Dermatol 99:647–654, 1978.

In four cases curettage was done after 4, 6, 12, and 20 weeks, and the lesions healed in 2 to 3 weeks without scarring, whereas five cases were not treated, and the lesions healed with local dark pigmentation after 26 weeks.

Behl PN: Practice of Dermatology, 2nd ed. Delhi, Oxford Printcraft India, in association with Arnold-Heinemann, 1972, 528 pp.

Curettage of lesions of orf is advised.

Lang HA: Human orf. Br Med J 2:1566, 1961.

After excision of sodden skin at the base of a necrotic papule of orf, the scissors used were cleansed in alcohol but not sterilized by boiling. Subsequent use of these scissors on the same day to remove sutures from another patient led to the appearance of orf at the suture site two to three weeks later.

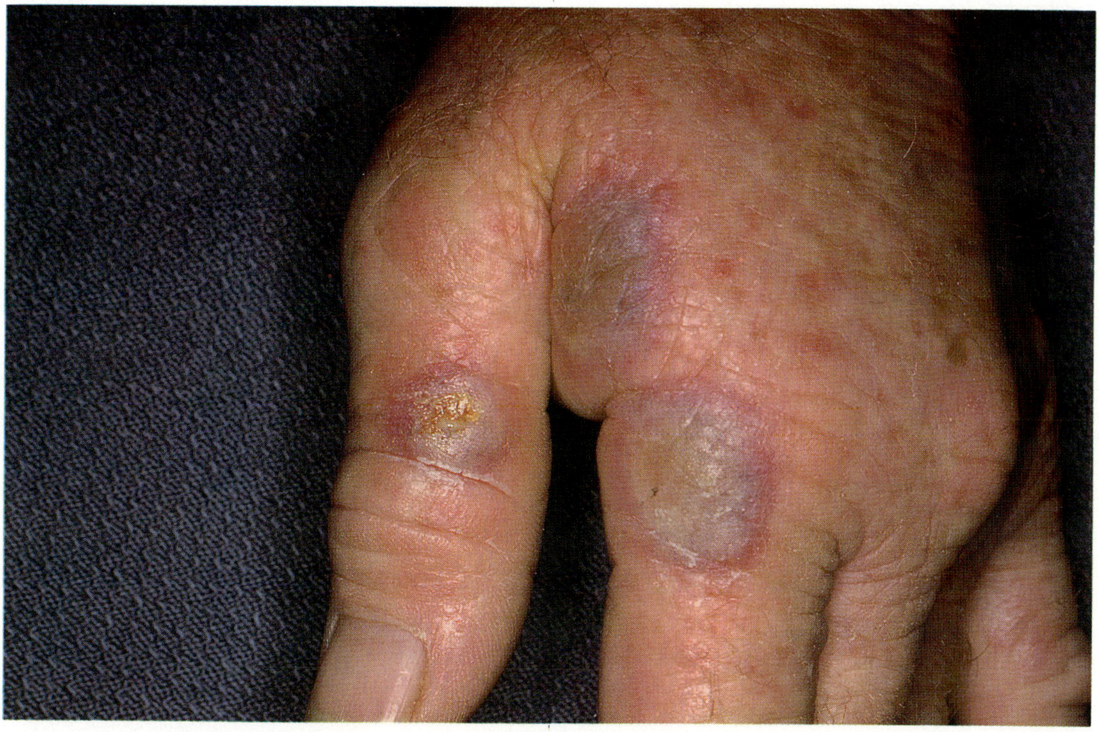

Hunskaar S: A case of ecthyma contagiosum (human orf) treated with iodoxuridine. Dermatologica 168:207, 1984.

Application of **iodoxuridine** (idoxuridine 40 per cent in DMSO three times a day for six days) produced definite improvement in a lesion of orf in a 53-year-old woman. The lesion completely healed in 18 to 20 days.

Savage J, Black MM: "Giant" orf of finger in a patient with a lymphoma. Proc R Soc Med 65:766–768, 1972.

Amputation of the finger was required in a 65-year-old man receiving chemotherapy for a lymphocytic lymphoma after an orf lesion enlarged over two months to 5 cm in diameter and 3 cm in depth.

Idoxuridine (20 per cent DMSO) was suggested as another treatment of orf (also good on infected sheep).

Reading a book on medical malpractice lets you know how a duck feels reading a book on duck hunting.

Ervin Epstein

Parapsoriasis en Plaques

Topical steroids PUVA Nitrogen mustard BCNU

The synonymy of parapsoriasis is unrivaled by any other disease in dermatology. However, even being in nosologic command grants no therapeutic edge to the clinician. None of the innumerable variants responds well to therapy.

The issue, and it is always decided histologically, is whether or not a T-cell lymphoma is evolving or mycosis fungoides is emerging. Although this transformation is rare, parapsoriasis patients at the very least need monitoring throughout the years of their often asymptomatic lesions. We are of the school that favors a conservative approach to parapsoriasis en plaques. We try to bring sunlight in the patients' lives in more than one way. We try to reassure them, but ask for annual "birthday" checkups, as well as "stat" review if noticeable changes occur. We explain that we have two patients who have coexisted pleasantly with their large brown plaques for 40 and 50 years respectively.

We recommend a mild steroid cream if the plaques are pruritic, but generally our role is more that of a safety officer than a fireman. We do not use topical nitrogen mustard until there is a fire.

Lambert WC, Everett MA: The nosology of parapsoriasis. J Am Acad Dermatol 5:373–395, 1981.

All forms of this confusing, confused, confounding, and confounded complex respond poorly to treatment.

Shelley ED, Shelley WB: Chronic dermatitis simulating small-plaque parapsoriasis due to cyanoacrylate adhesive used on fingernails. JAMA 252:2455–2456, 1984.

Cure of a parapsoriasis-like eruption in a 66-year-old woman was achieved by avoidance of an ethyl cyanoacrylate adhesive (Krazy Glue) she had been using to strengthen her brittle fingernails.

Powell FC, Spiegel GT, Muller SA: Treatment of parapsoriasis and mycosis fungoides: The role of psoralen and long-wave ultraviolet light A (PUVA). Mayo Clin Proc 59:538–546, 1984.

PUVA therapy produced excellent results in 12 patients with parapsoriasis. Complete clearing was achieved in all 7 patients with the en plaques type (average dose 406 joules/sq cm [range 118 to 1665] given in 57 sessions [range 29 to 147]). Of three patients with pityriasis lichenoides acuta and chronica one showed complete clearing, while the other two had greater than 80 per cent clearing (average dose 281 joules/sq cm [range 189 to 307] given in 39 sessions [range 26 to 57]). One case of atrophic parapsoriasis and one case of digitate parapsoriasis also showed considerable improvement.

Fischer T, Skogk M: Treatment of parapsoriasis en plaques, mycosis fungoides and Sezary's syndrome with trioxsalen baths followed by ultraviolet light. Acta Derm Venereol 59:171–173, 1979.

In three patients with parapsoriasis en plaques, **trioxsalen** baths and UVA therapy (dysprosium lamps) for two to six months completely or almost completely healed the lesions. UVA light therapy (five days per week for two months, then two days per week for two months, then once weekly maintenance) was preceded by a 15-minute bath containing the photosensitizer trioxsalen (0.1 liter of 0.05 per cent in 70 per cent ethanol added to 150 liters of 37°C water).

Zackheim HS, Epstein EH Jr, McNutt NS, et al: Topical carmustine (BCNU) for mycosis fungoides and related disorders: A 10-year experience. J Am Acad Dermatol 9:363–374, 1983.

Two patients with parapsoriasis en plaques responded well to the application of the nitrosourea compound **carmustine** (BCNU 10 mg/60 ml of 95 per cent ethyl alcohol applied daily for two months).

Wiskemann A: Radiation therapy of psoriasis and parapsoriasis. Z Hautkr 57:1317–1324, 1982.

The author prefers the milder UVB therapy for treating pityriasis lichenoides chronica, but PUVA for parapsoriasis en plaques and parapsoriasis variegata. Of 36 PUVA-treated parapsoriasis patients 30 were clear after an average of 26 treatments.

Vella Briffa D, Warin AP, Calnan CD: Parakeratosis variegata: A report of two cases and their treatment with PUVA. Clin Exp Dermatol 4:537–541, 1979.

Two patients with this rare retiform parapsoriasis responded well to PUVA therapy, but the cosmetically disturbing reticulate hyperpigmentation was not altered.

Outdated magazines belong in the Boy Scout paper drive—not in your waiting room.

Pediculosis

Kwell	Prioderm
RID	Bactrim
Eurax	Nix

The ad reads, "The only disease you can cure in 4 minutes." And it is true. But just to be sure, in actual practice we leave the insecticidal shampoo (Kwell) on for 10 minutes before washing it out. A second 10-minute treatment is also necessary in seven days to kill newly hatched larvae, which were protected from the first dose by an egg casing coated with an impermeable cement substance.

It is impressive therapy and a public health triumph. Lice are more than a cosmetic problem and more than a source of pruritus. They are carriers of diseases, many of which we know and others we probably do not even suspect. Their eradication is important for both the private health of the individual and the public health of the community.

We not only have Kwell or Scabene (gamma benzene hexachloride, i.e., lindane) to kill lice, but also a number of equally effective and safe alternates. The insecticidal pyrethrins from the chrysanthemum plant are available over the counter (RID, A-200 Pyrinate), and a 10-minute application, repeated in a week, here too is curative.

And the list of therapeutic weapons grows. Now it is possible to kill the louse by paralyzing his cholinesterase, using the cholinesterase inhibitors malathion (Prioderm lotion) or the carbamates.

DDT, the wonder "delousing drug" of World War II, is no longer used because it is an environmental hazard and because of the fact that lice grew indifferent to it. Fortunately there is no evidence of resistance of the community or the louse to the new spate of sophisticated insecticides being used today. We suspect that treatment for pediculosis has reached its climax stage.

But treatment of your private patient and his contacts is the easy part. The challenge is eradication of the infestational pool. At least five million children in the United States have pediculosis capitis. The constant "pollination of pathogens" from head to head has to be a health threat in the transmission of systemic disease. The public must be educated to this hazard and how it can be eliminated. It is a problem for which we know the cause, the epidemiology, and the cure. We must not let the louse, which brought us typhus, continue to bring us disease.

The time has come to make *Pediculus humanus* not merely an endangered species but an extinct species. Let's do it.

Buxton PA: The Louse: An Account of the Lice That Infest Man, Their Medical Importance and Control. Baltimore, Williams & Wilkins Co., 1940, 115 pp.

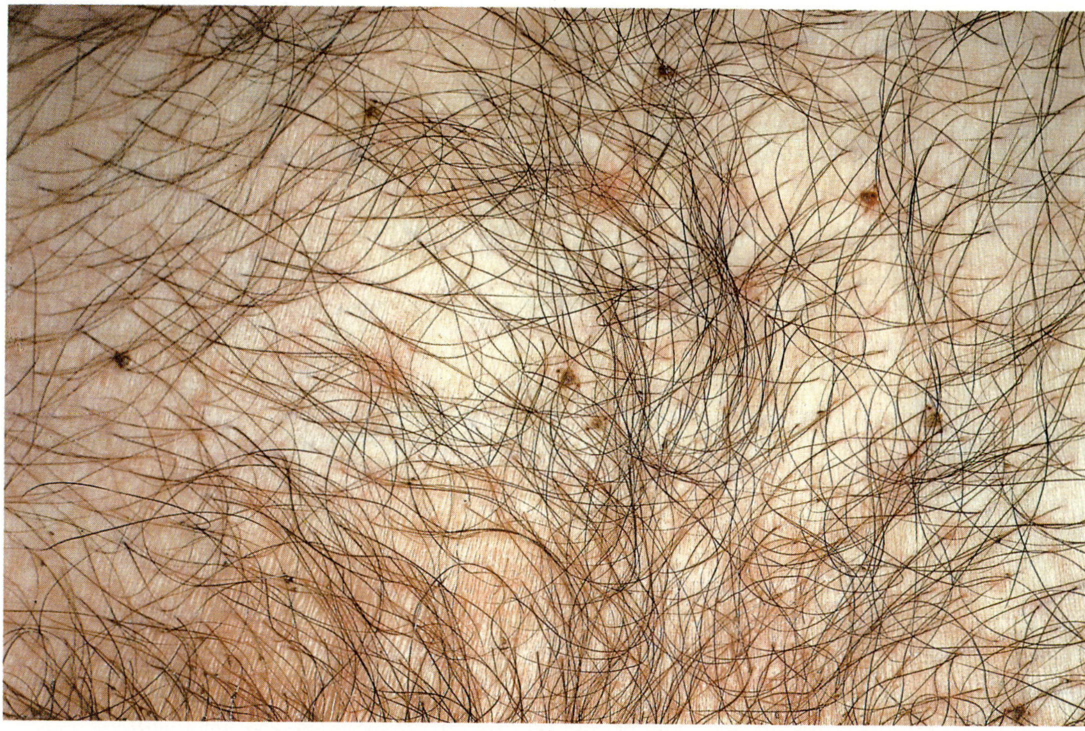

Use magnifying lens here—as well as in office.

A classic reference concerning the lowly louse that brought armies to their knees with disease (typhus, trench fever, relapsing fever). For nine centuries the louse had been brought to its knees with quicksilver (mercury) ointment, but at the time of this account (which predated DDT), the armies were using pure kerosene, 25 per cent gasoline in petrolatum, or 25 per cent xylene in Vaseline and lanolin, to do battle with this little enemy.

Rasmussen JE: Pediculosis and the pediatrician. Pediatr Dermatol 2:74–79, 1984.

All of the following treatments are truly effective:

1. Kwell or Scabene shampoo (1 per cent **lindane**): Leave on 10 minutes.
2. **Crotamiton** lotion 10 per cent (Eurax): Leave on 24 hours.
3. **Malathion** 0.5 per cent lotion (Prioderm lotion): Leave on 12 hours (cholinesterase inhibitor).
4. RID or A-200 Pyrinate gel (**pyrethrins** 0.3 per cent, usually combined with piperonyl butoxide 3.0 per cent and petroleum distillate 1.2 per cent in an inert vehicle): Apply for 10 minutes, then wash off with soap or mild shampoo (over the counter).

For pediculosis of the eyelashes—alternative treatments:

petrolatum (Vaseline three to five times daily).

physostigmine ophthalmic solution or ointment 0.25 per cent (Eserine several times a day for three days).

fluorescein drops to eyelids and eyelashes.

yellow oxide of mercury 0.1 per cent (now an outmoded treatment).

Fine BC: Pediculosis capitis. N Engl J Med 309:1461, 1983.

Eggs are laid and cemented to the hair just above the skin surface, thus providing warmth from the skin for hatching. As hair grows and the eggs hatch 10 days later, empty gray nits are carried outward. Use of a nit comb with fine teeth is a cosmetic maneuver only, since it debrides the distal empty egg capsules but not the viable lice eggs at the base of the hair.

To stop an epidemic, careful inspection must be made of others at home and at school. Regular brushing and combing at bedtime will injure and dislodge many lice acquired through direct head-to-head contact during the school day.

Karacic I, Yawalkar SJ: A single application of crotamiton lotion in the treatment of patients with pediculosis capitis. Int J Dermatol 21:611–613, 1982.

Crotamiton lotion (Eurax, 10 per cent crotonyl-N-ethyl-o-toluidine), a croton oil derivative toxic to lice, applied to the scalp for 24 hours cured 96 per cent of 49 patients with pediculosis capitis. After a shampoo, nits were removed each day thereafter for seven days using a fine-tooth comb dipped in 5 per cent acetic acid. A second treatment was rarely needed when patients were examined on the eighth day. Bedding and clothing were laundered or dry cleaned after completion of treatment.

Taplin D, Castillero PM, Spiegel J, et al: Malathion for treatment of *Pediculus humanus* var *capitis* infestation. JAMA 247:3103–3105, 1982.

Prioderm lotion (0.5 per cent **malathion** in isopropyl alcohol), an organic phosphate insecticide, provides a powerful alternate to lindane. Used in a double-blind study of 115 children with head lice on the San Blas Islands in Panama, it cured 95 per cent when applied for 12 hours. It is ovicidal as well as pediculocidal. It is hoped that a resistant strain of louse will not emerge if reinfestation can be stopped by the residual effect of malathion.

Mathias RG, Huggins DR, Leroux SJ, Proctor EM: Comparative trial of treatment with Prioderm lotion and Kwellada shampoo in children with head lice. Can Med Assoc J 130:407–409, 1984.

Prioderm lotion (0.5 per cent **malathion** in isopropanol, applied for two hours) and Kwellada shampoo (1 per cent **lindane** applied for five minutes) were compared in a study of 62 children with pediculosis capitis. Both preparations killed all lice present, but at seven days live lice were found on the scalps of 2 of 29 patients treated with Prioderm and in 4 of 33 treated with Kwellada. This supports the view that these regimens are not completely ovicidal and that all patients should be retreated after seven days to kill the second generation before further eggs are laid.

Maunder JW: Clinical and laboratory trials employing carbaryl against the human head-louse, *Pediculosis humanus capitis* (de Geer). Clin Exp Dermatol 6:605–612, 1981.

Carbaryl 0.5% (naphthyl-1-yl methylcarbamate) used as a lotion kept on 24 hours or a shampoo kept on 3 minutes gave a 98 per cent cure rate in 81 children with pediculosis capitis. The reinfection rate at one month was 2.5 per cent. This compound is not available in the United States (except as the agricultural insecticide Sevin), but is marketed in the United Kingdom as Caryl Derm and also as Derbac.

Fine BC: Controversy about pediculosis capitis. N Engl J Med 311:801, 1984.

An articulate informal plea for using **malathion** and licensing **carbaryl** in the United States for treating pediculosis capitis. Malathion has great residual pediculocidal activity in the hair up to five weeks after treatment.

Smith DE, Walsh J: Treatment of pubic lice infestation: A comparison of two agents. Cutis 26:618–619, 1980.

Ten minutes of contact with RID (a **pyrethrin**-based pediculocide made from chrysanthemums, an over-the-counter product) was as effective as four minutes' contact with Kwell shampoo (1 per cent lindane or **gamma benzene hexachloride**) in eradicating pediculosis pubis in 30 patients. No recurrence was seen at seven days.

Couch JM, Green WR, Hirst LW, De La Cruz ZC: Diagnosing and treating *Phthirus pubis* palpebrarum. Surv Ophthalmol 26:219–225, 1982.

Do not get Kwell or A-200 Pyrinate near the eyes.

Ideal treatment of lice infestation of eyelids: Mechanical removal of lice and nits.

Alternate treatments:

1. **Yellow oxide of mercury** 1 per cent ophthalmic ointment (twice daily for one week)
2. **Ammoniated mercury** 3 per cent ophthalmic ointment (twice daily for one week)
3. Eserine (**physostigmine**) 0.25 per cent in petrolatum ointment twice daily for 10 days.

Check for pediculosis pubis in the patient, family, sexual contacts, or close companions.

Discard used cosmetics.

Heat-disinfect clothing at 50°C for 30 minutes (accomplished with high settings on home washers and dryers).

Mathew M, D'Souza P, Mehta DK: A new treatment of phthiriasis palpebrarum. Ann Ophthalmol 14:439–441, 1982.

Application of freshly prepared 20 per cent **fluorescein** eye drops (one or two drops) to the lid margins is instantly lethal to the *Phthirus pubis* louse and nits. Reapply once 10 days later to kill any new generation lice. The dead lice and nits may be removed with forceps or a cotton swab.

Awan KJ: Cryotherapy in phthiriasis palpebrarum. Am J Ophthalmol 83:906–907, 1977.

An ingenious use of a cryoprobe to kill each louse roosting on an eyelash. Slit-lamp illumination was used and the eyelashes were moistened with normal saline prior to freezing each louse. Must avoid freezing the eyelid skin. (What next—the laser?)

Scott MJ, Esterly NB: Eyelash infestation by *Phthirus pubis* as a manifestation of child abuse. Pediatr Dermatol 1:179, 1983.

The crab louse on the eyelash led to the "pubic louse" responsible for sexually abusing this four-year-old girl.

Shashindran CH, Gandhi IS, Krishnasamy S, Ghosh MN: Oral therapy of pediculosis capitis with cotrimoxazole. Br J Dermatol 98:699–700, 1978.

A serendipitous discovery that lice that feed on patients who are taking Bactrim leave the patient within 12 to 48 hours and are found dead in the bed clothes. A study of 20 patients with pediculosis capitis who took **cotrimoxazole** (Bactrim or Septra 1 tablet bid for three days) proved this systemic therapy to be regularly effective. Since medication in the blood has no effect on the eggs, the course of treatment must be repeated after 10 days. Neither **trimethoprim** 80 mg nor **sulfamethoxazole** 400 mg alone was effective.

Brenner S, Ophir J, Krakowski A: Pediculid—An unusual -id reaction to pediculosis capitis. Dermatologica 168:189–191, 1984.

Treatment of pediculosis capitis cleared two children of a fine generalized pruritic skin-colored papular rash, which represented a pediculid.

Munkvad IM, Klemp P: Co-existence of venereal infection and pediculosis pubis. Acta Derm Venereol 62:366–367, 1982.

During a five-year study of 69 women and 167 men with pediculosis pubis, 5 per cent of the men were found to have syphilis. Gonorrhea was also found in 7.2 per cent of the men and 15.3 per cent of the women.

Moral: Every patient with pediculosis pubis should have tests for gonorrhea and syphilis.

Hoffman G: Epidemiology and control of pediculosis capitis infestation in the Federal Republic of Germany. J R Soc Health 103:88–92, 1983.

Disinfection of rooms, upholstered furniture, and carpets is not necessary except in rare instances, since eggs dropping to the floor will not develop and hatch into larvae if the temperature is below 22°C. Lice on fomites may also be killed by cooling (−10 to −15°C for one day), heating (45°C hot air for 16 minutes—e.g., shawls, caps, wigs in drying hood), and starvation by isolation of the object.

The increase in head louse infestation is shown to be due to:

1. Increased communal facilities—holiday camps, kindergartens, day homes for children, sports centers
2. Bus transportation
3. Vacation tourism

There is no evidence that lice have acquired resistance to any medications. 35 valuable references.

Sinniah B, Shekhar C, Ramphal L, Senan P: Pediculosis among rural school children in Kelang, Selangor, Malaysia and their susceptibility to malathion, carbaryl, perigen and kerosene. J R Soc Health 104:114–115, 118, 1984.

In a primary school population of 1243 children (41.5 per cent of whom had pediculosis capitis), the following insecticides gave these cure rates:

Insecticide	***Application time***	***Cure rate (%)***
Carbaryl (0.6 per cent)	15 min	100.0
Permethrin (0.1 per cent)	15 min	97.6
Malathion (0.5 per cent)	24 hr	91.5
Kerosene (undiluted)	24 hr	87.5

None of these agents affected the eggs.

Long hair favors spreading of lice.

Unless the infested members of the family, friends, and schoolmates are treated, recurrence is the rule.

Meinking TL, Taplin D, Kalter DC, Eberle MW: Comparative efficacy of treatments for pediculosis capitis infestations. Arch Dermatol 122:267–271, 1986.

Using viable eggs and head lice from infested children, six pediculicides were tested:

Agent	***Time Required to Kill Lice***	***Per cent of Eggs That Hatched***
Prioderm Lotion (malathion)	5 minutes	5%
Synergized pyrethrin products (Rid, R&C Shampoo, A-200 Pyrinate Shampoo, A-200 Pyrinate Liquid)	10 to 23 minutes	23 to 32%
Kwell shampoo (1% lindane)	180 minutes	30%

These in vitro results were validated by clinical trials.

Happiness is seeing that new drug work on that old patient.

Pemphigus Erythematosus

Corticosteroids	Sunscreens
Sulfapyridine	Chloroquine
Azathioprine	Beta-blockers
Cyclophosphamide	
Methotrexate	

This is a hybrid disease, part pemphigus and part lupus erythematosus, which calls for hybrid therapy. The keystone is prednisone, but the arch must be completed with the supporting stones of cyclophosphamide or azathioprine. Topically our favorite is Diprolene ointment (betamethasone 0.05 per cent applied at bedtime) on discrete crusted lesions. An SPF 15 sunscreen (Solbar Plus 15) must be used during the day.

We regularly hybridize the systemic therapy as well, by prescribing chloroquine (250 mg daily). If flushing is a major factor, we also prescribe the beta-blocker propranolol hydrochloride (Inderal 20 mg tid). For milder cases we favor the injection of ACTH (Acthar gel 40 U IM at increasing intervals determined by the response).

All patients must be alert to the hazards of sunlight, thermal burns, and specific drugs such as penicillamine, captopril, and photosensitizers (e.g., thiazides and naproxen). We regularly screen patients for the presence of malignant disease or tumors such as thymomas. Autoimmune parameters such as ANA and anti–skeletal muscle antibodies can be used to assess the therapeutic response to immunosuppressants, but we rely mainly on the clinical picture to judge progress.

Fortunately this strange mix of two potentially lethal diseases results in an entity that is usually mild. Accordingly, with a modern blend of therapy and the avoidance of sunburn, we can give these patients a good prognosis.

Amerian ML, Ahmed AR: Pemphigus erythematosus: Senear-Usher syndrome. Int J Dermatol 24:16–25, 1985.

A stunning review of the disease and all therapeutic regimens reported to date.

1. Corticosteroids used in conjunction with immunosuppressants provide the best help.
2. The disease can be induced by **penicillamine** (Cuprimine), **captopril** (Capoten), **propranolol** (Inderal), heroin, **pyritinol**, or **thiopronine**.

Jablonska S, Chorzelski T, Blaszczyk M: Immunosuppressants in the treatment of pemphigus. Br J Dermatol 83:315–323, 1970.

Triamcinolone (8 to 32 mg/day for up to four months) plus **methotrexate** (12.5 mg IM twice a week) cleared pemphigus erythematosus in six of seven patients.

Bean SF, Lynch FW: Senear-Usher syndrome (pemphigus erythematosus): Immunofluorescent studies in a patient. Arch Dermatol 101:642–645, 1970.

Sulfapyridine (500 mg qid) and **flurandrenolide** cream (Cordran) led to rapid resolution of lesions on the face and trunk in an 84-year-old man.

Chorzelski T, Jablonska S, Maciejowska E, Blaszczyk M: Visken as supplementary drug in the treatment of pemphigus. Dermatologica 150:360–365, 1975.

The beta-adrenergic blocking agent **pindolol** (Visken 7.5 to 15 mg/day for 3 to 12 months) combined with corticosteroids in decreasing dosage proved effective in treating three of five patients with pemphigus erythematosus. It was not helpful in pemphigus vulgaris. No complications were observed.

Livden JK, Naevdal A, Milde EJ: Pemphigus in rheumatoid arthritis treated with penicillamine. Scand J Rheumatol 10:95–96, 1981.

A 58-year-old woman with seropositive rheumatoid arthritis developed penicillamine-induced pemphigus erythematosus 18 months after starting **penicillamine** therapy (500 to 750 mg daily). The pemphigus continued after the stopping of penicillamine, but she underwent prompt remission when given **prednisone** (60 mg/day) and **azathioprine** (Imuran 100 mg/day). The dose was tapered after a few months with good control, but prednisone and topical steroids were still required.

Parfrey PS, Clement M, Vandenburg MJ, Wright P: Captopril-induced pemphigus. Br Med J 281:194, 1980.

Pemphigus erythematosus developed in a 45-year-old man receiving **captopril** (150 mg tid for six months).

Note: Captopril is similar in structure to **penicillamine**, which produces pemphigus in 7 per cent of patients taking it for six months or longer.

Schiff M: Jamarsan therapy of pemphigus erythematosus: Observations on 2 patients treated with Brazilian regimen. Arch Dermatol 84:103–108, 1961.

A heroic treatment for those who would avoid or who do poorly with steroids and immunosuppressants:

Iron, quinine, strychnine elixir NF (IQS elixir 4 ml tid)

Application (to entire body three times a week) of a black liquid paint, *Jamarsan* (named after a one-time medical student, Isadore Jamar, who devised it to cure Brazilian pemphigus)

Ingredient	***Amount***
sulfur ppt.	15.0
zinc oxide	12.0
boric acid	10.0
calcium hydroxide	10.0
turpentine	1.5
crude coal tar	300.0
cottonseed oil	150.0

Application is preceded by a cleansing bath with **hexachlorophene** (pHisoHex) to remove crusts and then a 30-minute bath containing 10 ml of **oil of eucalyptus** (one part) in 70 per cent ethyl alcohol (five parts).

Describes two patients with excellent response to this treatment used in conjunction with **chloroquine** (250 mg bid).

de Jong MCJM, Doeglas HMG, Dijkstra JWE: Immunohistochemical findings in a patient with penicillamine pemphigus. Br J Dermatol 102:333–337, 1980.

A more recent example of success with the Jamarsan treatment in a 57-year-old man with rheumatoid arthritis and penicillamine-induced pemphigus (having characteristics of both pemphigus erythematosus and pemphigus foliaceus).

Kudejko J, Buczkowska J, Trzebuchowska T: Pemphigus erythematosus confined to the post-burn scar. Dermatologica 147:174–178, 1973.

A 54-year-old man had pemphigus erythematosus arise precisely where he had been burned as an infant. The scarred site had remained a locus minoris resistentiae for 53 years.

Saikia NK, MacConnell LES: Senear-Usher syndrome and internal malignancy. Br J Dermatol 87:1–5, 1972.

Describes **prednisone** and **cyclophosphamide** therapy of pemphigus erythematosus in three patients who had internal malignant disease (bronchial carcinoma [two] and hepatic metastases [one]).

Basler RSW: Senear-Usher syndrome with parathyroid adenoma. Br J Dermatol 91:465–467, 1974.

Excision of a parathyroid adenoma in a 46-year-old man led to dramatic improvement of extensive pemphigus erythematosus within 48 hours, and this was sustained. His disease had previously not been controlled with **prednisone** (160 mg/day) coupled with **methotrexate** (25 mg IM/week) given for nearly six weeks.

Uhlin SR, Maiocco KJ, Bhatia SG: Pemphigus erythematosus and thymoma. Cutis 25:177–179, 182, 1980.

Avoidance of heat and sunlight was helpful in a 60-year-old woman with pemphigus erythematosus associated with a benign thymoma. Her skin lesions were controlled with topical steroids and **prednisone** (15 mg qid rapidly tapered to 5 mg every other day). She had no evidence of myasthenia gravis or skeletal muscle antibodies.

There are none so credulous as sufferers from disease.
PRESIDENT WILLIAM HOWARD TAFT (1911)

Pemphigus Vulgaris

Corticosteroids	Gold
Cyclophosphamide	Levamisole
Azathioprine	Cyclosporine
Methotrexate	Plasmapheresis
Dapsone	

Every cell in the entire epidermis is a target for immune rejection by these patients. Accordingly, treatment centers on suppression of these immune forces. In severe life-threatening cases this calls for hospitalization and corticosteroids in very high dosage.

Although prednisone is the steroid used, the range and style of dosage are matters of physician preference. The goal is to suppress new lesions, reverse the Nikolsky sign, and induce healing. This may take as much as 400 mg of prednisone a day, although generally we start with 100 mg daily, increasing as the need becomes evident. This protective steroid shield is continued for several months, at which time the prednisone is slowly tapered, again as the patient's response is watched.

If the maintenance dose proves to be high, the fear of pemphigus is replaced by the fear of side effects from the prednisone. In such individuals, adjuvant therapy with immunosuppressants is undertaken. Our favorite is cyclophosphamide (Cytoxan 50 mg tid). It has a steroid-sparing effect after a month, so that the maintenance dose of prednisone can be further reduced.

The patient also needs local treatment of erosive areas with a steroid ointment such as Synalar (0.025 per cent ointment) and erythromycin (250 mg qid) to reduce the possibility of bacterial infection. Likewise, close attention must be paid to electrolyte balance, nutrition, soft diet, IV hyperalimentation, antacid therapy, latent tuberculosis or deep fungal infection, and the possibility of adverse reactions to the prednisone and other immunosuppressant drugs used. Close hematologic and chemical monitoring is essential.

The duration of treatment is measured in years, rather than weeks or months, but the patient can be reassured that some day, somehow, he will be free not only of his lesions but of his medicines as well. The greater hope is that the new immunosuppressant drug cyclosporine, which dramatically permits organ transplants, will fulfill its early promise of permitting these patients to live with a skin that has strangely become as foreign to them as someone else's.

Lever WF, Schaumburg-Lever G: Treatment of pemphigus vulgaris. Results obtained in 84 patients between 1961 and 1982. Arch Dermatol 120:44–47, 1984.

Among 84 patients:

47 free of lesions and no longer receiving treatment
22 without lesions or treatment for more than 5 years

no disease- or treatment-related fatalities since 1976

Recommendation:

For severe cases: initial course of **prednisone** (200 to 400 mg daily for 6 to 10 weeks), then alternate-day prednisone (40 mg) plus daily **azathioprine** (Imuran 100 mg/day)

For mild cases: prednisone (40 mg every other day) and azathioprine (Imuran 100 mg/day)

Bystryn J-C: Adjuvant therapy of pemphigus. Arch Dermatol 120:941–951, 1984.

This comprehensive valuable review article concludes that the lack of controlled studies leaves doubt as to the value of adjuvants (immunosuppressants, **gold**, plasmapheresis, **dapsone**, intralesional corticosteroids).

Recommendation:

Hospitalization and corticosteroids in ascending daily bolus dosage (**prednisone** 80 mg/day given at 8 AM), increasing by 50 per cent every four to seven days as needed to prevent progression

If activity persists at levels above prednisone 240 mg/day, consider:
- IV **corticotropin** (ACTH 40 to 120 U/day in saline over 8 to 24 hours)
- changing to another steroid
- concurrent plasmapheresis
- pulse therapy: **methylprednisolone sodium succinate** (1 gm IV in 150 ml dextrose and water given in 90 minutes once a day at 8 AM for five days)
- immunosuppressant IM or **gold**

Once the bulk of the lesions has healed, decrease the steroids by 50 per cent every two weeks, leading to alternate-day therapy.

Levene GM: The treatment of pemphigus and pemphigoid. Clin Exp Dermatol 7:643–652, 1982.

Hospitalization on an urgent basis

Full explanation to the patient and family

Intensive nursing care
- air-pillow bed
- mechanical frame for moving self

Prednisone (150 mg/day); if not clearly better in 5 days:
- give double the dose or
- **methylprednisolone sodium succinate** (Solu-Medrol 1 gm/day IV for three days)

Concurrent immunosuppressant:
- **azathioprine** (150 mg/day)
- **gold**
- **cyclophosphamide** (100 mg/day)
- **methotrexate** (20 mg/week)
- **dapsone** (100 mg/day)

Concurrent systemic antibiotic—flucloxacillin (1.5 to 2.0 gm daily PO)

Oral care:
- **penicillin** or **metronidazole** tablets for halitosis (due to Vincent's organisms)
- **amphotericin B** lozenges (suck four times a day for candidiasis)
- **triamcinolone** in adhesive base (Kenalog in Orabase)

Savin JA: The events leading to the death of patients with pemphigus and pemphigoid. Br J Dermatol 101:521–534, 1979.

Respiratory tract infection and pulmonary embolism were the most common immediate causes of death among 210 patients with pemphigus or pemphigoid hospitalized in England and Wales from 1962 to 1969.

Treatment-induced diabetes mellitus, peptic ulcerations, and infections were also significant causes of death.

Krulig L, Jacobs PH, Loeffel D: Pemphigus vulgaris and disseminated coccidioidomycosis. Sabouraudia 14:5–9, 1976.

Patients with pemphigus vulgaris who are treated with long-term immunosuppressive agents should be carefully monitored for opportunistic systemic infections, including deep fungal infections. Unsuspected disseminated coccidioidomycosis was the cause of death in a 57-year-old Mexican-American man with widespread pemphigus vulgaris under treatment with high-dose steroids for approximately six months.

Fellner MJ, Mark AS: Penicillin- and ampicillin-induced pemphigus vulgaris. Int J Dermatol 19:392–393, 1980.

Drugs that can induce pemphigus vulgaris:

penicillamine (Cuprimine)	ibuprofen (Motrin)
rifampin (Rifadin)	heroin
isoniazid (INH)	practolol
ethambutol (Myambutol)	penicillin
phenylbutazone (Butazolidin)	ampicillin

Hempstead RW, Marks JG Jr: Pediatric pemphigus vulgaris: Treatment with topical adrenal steroids. Arch Dermatol 120:962–963, 1984.

Pemphigus vulgaris confined to the mouth in a 13-year-old girl was kept in good control for over four years by using **triamcinolone acetonide** 0.1 per cent in adhesive dental paste (Kenalog in Orabase—apply one to three times daily to eroded areas).

Moral: Systemic treatment is not always indicated. (Cut the cloth to fit the need.)

Lozada F, Silverman S Jr: Topically applied fluocinonide in an adhesive base in the treatment of oral vesiculoerosive diseases. Arch Dermatol 116:899–901, 1980.

Fluocinonide 0.05 per cent (Lidex, Topsyn) mixed with equal parts by weight of an adhesive base (gelatin, pectin, and sodium carboxymethyl cellulose in a polyethylene and mineral oil gel base) was applied three to six times daily after meals to oral lesions in 89 patients with assorted blistering diseases of the mouth. Most lesions responded favorably, with complete clearing in approximately 50 per cent. In one patient, pemphigus partially cleared.

Haim S, Abraham Z, Hirshowitz B: Surgical approach to the treatment of refractory lesions of pemphigus vulgaris. Int J Dermatol 23:279–280, 1984.

In a 38-year-old man with pemphigus vulgaris, **prednisone** (250 mg/day), **azathioprine** (Imuran 200 mg/day), and intralesional steroid (three times) cleared the oral lesions, but failed to induce healing of the lower lip. Cure was achieved by total vermilionectomy of the lower lip with advancement of buccal mucosa. Healing was nearly complete in 10 days, and 18 months later the patient required only small maintenance doses of **prednisone** (20 mg on alternate days).

Fellner MJ, Katz JM, McCabe JB: Successful use of cyclophosphamide and prednisone for initial treatment of pemphigus vulgaris. Arch Dermatol 114:889–894, 1978.

Excellent results were seen in five patients with pemphigus vulgaris by *initiating* treatment with both **prednisone** (100 to 200 mg/day) and **cyclophosphamide** (100 to 200 mg/day).

Haim S, Friedman-Birnbaum R: Dapsone in the treatment of pemphigus vulgaris. Dermatologica 156:120–123, 1978.

Control of oral pemphigus was achieved in two patients only after **dapsone** (100 mg/day) was substituted for **methotrexate** and added to high-dose

prednisone. Both patients could eventually be maintained on dapsone (100 mg/day) and low-dose prednisone (15 mg/day or 35 mg every other day).

Poulin Y, Perry HO, Muller SA: Pemphigus vulgaris: Results of treatment with gold as a steroid-sparing agent in a series of thirteen patients. J Am Acad Dermatol 11:851–857, 1985.

Gold (50 mg/week IM) induced complete remission in 7 of 13 patients with pemphigus vulgaris who were also receiving **prednisone**. The average dose of gold was 2374 mg given over 18.3 months. After four years, five cases remained in remission without treatment. Must watch for bone marrow toxicity and nephrotoxicity.

(Now consider using the new oral preparation, **auranofin** [Ridaura 3 mg bid].)

Lozada F, Silverman S, Cram D: Pemphigus vulgaris: A study of six cases treated with levamisole and prednisone. Oral Surg 54:161–165, 1982.

Levamisole (50 mg every other day or 50 mg/day for three consecutive days each week), an immune-potentiating anthelminthic, had a consistently marked steroid-sparing action within two to eight weeks in each of six patients with pemphigus vulgaris resistant to treatment except for steroids. With the addition of levamisole, the minimum effective dose range of **prednisone** was reduced from 40 to 80 mg/day to 5 to 35 mg daily.

Ruocco V, Astarita C, Pisani M: Plasmapheresis as an alternative or adjunctive therapy in problem cases of pemphigus. Dermatologica 168:219–223, 1984.

Weekly removal (for six weeks) of either 400 ml or 1200 ml of plasma, followed respectively by replacement with either 200 ml or 400 ml of 5 per cent human albumin solution and also 500 ml of physiologic saline solution with the large volume exchange, was very effective in treatment of six patients with treatment-resistant pemphigus vulgaris. A seventh patient also did well with massive volume plasma exchange (4000 ml of the patient's plasma were substituted with same amount of donors' plasma; then similar monthly 2500-ml exchanges for three months). In some cases, titers of pemphigus antibodies were significantly reduced.

Thivolet J, Barthelemy H, Rigot-Muller G, Bendelac A: Effects of cyclosporin on bullous pemphigoid and pemphigus. Lancet 1:334–335, 1985.

Cyclosporine (Sandimmune 6 mg/kg/day PO with plasma levels 80 to 180 μg/liter) cleared two cases of pemphigus vulgaris in 10 to 15 days. There was no relapse three months later after steroids were withdrawn, while the cyclosporine was continued. This drug has been very effective in suppressing T-cell immune rejection of transplants.

Think more about your patients and they'll think more of you.

Perifolliculitis Capitis

Topical and systemic antibacterials
Intralesional and systemic steroids
Dapsone
Surgery
Zinc

This deep, purulent, dissecting, scarring infection of the scalp defies conservative management. As in hidradenitis suppurativa, local excision of early fluctuant lesions is highly advisable to remove focal disease before it begins its insidious dissection throughout the scalp. For sinus tracts, excision without closure (marsupialization) is helpful. We suspect that the Mohs technique might be valuable in tracking and eradicating the disease. Severe cases call for more radical surgery. The ultimate successful surgery is complete removal of the scalp followed by skin grafting. Understandably, this is not something readily accepted by the patient in the early stage of the disease. However, it is probably the most reliable alternative to a psychologically and physically crippling malodorous disease that will persist for decades.

Less effective medical management includes systemic steroids or the injection of triamcinolone acetonide (40 mg/ml) into the lesions. Cultures of the lesions will help direct the choice of systemic antibiotics, which must be maintained at massive long-term dosages. We find dapsone helpful also, with prior assessment of G6PD and monitoring of blood counts in this black population. Daily shampooing with an antimicrobial such as Betadine serves a presumed prophylactic role. Finally, we attempt to augment the patient's immune response with daily oral zinc (45 mg elemental zinc tid with food).

Moyer DG, Williams RM: Perifolliculitis capitis abscedens et suffodiens. A report of six cases. Arch Dermatol 85:378–384, 1962.

Old standbys: incision, drainage, local and systemic antibiotics, epilating dose of x-rays.

Adrian RM, Arndt KA: Perifolliculitis capitis: Successful control with alternate-day corticosteroids. Ann Plast Surg 4:166–169, 1980.

In a 22-year-old black woman, **prednisone** (60 mg/day) caused rapid improvement and was slowly tapered to 5 mg every other day. At one year, control was still good. Antibiotics alone had been of no help.

Moschella SL, Klein MH, Miller RJ: Perifolliculitis capitis abscedens et suffodiens: Report of a successful therapeutic scalping. Arch Dermatol 96:195–197, 1967.

Total excision of scalp followed one week later by split-thickness grafts from thighs gave permanent cure.

Dellon AL, Orlando JC: Perifolliculitis capitis: Surgical treatment for the severe case. Ann Plast Surg 9:254–259, 1982.

Two cases: five-year cure by complete scalping therapy introduced by Moschella et al.

Curry SS, Gaither DH, King LE: Squamous cell carcinoma arising in dissecting perifolliculitis of the scalp. A case report and review of secondary squamous cell carcinomas. J Am Acad Dermatol 4:673–678, 1981.

A 47-year-old black male had been treated conservatively with incision and drainage, excision, and antibiotics. Eventually local squamous cell carcinoma developed, which was removed. Patient died of metastases.

Hazelrigg ED, William TE, Rudolph AH: Nodular granulomatous perifolliculitis. JAMA 233:270–271, 1975.

Not on the scalp. Erythematous nodules on the arm beneath a leather watchband proved to be perifolliculitis due to *Trichophyton rubrum*. Cleared in two months with **griseofulvin** (1 gm/day). Worth considering. Search for focus of fungal infection elsewhere (feet and nails in this case).

The difference between a clinician and an academician, basically, is the experience of 250 patient visits a week.

ERVIN EPSTEIN

Perioral Dermatitis

Tetracycline

Easy to acquire, easy to cure.

Wilkinson DS, Kirton V, Wilkinson JD: Perioral dermatitis: A 12 year review. Br J Dermatol 101:245–257, 1979.

A comprehensive analysis based on experience with 203 patients with perioral dermatitis:

1. Prolonged use of potent topical steroids is the most likely cause.
2. Tetracyclines are curative in the great majority of patients in six weeks *if* local corticosteroids are discontinued.
3. Relapses are rare.
4. The incidence is declining.

Sneddon I: Perioral dermatitis. Br J Dermatol 87:430–434, 1972.

A study of 73 patients suffering from perioral dermatitis showed that elimination of topical fluorinated steroids and use of **oxytetracycline** (Terramycin 250 mg bid for several months) produced complete recovery in all.

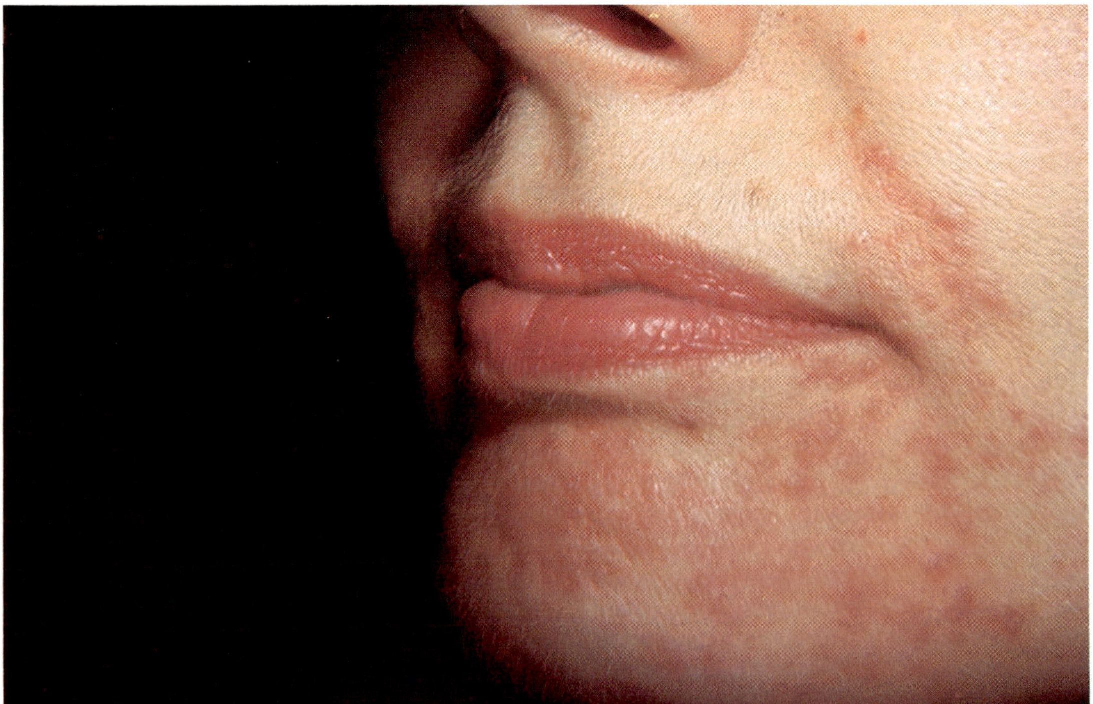

Weber G: Rosacea-like dermatitis: Contraindication or intolerance reaction to strong steroids. Br J Dermatol 86:253–259, 1972.

Nine patients were cured of perioral dermatitis by simply eliminating strong topical corticosteroids (**betamethasone valerate** and **fluocinolone acetonide**) and using a fat-free powder lotion for eight weeks. The author feels that a preexisting seborrheic diathesis is an important factor in developing the dermatitis.

Cotterill JA: Perioral dermatitis. Br J Dermatol 101:259–262, 1979.

Based on experience with 43 patients with this topical steroid-induced disease, the author recommends:

1. Alerting all doctors to the hazard
2. Instructing the public to avoid the seduction of easy cure of facial rashes by long-term usage of potent topical steroids
3. Printing a warning label on tubes of potent topical steroids about the hazards of long-term use on the face

Smith EB, Powell RF, Graham JL: Periorbital dermatitis. Arch Dermatol 112:563, 1976.

As observed in three patients reported here, this analogue of perioral dermatitis is also made worse by topical fluorinated steroids. It responds to **tetracycline** (250 mg qid for one week, then bid for seven weeks) with complete clearing in three weeks. The authors view it and perioral dermatitis as a rosacea-like dermatitis.

Try to learn about new drugs before the expiration date of their effectiveness.

Perlèche (Angular Cheilitis)

Lotrimin cream	Multivitamins
Clotrimazole lozenge	Zinc sulfate
Zinc oxide paste	Iron sulfate

Saliva is a digestive juice that should not be in prolonged contact with the skin. Cheilitis and angular cheilitis (perlèche) demonstrate the erosive power of saliva, which is loaded with enzymes and microbes. When saliva spills out over the skin at the corners of the mouth it has the capacity to induce disease. This is accentuated in individuals with furrows, which act as troughs that allow saliva to drain out and also favor constant maceration leading to overgrowth of *Candida* and bacteria.

Accordingly, the first principle of therapy is protection of the angles of the mouth from salivary overflow. This can be achieved in many instances with zinc oxide paste applied at night. In edentulous patients, new better-fitting dentures are often curative by providing a more physiologic facial contour.

In addition to bringing enzymatic damage to the skin, saliva carries a wide spectrum of microbes. Dominant among these are the *Candida* species. We regularly prescribe Lotrimin cream (three times a day) to the angles of the mouth and clotrimazole lozenges (Mycelex troche 10 mg—one in mouth tid). An alternative is to hold Mycostatin oral suspension in the mouth for two minutes (1 teaspoon tid) prior to swallowing.

At times the perlèche is due to bacteria, particularly *Staphylococcus aureus*, and here the use of an antibiotic topically, such as erythromycin ointment (Acnemycin) or gentamicin cream (Garamycin cream 0.1 per cent tid) is of value. It is well to use the topical antibiotic within the nares as well at bedtimes.

A few instances of angular cheilitis are due to contact sensitivity, so that cigarettes, toothpaste, lozenges, mouthwash, lifesavers, and cinnamon should be interdicted on a trial basis. Patch testing to the scout tray and to denture material (e.g., mercury amalgams or crown compounds) is advisable, especially if there is associated stomatitis. The patient must also be cautioned against holding bobby pins, metal pencils, cigarette holders, pipes, or other objects between the lips. Biting the fingernails is hazardous to those sensitive to nail polish.

Finally, all patients with persistent perlèche must be given full supplements of multivitamins, zinc, and iron. This is especially necessary in the older age group, in whom occult nutritional deficits first become manifest as angular cheilitis.

Makila E: Prevalence of angular stomatitis: Correlation with composition of food and metabolism of vitamins and iron. Acta Odontol Scand 27:655–680, 1969.

Angular cheilitis often develops with loss of teeth and the wearing of ill-fitting full dentures. It may be unilateral or bilateral. Overclosure of the mouth leads to deep furrows of the corners of the mouth, which become macerated with saliva. Of 339 edentulous individuals studied, 61 had angular stomatitis. In 77 per cent of these, healing occurred as soon as new dentures were in place.

Turrell AJW: Angular cheilosis and dentures. Br J Dermatol 79:331–338, 1967.

A careful, detailed study of 135 patients with angular cheilitis. In 71 per cent there was total clearing by keeping dentures completely out of the mouth for two weeks. New dentures gave permanent cure. If a burning sensation is present in the mouth, consider allergy to denture or cleansing compound, but this is rare. Recommends brushing dentures with soap and water after meals and nightly immersion of dentures in sodium perborate denture-cleansing solution. **Nystatin** powder (100,000 U/gm in Orahesive) can also be sprinkled on the fitting surface of the upper denture after meals and at bedtime to act as a fungistatic denture fixative. Dentures should be checked for fit every year, as resorption of alveolar bone usually leads to poor fitting within five years.

Schoenfeld RJ, Schoenfeld FI: Angular cheilitis. Cutis 19:213–216, 1977.

Details 21 different causes, but stresses that candidal infection is almost always present and deserves treatment. Must try to stop drooling, which is promoted by sucking on pipes, pencil, or thumb in the corner of the mouth.

MacFarlane TW, Helnarska SJ: The microbiology of angular cheilitis. Br Dent J 140:403–406, 1976.

Staphylococcus aureus may be more common than *Candida albicans* in causing angular cheilitis. Look for yellow crusts resembling impetigo. Suspect nasal carriage of *S. aureus* and treat anterior nares and angles of mouth with an antimicrobial cream (e.g., Neosporin ointment).

A microbiologic study of 100 patients with angular cheilitis sometimes associated with stomatitis revealed the following:

68 patients
- *Staphylococcus aureus* 79 per cent
- *Candida* spp. 44 per cent
- beta-hemolytic streptococci 15 per cent

32 patients
- no infective agent

Control group—45 individuals
- *Staphylococcus aureus* 7 per cent
- *Candida* spp. 22 per cent
- beta-hemolytic streptococci 0 per cent

Fisher AA: Contact stomatitis, glossitis, and cheilitis. Otolaryngol Clin North Am 7:827–843, 1974.

Angular cheilitis may result from allergy to:

denture materials (acrylic resins)
metals
- mercury
- nickel
- copper
- gold
- chrome
- cobalt
- platinum
- amalgams

denture adherents
toothpaste, dentifrices, mouthwashes
nailpolish
lipstick
menthol

Cinnamon-sensitive patients should avoid dry vermouth.

Suggested treatment:

petrolatum
ice water compresses
erythromycin ointment
Kenalog in Orabase
viscous Xylocaine (2 per cent lidocaine)
Kenalog 40 mg IM

Rose JA: Folic-acid deficiency as a cause of angular cheilosis. Lancet 2:453–454, 1971.

Two men with angular cheilitis of 10 and 20 years respectively and low folate levels were given **folic acid** (10 mg/day). Their lesions disappeared within a month.

Rose JA: Aetiology of angular cheilosis: Iron metabolism. Br Dent J 125:67–71, 1968.

In four patients with angular cheilitis and low plasma iron levels, there was clearing with systemic **iron** therapy only. Such iron deficiency, not apparent as anemia, was disclosed only by serum iron determinations.

Murphy NC, Bissada NF: Iron deficiency: An overlooked predisposing factor in angular cheilitis. J Am Dent Assoc 99:640–641, 1979.

Ferrous sulfate (2 capsules bid) cured angular cheilitis in a pregnant 25-year-old white woman. Patients with angular cheilitis deserve a CBC and determination of serum iron and total iron-binding capacity (TIBC) to check for latent iron deficiency. Must also rule out megaloblastic anemia due to folic acid deficiency or pernicious anemia (vitamin B_{12} deficiency) as causes of angular cheilitis.

Chernosky ME: Collagen implant in the management of perleche (angular cheilosis). J Am Acad Dermatol 12:493–496, 1985.

Ingenious correction of "saliva trap" by local injection of bovine **collagen** (Zyderm) into angles of the mouth was followed by cure of angular cheilitis.

Details are also given for measuring the face with a millimeter ruler and tongue blade to see if a decreased vertical facial dimension of the lower third of the face is responsible for the perlèche. The mouth appears slitlike and horizontal.

Rule: If B is 6 mm shorter than A, the vertical dimension is decreased.

distance A: center of eye pupil to parting line of lips (rima oris)
distance B: base of nose to lower edge of mandible

Dentists may help restore the loss of vertical dimension by capping teeth, replacing lost teeth, or increasing denture height to compensate for bone resorption.

Some patients, like some bacteria, are drug resistant.

Photosensitivity

Sun screens	Nicotinic acid
Steroids	PUVA
Beta-carotene	Azathioprine
	See specific disease

At the dawn of civilization, the sun was worshipped as a god. Now at high noon, the sun is regarded as a devil: the cause of skin cancer, photosensitivity, and heat stroke. What can be done to stay out of the hands of this devil? For individuals who are photosensitive, this is a real problem.

The simplest answer is to stay indoors. But for those who must be out of doors for work or play, the modern topical sun screens are a blessing. Rated on a sun protection factor (SPF) scale of 1 to 15, they offer in their most effective form, SPF 15, the chance of increasing one's time tolerance for the sun's rays by a factor of 15. The photosensitive patient must use these SPF 15 sun screens on all exposed skin. We usually recommend Bain de Soleil 15 or Solbar Plus. For the PABA-sensitive patient we advise RVP (red veterinary petrolatum) or Solbar PF (PABA free).

But these patients need more than a sun screen. They require diagnostic study. Most of the patients seen by us are photosensitive as a result of a drug. The most recent drugs implicated are naproxen (Naprosyn), captopril (Capoten), and etretinate, while hydrochlorothiazide (HydroDIURIL) and quinidine have long been recognized as photosensitizers. We rarely see contact photosensitivities, but herbal shampoos remain high on our list of suspects. We check for porphyria in all patients, the most common example being porphyria cutanea tarda. We also screen for lupus erythematosus, since it may begin with photosensitivity.

In the patients who come in the spring with newborn photosensitivity, the most likely diagnosis is polymorphous light eruption. In these patients the problem may vanish with the "hardening" that occurs once tanning has come. Most dreaded is the fearsome idiopathic problem of actinic reticuloid, in which the patient, after years of sun sensitivity, shows lymphoma-like changes in the skin.

The specific measures for management of particular photosensitivity states are presented elsewhere under the appropriate diagnostic headings. However, all of these patients must be given an education concerning photoprotection. They must be aware of the gravity and chronicity of their problem and of the need of eliminating any suspect drugs. Unfortunately, elimination of a causal drug and its congeners does not bring as rapid relief to the patient as in a simple drug eruption. It is an essential step, but often topical and systemic steroids are necessary to bring prompt relief. Chloroquine is dramatically helpful in lupus

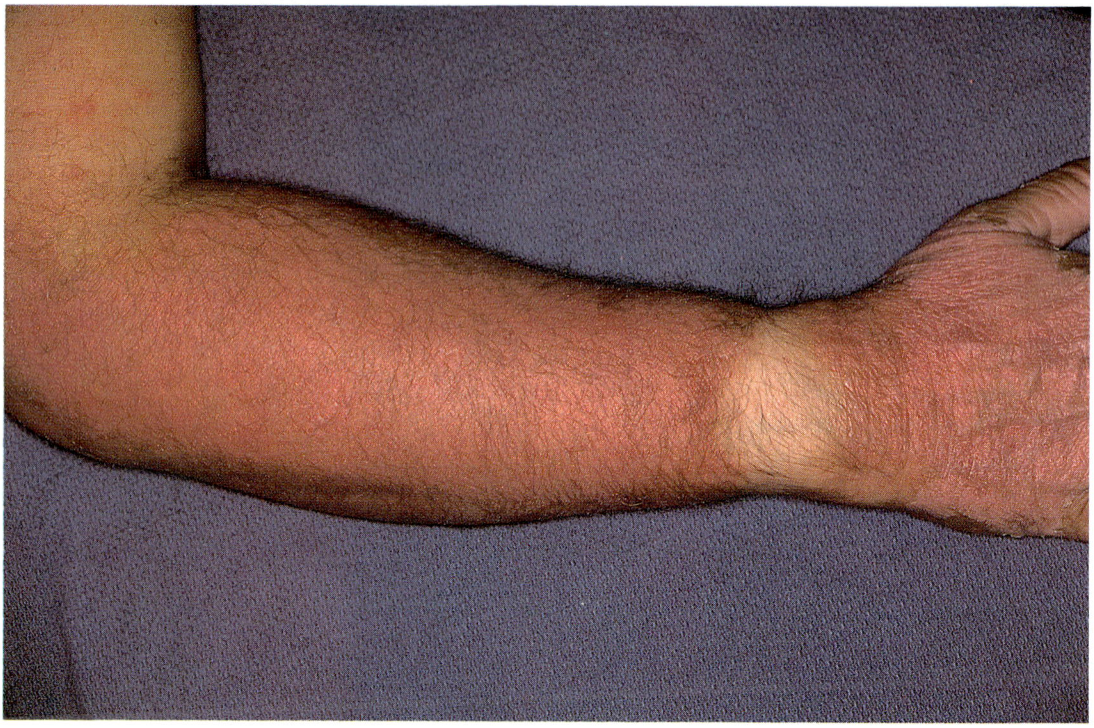

erythematosus, as is beta-carotene in erythropoietic protoporphyria. Still, there is no systemic drug or compound that provides photoprotection for the ordinary photosensitivity state.

Accordingly, the patient must use common sense in minimizing ultraviolet and short-wave visible light exposure. Some of the effective specific maneuvers employed by our patients include:

1. Being outdoors only before 9 AM and after 4 PM
2. Wearing clothing and a broad-brimmed hat that does not allow light to penetrate
3. Avoiding prolonged exposure to fluorescent lamps
4. Standing within the church instead of outside chatting with friends after Sunday services
5. Sitting on the shady side of the football stadium
6. Wearing a leather face mask and glasses
7. Changing the occupation from farmer to miner
8. Placing plastic UV opaque sheets on the inside of car windows and windshields
9. Vacationing in Canada instead of Florida
10. Camping in the woods instead of at the seashore

Each visit gives you a chance to reinforce the patient's awareness of the hazards of sunlight in the months and even years to come. These patients need frequent monitoring as well as emotional support. They need sequential instruction that new drugs may be photosensitizers and that sun screens can turn on them, becoming pathogenic instead of protective. They must be taught that celery, carrots, figs, and parsnips contain phototoxic chemicals. They need to know that the oils of the skin of citrus fruits, the herbs of shampoos, and the fragrances of colognes and after-shave lotions all are potential photosensitizers. Even their soap should be perfume free, e.g., Neutrogena unperfumed soap. No patient needs more continued observation and evaluation than the persistent light reactor. He must be shadowed indefinitely.

Harber LC, Bickers DR: Photosensitivity Diseases: Principles of Diagnosis and Treatment. Philadelphia, WB Saunders Co, 1981, 372 pp.

The standard reference work on all aspects of treatment for patients who have unique hypersensitivity to ultraviolet or visible light.

Note that **atabrine**, **beta-carotene**, and **chloroquine** do not protect against ordinary sunburn.

Appendices give useful details for the following:

1. Goeckerman therapy
2. PUVA therapy
3. Sun screens and sun-blocking agents
4. Phototesting and photopatch testing
5. Phytophotodermatitis

Pathak MA, Fitzpatrick TB, Greiter FJ, Kraus EW: Principles of photoprotection in sunburn and suntanning, and topical and systemic photoprotection in health and diseases. J Dermatol Surg Oncol 11:575–579, 1985.

This valuable comprehensive source of data includes a table of 28 currently available sun screens with sun protection factor (SPF) ratings as well as evaluations of resistance to sweating and swimming. Among the most effective are PreSun 15 (clear lotion), Sundown 15 (milky lotion), and Total Eclipse 15 (milky lotion). These **PABA**-containing sun screens, however, are not to be used by patients receiving **chlorothiazide** diuretics since cross-reactions occur. Such patients should use UVAL or Solbar PF, which contain **benzophenones**.

PABA causes yellow discoloration of clothes, especially with sun exposure. It also may cause allergic reactions in people already sensitized to **benzocaine**, **procaine**, **paraphenylenediamine**, and **sulfanilamide**. Impurities in the form of ortho and meta esters of PABA may cause contact and photocontact dermatitis.

Patients with polymorphic photodermatitis may be able to be outdoors as long as 30 to 60 minutes if they apply a first coat of 5 per cent PABA in alcohol (PreSun) (check that photopatch test is negative) and a second coat of UVAL or Solbar, in addition to taking **beta-carotene** (Solatene 120 to 180 mg/day for adults, 30 to 90 mg/day for children under the age of 12 years).

Schauder S, Ippen H: Photodermatoses and light protection. Int J Dermatol 21:241–247, 1982.

Severely reacting light-sensitive skin may not tolerate topically applied sun screens. Use topical steroids first.

Emmett EA: Drug photoallergy. Int J Dermatol 17:370–379, 1978.

Protocol:

Vigorous search for a contact or systemic photoallergen
Rigorous elimination of it and cross-sensitizers
Minimize ultraviolet radiation until the hyperactivity has passed
Educate the patient that this may take weeks, months, or even years
Advise the wearing of closely woven dark clothing, wide-brimmed hat, and gloves

Plastic (clear and colored), not window glass, protection
PABA sun screens ineffective
Advise **benzophenone** sun screen (**titanium dioxide** screens [Covermark] also effective)
Cautious attempt of **8-methoxypsoralen** induction of a tan
Avoid new photosensitizers
Remember that clouds are not a sun screen

Robinson HN, Morison WL, Hood AF: Thiazide diuretic therapy and chronic photosensitivity. Arch Dermatol 121:522–524, 1985.

In four patients **hydrochlorothiazide** produced debilitating photosensitivity that lasted from 1 to 20 years after stopping the diuretic. Three cases were successfully cleared in the hospital with **methoxsalen** plus UVA radiation (1 to 3 weeks of PUVA, as for psoriasis) while the photosensitivity was controlled with **prednisone** (100 mg/day). Subsequent weekly maintenance treatments kept the patients free of photosensitivity. Note that the photosensitivity promptly recurred whenever PUVA therapy was stopped. Sun screens, **beta-carotene**, and **chloroquine** were of no value. The one patient who refused PUVA therapy subsequently developed actinic reticuloid.

Burry JN: Unusual skin manifestations of drug photosensitivity. Australas J Dermatol 25:115–117, 1984.

The following drugs were observed by the author to induce transient light reactions:

carbamazepine (Tegretol)
chlorpromazine* (Thorazine)
chlorpropamide (Diabinese)
cyclopenthiazide*
diazepam (Valium)
diphenhydramine (Benadryl)
estrogens
furosemide* (Lasix)
hydrochlorothiazide* (HydroDIURIL)
methyldopa (Aldomet)
prochlorperazine (Compazine)
promethazine* (Phenergan)
quinethazone (Hydromox)
quinine
sulfonamides
tamoxifen (Nolvadex)
thioridazine (Mellaril)
trimeprazine (Temaril)

---

* cross-reactive

Ramsay CA: Transient and persistent photosensitivity due to musk ambrette. Clinical and photobiological studies. Br J Dermatol 111:423–429, 1984.

Contact photosensitivity resulting in persistent light reactivity is less common now that many of the responsible chemicals (e.g., halogenated salicylanilides in soaps) have been removed from the market. However, new photosensitizers are still being introduced, including musk ambrette found in many cosmetics. Fluorescent light exposure caused exacerbation of the eruption in one of the five male patients reported here.

Kaidbey KH, Messenger JL: The clinical spectrum of the persistent light reactor. Arch Dermatol 120:1441–1448, 1984.

An analysis of eight men with photodermatitis of 5 to 19 years' duration revealed:

five had positive photopatch tests to musk ambrette (1 per cent in petrolatum).
three had positive photopatch tests to halogenated salicylanilides (1 per cent in petrolatum).

Treatment that helped most of the patients:

avoidance of contact with colognes and after-shave lotion
corticosteroids locally
sunblocking agents

LeVine MJ: Idiopathic photodermatitis with a positive paraphenylenediamine photopatch test. Arch Dermatol 120:1488–1490, 1984.

A 61-year-old man with eczematous dermatitis of the forearms and face, recurrent each summer for 13 years, proved to have strongly positive photopatch tests to both paraphenylenediamine and the caine mix (which cross-react).

Treatment: Avoidance of the sun and use of sun screens prevented recurrence.

Maurer T: Contact and Photocontact Allergens. A Manual of Predictive Test Methods. New York, Marcel Dekker, 1983, 179 pp.

How to detect contactants responsible for your patient's photosensitivity.

Herman PS, Sams WM Jr.: Soap Photodermatitis. Photosensitivity to Halogenated Salicylanilides. Springfield, Ill., Charles C Thomas, 1972, 181 pp.

Manufacturers eliminated salicylanilides from soaps when they were shown to be a major cause of photosensitivity, but the light sensitivity initiated by them lingers on.

Hjorth N, Roed-Petersen J, Thomsen K: Airborne contact dermatitis from Compositae oleoresins simulating photodermatitis. Br J Dermatol 95:613–620, 1976.

Seven patients in Denmark with the diagnosis of photodermatitis, and treated for many years, were eventually shown to be suffering from ragweed contact dermatitis. Since there is no effective treatment for airborne allergen contact dermatitis, these patients now had a new diagnosis, but still no cure.

Hölzle E, Hofmann C, Plewig G: PUVA-treatment for solar urticaria and persistent light reaction. Arch Dermatol Res 269:87–91, 1980.

PUVA therapy (four times weekly) resulted in symptom-free, normal outdoor lives for the first time in years for two patients (ages 22 and 76 years) who were persistent light reactors. Initial UVA doses were very low (0.1 to 0.25 J/sq cm), and only parts of the body were exposed. When the initial dose was tolerated on the entire body, UVA doses were increased by 0.25 to 0.5 J/sq cm to induce a tan without precipitating photodermatitis. Patients become free from symptoms at cumulative doses of 60 J/sq cm (33 treatments) and 49 J/sq cm (37 exposures) respectively. Maintenance dosage (one to two times weekly) was required to sustain protection.

Morison WL, White HAD, Gonzalez E, et al: Oral methoxsalen photochemotherapy of uncommon photodermatoses. Acta Derm Venereol 59:366–368, 1979.

PUVA therapy (psoriasis therapy protocol, three times a week until tanned), greatly helped two photosensitive atopic patients, one thiazide photosensitivity patient, and one patient with actinic reticuloid. Maintenance PUVA therapy (once a week for two years) was required for the patient with actinic reticuloid, while the remaining three patients utilized summer sunshine (midday, three hours/week) to maintain clearing.

Rothschild CJ: Photosensitivity reaction treated with diphenhydramine. Can Med Assoc J 125:1085–1087, 1981.

In a 10-year-old boy taking phenothiazines (**thioridazine** [Mellaril], **promazine** [Sparine], and **methylphenidate** [Ritalin]), **diphenhydramine** (Benadryl 25 mg) was of great benefit in treating and preventing marked photosensitivity.

Kaufmann G: Pyridoxine against amiodarone-induced photosensitivity. Lancet 1:51–52, 1984.

In three patients, **pyridoxine** (40 to 300 mg/day) ameliorated photosensitivity induced by the cardiac drug **amiodarone**.

Mulrow JP, Mulrow CD, McKenna WJ: Pyridoxine and amiodarone-induced photosensitivity. Ann Intern Med 103:68–69, 1985.

Seventy-five per cent of patients receiving the antiarrhythmic agent **amiodarone** develop photosensitivity despite use of sun screens. In a double-blind controlled study of 46 patients, **pyridoxine** (100 mg with each amiodarone dosage) did not afford any sun protection. A surprising 70 per cent of patients taking the placebo (**lactase**, talcum, and **magnesium stearate**) claimed improved sun tolerance, which suggested that in the other group the pyridoxine perhaps enhanced amiodarone-induced photosensitivity.

Shelley WB, Shelley ED: Nicotinic-acid-responsive photosensitivity. Lancet 2:576, 1984.

Nicotinic acid (100 mg bid) rapidly and totally eliminated the severe erythematous reaction to sunlight that had condemned a 59-year-old man to seven years of hermetic indoor existence. It was considered that the patient had a forme fruste of pellagra due to a gastrectomy and poor diet, with photosensitivity as its only sign.

Isaacson D, Elgart M, Turner ML: Anti-malarials in dermatology. Int J Dermatol 21:379–395, 1982.

Chloroquine and its variants, as well as its antecedent, **quinacrine** (Atabrine), are uniquely valuable in controlling the photosensitivity of lupus erythematosus.

Drug names:

amodiaquine (Camoquin, Miaquin)
chloroquine (Aralen, Avochlor, Resochin)
hydroxychloroquine (Plaquenil)
quinacrine (mepacrine, Atabrine, Atebrin)
quinacrine, chloroquine, hydroxychloroquine (Triquin)

Leigh IM, Hawk JLM: Treatment of chronic actinic dermatitis with azathioprine. Br J Dermatol 110:691–695, 1984.

Azathioprine (100 to 200 mg/day for one year) cleared or markedly improved 9 of 14 patients with chronic unexplained photosensitivity; two did not tolerate the medication, two showed no response, and in one there was relapse after initial improvement. The nine patients experienced clearing within two weeks to two months of starting therapy. During a two-year follow-up period there was no relapse after the azathioprine was stopped.

Roed-Petersen J, Thomsen K: Azathioprin in the treatment of airborne contact dermatitis from Compositae oleoresins and sensitivity to UVA. Acta Derm Venereol 60:275–277, 1980.

A 57-year-old farmer sensitive to ragweed-type oleoresins and UVA showed remarkable clearing shortly after starting **azathioprine** (Imuran 50 mg bid). Another working man, 62 years old, with similar photosensitivity also did well with azathioprine (150 mg daily for five months), although his skin did not clear completely.

Frain-Bell W: Management of the photodermatoses. Clin Exp Dermatol 7:565–571, 1982.

May need to hospitalize the patient in a light-protection cubicle, with clear plastic curtains hung around the patient's bed, to block out the responsible wavelengths and enable the skin to heal. As the skin heals with the use of topical corticosteroids, a topical sun screen may be added to protect the skin from the responsible wavelengths.

Phototesting should be done to determine the causative wavelengths and confirm the exact diagnosis.

Shelley WB: Immediate sunburn-like reaction in a patient with formaldehyde photosensitivity. Arch Dermatol 118:117–118, 1982.

A rare case of photosensitivity traced by photo-patch testing to its source: formaldehyde.

Piomelli S, Poh-Fitzpatrick MB, Seaman C, Skolnick LM, Berdon WE: Complete suppression of the symptoms of congenital erythropoietic porphyria by long term treatment with high level transfusions. N Engl J Med 314:1029–1031, 1986.

The severe disabling photosensitivity of a young boy was virtually eliminated by long-term transfusion therapy with packed red cells. By maintaining the hematocrit above 39 per cent, nearly complete suppression of erythropoiesis and excessive production of photoactive porphyrins occurred. Following splenectomy the transfusion requirement of packed red cells dropped from 278 to 174 ml per kilogram of body weight per year. The iron overload was mitigated by slow subcutaneous infusion of the chelator, **deferoxamine mesylate** (Desferal 40 mg per kilogram). The child, now age 10 after four years of this therapy, is able to go to camp, swim, and tan. Prior to transfusion therapy he had marked photosensitivity requiring complete avoidance of outdoor activity in addition to use of a sun-blocking cream, protective clothing, and oral beta-carotene.

The secret of being well read is not speed reading, but speed scanning.

Pityriasis Rubra Pilaris

Aquasol A	Stanozolol
Accutane	Vitamin C
Steroids	Thyroid
Methotrexate	Penicillin
Azathioprine	INH-PAS
Erythromycin	

This strange abnormality of follicular keratinization has been most responsive to the vitamin A class of drugs and to immunosuppressants. Topical measures remain largely emollient, with our preference being either 20 per cent urea cream (Carmol 20) or Synalar ointment (0.025 per cent).

Our long-term favorite systemic therapy has been Aquasol A (water-soluble vitamin A 50,000 IU tid). It probably will be supplanted by Accutane (13-*cis*-retinoic acid), which has a more powerful effect on the keratinization process. We prescribe 40 mg bid as the usual adult dose, and this must be continued for months. The patient failing to respond to vitamin A or Accutane may be helped by the addition of vitamin C or thyroid hormone. Methotrexate, azathioprine, and stanozolol also deserve a trial.

Many patients with pityriasis rubra pilaris are photosensitive, so that ultraviolet light therapy is to be avoided. Sun screens and even oral chloroquine (250 mg/day) may be advisable. Despite lack of evidence of underlying infection, some patients respond dramatically to either penicillin, erythromycin, or INH-PAS.

Although total clearing may take months to years, a patient should show appreciable improvement in a therapeutic trial within one month, which allows for complete epidermal turnover. If there is no improvement after one month, alternate treatments should be undertaken. While patience is an essential ingredient in treating chronic disease, it must not lull us into mindless acceptance of a worthless regimen.

Griffiths WAD: Pityriasis rubra pilaris. Clin Exp Dermatol 5:105–112, 1980.

Most informative review of 100 cases with division into type of therapeutic response:

Therapy	***Good Response***
Azathioprine	7 of 8
Methotrexate (dosage as for psoriasis)	17 of 44
Vitamin A (150,000 to 300,000 IU/day)	1 of 3
Corticosteroid (prednisolone, up to 90 mg/day PO)	5 of 14
Favors yellow soft paraffin (Vaseline) topically	

Griffiths WAD: Vitamin A and pityriasis rubra pilaris. J Am Acad Dermatol 7:555, 1982.

Clearing occurred in 12 of 37 patients treated with **vitamin A** (25,000 to 1,000,000 IU/day), but there was relapse on stopping medication.

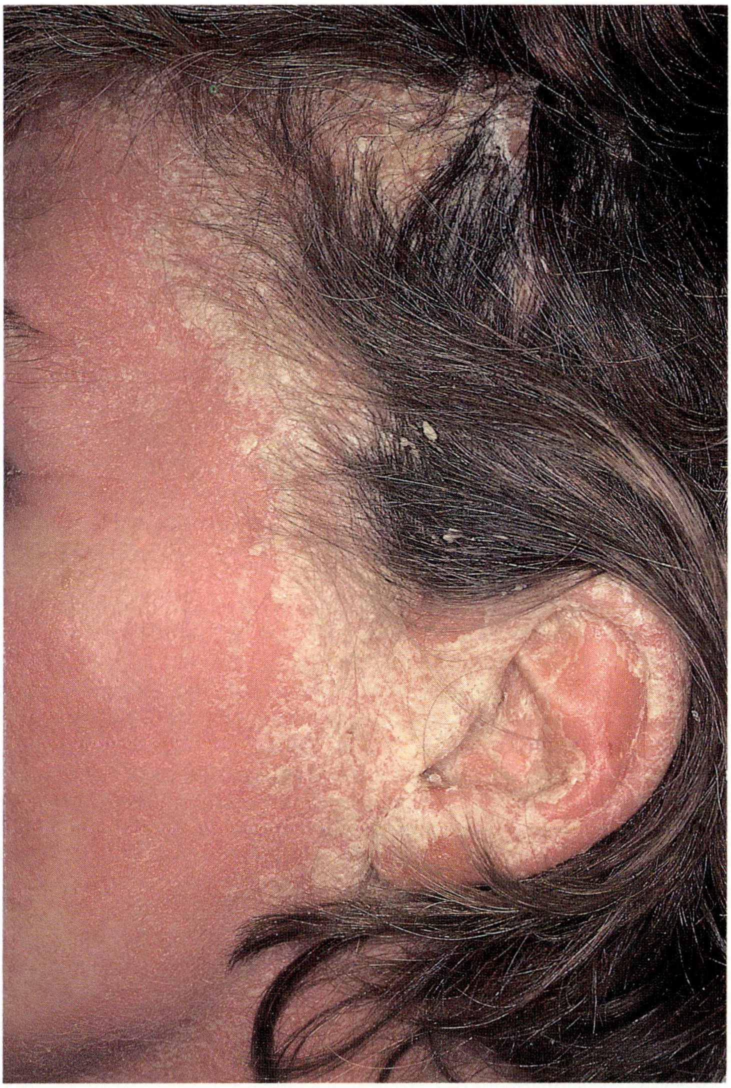

Dolezal JF: Pityriasis rubra pilaris. A case report and photo essay. Cutis 26:37–40, 1980.

Lesions were present for three months in a 12-year-old boy.
Treatment:
systemic:
vitamin A (50,000 IU tid orally)
topical:
scalp: daily tar shampoo and **flurandrenolone** lotion after shampoo
palms and soles: **salicylic acid** (5 per cent in petrolatum)
body: **retinoic acid** with two-hour occlusive dressing; **flurandrenolone** ointment (Cordran 0.05 per cent) under occlusive dressing at bedtime
Clearing time, 6 months. No recurrence in subsequent 18 months.

Randle HW, Diaz-Perez JL, Winkelmann RK: Toxic doses of vitamin A for pityriasis rubra pilaris. Arch Dermatol 116:888–892, 1980.

Vitamin A (1 million IU/day) given for 5 to 14 days cleared six of seven cases with no relapses. Exfoliation occurs within three days, and skin remains red for three months.

Winkelmann RK, Thomas JR, Randle HW: Further experience with toxic vitamin A therapy in pityriasis rubra pilaris. Cutis 31:621–629, 1983.

Vitamin A (1 million units) was given orally for eight days to an adult woman. The eruption disappeared on the fifth day. Recurrence six months later was limited to previously uninvolved sites!

Murray JC, Gilgor RS, Lazarus GS: Serum triglyceride elevation following high-dose vitamin A treatment for pityriasis rubra pilaris. Arch Dermatol 119:675–676, 1983.

A dissenting vote for megadose **vitamin A**. Two patients given 1 million IU vitamin A for 10 to 14 days received minimal help.

Goldsmith LA, Weinrich AL, Shupack J: Pityriasis rubra pilaris response to 13-cis-retinoic acid (isotretinoin). J Am Acad Dermatol 6:710–715, 1982.

Improvement was shown by 90 per cent of 45 patients (at 16 centers) when given oral **13-*cis*-retinoic acid** (1.63 to 2.13 mg/kg/day). Some had complete clearing and no relapse on stopping the drug.

Prior treatments had included **penicillin**, **hydroxychloroquine**, **isoniazid**, and **para-aminosalicylic acid**.

Kanerva L, Lauharanta J, Niemi K-M, Lassus A: Ultrastructure of pityriasis rubra pilaris with observations during retinoid (etretinate) treatment. Br J Dermatol 108:653–663, 1983.

Etretinate (0.75 to 1.0 mg/kg/day) helped five patients with pityriasis rubra pilaris, evident within four weeks. There was clearing in one patient; one patient quit because of side effects (alopecia plus cheilitis); and three were receiving maintenance etretinate (0.3 to 0.9 mg/kg/day). PUVA had produced exacerbation of pityriasis rubra pilaris in three patients.

Braun-Falco O, Ryckmanns F, Schmoeckel C, Landthaler M: Pityriasis rubra pilaris: A clinic-pathological and therapeutic study with special reference to histochemistry, autoradiography, and electron microscopy. Arch Dermatol Res 275:287–295, 1983.

Three patients received significant help from the new retinoid, **etretinate** (Tigason 50 to 75 mg/day). Not available in the United States. One improved moderately with 13-*cis*-retinoic acid (Accutane 0.5 mg/kg/day) with 20 mg/day long-term treatment still being studied.

Knowles WR, Chernosky ME: Pityriasis rubra pilaris: Prolonged treatment with methotrexate. Arch Dermatol 102:603–612, 1970.

Six men with severe disabling pityriasis rubra pilaris responded to **methotrexate** given in a variety of ways (PO, IM, IV). The best regimen was alternate oral daily doses of 5 mg and 2.5 mg. Three of the six cases cleared within four months, and all six remained clear after long-term treatment.

Hanke CW, Steck WD: Childhood-onset pityriasis rubra pilaris treated with methotrexate administered intravenously. Cleve Clin Q 50:201–203, 1983.

A 24-year-old man had had incapacitating pityriasis rubra pilaris since the age of three weeks. All modes of therapy, including oral **methotrexate** (25 mg once/week), had been unsuccessful. Clearing occurred within three weeks of starting IV methotrexate (50 mg once a week), with maintenance of 30 to 50 mg IV required every one to three weeks. Interruption of therapy on five occasions during a five-year period was followed by erythroderma within three weeks. Minimal changes were noted in sequential liver biopsies taken every 12 to 18 months. A dramatic example of the significance of the delivery route!

Hunter GA, Forbes IJ: Treatment of pityriasis rubra pilaris with azathioprine. Br J Dermatol 87:42–45, 1972.

Four of five cases cleared completely when **azathioprine** (Imuran 100 to 200 mg daily) was given. Response obvious within one to four weeks. No relapse in two patients on stopping the drug after one to two years.

Anthony TC: Brief clinical reports of two cases of pityriasis rubra pilaris. Aust J Dermatol 5:185–186, 1960.

Penicillin (600,000 U IM daily for 10 days) greatly helped two women with pityriasis rubra pilaris within one week.

Watt TL, Jillson OF: Pityriasis rubra pilaris: Penicillin and antituberculous drugs as possible therapeutic agents. Arch Dermatol 92:428–430, 1965.

In three cases, **phenoxymethyl penicillin** (penicillin V 1 to 3 million units daily PO or IM) caused complete clearing within one month. In another case unresponsive to **vitamin A** and **hydroxychloroquine**, **isoniazid** and **aminosalicylic acid** resulted in complete clearing in 1 month.

Ashurst PJC: The treatment of pityriasis rubra pilaris with Dipasic. Br J Dermatol 74:372–375, 1962.

Dramatic response within two weeks in three cases of pityriasis rubra pilaris given **isonicotinic acid hydrazide para-aminosalicylate** (INH-PAS 100 mg qid). The drug was continued for eight months to achieve total clearing. None of the patients had tuberculosis.

Binnick SA: Pityriasis rubra pilaris responding to aminonicotinamide. Arch Dermatol 114:1348–1349, 1978.

One case. Paired comparison-controlled study of topical 1 per cent **aminonicotinamide** in hydrophilic ointment applied once daily to the right half of the body showed almost complete clearing of the treated side but no improvement of the untreated side after two weeks. Clearing was complete after an additional two weeks of treatment to all involved areas. Side effect: minimal facial burning after sun exposure.

Tunnessen WW, Nieburg PI, Voorhess ML: Hypothyroidism and pityriasis rubra pilaris response to thyroid hormone. J Pediatr 88:456–458, 1976.

In a four-year-old girl with hypothyroidism and pityriasis rubra pilaris, there was complete clearing after four months of **thyroid** replacement therapy. Thyroid hormone is necessary to convert ingested carotenes to vitamin A, with nearly complete blockage in hypothyroidism.

Irgang S: Pityriasis rubra pilaris responsive to ascorbic acid. Aust J Dermatol 9:211–217, 1968.

Ascorbic acid (500 mg/day PO and 500 mg/week IM) given to an elderly scorbutic black woman was associated with excellent clearing of her pityriasis rubra pilaris in five months. Addition of **vitamin A** (100,000 IU/day) for three months terminated a mild relapse. **Vitamin C** is known to counteract follicular hyperkeratosis, and epidermal deficiency of vitamin C leads to abnormal keratin production.

Bergamaschini L, Tucci A, Colombo A, Agostoni A, Finzi AG, Altomare GF, Pigatto PD: Effect of stanozolol in patients with pityriasis rubra pilaris and retinol-binding protein deficiency. N Engl J Med 306:546–547, 1982.

Stanozolol (Winstrol, 4 to 6 mg/day for two to four weeks) resulted in distinct improvement of pityriasis rubra pilaris in three patients with correction of low serum retinol-binding protein levels. Pityriasis rubra pilaris may be a genetic disease with protein defects correctable with 17α-alkylated androgens (analogous to hereditary angioedema).

Pavlidakey GP, Hashimoto K, Savoy LB, et al: Stanozolol in the treatment of pityriasis rubra pilaris. Arch Dermatol 121:546–548, 1985.

Stanozolol (2 mg tid) gave rapid improvement within one week and complete clearing after four months in a 26-year-old man. No recurrence in eight-month follow-up.

Brenner W, Gschnait F, Hönigsmann H, Fritsch P: Erprobung von PUVA bei Verschiedenen Dermatosen. Hautarzt 29:541–544, 1978.

PUVA in one case of pityriasis rubra pilaris induced complete remission.
dosage: 8-MOP (0.6 to 0.8 mg/kg)
number of treatments: 28 over two-month period
total UVA: 244.5 J/sq cm

If you are not thinking about some of your patients' problems after office hours, those patients have a problem.

Polymorphous Light Eruption

Sunscreens	Carotenoids
Trisoralen	Thalidomide
PUVA	

Polymorphous light eruption is a potpourri of photosensitivity. It's the diagnosis when you've ruled out drugs, contactants, porphyrias, and lupus. There is no biochemical marker for it, and, as its name indicates, its clinical presentation is not monomorphic.

It is not rare, and assuredly many of the patients never consult a physician, since tanning acts as a unique servomechanism that shuts off the disease. At least half of the patients experience this. For them, it is a disease of Maytime. By the summer solstice they are safe under their melanin umbrella.

We use this paradox of the sun curing sun sensitivity in treating the patients who come to see us. We "harden" their skin by prescribing trioxsalen (Trisoralen 20 to 30 mg) to be taken two hours before gradually increasing exposures of sunlight. Once a tan is achieved, the treatment can be discontinued until the new epidermis a month later needs hardening. It is the poor man's PUVA.

Our favorite alternate treatment is chloroquine, but we tend to restrict its use to those patients with serious sun sensitivity that does not respond to vigorous avoidance of unnecessary sun exposure, use of sun screens, and use of protective clothing. We do not use it in children.

Fortunately, in most patients this sun sensitivity is mild, and much is accomplished once the patient understands the need for developing his own melanin sun screen. Each spring, with or without Trisoralen, sun exposure must be precisely graded so as to stimulate the melanocyte yet not kill the keratinocytes.

Jansen CT: The natural history of polymorphous light eruptions. Arch Dermatol 115:165–169, 1979.

A study of 138 patients revealed:

Mean age of onset	26 years
Duration	10 years
Annual onset	March
Diminution in symptoms as summer progressed	51 per cent
Spontaneous remission	10 per cent

Many (69 per cent) had some degree of associated chills, fever, headache, or nausea following sun exposure.

Epstein JH: Polymorphous light eruption. J Am Acad Dermatol 3:329–343, 1980.

In those patients who do not develop "hardening" as the summer progresses, reemphasize their use of protective clothing, sunblocks, sunscreens, and common sense. **Chloroquine** is effective in many patients, but **beta-carotene** and PUVA have not been helpful.

Jansen CT: Photosensitivity in childhood. Acta Derm Venereol Suppl 95:54–57, 1981.

Childhood-onset photodermatosis, 95 cases:

Polymorphous light eruption	78
Xeroderma pigmentosum	13
Erythropoietic protoporphyria	2
Systemic lupus erythematosus	1
Pellagra*	1
Drugs	0
Contactants	0

* Due to isoniazid (INH) taken for two months as tuberculosis prophylaxis by a three-year-old boy.

Approximately 10 per cent of atopic patients are photosensitive.

Jillson OF: Treatment of polymorphous light eruption with Trisoralen and natural sunlight. Cutis 27:592, 598, 1981.

Trioxsalen (Trisoralen 5 or 6 tablets (5 mg) two hours before sunning, daily for three weeks) is the most effective treatment for polymorphous light eruption. Patient gratitude is limitless, since it enables the patient to swim, sail, and sun normally. Avoid 8-methoxypsoralen (Oxsoralen), as it is too potent a photosensitizer and causes flares. Sun glasses are worn as usual. Repeat every month. The beneficial effect comes on in three weeks and lasts six weeks.

Birt AR: Polymorphous light eruption. J Am Acad Dermatol 4:610–611, 1981.

Trimethylpsoralen (Trisoralen 5 to 10 mg/day) is the most effective treatment for the hereditary type of polymorphous light eruption and actinic cheilitis seen in North American Indians.

Gschnait F, Hönigsmann H, Brenner W, et al: Induction of UV light tolerance by PUVA in patients with polymorphous light eruption. Br J Dermatol 99:293–295, 1978.

In five patients who for at least three years had problems every summer, getting a tan induced by PUVA (**8-methyoxypsoralen** + UVA 4 times a week, 6 to 10 exposures, total 20 J/sq cm, given in May and June) proved to be an effective photoprotective sun screen for the entire summer.

Parrish JA, Le Vine MJ, Morrison WL, et al: Comparison of PUVA and beta-carotene in the treatment of polymorphous light eruption. Br J Dermatol 100:187–191, 1979.

PUVA: Complete remission in 9 of 10 patients treated with PUVA (**8-methoxypsoralen** 0.6 mg/kg taken two hours before UVA 1.5 to 4.5 J/sq cm, three times weekly for 4 to 12 weeks in spring).

Beta-carotene: Complete remission in 6 of 19 treated with beta-carotene (Solatene 3 mg/kg bid for entire summer).

Corbett MF, Hawk JLM, Herxheimer A, Magnus IA: Controlled therapeutic trials in polymorphic light eruption. Br J Dermatol 107:571–581, 1982.

A double-blind study of 120 patients: No consistent help from either **beta-carotene** (200 mg/day for 15 weeks) or **chloroquine sulfate** (400 mg/day for 12 weeks).

Suhonen R, Plosila M: The effect of beta-carotene in combination with canthaxanthin, Ro 8-8427 (Phenoro) in treatment of polymorphous light eruptions. Dermatologica 163:172–176, 1981.

A double-blind study of 50 patients with polymorphous light eruption taking Phenoro (100 mg/day: 2 capsules bid of 10 mg **beta-carotene** + 15 mg **canthaxanthin**) for five weeks gave excellent results in 27 cases. Note that the placebo was effective in 16 cases. There was good patient acceptance of skin staining (carotenodermia).

Wennersten G: Carotenoid treatment for light sensitivity: A reappraisal and six years experience. Acta Derm Venereol 60:251–255, 1980.

Oral carotenoid therapy (four capsules a day, each containing **beta-carotene** 10 mg and **canthaxanthin** 15 mg, for six months per year for at least two years) gave good to excellent results in 20 of 31 cases of polymorphous light eruption. It had no effect in persistent light reaction, actinic reticuloid, or solar urticaria.

Saul A, Flores O, Novales J: Polymorphous light eruption: Treatment with thalidomide. Australas J Dermatol 17:17–21, 1976.

Thalidomide (100 to 200 mg daily for 45 to 150 days) resulted in complete healing in 13 of 25 patients (age 18 months to 52 years) with polymorphous light eruption. Lichenified pruritic plaques as well as lesions of prurigo that had been present for six months to seven years disappeared, even though the patient was in sunlight. Improvement was first noted within 8 to 30 days; 12 of the 20 patients in whom the drug was stopped remained asymptomatic for more than 1 year. Only five patients needed maintenance thalidomide (25 mg/day). There were no serious side effects, although this drug is a powerful teratogen.

There are no reproductions of disease. Every patient is an original canvas.

Porphyria Cutanea Tarda

No ethanol
No estrogens
Chloroquine
Venesection

Nearly all of our patients with porphyria cutanea tarda do well with a sermon on the "evils of ethanol and estrogen." It must be given seriously, and repeatedly, because this is a disease to cure by taking something away rather than giving something. Patients must know that the cause is a chemical that will keep on forming until they eliminate the alcohol, estrogens, or both that cripple their liver. And they must eliminate all other drugs not essential to them. The interdiction extends to occupational hazards such as pesticides and herbicides. Even a job change may be necessary. Continual review of the patient's environmental exposures and drug intake is necessary. But above all, encourage total abstinence from all alcoholic beverages.

The two excellent alternate treatments are low-dose chloroquine and venesection. We have used both with success. Indeed, one of our patients shortly after his first sermon on alcohol and the avoidance of sunlight left for Jamaica on vacation. We were astonished to see him absolutely clear of lesions on his return. He honestly admitted to having had a good vacation with sun and alcohol. It was not until we noted a fresh long scar across his bald head that the answer was forthcoming. "Yes, doc, I fell getting off the plane and like to bled to death from the gash on my head; had to go to the hospital for stitches."

Rorsman H, Harber LC (eds): Cutaneous porphyrias. Acta Derm Venereol Suppl 100:1–131, 1982.

Eighteen authorities participated in a symposium in Lund, Sweden, in May, 1981. Here they cover every aspect of every form of this biochemically defined area of photosensitivity, with presentations ranging from eyelid hypermelanosis to scarring alopecia, hypertrichosis, and blisters on the toes. Detailed data are given for laboratory differentiation of responsible abnormalities in heme synthesis in the bone marrow or liver.

Grossman ME, Bickers DR, Poh-Fitzpatrick MB, et al: Porphyria cutanea tarda: Clinical features and laboratory findings in 40 patients. Am J Med 67:277–286, 1979.

A complete clinical review, stressing that ethanol and estrogens are the most common causes of porphyria cutanea tarda, and venesection is the most common treatment (with average remission of $2\frac{1}{2}$ years).

Topi GC, Amantea A, Griso D: Recovery from porphyria cutanea tarda with no specific therapy other than avoidance of hepatic toxins. Br J Dermatol 111:75–82, 1984.

A careful detailed study of 16 patients in whom complete elimination of alcohol and exposure to other hepatotoxins resulted in complete clinical clearing of bullae and skin fragility in a period of two months to two years, showing that the metabolic defect is reversible. Patients were observed every three months for 3 to 13 years. In other patients phlebotomy and **chloroquine** therapy were used.

Specific hepatotoxins to be avoided:

- alcohol
- sulfa drugs
- nonsteroidal anti-inflammatory agents
- isoniazid
- herbicides
- pesticides
- sulfonylureas (Dymelor, Diabinese, Tolinase, Orinase)
- antiparasitic agents
- diazepam (Valium)
- norgestyl
- estradiol
- indomethacin (Indocin)
- ketoprofen
- testosterone
- aminopyrine

Ashton RE, Hawk JLM, Magnus IA: Low-dose oral chloroquine in the treatment of porphyria cutanea tarda. Br J Dermatol 111:609–613, 1984.

Low-dose **chloroquine phosphate** (125 mg twice a week until the uroporphyrin excretion is below 100 nmol/24 hours) proved to be a safe, effective, and convenient treatment for porphyria cutanea tarda. The mean treatment time was 14.9 months (range 10 to 23 months). Each of the seven patients treated had a sustained clinical and biochemical remission, although four had relapses 3 to 35 months (mean 17 months) after treatment was stopped.

Rogers M, Kamath KR, Poulos V: Porphyria cutanea tarda in a seven year old child. Australas J Dermatol 25:107–112, 1984.

Chloroquine (75 mg twice a week for five doses, then every 10 days for three months) cleared the condition in a seven-year-old girl after an initial flare of blisters and elevation of liver enzymes at three weeks. Long-term maintenance with chloroquine (75 mg every 10 days) was planned, since the problem is familial. Sun exposure was minimized as well, and her parents were advised that she must avoid estrogens and alcohol.

Ramsay CA, Magnus IA, Turnbull A, Baker H: The treatment of porphyria cutanea tarda by venesection. Q J Med 43:1–24, 1974.

Of 16 patients with porphyria cutanea tarda 15 showed an excellent response to repeated venesections (remove 400 to 500 ml blood every two to four weeks until the hemoglobin level falls to 12 gm/100 ml). The total blood volume removed varied from 2650 to 6500 ml over 2 to 10 months. Clinical improvement lagged behind the drop in urinary uroporphyrin excretion, but spontaneous blistering was the first sign to disappear. Remarkable clearing was seen of milia, scars, and in one case pseudoscleroderma. The authors consider phlebotomy to be the treatment of choice for porphyria cutanea tarda. It probably works through alteration of iron metabolism and subsequent reduction of uroporphyrin synthesis.

Attending to the minor details of your patient's care is a major accomplishment.

Prurigo Nodularis

Occlusion	Metronidazole
Corticosteroids	Benoxaprofen
Drysol	Phototherapy
Antihistamines	Cryotherapy
Erythromycin	Thalidomide

The "ecstasy and agony" of itch creates a work of art in the prurigo nodularis patient. Each lesion evolves into a supersensitive organoid itch receptor that self-renews through the reflex scratch it induces and becomes a perpetual itch machine. Most of these patients present with years filled with thousands of scratch hours. One of our patients had this megascratch problem for 34 years.

Although some of these patients are atopic and have elevated IgE levels, we have not been successful in finding a specific allergen. Our approach is to have the patient bring the scratch to the level of consciousness, so that Diprolene ointment or Drysol can be applied whenever there is a new wave of itching. The Diprolene is soothing, and the Drysol (aluminum chloride hexahydrate 20 per cent in anhydrous ethyl alcohol) substitutes a tingling pain for the itch and aborts the scratch reflex. Another aid is the use of Cordran tape over the lesions to protect nodules from the trauma of scratching and reduce the inflammatory element. The fingernails should be cut short.

We regularly prescribe erythromycin (250 mg qid) to reduce the pruritogenic bacterial component that commonly occurs when the lesions are denuded by scratching. If this gives no help we prescribe Flagyl (250 mg tid). A third helpful measure is the tedious injection of each lesion with Kenalog suspension (10 mg/ml diluted with equal parts of 2 per cent lidocaine). Some patients prefer focal cryotherapy with liquid nitrogen, used much as one would treat a wart.

In no instance is progress rapid. In a disease that has taken years to reach its climax form, one needs months to effect a cure. But it can be done!

Jorizzo JL, Gatti S, Smith EB: Prurigo: A clinical review. J Am Acad Dermatol 4:723–728, 1981.

Advises:

- cutting fingernails
- having professional exterminators disinfest patient's home
- antihistamines at bedtime
- 0.5 per cent **menthol** in emollient
- topical anesthetic—**pramoxine hydrochloride** (Tronothane 1 per cent cream)
- topical or intralesional steroids
- prolonged systemic antibiotics
- occlusive bandages
- phototherapy

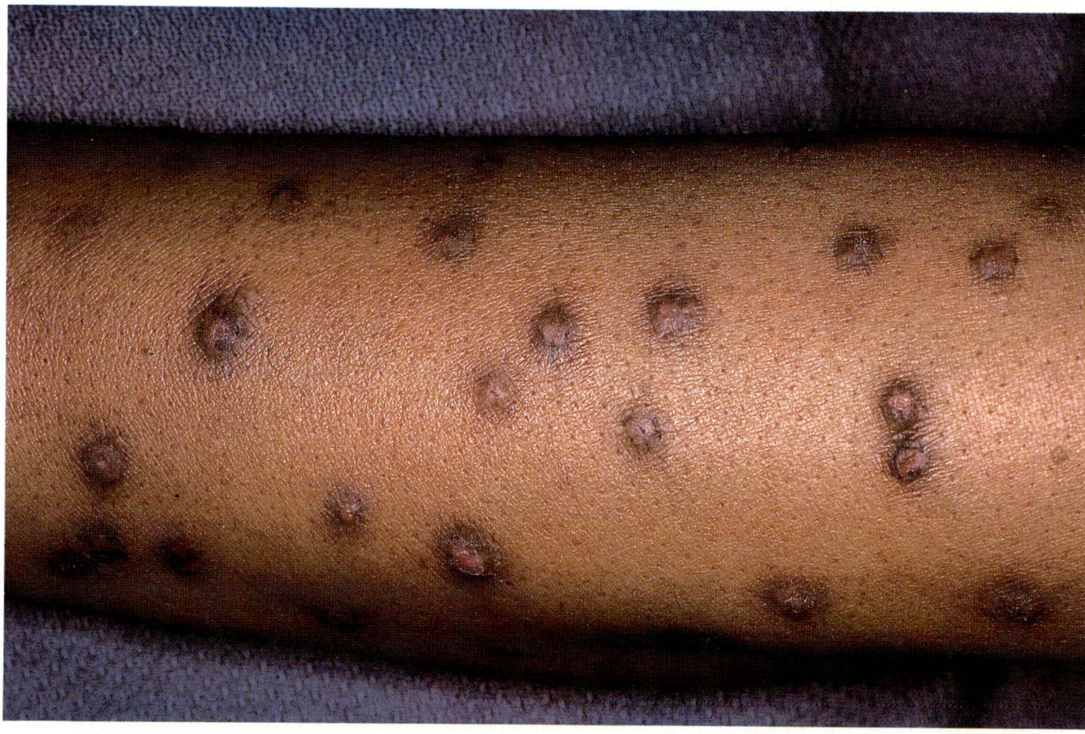

Runne U, Orfanos CE: Cutaneous neural proliferation in highly pruritic lesions of chronic prurigo. Arch Dermatol 113:787–791, 1977.

Nodular lesions of prurigo nodularis correspond to highly sensitive areas of neural proliferation as a result of the trauma of scratching. Occlusion with elastic bandages for four weeks betters both the clinical and histologic picture.

Suárez C, Pereda JM, Moreno LM, et al: Prurigo nodularis associated with malabsorption. Dermatologica 169:211–214, 1984.

A gluten-free diet supplemented with vitamins and iron induced complete clearing of all lesions within five months in a 72-year-old woman who had had prurigo nodularis for 16 years. Studies had previously ruled out biliary obstruction, diabetes, drug reaction, leukemia, lymphoma, parasitosis, polycythemia vera, renal insufficiency, thyroid disease, and tumors.

Goodwin PG: Nodular prurigo associated with gluten enteropathy. Proc R Soc Med 70:140–141, 1977.

Another example of prurigo nodularis that cleared with use of a gluten-free diet. Lesions that had been present for one year became much less pruritic within two months, and the 45-year-old woman was symptom free after one year, with only a few fibrotic nodules remaining on the skin.

Wood SM, Joseph S, Chalstrey LJ: A "side benefit" of metronidazole? Br Med J 1:552, 1979.

Treatment-resistant prurigo nodularis itch, present for 15 years, vanished within 24 hours of **metronidazole** prescribed for bowel sterilization in an 81-year-old man.

Hindson C, Lawlor F, Wacks H: Treatment of nodular prurigo with benoxaprofen. Br J Dermatol 107:369, 1982.

Benoxaprofen (ibuprofen—Motrin 600 mg/day) completely cleared two patients of nodular prurigo within two months.

Väätäinen N, Hannuksela M, Karvonen J: Local photochemotherapy in nodular prurigo. Acta Derm Venereol 59:544–547, 1979.

Good results were seen in 13 of 15 patients treated with PUVA, consisting of a **trioxsalen** bath (50 mg in 150 liters) and daily UVA in incremental dosage (total 14.6 J/sq cm). Pruritus abated within one week, and lesions subsided within one month. Maintenance doses were given every one to two months for two to four consecutive days.

Waldinger TP, Wong RC, Taylor WB, Voorhees JJ: Cryotherapy improves prurigo nodularis. Arch Dermatol 120:1598–1600, 1984.

Blistering cryotherapy (liquid N_2 10 to 30 seconds, two to four freeze-thaw cycles) cleared lesions in a 55-year-old black woman with prurigo nodularis for eight years. It had been resistant to **coal tar** and steroid creams, intralesional steroids, Atarax, and phototherapy. Complete hospital studies revealed no etiologic factor.

Stoll DM, Fields JP, King LE Jr: Treatment of prurigo nodularis: Use of cryosurgery and intralesional steroids plus lidocaine. J Dermatol Surg Oncol 9:922–924, 1983.

Two white men with prurigo nodularis were cured with this protocol:

1. Freeze with liquid N_2 cotton-tipped applicator.
2. Thaw for 10 seconds.
3. Inject lesion with a **triamcinolone acetonide-lidocaine** mixture (Kenalog 40 mg/ml diluted with three parts lidocaine hydrochloride 1 per cent). Note that lidocaine (Xylocaine) prevents flocculation of triamcinolone acetonide.
4. Repeat at monthly intervals, four to eight times.

Lovell CR, Hawk JLM, Calnan CD, Magnus IA: Thalidomide in actinic prurigo. Br J Dermatol 108:467–471, 1983.

Thalidomide (100 to 200 mg/day in adults, 50 to 100 mg/day in children), possibly acting as an immune suppressant, produced lasting improvement in 11 of 14 patients with actinic prurigo. Improvement was evident within two weeks. Maintenance therapy (50 to 100 mg/week up to 100 mg/day) was needed by eight patients.

Winkelmann RK, Connolly SM, Doyle JA, Padilha-Goncalves A: Thalidomide treatment of prurigo nodularis. Acta Derm Venereol 64:412–417, 1984.

Thalidomide (100 mg bid or tid) remarkably improved two patients within two to four weeks. Control was achieved with lower doses. Confirmatory evidence from six other patients is cited. Long-term benefit requires six months of therapy. Markedly elevated IgE levels decreased during treatment.

Unfortunately, some of the best therapists never write or never tell how they do it.

Pruritic Urticarial Papules and Plaques of Pregnancy (PUPPP)

Emollients Bandage Topical corticosteroids Prednisone

This is not an area in which to demonstrate one's therapeutic virtuosity. One's diagnostic skill should express itself in the good tidings: The baby will be normal, and the itch will go when the baby comes.

In our experience most of these women need only Synalar ointment 0.025 per cent applied once daily to the affected areas. Other emollients such as Acid Mantle cream or Eucerin aid in reducing the itch. We also caution against hot baths and overbathing. The usual sites of involvement are the stretched areas of the abdomen and thighs, so that part of the itch may come from simple pull on the epidermal nerve endings. Accordingly, every effort must be made to avoid excessive salt or caloric intake. If the patient cannot sleep we generally prescribe Benadryl (25 or 50 mg at hs).

We have not had to resort to systemic steroid therapy, but on occasion prednisone may be necessary and can be very effective. It is prudent to use minimal doses for short periods, but fortunately, this specific dermatosis occurs late in pregnancy so that systemic drugs do not pose the hazard they do in the early months.

Any form of vaginitis that may be present deserves appropriate local treatment as well. Similarly, diet should be adjusted for food intolerances such as eggs, pork, or chocolate, since in some women the problem may represent a form of urticaria localizing in the stretch marks.

With optimism, emollients, and empathy, these patients can be assisted through this uncommon trial of the last trimester of pregnancy. The good news is that, like pregnancy, these pruritic papules and plaques are a self-limiting problem.

Holmes RC, Black MM: The specific dermatoses of pregnancy. J Am Acad Dermatol 8:405–412, 1983.

Synonyms for pruritic urticarial papules and plaques of pregnancy:

- toxemic rash of pregnancy
- toxic erythema of pregnancy
- erythema multiforme of pregnancy
- polymorphic eruption of pregnancy
- urticarial eruptions of pregnancy
- late-onset prurigo of pregnancy

Yancey KB, Hall RP, Lawley TJ: Pruritic urticarial papules and plaques of pregnancy. J Am Acad Dermatol 10:473–480, 1984.

A careful study of 25 patients showed:

most frequent in primigravidas
no fetal problems
no spontaneous abortions
no prematurity or postmaturity
no recurrence in postpartum period
no recurrence with subsequent pregnancies
no recurrence with contraceptive use

Best treatment: Frequent application of high-potency corticosteroid gave relief of pruritus and arrest of new lesions in 13 of 14 patients.

Ahmed AR, Kaplan R: Pruritic urticarial papules and plaques of pregnancy. J Am Acad Dermatol 4:679–681, 1981.

Two examples of primigravidas in whom oilated Aveeno baths, **hydrocortisone** cream 1 per cent, and Benadryl (50 mg tid) were associated with complete disappearance of the rash in 7 and 10 days respectively. Both women delivered healthy baby girls.

Uhlin SR: Pruritic urticarial papules and plaques of pregnancy. Arch Dermatol 117:238–239, 1981.

Westcort cream (**hydrocortisone valerate** 0.2 per cent tid) cleared the pruritic eruption in 10 days in a 19-year-old primipara whose rash persisted after delivery. The infant son had a similar eruption that cleared in 10 days without treatment.

Callen JP, Hanno R: Pruritic urticarial papules and plaques of pregnancy (PUPPP): A clinicopathologic study. J Am Acad Dermatol 5:401–405, 1981.

Systemic steroids (**prednisone** 40 mg/day) were needed in only 1 of 15 patients in this study. Benadryl and topical steroids (applied three or four times daily) controlled the symptoms in most patients.

Cooper AJ, Fryer JA: Prurigo of late pregnancy. Australas J Dermatol 21:79–84, 1980.

Since mild topical steroids were ineffectual in five patients, the authors recommend **betamethasone valerate** cream 0.1 per cent (Valisone) under occlusion. If this is not successful, the treatment of choice is **prednisone** (20 mg/day for 2 to 4 days, tapered over 10 days, i.e., total dose 150 mg).

Stoller HE: Pruritic urticarial papules and plaques of pregnancy. JAMA 243:2156, 1980.

Three examples showing prompt resolution following **prednisone** therapy.

Holmes RC, McGibbon DH, Black, MM: Polymorphic eruption of pregnancy with subepidermal vesicles. J R Soc Med 77 (Suppl 4):22–23, 1984.

Two cases are recorded of spontaneous cures two and three weeks post partum, respectively. Lesions began within striae on the abdomen and consisted of papules surrounded by tiny vesicles. Direct and indirect immunofluorescent studies were negative. The subepidermal vesicles had numerous eosinophils.

The patient who sees many doctors for the same problem is basically a gambler.

Pruritus

Emollients	UVL
Antihistaminics	Naloxone
Anti-inflammatory agents	Charcoal
Antidepressants	Iron
Tranquilizers	Cholestyramine
Sedatives	Aspirin
Cooling	Lidocaine IV

Pruritus yields to the therapist who can discern and eliminate its cause. The diagnostic eye must thus focus on the dryness of overbathing, the little cluster of unroofed DH vesicles around the elbows, and the barely jaundiced conjunctivae. The diagnostic mind must suspect a drug, a soap, or the work place. And the diagnostic laboratory must screen the red and white cell count as well as the serum glucose, bilirubin, and iron, BUN, and thyroid levels.

Persistence of the pruritus coupled with the failure to detect a cause should lead to even more detailed studies and review. Look again for evidence of "bite and run" mites or fleas. Have the patient live in a new, animal-free environment for one week. Urge the patient to avoid bathing and to rub, instead of claw, itchy areas for one week. This will often allow a burrow to remain intact long enough to be seen by you. Examine the patient's clothing for mites or lice. Look for fiber glass insulation or fabrics in the environment. Check for use of antistatic compounds in the dryer.

With no objective findings other than excoriations, the search must continue within. Did the patient really stop all drugs? Are there any symptoms or signs that suggest a lymphoma or tumor? Any lymphadenopathy? A chest roentgenogram is always indicated. Serum protein electrophoresis, CEA, gastrointestinal series, and prostate and gynecologic examinations should extend the search. Examination of stools for ova and parasites is most valuable at times. Computed tomography and nuclear medicine studies remain the ultimate in diagnostic probing for an underlying tumor or occult cerebral infarct.

The quest must always be a steady, continuing one. As the data base expands and the disease state matures, further understanding of the pruritus may come. We recall vividly a 26-year-old school teacher hospitalized for intractable pruritus felt by a number of observers to be due to psychologic stress. Exhaustive studies ranging from sweat gland functioning to comprehensive neurologic examination failed to reveal any cause. Yet, in less than a year the true cause, Hodgkin's disease, became evident, and appropriate therapy could be initiated.

But what do we do until the cause goes away, is detected, or proves to be uncorrectable? Our preference is to advise daily inunctions with Eucerin, Acid Mantle creme or Synalar ointment (0.025 per cent). We interdict bathing except

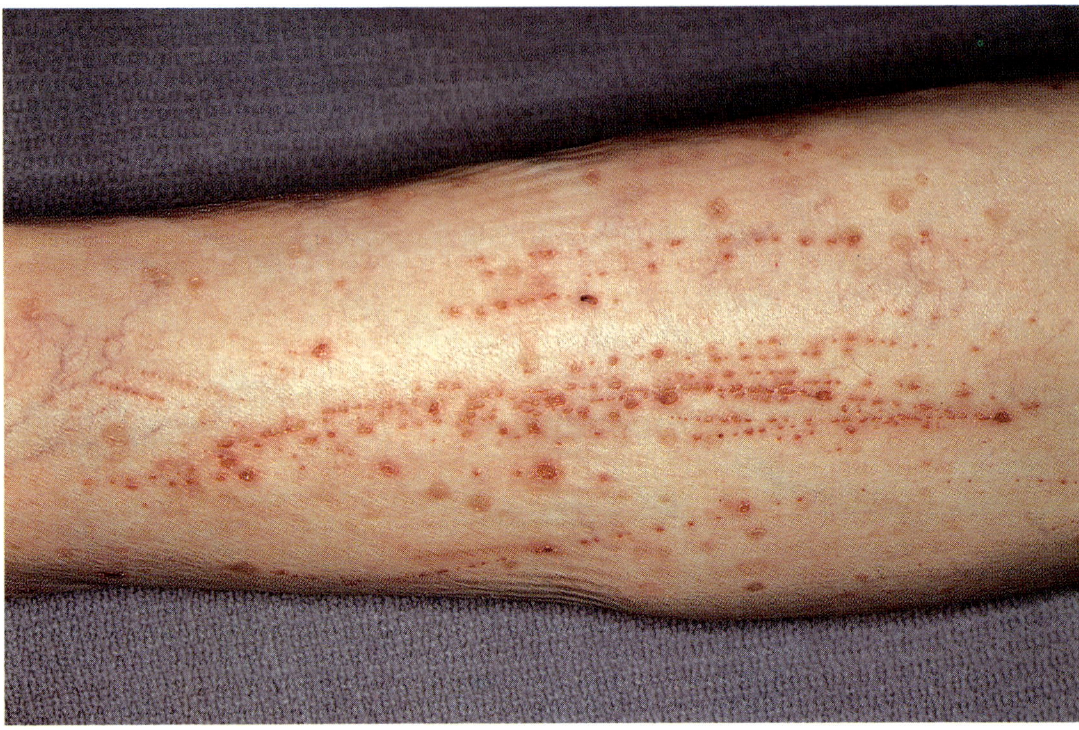

on "Saturday night." We ask the patient to wash with soap only in the intertriginous areas, using Neutrogena soap (marvelously water soluble and expensive enough to discourage excessive use). The use of washrags, Buf Puf, assorted back scratchers, alcohol, and hot water is frowned upon. The patient must clearly understand that the itch receptors are in the outermost part of the skin, much more superficial than the pain receptors. Anything that touches the skin virtually touches these itch nerves. All this mandates "hands off the itch trigger" (no touchy, no itchy).

Much help can be given to the patient with antihistaminics, which blunt the effect of histamine as an itch mediator in the skin. We favor Chlor-Trimeton (available OTC—chlorpheniramine maleate 4 mg). The dose must be adjusted carefully to the patient's tolerance and we generally avoid using it in the aged. Another favorite is Temaril (trimeprazine tartrate 2.5 mg qid). Here the dose range is phenomenal. We have achieved complete control in some patients only by using a dose of 25 mg qid. Terfenadine (Seldane 60 mg bid), cyproheptadine, and hydroxyzine complete our quintet of antipruritics. Seldane is the newest member, remarkable for its effectiveness and absence of the common side effect drowsiness.

For more specific help in patients with excoriations, and especially for the atopic, we prescribe an antibiotic, commonly erythromycin. This acts, we feel, by reducing the pruritogenic proteases released by clinically occult bacterial overgrowth.

We encourage the patient to avoid hot work places and overheated bedrooms and to use cooling compresses during acute attacks. The acquisition of a tan at the beach or in a tanning parlor or our office is of real benefit for these patients as well. Finally, but not as a therapy of despair, we ask that the fingernails be kept very short.

The fact that pharmacologists have never found a specific drug for stopping the torment of itch serves to spur us on to find the specific cause for itching. Each individual patient thus remains a wonderfully specific challenge we cannot resist. Here is an articulate novelist's rendering of this challenge:

I Wanted to Write by Kenneth Roberts, Garden City, NY, Doubleday & Company, Inc., 1949, pp 303–315.*

Porto Santo Stefano, Italy

January 16, 1936: Don't know what to do for the three bites I got on November 15, and they are not only swelling, but itching like Billy-be-damned.

January 25: Worried beyond expression by the violent itching of those three swollen bites. Can't understand why, in spite of constant application of S.T. 37, they grow larger and larger, itchier and itchier, and more and more inflamed.

January 26: Those damnable bites now have white cores, like miniature Vesuviases. Feel as if the damned things might suddenly explode, covering me with a mass of eruptions.

January 27: Dr. Polvani, dean of Porto Santo Stefano's Medical Corps, came up to examine the three bites and pustules that are radiating from them to legs, arms, back, hands, shoulders. . . . They were, he said, urticaria, brought on by eating shellfish. I must stop eating fish and eggs, stop drinking *vino*, and in a week all would go away. That would be fifty lire.

February 10: The pustules so thick and inflamed that they burst, gluing my shirt to my back . . . to the hot and airless office of Dottore Vincenzo Montesano. After using a magnifying glass on my eruptions, he stated unequivocally that the pustules were caused by zeccas, or ticks, which had embedded themselves in me while I was carrying some sort of tick-bearing animal, such as a rabbit, a lark, or a howl—meaning owl. . . . I must rub the pustules with lanolin salve, which he guaranteed would alleviate the itching immediately. He provided me with two small pots of salve. When I had used both pots, he said, I'd be cured. That would be two hundred lire . . . his insistence that I must have played host to a dead animal infested with zeccas, or ticks, convinced me that he didn't know what he was talking about, and that I would do well to check up on his diagnosis.

March 3: A miserable day of burning and itching. Smeared myself so thickly with lanolin that I had to put on two pajama tops under my clothes. Haven't smoked for days; but all my non-smoking, non-drinking, non-bathing, bidet-ing, injecting, purging, cal-

* Printed by permission of the Estate of Kenneth Roberts.

	cium taking, milk of magnesia-ing, castor-oiling, and greasing have done me no good whatever.
March 6:	Exasperated beyond words at the inability of these damned doctors to agree on what I've got or to prescribe anything that will cure it.
March 18:	I have now used thirty-six jars [of ointment], and today sent to Florence for ten more.
Boston, April 30:	Called on Dr. Emery at the Harvard Medical School. He could only guess that I'd picked up a fungus growth—some sort of tropical disease, and that it would be a waste of time and money to see specialists. His recommendation was to return to good Maine foods and good Maine customs with no loss of time.
	Since doctors had been unable to supply me with remedies to cure eruptions, I turned to household cures recommended by state-of-Mainers . . . application of brine from a pickle barrel . . . gallons of orange juice . . . swallow a few lead pellets from a shotgun shell every few days . . . a bottle of mange cure that a Sanford veterinarian insisted would cure any sort of human eczema.

Champion RH: Generalized pruritus. Br Med J 289:751–753, 1984.

Presents a marvelous two-page algorithm for treatment of pruritus:

Advice for doctors:

favorite drug: Phenergan (**promethazine hydrochloride**)
avoidance of:
- topical anesthetics and topical antihistaminics (these may sensitize)
- topical corticosteroids if the skin is normal (they simply do not penetrate)

Advice for patients:

avoidance of:
- calamine lotion (too drying)
- overheating
- hot baths
- harsh clothing
- alcohol

Psychogenic pruritus should be a "reluctant" diagnosis made only by exclusion of other causes and only if psychiatric abnormalities are present.

Savin J: Itching. *In* Rook A, Savin J (eds): Recent Advances in Dermatology, Number 5. London, Churchill Livingstone, 1980, pp 222–235.

A delightfully erudite synthesis of all we know about what itching means.

"Itching lies neglected in the shadow of pain. It is just as intolerable and an every-day problem in all skin clinics. . . . The similarities between the physiology of itching and pain are very close."

Itching may be abolished by pinpricks in the same dermatome and by electrical transcutaneous nerve stimulation for one to two minutes.

Lyell A: The itching patient: A review of the causes of pruritus. Scott Med J 17:334–347, 1972.

The best basis for management is identification of the cause. A three-year study of 74 cases showed that 23 were due to cutaneous problems, 23 were psychologic in nature, 18 were of systemic origin, and 10 were never explained.

Some unusual causes include:

- acquired anhidrosis
- erythropoietic protoporphyria
- electrostatic charge
- red-rust flower beetle (*Tribolium castaneum*)
- diatoms
- seaweed
- *Alconydium hirsutum* (a colonial animal in water)

Always check for hyperthyroidism and Hodgkin's disease.

Gilchrest BA: Pruritus: Pathogenesis, therapy, and significance in systemic disease states. Arch Intern Med 142:101–105, 1982.

A good screen for underlying disturbances includes checking for:

- drugs (opiates, **methoxsalen**)
- parasites
- hepatic disease (in primary biliary cirrhosis 50 per cent have itching)
- renal failure
- diabetes mellitus
- hypothyroidism or hyperthyroidism
- tumors

Kantor GR, Lookingbill DP: Generalized pruritus and systemic disease. J Am Acad Dermatol 9:375–382, 1983.

Simple correctable xerosis accounted for long-term pruritus in 7 of 44 patients studied.

Camp R: Generalized pruritus and its management. Clin Exp Dermatol 7:557–563, 1982.

Many patients with pruritus are placebo responders. The following treatments, initially acclaimed, failed to provide specific help under controlled evaluation:

- subtotal parathyroidectomy, **cholestyramine,** or UVB in uremic itch
- **naloxone** or **cimetidine** in pruritus of biliary cirrhosis

However, subgroups of patients appear to exist who do respond to these various treatments, and attempts should be made to identify them.

Winkelmann RK: Pharmacologic control of pruritus. Med Clin North Am 66:1119–1133, 1982.

A comprehensive review with 115 references.

Antihistamines should be tried in full dosage in all patients with pruritus, since histamine is the most common mediator known. Other antipruritics include antidepressants, tranquilizers, and sedatives. Simple cooling of the skin is another powerful way of allaying pruritus.

Hägermark Ö: Pruritus: Pathogenesis and therapeutic trials. *In* Kukita A, Seiji M (eds): Proceedings of the 16th International Congress of Dermatology. Tokyo, University of Tokyo Press, 1983, pp 61–67.

The H_1 receptor, but not the H_2 histamine receptor, mediates itch. Hence, **cimetidine** is without any effect other than as a placebo. Sunlight, UVA, UVB, and PUVA have significant ameliorative effects on standardized experimental itch induced by the histamine liberator compound 48/80.

Smitz S, Legros J-J, Le Maire M: Naloxone, itch, asthma, urticaria, and angioedema. Ann Intern Med 97:788–789, 1982.

A five-year itch of unknown origin in a 54-year-old woman was eliminated for more than six months by a single intravenous infusion of **naloxone** (1.6 mg/hour for four hours). A 39-year-old woman with asthma, chronic urticaria, and recurrent angioedema, who had taken systemic steroids for 10 years, was able to discontinue steroids after a similar **naloxone** infusion.

Summerfield JA: Naloxone modulates the perception of itch in man. Br J Clin Pharmacol 10:180–183, 1980.

In a double-blind study, 20 patients with cholestasis and protracted pruritus were given the opiate antagonist **naloxone** (Narcan 2 mg IV). Although scratching (a spinal reflex) was not affected, pruritus was significantly reduced. This observation (the reduced perception of itch) could only be made by the author's ingeniously removing the placebo reactors from the study (as the placebo responders felt that itching was worse when they were given naloxone).

Jillson OF: Pruritus. Cutis 28:335–339, 1981.

For winter itch (pruritus hiemalis):

Restrict soap to essential areas.
Bathe in a tub with one cup of table salt added to the warm bath.
Lubricate the skin daily.

Jorizzo JL: The itchy patient: A practical approach. Primary Care 10:339–353, 1983.

Use of emollients is extremely important, as xerosis often exacerbates pruritus. **Triamcinolone** cream 0.1 per cent or another middle-strength corticosteroid may also be needed.

Pederson JA, Matter BJ, Czerwinski AW, Llach F: Relief of idiopathic generalized pruritus in dialysis patients treated with activated oral charcoal. Ann Intern Med 93:446–448, 1980.

In 10 of 11 patients undergoing hemodialysis, **activated charcoal** (6 gm/day for eight weeks) relieved pruritus presumably due to enteric absorption of pruritogens.

Shaw D, Trotter JM, Calman KC: Plasma exchange to control sweats and pruritus in malignant disease. Br Med J 281:1459, 1980.

In a 54-year-old woman with non-Hodgkin's lymphoma, plasma replacement (4.9 liters and 4.3 liters done eight days apart) provided several weeks of relief from generalized pruritus.

Salem HH, Van der Weyden MB, Young IF, Wiley JS: Pruritus and severe iron deficiency in polycythaemia vera. Br Med J 285:91–92, 1982.

Ferrous gluconate (300 mg tid) or **ferrous sulfate** (300 mg daily) had the dramatic effect of abolishing generalized itching in six iron-deficient polycythemia patients. Improvement was noted within 2 to 14 days. Pruritus recurred when the iron supplement was discontinued. Treatment with iron should be continued for only two to three weeks after pruritus has abated to avoid progressive increases in the red cell mass.

Fjellner B, Hägermark Ö: Pruritus in polycythemia vera: Treatment with aspirin and possibility of platelet involvement. Acta Derm Venereol 59:505–512, 1979.

Itching triggered by the sudden cooling of skin after a hot bath or shower was relieved in 15 of 17 patients with polycythemia vera by taking aspirin (500 mg tid for seven days). However, the relief was complete in only 1 of the 15.

Valsecchi R, Cainelli T: Generalized pruritus: A manifestation of iron deficiency. Arch Dermatol 119:630, 1983.

In a 68-year-old man with unremitting pruritus for three years, raising the serum iron from 27 μg/dl to 58 μg/dl with an iron supplement led to complete disappearance of itching in 10 days.

Heyl T: Brachioradial pruritus. Arch Dermatol 119:115–116, 1983.

Intense pruritus of one or both arms may be due to cervical vertebral osteoarthritis and nerve compression. In three of five patients relief was obtained by manipulation, cervical traction, and physiotherapy. Anti-inflammatory drugs also provided some relief, although topical steroids were useless.

Osterman PO: Paroxysmal itching in multiple sclerosis. Br J Dermatol 95:555–558, 1976.

Recurrent short attacks of segmental paroxysmal itching were completely prevented in three women with multiple sclerosis by prescribing **carbamazepine** (Tegretol 200 to 400 mg tid). Such itching may be the first sign of MS.

Yamamoto M, Yabuki S, Hayabara T, Otsuki S: Paroxysmal itching in multiple sclerosis: A report of three cases. J Neurol Neurosurg Psychiatry 44:19–22, 1981.

Be alert to the need for neurologic consultation if a patient describes short bursts of severe localized pruritus, as this may be the only initial symptom of multiple sclerosis.

Arnold HL: Paroxysmal pruritus. Its clinical characterization and a hypothesis of its pathogenesis. J Am Acad Dermatol 11:322–326, 1984.

An instructive example of how questioning can reveal a psychic stress that is recognized, but not identified, by the patient as triggering severe pruritus. The cure was the simple revelation that a 35-year-old divorcee's paroxysmal attacks of pruritus began when her children returned to their father's custody.

King CA, Huff FJ, Jorizzo JL: Unilateral neurogenic pruritus: Paroxysmal itching associated with central nervous system lesions. Ann Intern Med 97:222–223, 1982.

A capsular infarction on the right side of the brain (seen on CT) was the cause of itching of the lower part of the left leg in a 58-year-old woman. Effective treatment: Tegretol.

Massey EW: Unilateral neurogenic pruritus following stroke. Stroke 15:901–903, 1984.

Nine stroke patients with excoriations of the involved side received relief from **glycerin** and **olive oil** lotion locally and oral **carbamazepine** (Tegretol) or **amitriptyline** (Elavil 50 mg at bedtime).

Harries AD, Tredree R, Heatley RV, et al: Pruritus as a manifestation of the dumping syndrome. Br J Dermatol 107:707–709, 1982.

A 62-year-old postgastrectomy patient had had generalized itching for six months, which appeared 30 minutes after each meal and lasted for two hours.

Cure: **Pectin** capsules (2 gm before and after each meal). Presumably, pectin increased the viscosity of the intraluminal contents, slowed passage of carbohydrates through the bowel, and delayed small-intestinal absorption. (An apple a day made the itch go away!)

Greaves MW, Black AK, Eady RAJ, Coutts A: Aquagenic pruritus. Br Med J 282:2008–2010, 1981.

Conjoint **cimetidine** (200 mg qid) and **chlorpheniramine** (8 mg qid) completely prevented itching from skin contact with water in two patients.

Johannessen H, Bergan-Skar B: Itching problems among potroom workers in factories using recycled alumina. Contact Dermatitis 6:42–43, 1980.

Skin problems, particularly itching on the legs, occurred in 46 of 123 workers. Cure: One week away from work and application of steroid creams.

Verbeck SJA, Buise-van Unnik EMM, Malten KE: Itching in office workers from glass fibres. Contact Dermatitis 7:354, 1981.

Thirteen office workers in a new building were cleared of itching within two weeks of sealing off the ceiling with plastic foil and thereby preventing long glass fibers of insulation material from entering the air ducts.

Brenner S, Ophir J, Krakowski A: Pediculid: An unusual -id reaction to pediculosis capitis. Dermatologica 168:189–191, 1984.

Two patients were cured of "idiopathic" pruritus and a widespread skin-colored papular eruption simply by treating occult pediculosis capitis.

Krass ME: Diagnosis and management of hypochrondriacal psychosis. Can Med Assoc J 124:968, 1981.

An elderly husband, wife, and blind sister each had severe generalized pruritus they attributed to mite or insect infestation. No ectoparasites could be found in a shopping bag full of samples they had collected.

Cure: Orap (**pimozide** 4 mg bid for three weeks). (This drug has proven to be of specific value in many other examples of delusions of parasitosis.)

Bingham EA, Burrows D, Sandford JC: Prolonged pruritus and bullous pemphigoid. Clin Exp Dermatol 9:564–570, 1984.

Eight elderly patients experienced unexplained prolonged (mean 10 months) generalized pruritus as the initial sign of bullous pemphigoid. Immunofluorescent studies of skin helped confirm the diagnosis in three patients without blisters, but detection of serum antibasement membrane antibody (IgG) was not specific for pemphigoid.

Treatment: **prednisone, ACTH, azathioprine.**

Soter NA, Austen KF, Wasserman SI: Oral disodium cromoglycate in the treatment of systemic mastocytosis. N Engl J Med 301:465–469, 1979.

Disodium cromoglycate (100 mg qid for 1 to 10 months) greatly reduced the pruritus, whealing, flushing, diarrhea, and abdominal pain associated with systemic mastocytosis. Improvement was noted after two to three weeks. (Oral form not available in the United States.)

Kligman AM, Greaves MW, Steinman H: Water-induced itching without cutaneous signs: Aquagenic pruritus. Arch Dermatol 122:183–186, 1986.

This problem is reversible in the elderly patient by following these rules:

1. Sponge baths or quick warm showers only.
2. Hydrophobic moisturizers applied twice daily.
3. Avoid topical corticosteroids.
4. Avoid moisturizers with such potential irritants as propylene glycol, salicylic acid, coal tar, or urea.

Denman ST: A review of pruritus. J Am Acad Dermatol 14:375–392, 1986.

An excellent survey of 142 articles. Physicians who treat pruritus must consider all contributing factors, including dry skin, the psyche, and any underlying disease. Basic evaluation demands careful history, physical examination, chest x-ray, CBC and differential, blood chemistry profile, and stool for occult blood. Therapy centers on the H_1 histamine blockers hydroxyzine and doxepin.

A good doctor can do a good deal for a good patient.

Pruritus Ani

Cleansing	Charcoal
Hydrocortisone cream	Cholestyramine
Diet	

These patients do not come to you with a trivial itch. They come with a terrible itch. They want a serious appraisal of their problem and medical health.

Our first effort is careful inspection of the area. Is there evidence of any skin disease that allows fecal material to be more irritating or more resistant to removal? We look for psoriasis, erythrasma, intertrigo, and contact dermatitis, as well as warts, hemorrhoids, and fissures. Is there evidence of lichen simplex chronicus? We check elsewhere on the skin for evidence of psoriasis or atopic dermatitis. Any disease found needs corrective measures, and we are particularly alert to specific anorectal problems such as prolapsing internal hemorrhoids, mucosal prolapse, and chronic anal fissures. Proctoscopy is always necessary in recalcitrant pruritus ani, as it may reveal underlying proctitis or a secretory villous polyp leading to mucoid leakage and skin irritation. Likewise, a 2-AM stool collection on "double-stick" Scotch tape touched to the anal area may, on rare occasions, reveal a pinworm infection.

Given an absence of skin lesions, aside from excoriations, we focus our attention on the obvious cause of irritation, feces. We instruct the patient that in the treatment of pruritus ani, cleanliness is "godliness." Any feces not removed remains as a real threat to comfort. If it remains in that "closed patch-test" environment it will surely cause itch. It will keep the skin wet, alkaline (may reach pH 10), and exposed to allergens (foods), as well as bacterial toxins and proteases (25 per cent of feces is bacteria).

Accordingly, the patient must cleanse the area after every bowel movement and also whenever he feels itching. Too often a bowel movement is considered the only source of fecal soiling. Many times soiling comes from the passage of gas, a momentary relaxation of the anal sphincter, the stress pressure of physical exercise, or a long peristaltic wave. Ideally, cleansing should be done with unscented Neutrogena soap and water or a cleansing lotion such as Balneol. However, gentle use of soft white toilet paper (and there are differences!) or Kleenex is often sufficient.

We instruct the patient that his anal sphincter is the guard protecting the outside from what is inside. Its tone must be optimal, kept that way by the patient eliminating the pharmacologic foods that relax the sphincter. Thus, he must avoid all coffee, tea, cola drinks, chocolate, and alcoholic beverages. He also should avoid medicines in general, especially antibiotics, laxatives, and mineral oil, all of which give the feces a fluidity permitting anal leakage. Foods that cause excessive gas in the colon are likewise to be avoided. Since food allergens may cause no sign of intolerance other than pruritic contact dermatitis of the anal area, we ask the patient to avoid all milk, pork, tomatoes, corn, and nuts on a trial basis.

If the patient has continuing difficulty we prescribe Mycostatin oral tablets (500,000 U tid) or Nizoral (200 mg/day) to reduce the yeast content of the bowel, another source of irritation in the *Candida*-sensitive patient. Nonspecific absorption of allergens may be achieved with the ion exchange resin cholestyramine (Questran 9 gm tid), or activated charcoal (780 mg tid) for two weeks.

The patient must also be aided in achieving regular, formed bowel movements by the use of bulk laxatives containing psyllium hydrophilic mucilloid (Metamucil, Konsyl). Checking the underwear for wetness or soiling helps monitor the patient's progress.

We are especially careful to make the patient aware of the hazards of using certain medications in the anal area such as fluorinated steroid creams, which are atrophogenic, and potentially sensitizing preparations such as local anesthetics and some home remedies (topical vitamin E, Noxzema).

Finally, we reassure the patient that he does not have cancer and that in the end all will be well.

Smith LE, Henrichs D, McCullah RD: Prospective studies on the etiology and treatment of pruritus ani. Dis Colon Rectum 25:358–363, 1982.

Exquisite study of 75 patients:

1. Soiling due to poorly formed stools or incomplete stool evacuation occurred in 50 per cent.
2. Most tended to worsen the pruritus ani by overzealous cleansing and medication.
3. The condition responds well to anal cleanliness, dietary discretion, bowel habit regulation (always answer "the call"), and **hydrocortisone** cream or ointment 1 per cent.
4. Partial to complete relief was achieved in 27 of 50 patients by total elimination of:
   coffee, tea, cola, chocolate
   alcohol (especially beer), tobacco
   milk, nuts, pork, ketchup
   citrus fruits, spices
5. Laboratory studies were not helpful in management.
6. Reassure the patient that the perianal itching is not a sign of cancer.
7. Avoid girdles and corsets that bind the buttocks together.
8. Add no salts or antiseptics to the bath water.
9. Use bran or a bulk stool softener taken at the same time daily to promote regularity and eliminate diarrhea or leakage.

Verbov J: Pruritus ani and its management—A study and reappraisal. Clin Exp Dermatol 9:46–52, 1984.

A careful study of 47 patients with pruritus ani (1.6 per cent incidence in a survey of 3000 dermatologic outpatients) revealed:

1. In 55 per cent pruritus was secondary to:

psoriasis	excessive hair
eczema	anal warts
intertrigo	diarrhea
candidiasis	threadworms
tinea	

2. In 45 per cent there were no signs of skin disease; these patients tend to enjoy a number of minor ills and disabilities, but live to a ripe old age. Relapse is common with adversity.

3. Best treatment regimen:
    When moving the bowels
        avoid straining
        sit for 3 to 4 minutes on the toilet afterward prior to wiping with soft toilet paper.
        "rushing in and out of the toilet is ill advised"
    anal cleansing
    cotton underpants (loose fitting)
    silver nitrate solution (0.25 per cent aqueous bid)—apply and let dry
    1 per cent **hydrocortisone** cream (bid or after each bowel movement [after application of silver nitrate])
    avoidance of coffee, alcohol, spices
    warm bath with 1 to 2 teaspoons of salt
    Atarax at bedtime

The dermatologist should:

- spend time talking to the patient
- remember to check the feet for tinea
- watch out for overuse of topical steroids (especially potent ones)
- patch test if many topical preparations have been applied

Bowyer A, McColl I: A study of 200 patients with pruritus ani. Proc R Soc Med 63(Suppl):96–98, 1970.

Pruritus ani should never be accepted as a diagnosis, since erythrasma, contact dermatitis, candidiasis, hemorrhoids, and anal fissures are significant etiologic factors that should be determined. Many patients have three or more separate causes of itching, each of which must be eliminated to achieve a cure.

Sullivan ES, Garnjobst WM: Pruritus ani: A practical approach. Surg Clin North Am 58:505–512, 1978.

Be certain that the patient is not taking drugs that irritate the gut, resulting in inadvertent perianal seepage. These include mineral oil, **quinidine**, and **colchicine**. Misuse of premoistened witch hazel (50 per cent)–glycerin (10 per cent) pads (Tucks) with prolonged contact with the anus will also induce intense maceration, itching, and burning.

Popcorn may cause mechnical and chemical irritation of the gut, with fecal drainage due to increased mucous production and increased colonic motility.

Menopausal women may have perianal burning or soreness due to estrogen deficiency. Treatment should include systemic estrogen initially, followed by a topical estrogen cream.

If furuncles or purulent discharge is present, add ½ to 1 ounce of Purex or Clorox to the sitz bath to satisfy the need of the patient to "medicate" the water.

Rectal irrigations with a bulb syringe and 6 to 8 ounces of lukewarm water may help prevent afterdrainage, which usually causes perianal itching within an hour after defecation (often seen in milk drinkers with pasty or constipated stools).

Adult athletes with perianal hirsutism may develop friction injury from hair trauma. They are helped by lubricating-ointment–based preparations.

If pruritus occurs during the night, apply a **lidocaine**-containing water-soluble cream with an acid pH at bedtime (Lida-Mantle cream 1 per cent).

A hydrophilic stool-conditioning preparation such as Konsyl (**psyllium hydrophilic mucilloid**) helps patients with diarrhea or constipation.

Surgery may be necessary in about one of six (16 per cent) patients with pruritus ani to eliminate causes of mucous or purulent discharge.

Remember that Paget's disease is notoriously pruritic, so that any unilateral lesions unresponsive to treatment should have an early biopsy.

Alexander-Williams J: Pruritis ani. Br Med J 287:159–160, 1983.

Perianal polypharmacy perpetuates pruritus.

Aging anal sphincters allow leakage of mucus and feces.

The author recommends cleansing with wet wipes or a moist cloth to remove fecal material frequently missed by dry wiping.

The author uses **silver nitrate** (0.5 per cent aqueous) to maintain perianal dryness.

Caplan RM: The irritant role of feces in the genesis of perianal itch. Gastroenterology 50:19–23, 1966.

Rabelais wrote that wiping the perianal skin with the neck of a plump, downy, warm goose was unquestionably "the most lordly, excellent, and expedient technique ever seen." In lieu of a goose, wipe gently with soft white toilet paper to remove feces that, in this study of 27 subjects, proved on patch testing to be of the same irritancy in patients and in controls.

Alexander-Williams J: Causes and management of anal irritation. Br Med J 287:1528, 1983.

Ten rules for the patient with pruritus ani:

1. Keep the area clean—wash night and morning and after every bowel action.
2. Avoid rubbing with a bar of soap or washcloth.
3. If away from home, use medicated baby wipes.
4. Keep the area dry—a hair dryer is the best aid.
5. Avoid garments that press the buttocks together and cause excessive moisture.
6. Place cotton dusted with powder against the anus—change after each washing.
7. Avoid perfumed talcum powder. The author advises use of Zeasorb powder on the cotton pledget.
8. Avoid ointments and creams. Use **silver nitrate** (0.5 per cent aqueous) or Castellani's paint (50 per cent aqueous) as antiseptic drying lotions.
9. Keep bowels regular with fiber (roughage, bran) in diet.
10. Wear cotton gloves at night if you scratch during sleep.

Goldman L: A cream cleanser for anal hygiene in the treatment of pruritus ani. Arch Dermatol 116:1346, 1980.

Recommends a copper-containing cream (Harper's cleanser cream) for thorough anal cleansing after each bowel movement. Apply and remove with moistened toilet paper, pat dry, and powder.

Kocsard E: Pruritus ani: A symptom of fecal contamination. Cutis 27:518, 1981.

Advises patients to stop using toilet paper, Instead, wash the perianal skin *and the anal canal* (use finger!) with water and a mild soap after every bowel movement. Gently dry and apply **hydrocortisone** cream 1 per cent around the anal opening and inside the anal canal. Must avoid rubbing and scratching during the cleansing procedure.

Friend WG: The cause and treatment of idiopathic pruritus ani. Dis Colon Rectum 20:40–42, 1977.

The most common cause of "idiopathic" pruritus ani is coffee. To persuade the patient, eliminate coffee for two weeks, then challenge with increasing amounts (1 to 3 cups a day). The delay before symptoms return following a threshold dose is 24 to 48 hours. Other foods implicated in pruritus ani are tea, cola, beer, chocolate, and tomatoes (ketchup). They should also be eliminated for two weeks before being added back one by one to test threshold amounts.

Jillson OF: Pruritus ani: Disputing the passage. Cutis 33:537–548, 1984.

Be sure to look at the perianal area under the Wood's light for erythrasma. If present, treat with **erythromycin** (250 mg qid for 10 days). Use topical erythromycin and **miconazole** cream to prevent relapses.

A pledget of cotton applied to the anal area at bedtime gives relief by absorbing drainage and stifling itch.

Detrano SJ: Cryotherapy for chronic nonspecific pruritus ani. J Dermatol Surg Oncol 10:483–484, 1984.

Relief of pruritus ani in 15 of 18 patients was achieved by using a liquid nitrogen spray of the entire area for 2 to 3 seconds (with a C.S. 76 or C.E. 4 Frigitronics unit). Repeat once after a complete thaw. Alert the patient that drainage will last for five days and that complete healing will take two weeks.

Ely PH: "Sure-fire-success-guaranteed" treatment for pruritus ani. Schoch Letter 35(4):16, 1985.

1. Examine the axillary and perirectal areas with Wood's light to rule out erythrasma.
2. Wash the perirectal skin with a **benzoyl peroxide** wash (Oxy Wash, Desquam-X 10 wash) at bedtime followed by a small dab of Vytone cream (**hydrocortisone-iodoquinol**).
3. **Activated charcoal** (Charcocaps, OTC, 260-mg capsules, three with each meal). Note: This activated charcoal USP can also adsorb medications such as oral contraceptives.
4. Eliminate cinnamon from diet, if patch test is positive.

Count that day lost that has not presented you with a therapeutic challenge.

Pruritus of Uremia and Cholestasis

Eurax cream	Heparin IV
Cholestyramine	Vitamin K
Charcoal	Hemodialysis
UVB	Plasma perfusion
Lidocaine IV	

See Pruritus section also.

Rosen T: Uremic pruritus: A review. Cutis 23:790–792, 1979.

The cornerstone of therapy of uremic pruritus is hemodialysis. Adjuncts include **cholestyramine** (5 gm bid), IV lidocaine (200 mg in 100 ml saline, 20-minute drip, repeat in one hour if itching persists), and IV **heparin** (100 mg q12h for three weeks). Sauna baths may also help pruritus.

Bourlod AE: Ultraviolet phototherapy. Int J Dermatol 19:223, 1980.

For uremic patients in whom UVB phototherapy may not be used, 10 per cent **crotamiton** in a shake lotion or hydrophilic ointment (Eurax cream bid or tid) helps combat pruritus.

Silverberg DS, Iaina A, Reisin E, et al: Cholestyramine in uraemic pruritus. Br Med J 1:752–753, 1977.

In a controlled double-blind study of 10 patients with severe uremic pruritus who were undergoing chronic hemodialysis, **cholestyramine** (5 gm bid in juice) greatly improved pruritus in four of five patients, clearing one completely. The fifth patient improved with an increased dose of cholestyramine (5 gm qid). In contrast, only one of five patients receiving a placebo was helped.

Pederson JA, Matter BJ, Czerwinski AW, Llach F: Relief of idiopathic generalized pruritus in dialysis patients treated with activated oral charcoal. Ann Intern Med 93:446–448, 1980.

In a double-blind study, 10 of 11 hemodialysis patients with pruritus were helped by taking **charcoal** (6 gm daily for eight weeks). Compliance was monitored through observation of stool discoloration.

Gilchrest BA, Rowe JW, Brown RS, et al: Ultraviolet phototherapy of uremic pruritus: Long-term results and possible mechanism of action. Ann Intern Med 91:17–21, 1979.

After a course of six to eight UVB exposures 32 of 38 patients improved. The pruritus recurred in half the patients after a mean remission period of three months. Patients received one to three treatments per week, with an initial dose of 75 per cent of the estimated minimal erythema dose (MED). Subsequent treatments stayed just below the MED. If a second course of treatment was necessary, the itching responded even more rapidly. A beneficial response was sometimes delayed until two weeks after therapy was completed.

Shultz BC, Roenigk HH Jr: Uremic pruritus treated with ultraviolet light. JAMA 243:1836–1837, 1980.

Of 10 patients studied 8 had nearly complete relief of itching for at least one month after completing 7 to 20 treatments (three times a week) with ultraviolet B (290 to 320 nm) light. Treatments were given in a box with 24 122-cm Westinghouse FS40 fluorescent bulbs mounted on four reflecting walls. In 6 patients relief persisted for more than six months after the course of UVB light therapy.

Taylor R, Taylor AEM, Diffey BL, Hindson TC: A placebo-controlled trial of UV-A phototherapy for the treatment of uraemic pruritus. Nephron 33:14–16, 1983.

A significant reduction of itching occurred in *both* the visible blue-light–treated group and the UVA–treated group of 11 patients given phototherapy (three times a week for six weeks). Patients receiving blue light (wavelength 400 to 450 nm) received exposure approximately six times stronger than that of normal sunlight.

Tapia L, Cheigh JS, David DS, et al: Pruritus in dialysis patients treated with parenteral lidocaine. N Engl J Med 296:261–262, 1977.

Lidocaine (200 mg in 100 ml of physiologic saline given intra-arterially over 20 minutes during hemodialysis, repeat in one hour if no help) aided in relieving pruritus for more than 24 hours in all 20 patients in this double-blind study.

Gilchrest BA, Stern RS, Steinman TI, et al: Clinical features of pruritus among patients undergoing maintenance hemodialysis. Arch Dermatol 118:154–156, 1982.

Changing the type of **heparin** used in hemodialysis may eliminate pruritus caused by allergy to the bovine or porcine component. In many patients pruritus occurs only during or shortly after dialysis.

Graf H, Kovarik J, Stummvoll HK, Wolf A: Disappearance of uraemic pruritus after lowering dialysate magnesium concentration. Br Med J 2:1478–1479, 1979.

Lowering the **magnesium** concentration in the dialysate from 2.4 mg/dl to 0.48 mg/dl gave prompt disappearance of pruritus in a 59-year-old man who had been undergoing dialysis for two years. There was no recurrence of pruritus in the following eight months. Lowering the dialysate magnesium concentration is known to restore nerve conduction velocity toward normal.

Andersen LW, Friedberg M, Lokkegaard N: Naloxone in the treatment of uremic pruritus: A case history. Clin Nephrol 21:355–356, 1984.

A single injection of **naloxone** (Narcan 0.8 mg IV) abolished pruritus within five minutes and for more than two hours in a 65-year-old woman with terminal uremia.

Yatzidis H, Digenis P, Tounts C: Heparin treatment of uremic itching. JAMA 222:1183, 1972.

Heparin (IV 100 mg q12h for two to three weeks) stopped itch in four of five patients for several weeks.

Massry SG, Popovtzer MM, Coburn JW, et al: Intractable pruritus as a manifestation of secondary hyperparathyroidism in uremia: Disappearance of itching after subtotal parathyroidectomy. N Engl J Med 279:697–700, 1968.

This series of seven patients with advanced uremia, marked hyperparathyroidism, osteitis fibrosa, and severe intolerable pruritus had complete disappearance of itching within a few days of subtotal parathyroidectomy. No controls.

Duncan JS, Kennedy HJ, Triger DR: Treatment of pruritus due to chronic obstructive liver disease. Br Med J 289:22, 1984.

Pruritus of chronic obstructive liver disease is difficult to treat. A single-blind controlled crossover study of eight patients over a 10-day period underscored the value of **cholestyramine** (4 gm/day).

Terfenadine, the new nonsedating antihistamine (Seldane 60 mg hs or bid), also had a significant antipruritic effect. In contrast, **chlorpheniramine** (4 mg tid) was no better than **lactose**.

Ryatt KS, Cotterill JA, Littlewood JM: Generalized pruritus in a baby as a presenting feature of the arteriohepatic dysplasia syndrome. Clin Exp Dermatol 8:657–661, 1983.

Cholestyramine (3 gm/day) dramatically reduced pruritus in a two-year-old boy who had scratched since birth despite topical steroids, antihistamines, and an elimination diet. A needle biopsy of the liver revealed hypoplastic bile ducts as the cause. The itch returned if the cholestyramine dose was less than 2.5 gm/day. **Vitamin D** (400 U/day) and other fat-soluble vitamin supplementation was necessary.

Greaves MW: The nature and management of pruritus. Practitioner 226:1223–1225, 1982.

Naloxone (Narcan), an opiate antagonist, relieves itching in patients with cholestatic jaundice, suggesting that endorphins have a central modulating effect on itch in man. (The endorphins thus could be the physiologic basis for the placebo-responsive patient.)

Carey WD, Smith J, Asanuma Y, et al: Pruritus of cholestasis treated with plasma perfusion. Am J Gastroenterol 76:330–337, 1981.

Use of a $1600 plasma-perfusion unit (cellulose acetate filter, an ion exchange resin, activated charcoal cartridge) gave long-lasting improvement (1 to 12 weeks) in the five of six patients in whom bile acid levels were reduced. Each patient received nine courses of treatment (three perfusions each course).

Hoek FJ, Grijm R, Sanders GTB, et al: Removal of bile acids from the blood by hemodialysis with a polyacrylonitril membrane: Treatment of pruritus of cholestatic disease. Digestion 23:135–140, 1982.

Good results were seen in a single patient after 30 dialysis sessions (six hours each over nine months). Bile acids were removed by a new polyacrylonitril filter used in the hemodialysis.

Snyder D, Merrill JP: Sauna baths in the treatment of chronic renal failure. Trans Am Soc Artif Intern Organs 12:188–192, 1966.

Uremic pruritus was completely relieved in eight patients after a series of five or six **sauna baths**. Each bath consisted of two 15-minute periods at 75°C separated by a 10-minute break out of the sauna. Sauna baths were given daily except on the day of dialysis. Profuse sweating helped to eliminate urea and other metabolic products. All patients experienced an increased sense of well-being.

Garden JM, Ostrow JD, Roenigk HH: Pruritus in hepatic cholestasis: Pathogenesis and therapy. Arch Dermatol 121:1415–1420, 1985.

A complete review of all therapeutic avenues (79 references):

Cholestyramine resin (Questran 4 grams one to three times/day, available in 378 grain cans) remains the agent most widely accepted for treatment.
Phenobarbital (3 to 4 mg/kg/day) is beneficial, possibly owing to its effect on hepatic metabolism.
Diets rich in polyunsaturated fatty acids reduce the pruritus.
Extracorporeal plasmapheresis, intravenous **albumin**, or **lidocaine** are other approaches.

If much of what you do in your office today is the same as you did in your residency, you really need a tune-up.

Pruritus Vulvae

Synalar ointment	Flagyl
Erythromycin	Atarax
Nizoral	

The causes of pruritus vulvae are as legion as the causes of pruritus. And it is the cause we seek. But what is our focus?

First, we eliminate skin disease by inspection and biopsy. Hidden in the inflamed skin may be the histologic signs of lichen sclerosus et atrophicus, psoriasis, neurodermatitis, or even Paget's disease. Each has its appropriate treatment.

If the pruritus still remains idiopathic, we center our initial attack on vaginal secretions. If there is clinical or laboratory evidence of candidiasis, trichomoniasis, or nonspecific vaginitis, we use appropriate therapy. In the absence of these conditions, we initially prescribe a two-week course of erythromycin (250 mg qid). If there is no improvement, this is followed by two weeks of Nizoral (200 mg/day). Again if there is no success, we give two weeks of Flagyl (250 mg tid). All cases refractory to this regimen need expert gynecologic review.

Meanwhile a serious effort is made to eliminate contact sensitizers. No topical preparations are allowed in the area except Synalar ointment (0.025 per cent), which is devoid of preservatives, perfumes, and irritants. The patient must not wear any nail polish ("no, not even colorless"). Douches, spermicidal gels, perfumed tampons, panty liners, and sanitary napkins are also interdicted.

If the problem is extremely discomforting we give ACTH (40 U IM) every few days or Kenalog 40 mg IM every three weeks until the acute phase is over.

We advise careful washing of the area with unscented Neutrogena soap, the wearing of loose clothing, and the use of an unscented talcum powder after bathing.

Most of the patients need long-term supportive care and assurance, since the heightened itch sensitivity remains long after the cause is eliminated. Awareness of this physiologic hyperalgesia and its anatomic basis of proliferation of new itch receptor nerve terminals helps the patient through the usually prolonged convalescence. It is during this phase that the use of Atarax is particularly advantageous. But in all phases, these patients need a sympathetic physician with an inquiring mind.

Pumpianski R, Sheskin J: Pruritus vulvae: A five year survey. Dermatologica 131:446–451, 1965.

A study of 1104 patients with a chief complaint of vulvar itching (11 per cent of all new gynecologic patients seen in five years at Hadassah University Hospital):

Vaginal origin of itching:

candidiasis	503 patients
trichomonas	414
bacillary	17
senile	18
total	952 patients (86 per cent)

Extravaginal source of itching

vulvar candidiasis	29 patients
lichen sclerosus et atrophicus	16
*Enterobius vermicularis**	17
diabetes (without candidiasis)	18
dermatitis	13
neurodermatitis	13
tinea inguinalis	7
miscellaneous	46
total	152 (14 per cent)

Overall causes of vulvar itching

candidiasis	48 per cent
trichomonas	38 per cent
total	86 per cent

Friedrich EG: Vulvar pruritus: A symptom, not a disease. Postgrad Med 61(6):164–171, 1977.

Recommends:

Treat vaginitis.
Use hair dryer to dry vulvar skin after bathing.
Apply Eurax cream locally.
Wear 100 per cent cotton underwear.
Use tranquilizer at night.

Rees RB: The importance of biopsy in pruritus vulvae. Int J Dermatol 16:408, 1977.

Case 1. A 75-year old woman with "nondescript" lesions of the labia majora, minora, and mons.

biopsy: extramammary Paget's disease
treatment: vulvectomy and search for underlying malignant disease (none found)
follow-up: no problem in the remaining ten years of her life

Case 2. A 56-year-old woman with white thickened areas on the labia majora and minora.

biopsy: lichen sclerosus et atrophicus
treatment: vitamin E 1600 U/day for three months
follow-up: lesions involuted

Greaves MW: The nature and management of pruritus. Practitioner 226:1223–1225, 1982.

For pruritus vulvae:

Careful patch testing for allergic sensitization due to application of a wide variety of topical medications. Common culprits: local anesthetics, balsam of Peru, lanolin, and EDTA (edetic acid; ethylenediamine).

The contact element is important if systemic and local diseases are ruled out. Improved local hygiene should include washing several times daily and use of talcum powder.

---

* Eggs of *E. vermicularis* were found in skin scrapings from the vulva, perianal, inguinal, suprapubic, and umbilical areas. Most patients were older with good hygiene and were not taking care of young children.

Woodruff JD, Babaknia A: Local alcohol injection of the vulva: Discussion of 35 cases. Obstet Gynecol 54:512–514, 1979.

Thirteen patients had complete relief of chronic vulvar pruritus for more than three years after absolute alcohol injections (0.2 cc subcutaneously) into each square centimeter of the vulva; 90 per cent of the entire group of 35 patients had relief for more than one year.

Sutherst JR: Treatment of pruritus vulvae by multiple intradermal injections of alcohol. A double-blind study. Br J Obstet Gynaecol 86:371–373, 1979.

These 17 patients had intractable pruritus vulvae for an average of 10 years each. With the patient under general anesthesia, absolute alcohol (0.1 to 0.2 ml) was injected 5 mm below the skin surface of the vulva in each square centimeter in a grid fashion. The control side was injected with water. No sloughing of skin occurred, but sensation was lost for six weeks as the nerve endings in the skin were temporarily destroyed. At the two-month follow-up, 14 of 17 sides treated with the alcohol were free of itch.

Ovadia J, Levavi H, Edelstein T: Treatment of pruritus vulvae by means of CO_2 laser. Acta Obstet Gynecol Scand 63:265–267, 1984.

Laser beam therapy to the entire vulvar area (depth of 3 mm) gave excellent results, and there was disappearance of all itch for more than one year in four patients. Post-treatment care included saline sitz baths and analgesics. Reepithelialization was complete after six weeks, with mild scarring.

Zelle K: Treatment of vulvar dystrophies with topical testosterone propionate. Am J Obstet Gynecol 109:570–573, 1971.

Testosterone propionate ointment (2 per cent in petrolatum tid for six weeks, then bid for four weeks, then once daily for maintenance) relieved chronic vulvar pruritus and dyspareunia in 15 women with either lichen sclerosus et atrophicus or hyperplastic dystrophies. Post-treatment biopsies showed histologic change toward a more normal epithelium. Symptoms recurred after six to seven weeks without treatment but could eventually be controlled with applications of ointment once or twice weekly.

Jasionowski EA: Topical progesterone in treatment of vulvar dystrophy: Preliminary report of five cases. Am J Obstet Gynecol 127:667–670, 1977.

Progesterone ointment (200 mg in 2 ounces hydrophilic ointment or Unibase applied bid for six to nine months) helped three of five women with chronic vulvar dystrophy by relieving pruritus and dyspareunia.

Patient instructions: Writing them once is worth more than telling them twice.

Pseudofolliculitis Barbae

Magic Powder
Nair
Retin-A
Surgery

This is a factitial dermatitis! Induced by shaving, it results from the razor transecting curved hairs at an angle to produce needle-sharp beveled hair tips. As the curved hairs continue to grow, the pointed tips pierce into the perifollicular skin where they act as foreign bodies (pili incarnati). Three factors account for this problem occurring almost exclusively in black men: (1) their beard hair more commonly grows out in a loop; (2) their follicles grow at a more acute angle to the skin surface; (3) their hair is stiffer.

Simple abstinence from shaving for a month is curative, since the unshaved hair loop acts like a coiled spring, snapping the hair tip out of the skin. Rapid resolution of inflammation follows, as this is not a bacterial or fungal infection. The problem is thus simply solved if wearing a beard is acceptable.

All other therapy is based on ways to reinstitute removal of the beard hair in such a fashion as to prevent the hair from curving back into the skin. Each treatment must be tailored to the specific patient. If a short stubble is tolerable to the patient and his mate, the barber's electric clipper is the best answer. Hair clipped this way never "hairpin curves" back into the skin.

For those who can tolerate depilatories (Magic Powder or Nair), this removal technique leaves a blunt hair tip incapable of piercing the skin. If shaving with a safety razor or the Norelco black electric shaver is the patient's choice, he must be cautioned to avoid cutting the hairs very short. He must not (1) pull the skin taut for a closer shave; (2) shave against the grain; (3) shave back and forth over the same area. He must also use a sharp new disposable safety razor or blade each time.

Before each shave, ingrown hairs should be freed with a fine needle, using a magnifying mirror and good lighting.

Finally, plucking and wax epilation should be avoided, since they commonly result in hair breakage within the follicle, increasing the likelihood of the shaft piercing the follicular wall.

Brown LA: Pathogenesis and treatment of pseudofolliculitis barbae. Cutis 32:373–375, 1983.

Classic review of all therapies for a problem in which patient instruction is more important than prescriptions.

The author favors growing a beard for one month to bring ingrown hairs to the surface, then using electric barber clippers. If secondarily infected, use topical and systemic antibiotics (Cleocin T, **erythromycin**).

Strauss JS, Kligman AM: Pseudofolliculitis of the beard. Arch Dermatol 74:533–542, 1956.

Untreated, can lead to scarring
In 26 subjects, spontaneous clearing after not shaving for one month.
Favor a chemical depilatory rather than shaving in an experimental study of 43 black men with pseudofolliculitis.

Kenney JA: Management of dermatoses peculiar to Negroes. Arch Dermatol 91:126–129, 1965.

First, try depilatory creams. Afterward (to prevent irritation) use lukewarm wet compresses for a few minutes followed by Neosporin cream. If shaving is necessary do not shave as closely as usual, and use mechanical means to prevent hairs from becoming ingrown.

De La Guardia M: Facial depilatories on black skin. Cosmet Toilet 91:37–38 (July), 1976.

Black men with "razor bumps" prefer powder depilatories containing **barium sulfide**, which act rapidly (5 minutes) and give the smoothest shave for a tough beard.

Disadvantage: odor of sulfide.

Instructions:

Do not wash face first.
Mix powder with water to make paste.
Apply with wooden spatula and leave on three to seven minutes.
Gently remove with blunt edge of spatula.
Rinse face thoroughly with cool water.
Apply emollient cream with acidic pH (to help neutralize residual alkalinity—depilatory products have pH of 12.0 to 12.6).
Avoid alcoholic lotions.

Note: Use only every other day to decrease irritation. As one keeps using it, skin gets "tougher." Depilatories soften the tips of hair, decreasing the penetration of follicle walls. Cream and aerosol depilatories take longer (15 to 20 minutes).

Alternative: **Calcium thioglycolate**. Shave is not as smooth, but mercaptan odor can be masked with fragrance.

Conte MS, Lawrence JE: Pseudofolliculitis barbae: No "pseudoproblem." JAMA 241:53–54, 1979.

Affects 45 per cent of all black servicemen, who run into trouble with military grooming codes. In 96 cases, 96 per cent cure rate with this routine: no shaving for first month, use polyester cleansing pad twice daily, cut hairs no shorter than 1 mm with electric clippers (with triple "O" head).

Brauner GJ, Flandermeyer KL: Pseudofolliculitis barbae: Medical consequences of interracial friction in the U.S. Army. Cutis 23:61–66, 1979.

Complete cessation of shaving (against Army regulations) is first required, followed by lotion depilatories or hair clippers and simple routine freeing of ingrowing hairs. Do not epilate.

Garcia RL, Henderson R: The adjustable rotary electric razor in the control of pseudofolliculitis barbae. J Assoc Milit Dermatol 4(1):28, 1978.

The Norelco adjustable three-headed rotary electric **razor** gave satisfactory results in more than 300 cases of mild to moderate pseudofolliculitis barbae.

Must follow careful instructions:

Apply preshaving lotion and allow to evaporate.
Use trimming clipper part of razor to cut hair to $\frac{1}{16}$ inch.
Shave beard with rotary heads in slow circular motion just above the surface of the skin. Do *not* press the razor against the face.

Wash the face with cool water; rinse thoroughly.
Optional: Use aftershave lotion and face cream.
Loosen ingrown hairs with a toothpick.

Alexander AM: Evaluation of foil-guarded shaver in the management of pseudofolliculitis barbae. Cutis 27:534–542, 1981.

Improvement occurred in 86 per cent of 22 black men following use of a serrated foil guard on a disposable safety razor blade to prevent an ultraclose shave. (PFB Shaving System, American Safety Razor Co., Staunton, VA.) Electric razors are generally not favored by blacks, and clippers leave uncomely stubble, uninviting to the opposite sex.

Kligman AM, Mills OH Jr.: Pseudofolliculitis of the beard and topically applied tretinoin. Arch Dermatol 107:551–552, 1973.

In 38 cases, Retin-A (0.05 per cent solution applied at bedtime for two months) was uniformly successful in mild cases, but relapse occurred two weeks after stopping treatment. It was uniformly unsuccessful in severe cases. May be irritating, but reduction of application to twice weekly was often helpful.

Hall JC, Goetz CS, Bartholome CS, Livingood CS: Pseudofolliculitis-revised concepts of diagnosis and treatment. Report of three cases in women. Cutis 23:798–800, 1979.

Examples of a rarely reported but possibly common problem in black women. Pseudofolliculitis developed in the axillae, pubic areas, neck, and face after shaving or use of depilatories. **Tretinoin** cream (Retin-A 0.05 to 0.1 per cent applied at bedtime) was the treatment of choice.

Bouman FG: Surgical depilation for treatment of pseudofolliculitis or local hirsutism of the face. Plast Reconst Surg 62:390–395, 1978.

Surgical treatment for pseudofolliculitis on the sides of the neck (where straight hairs grow obliquely and may pierce follicle walls after shaving).

1. Incise center of area and undermine in all directions close to the dermis.
2. Evert skin on a fingertip hook, revealing hair roots as black dots in the subcutaneous fat.
3. Cut roots with sharp (serrated) scissors and remove.
4. Pull out hair shafts (do not try to cut out).

Recurrences are usually due to hairs in the telogen (resting) phase during surgery (about 10 per cent of beard hairs) whose roots do not extend into the subcutaneous fat. Electrical depilation is used to remove these regrowing hairs.

Dermatologists are most admired by other dermatologists—and their mothers.

Psoriasis

Sunlight	Photochemotherapy
Tar	Methotrexate
Anthralin	Retinoids
Topical steroids	Antibiotics
Phototherapy	

Treatment of psoriasis centers on slowing down the fantastically accelerated overgrowth of keratinocytes that occurs in this disease. A variety of means has been discovered for rather selectively and safely applying a "metabolic brake" to these rapidly dividing cells. No longer do we use the poisons such as mercury and arsenic; nonetheless, caution must be observed in using our current growth-rate inhibitors. The continued use of tar and ultraviolet light for decades can lead to some cells escaping the growth suppression and becoming truly malignant.

Not only should one try to slow down the growth rate of the keratinocytes, but one should look for the cause of this. Here the paradigm is guttate psoriasis. In this variant, streptococcal pharyngitis is a common antecedent, and elimination of the streptococcal antigen is often curative. We feel that many other types of psoriasis vulgaris are also the result of infection, be it occult or otherwise. Accordingly, we routinely look for infection and treat it appropriately. If none is found we still prescribe erythromycin 250 mg qid on a trial basis. If no improvement is seen in two weeks, or if progress lags at any time, we prescribe an alternate such as ampicillin.

Infection as a triggering factor need not be bacterial. In some instances yeast infections are present and ketoconazole (200 mg/day) is then effective. We also employ metronidazole (250 mg tid) in our effort to eradicate occult yet significant infections such as a prostatitis, cystitis, or vaginitis. In this regard, careful dental evaluation should rule out periapical abscesses. Sinusitis, bronchitis, and diverticulitis are less easily controlled, but again may require long-term antibiotic therapy.

The growth rate of the keratinocyte can be curbed by fasting. We urge our overweight patients to reduce their caloric intake and record their weights at each visit. Some have benefited from joining Weight Watchers. We have not found any specific food factors to be significant and suspect that the many specialized diets proposed for psoriasis treatment owe their efficacy to caloric restriction. The most dramatic example we can cite to our obese patients is the fact that psoriasis became an uncommon disease in Germany after World War I, a period of terrifying food shortages. Conversely, the worst example of psoriasis we have seen was in a woman who gained 90 pounds during the nine months of her pregnancy. The psoriasis, which began early in the pregnancy, completely disappeared once the patient lost the excess weight. As a corollary, we recommend that patients with significant psoriasis refrain from all alcohol,

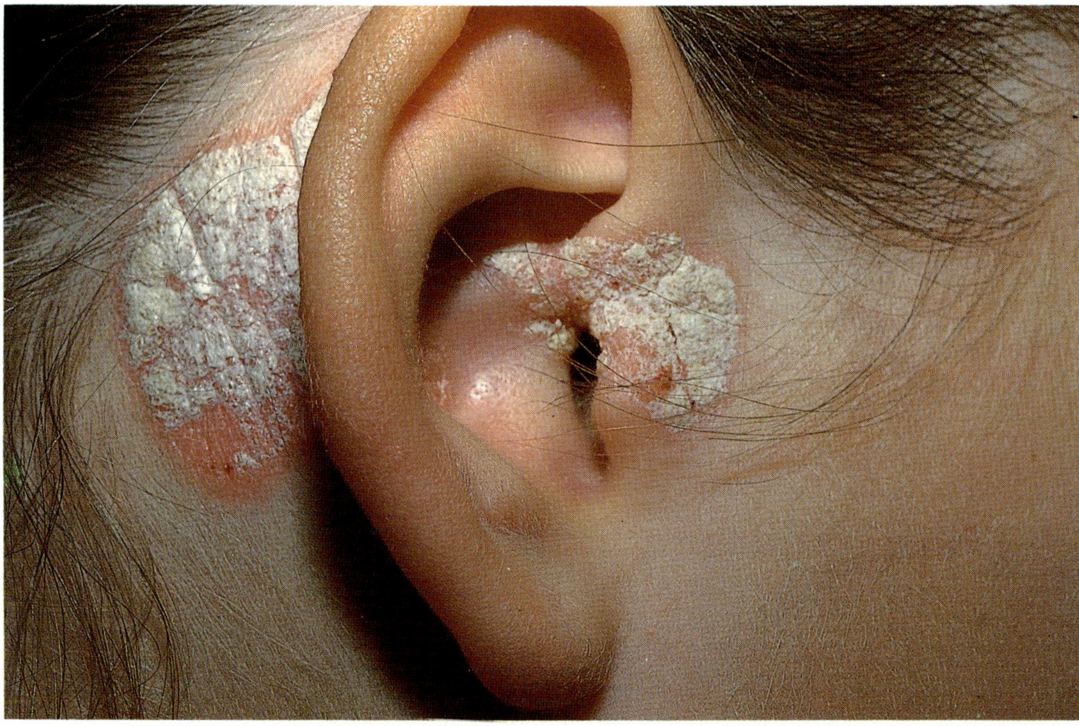

as it can be an overlooked source of calories and has potentially deleterious effects on the liver.

Stress is another trigger factor, but one over which we have little control. We are convinced of its role, having seen a perfectly healthy 16-year-old girl develop florid generalized psoriasis just two weeks after having seen her father die suddenly as blood gushed out from his esophageal varices over the white tablecloth in front of the entire family seated at dinner.

We always instruct the patient that such local trauma as vigorous hair combing, scratching, leaning on elbows, or wearing an arch support can lead to local lesions of psoriasis. Sometimes simple awareness of this can be curative. We had one patient whose psoriasis of the palms was the result of catching parcels coming down a postal chute. Assignment to another job was curative. Another woman had psoriasis of the fingers simply due to the trauma of twisting tight window latches.

Rarely do we see drugs as a trigger factor, but lithium may worsen psoriasis. Possibly this is due to its tendency to produce increased neutrophils, which are so critical in the developmental sequence of the psoriatic lesion. Chloroquine also can trigger severe psoriasis in some patients. If steroids are being taken, we emphasize the need to slowly taper their dose to avoid a rebound of psoriasis or the induction of pustular psoriasis. It is also preferable that patients with psoriasis not receive beta-blockers. We have additionally seen iodides flare psoriasis.

For topical treatment of small localized lesions we favor the use of Diprolene ointment. For larger areas we use Synalar ointment (0.025 per cent) or triamcinolone cream (0.1 per cent) and liquor carbonis detergens (LCD 5 per cent in cold cream or Aquaphor). If the lesion is unresponsive we then prescribe anthralin ointment in ascending strengths (0.1 to 1.0 per cent). Whenever there is fissuring, such as on the palms and soles, we apply Castellani's paint in the office and prescribe Cordran tape, which is left in place, being replaced only when it comes off.

For the scalp we regularly use a daily tar shampoo such as Zetar shampoo, followed immediately by Synalar solution. For more recalcitrant plaques on the scalp we have the patient use anthralin (Dritho-Scalp 0.25 per cent or 0.5 per cent once daily). Alternates are P&S Plus (tar and salicylic acid) and that time-honored powerful topical remedy "20-10-5" (20 per cent oil of cade, 10 per cent finely precipitated sulfur, and 5 per cent salicylic acid in petrolatum). Internally, ketoconazole (200 mg/day) has proven beneficial for scalp psoriasis.

Commonly, we prescribe Aquasol A 50,000 IU tid in conjunction with a systemic antibiotic to reduce the scaling. In the event that noticeable improvement does not occur, we move to the next step up, which is methotrexate. We give it either 25 mg IM once a week or have the patient take 2.5 to 5.0 mg q12h for three doses once a week. We monitor hepatic function by blood samples, but not liver biopsy unless the patient has a history of liver problems. Alcohol is absolutely contraindicated in all of these patients. Methotrexate is not used if there is evidence of hepatic disease.

We always stress the benefits of sun. If the patient has had good summer remissions we suggest use of ultraviolet (UVB) light for maintenance during the winter months, as well as a scheduled winter vacation in the South.

Our favorite approach for severe recalcitrant psoriasis still remains the Goeckerman regimen with hospitalization for 10 to 14 days, using crude coal tar (5 per cent in ointment) and daily UVB to the point of erythema. There is still no ideal treatment (witness the multiple combinational approaches), but much can be done to cut down on the cell proliferation that can literallly produce a dustpanful of scales in a day.

These patients need your reassurance as well as your supportive and adjunctive therapy, such as Atarax for itching and Castellani's paint for gluteal fissures. They need to know of the bright promise around the corner of the retinoids, such as Tigason for psoriasis of the nails. They need to know that their disease is not contagious, that it is not a sign of cancer, and that it often can be ignored without risk. They need to know that there are millions of others with the same problem and that there is a foundation, the National Psoriasis Foundation (6415 S.W. Canyon Court, Portland, OR 97221), which pleads their cause in education and research funding. It deserves their support.

Updike J: Personal history: A war with my skin. The New Yorker, Sept. 2, 1985, pp 39–57.

"Psoriasis keeps you thinking. Strategies of concealment ramify, and self examination is endless . . . I cannot pass a reflecting surface on the street without glancing in, in hopes that I have somehow changed . . . One hates one's abnormal, erupting skin but is led into a brooding, solicitous attention to it . . . one struggles for philosophy, for thoughts that are more than skin deep. What could matter less than the integument a skeleton once wore?"

In this essay, one of America's greatest writers takes us into his private tortured world of skin disease. Afflicted with extensive psoriasis since the age of six, he is able to evoke the fears, the anguish, and the triumphs of a life-long war with this disease. His was a life of fear of being seen taking off his shirt or even rolling up his sleeves, or of being in a swim suit. His was a life of rejection, separation, and pariah-like solitude.

No physician can read these poignant confessions and not search for new ways to bring sunshine and sunlight into the lives of his psoriatic patients.

Farber EM, Nall ML: The natural history of psoriasis in 5600 patients. Dermatologica 148:1–18, 1974.

Complete remissions were experienced by 39 per cent of these patients. Expect improvement with hot weather, sunlight, and pregnancy.

Krueger GC, Eyre RW: Trigger factors in psoriasis. Dermatol Clin 2:373–381, 1984.

Infections, stress, and local trauma are common antecedents.

Olsen TG: Chloroquine and psoriasis. Ann Intern Med 94:546–547, 1981.

A vacation in Brazil was aborted by a severe flare of psoriasis induced by **chloroquine phosphate** (Aralen 500 mg, 1 tablet/week for two weeks) given for chemoprophylaxis of malaria.

Kuflik EG: Effect of antimalarial drugs on psoriasis. Cutis 26:153–155, 1980.

A study of 48 U.S. Army patients with psoriasis in Vietnam showed that prophylactic **chloroquine** did not cause severe exacerbations of psoriasis. Although 42 per cent showed some worsening, only 6 per cent had significant flares of skin lesions, and most were well controlled with topical medications.

Patients with psoriasis needing chloroquine for treatment of rheumatoid arthritis or systemic lupus erythematosus or for travel to endemic areas of malaria should not be discouraged from a trial of chloroquine.

Farber EM, Abel EA, Charuworn A: Recent advances in the treatment of psoriasis. J Am Acad Dermatol 8:311–321, 1983.

The systemic treatment of streptococcal or other infections is one of the helpful approaches mentioned in this comprehensive review. 88 references.

Halprin KM: Treatments of psoriasis. J Dermatol (Tokyo) 11:419–424, 1984.

This thoughtful overview of today's therapy and its rationale stresses the fact that the drugs used may act by inhibiting mitoses, counteracting inflammatory mediators, or rendering neutrophils indifferent to chemotactic stimuli in the epidermis. Of the internal drugs, **methotrexate** is probably the most effective single agent, although 10 per cent cannot tolerate it because of nausea and fatigue. Furthermore, methotrexate treatment, which must be continued indefinitely, is contraindicated if the patient drinks any alcohol or is pregnant. In contrast, none of these strictures hold for the most commonly used external therapy, i.e., ultraviolet light (UVB).

Jillson OF: Psoriasis. Cutis 29:230–242, 1982.

Some Jillson gems:

1. Explain to the patient:
   His disease is noncontagious.

The cause is not known.
The tendency is inherited.
Six million other Americans have it.
He should avoid alcohol and obesity.

2. Encourage the patient to soak and scrub off scales and then apply 10 per cent crude **coal tar** in petrolatum.
3. Tanning salons help when the summer sun is gone.
4. Tonsillectomy is indicated in patients with recurrent guttate psoriasis.
5. Disabling hypertrophic psoriatic great toe nails are best permanently removed by surgery. This may help prevent future pain from the commonly associated arthritis of the distal toe joint.

Nyfors A: Psoriasis in children: Characteristics, prognosis and therapy. A review. Acta Derm Venereol Suppl 95:47–53, 1981.

A study of 245 psoriatic children showed lesions more often triggered by infections and psychic stress, more often localized to the face and scalp, and more pruritic than in adults. Do not use **methotrexate** or PUVA therapy in children.

Loeffel ED: Psoriasis in adolescence. *In* Solomon LM, Esterly NB, Loeffel ED (eds): Adolescent Dermatology. Philadelphia, WB Saunders Co, 1978, pp 143–162.

Helpful hints:

Tailor treatment to allow continuation of normal school activities.
Make treatment cosmetically acceptable.
Put the teenager in charge of the treatment (parents should not nag).
Look for underlying beta-hemolytic streptococcal infection (throat culture, ASO titer, urinalysis). Consider tonsillectomy.
Look for precipitating activities (athletics, cosmetic, hobbies, work, study, etc.) that can injure the skin and induce a Koebner response.
Try to anticipate and prevent social and emotional crises at school. Educate parents and teachers about the disease and its noncontagious nature. Insist that certain rules be relaxed, such as taking swimming or participating in group showers after athletics.
Consider **methotrexate** as a temporary crutch in times of serious emotional trouble. Remember that embarrassment and anger about the disease and loss of self-image due to disfigurement may lead to severe depression and suicide.
Discuss vocational plans that might be influenced by psoriasis.
Consider hospitalization for the Goeckerman treatment—good for educating the patient and helping combat discouragement.

Lukovsky LA, Nesterenko GB, Tytar GM, Bashmakov GV: The immediate and remote results of tonsillectomy in patients with chronic tonsillitis and psoriasis. Vestn Otorinolaringol 32(6):23–26, 1970.

The effect of tonsillectomy on psoriasis in 57 patients 7 to 15 days after surgery:

complete clearing	21 (36.8 per cent)
partial improvement	30 (52.6 per cent)
no effect	6 (10.5 per cent)

Nyfors A, Rasmussen PA, Lemholt K, Eriksen B: Improvement of refractory psoriasis vulgaris after tonsillectomy. Dermatologica 151:216–222, 1975.

A retrospective study in Denmark of 74 patients (ages 4 to 33 years) found improvement in 71 per cent following tonsillectomy; 66 of the patients had tonsillitis.

Results:	
cleared	24 (32 per cent)
improved	29 (39 per cent)
unchanged	16 (22 per cent)
worsened	5 (7 per cent)

Comaish JS: Tar and related compounds in the therapy of psoriasis. Clin Exp Dermatol 6:639–645, 1981.

A complete review of this mainstay of local therapy points out that tars should be avoided:

- if psoriasis is acutely inflamed
- if of no benefit previously
- if the patient is sun sensitive or taking photosensitizing drugs at the time
- if folliculitis or acne is present in the area

Ashton RE, Andre P, Lowe NJ, Whitefield M: Anthralin: Historical and current perspectives. J Am Acad Dermatol 9:173–192, 1983.

Included are 161 references that attest to the value of this century-old irreplaceable compound. The authors recommend spot use of **anthralin** cream (Drithocreme) or ointment (Anthra-Derm) bid in ascending concentrations (0.1, 0.25, 0.5, 1.0 per cent) as tolerated. The stratum corneum stain exfoliates within two weeks of stopping therapy.

Lowe NJ, Ashton RE, Koudsi H, et al: Anthralin for psoriasis: Short-contact anthralin therapy compared with topical steroid and conventional anthralin. J Am Acad Dermatol 10:69–72, 1984.

A study of 26 patients showed that **anthralin** (0.3 per cent in petrolatum) could be washed off 10 minutes after application and still be as effective as anthralin (0.1 to 0.5 per cent in petrolatum) or steroid ointment (**diflorosone diacetate** 0.05 per cent) left on for 8 hours.

Pearlman DL, Burns J, Cannon TC, Engelhard CS: Paper-tape occlusion of anthralin paste: A new outpatient therapy for psoriasis. Arch Dermatol 120:625–630, 1984.

The classic anthralin "stiff" paste:

anthralin	0.2 to 0.8 per cent
salicylic acid	0.4 to 0.8 per cent
hard paraffin (candle wax)	5 per cent
zinc oxide paste, petrolatum	equal parts to make 100 per cent

When this paste was applied to plaques and covered with semipermeable paper adhesive tape each night for three months, 90 per cent clearing of psoriatic lesions occurred in 6 of 12 patients; two other patients had 70 per cent clearing, while four others showed no response. The anthralin was removed each morning with a cloth containing mineral oil.

Broughton R: Corticosteroid injections into the hands and feet. Cutis 33:575–577, 1984.

Describes remission of palmar psoriasis for many months following intralesional injection of **triamcinolone diacetate** suspension (Aristocort Forte 40 mg/ml, 0.25 cc diluted with 2 per cent **lidocaine** 0.75 cc). Use a tuberculin syringe, 30-gauge needle, and 0.5 ml in each site. No value in pustular psoriasis of the hands and feet.

Lowe NJ: Therapy of scalp psoriasis. Dermatol Clin 2:471–476, 1984.

Favors preparations that are easy to apply and remove, usually in vehicles that are gels or lotions:

phenol and saline (Baker's P & S lotion)

salicylic acid (2 to 5 per cent in lotion)
crude **coal tar** (2 to 10 per cent in lotion) } combination

salicylic acid (5 to 10 per cent in petrolatum overnight)
steroid solution (Cordran, Synalar, Diprosone, Valisone)

oil of cade (6 per cent)
sulfur (Ppt) (2 per cent)
salicylic acid (2 per cent) } in emulsifying ointment

anthralin cream (0.5 per cent—30-minute contact followed by tar shampoo)
LCD 5 to 15 per cent
Zetar or T gel shampoo daily
Accutane
ketoconazole
PUVA if bald!
Purified tar preparations—Estar gel, Fototar cream, P&S Plus tar gel, Psorigel, T-Derm tar oil

Zaias N: Psoriasis of the nail unit. Dermatol Clin 2:493–505, 1984.

Avoidance of Koebner-like insults from nail cutting, cleaning, or tampering with subungual debris
Dermojet injection of steroid (1 mg/ml) into matrix or nail bed
Methotrexate
Treatment of secondary candidiasis
No help from 5-FU, **anthralin**, **retinoic acid** or steroids because of barrier of nail plate

Rabinovitz HS, Scher RK, Shupack JL: Response of psoriatic nails to the aromatic retinoid etretinate. Arch Dermatol 119:627–628, 1983.

Color plates show excellent response of two patients to **etretinate** (0.5 to 1.0 mg/kg/day). Crumbling subungual hyperkeratoses and onycholysis disappeared, but some pitting remained. Longitudinal splitting and breaking of the nails were side effects of the treatment.

Finnerty EF: Successful treatment of psoriasis of the nails. Cutis 23:43–44, 1979.

Three patients responded well to superficial x-ray (400 to 600 r, given in divided doses of 75 r every two weeks for four months 2-mm aluminum filtration). The treated areas include the nail and the adjoining 3 mm at the base of the nail. Improvement was not noted until two, four, and five months, respectively, after therapy.

Montgomery BJ: Bathing for psoriasis in the Dead Sea. JAMA 241:227–231, 1979.

Bathing in the Dead Sea's 30 per cent saline brine, basking in haze-enriched UVA sunlight, and relaxing with fellow patients with psoriasis at the lowest level of the earth's surface for four weeks has proven helpful for 95 per cent of more than 3000 patients in the past decade. Regrettably, 44 per cent relapsed within four weeks of returning home. The Dead Sea International Psoriasis Treatment Center is located in the village of Ein Bokek in Southern Israel.

Fischer T: UV-light treatment of psoriasis. Acta Derm Venereol 56:473–479, 1976.

Effective healing of psoriasis was obtained only with UV light of 313-nm band given in 1 and 2 MED daily for three weeks. UV light of the 334-, 365- and 405-nm bands did not produce healing of psoriatic lesions even in doses as high as 30 J/sq cm.

Analysis of a large group of psoriasis patients with ultraviolet light intolerance revealed four distinct groups:

- polymorphous light eruption
- photosensitizing drugs
- large alcohol intake
- pustular psoriasis in a labile state

Menter A, Cram DL: The Goeckerman regimen in two psoriasis day care centers. J Am Acad Dermatol 9:59–65, 1983.

Clearing occurred in 18 days in 270 of 300 patients with severe psoriasis and continued for more than eight months following this routine:

Crude **coal tar** (2 to 5 per cent with Tween 80 2.5 per cent in petrolatum) applied seven hours per day for six days a week. For thick plaques, **salicylic acid** (2 to 5 per cent) was added.

UVB (FS20 and FS40 Westinghouse bulbs), starting dose 2.85 to 5.70 millijoules/sq cm (15- to 30-seconds exposure), total dose 1.96 joules/sq cm achieved through incremental minimal erythema dosage.

Liquor carbonis detergens (LCD 10 to 20 per cent) in Aquaphor or Eucerin was applied overnight.

Individualized care

- extra dose on plaques
- plastic shower caps
- LCD lotion (10 per cent in oil) to scalp bid (e.g., Nivea oil)
- **triamcinolone acetonide** (Kenalog 0.025 per cent) or **fluocinolone acetonide** cream (Synalar 0.01 per cent) was applied sparingly bid to resistant sites on face, ears, axillae, and groin.

Diette KM, Momtaz-T K, Stern RS, et al: Role of ultraviolet A in phototherapy for psoriasis. J Am Acad Dermatol 11:441–447, 1984.

In 13 patients UVB plus tar gave the same clearing rate and the same relapse sequences with or without UVA. Despite the fact that UVA is the action spectrum for **coal tar** phototoxicity, no additional benefit was seen with UVA.

Baker H: PUVA therapy for psoriasis. J R Soc Med 77:537–539, 1984.

A decade after its introduction, PUVA therapy is well established as an effective, pleasant, and safe treatment that no dermatologist would want to be without. The English experience shows it to clear 60 per cent of cases completely, to improve 30 per cent, and to fail in only 10 per cent. It consists of giving 8-MOP (0.6 mg/kg) two hours prior to UVA (initially 1.0 J/sq cm total skin, eyes protected, three to four times/week, incremental increases to 7.0 J/sq cm). The average need is for 20 treatments (100 J/sq cm) followed by maintenance radiation every two weeks. The possibility of late carcinogenic sequelae remains under scrutiny. PUVA inhibition of DNA synthesis was made possible by industry's development of high-potency UVA light bulbs.

Roenigk HH, Farber EM, Storrs F, et al: Photochemotherapy for psoriasis: A clinical cooperative study of PUVA-48 and PUVA-64. Arch Dermatol 115:576–579, 1979.

The United States experience with 465 patients in 14 centers using cabinets with 48 tubular bulbs resulted in clearing in 85 per cent, with a mean total dose of 166 J/sq cm. Maintenance required either weekly follow-up treatments or treatment only as needed.

Epstein JH, Farber EM, Nall L, et al: Current status of oral PUVA therapy for psoriasis. J Am Acad Dermatol 1:106–117, 1979.

A bible filled with invaluable detailed advice on every aspect of PUVA therapy. Includes tables showing dosage as related to weight and skin type, and a patient interview check list.

Boer J, Hermans J, Schothorst AA, Suurmond D: Comparison of phototherapy (UV-B) and photochemotherapy (PUVA) for clearing and maintenance therapy of psoriasis. Arch Dermatol 120:52–57, 1984.

In a study of 183 patients, PUVA was better than UVB if more than 50 per cent of the skin surface was affected by psoriasis. There was no difference if less than 50 per cent of the skin was involved. If there is a good response to sunbathing, UVB is usually very helpful.

Salo OP, Lassus A, Taskinen J: Trioxsalen bath plus UVA treatment of psoriasis: Plasma concentration of the drug and clinical results. Acta Derm Venereol 61:551–554, 1981.

If oral 8-MOP is not tolerated, use a **trioxsalen** bath (50 mg in alcoholic solution added to 150 liters of water for 10 minutes) immediately prior to UVA (0.2 J/sq cm at start, increasing to a maximum of 2 J/sq cm per treatment session). Results were good in 67 per cent of 45 patients after an average of 19.4 J/sq cm.

Berns MW, Rettenmaier M, McCullough J, et al: Response of psoriasis to red laser light (630 nm) following systemic injection of hematoporphyrin derivative. Lasers Surg Med 4:73–77, 1984.

An intravenous bolus injection of hematoporphyrin derivative (3 mg/kg) followed 72 hours later by a single pulse of red laser light (40 J/sq cm) destroyed psoriatic epidermis in a single subject. The skin reepithelialized normally within two months. This may form the basis for a nonpsoralen photosensitization therapy, but the patient must avoid bright sunlight for one month while the hematoporphyrin is being eliminated. (Perhaps topical use of this powerful photosensitizer should be studied).

Roenigk HH: Commentary and update: Methotrexate for psoriasis—Two decades later. Cleve Clin Q 50:107–110, 1983.

Methotrexate has proven to be the best and safest of the antimetabolites (including **arsenic**, **hydroxyurea**, **azathioprine**, **azaribine**, and **mycophenolic acid**) in treating widespread recalcitrant psoriasis not responsive to topical therapy. It is given as a single 25-mg IM dose or 2.5 mg q12h for three times once a week. This review provides detailed guidelines, including liver biopsy desiderata.

Zackheim HS: Topical 6-aminonicotinamide plus oral niacinamide therapy for psoriasis. Arch Dermatol 114:1632–1638, 1978.

In a double-blind study of 99 patients, topical **6-aminonicotinamide** (1 per cent gel bid or tid for four weeks) was as effective as 0.1 per cent Kenalog cream in treating psoriasis. All patients took **niacinamide** (100 mg tid) to avoid possible systemic effects of absorbed 6-aminonicotinamide, as 6-aminonicotinamide is a powerful antagonist of the essential niacin.

Rosenberg EW, Belew PW: Improvement of psoriasis of the scalp with ketoconazole. Arch Dermatol 118:370–371, 1982.

Ketoconazole (Nizoral 200 mg/day for two to three months) cleared psoriatic lesions of the scalp in three out of four patients. No improvement was noted until after one month.

Crutcher N, Rosenberg EW, Belew PW, et al: Oral nystatin in the treatment of psoriasis. Arch Dermatol 120:435–436, 1984.

Nystatin (500,000 to 1,000,000 U PO qid) cleared four patients of psoriatic lesions within two to five months.

Skinner RB, Rosenberg EW, Belew PW, Marley WM: Improvement of psoriasis with cholestyramine. Arch Dermatol 118:144, 1982.

Cholestyramine (Questran 4 gm qid) induced rapid clearing of lesions in five patients. It may act by binding endotoxin in the gut, since this ion exchange resin is not absorbed.

Wahba A, Cohen H: Therapeutic trials with oral colchicine in psoriasis. Acta Derm Venereol 60:515–520, 1980.

Colchicine (0.02 mg/kg/day) virtually cleared psoriatic papules and thin plaques in eight of nine patients in two to four months. Thicker plaques were not cleared, but colchicine was helpful in maintaining remissions for 8 to 9 months in four patients whose plaques had been cleared with either **methotrexate** or Goeckerman therapy.

Weber G, Neidhardt M, Frey H, et al: Treatment of psoriasis with bromocriptin. Arch Dermatol Res 271:437–439, 1981.

Bromocriptine (Parlodel 2.5 mg qid), a dopamine agonist that inhibits human growth hormone, induced complete remission in 10 of 60 patients (17 per cent). A gradual remission was seen in an additional 19 patients (32 per cent).

Ward A, Brogden RN, Heel RC, et al: Etretinate: A review of its pharmacological properties and therapeutic efficacy in psoriasis and other skin disorders. Drugs 26:9–43, 1983.

Etretinate (Tigason 0.75 to 1.0 mg/kg/day for three months) gave consistently impressive results in several studies, especially in pustular and erythrodermic psoriasis. However, 70 per cent of patients showed relapse despite a maintenance dose. It may be used with PUVA for an enhanced therapeutic response. Plasma levels of the drug are detectable for three to four months after discontinuation of therapy. Hair loss is usually the primary reason for stopping the drug.

Wolff K, Fritsch PO: Retinoid-PUVA chemo-photochemotherapy. *In* Farber EM, Cox AJ (eds): Psoriasis: Proceedings of the 3rd International Symposium. New York, Grune & Stratton, 1982, pp 211–219.

Best results were seen in treating severe psoriasis when etretinate (1.0 mg/kg/day) was started 10 days before PUVA (standard dose four times a week) and was continued along with PUVA until clearing occurred.

Whittier FC, Evans DH, Anderson PC, Nolph KD: Peritoneal dialysis for psoriasis: A controlled study. Ann Intern Med 99:165–168, 1983.

Results of a six-month double-blind crossover study of five patients with disabling **methotrexate**-resistant plaque-type psoriasis: **Peritoneal dialysis** (48 hours/week for four weeks, 1.5-hour cycle time for 2-liter exchanges) induced complete clearing in two patients, more than 75 per cent clearing in two additional patients, and no change in one patient. The remissions lasted up to six months, and in one case dialysis for a second course gave remission of more than one year. Sham dialysis had no effect.

Guillot B, Guilhou JJ, Donadio D, Meynadier J: Plasma exchanges in psoriasis. Clin Exp Dermatol 9:42–45, 1984.

Improvement was noted in all five patients treated by plasma exchange (10 times in one month) by the end of the third treatment. Reduction of elevated circulating immune complex levels by 20 to 70 per cent may have contributed to the improvement noted. All patients showed relapse in lesions within one month.

Clemmensen OJ, Andersen R, Andersen E: Plasmapheresis in the treatment of psoriasis: A controlled clinical study. J Am Acad Dermatol 8:190–192, 1983.

A double-blind study of six patients having plasma exchange once a week for seven weeks found no effect on psoriasis.

Bohm M, Voorhees J, et al: White paper on hospitalization for psoriasis care. J Am Acad Dermatol 10:842–851, 1984.

An authoritative position paper for public enlightenment of what can and cannot be done for patients with psoriasis. It clearly defines both benefits and risks.

Alper JC, Weimann MC, Kegel M, et al: Outpatient 5-fluorouracil therapy for resistant psoriasis. Clin Res 33:622A, 1985.

5-Fluorouracil (300 mg/sq m, IV bolus once/week) induced 75 to 100 per cent clearing of recalcitrant psoriasis in 5 of 16 patients. In 6 of the 16, there was 50 to 75 per cent clearing, while 5 failed to respond.

Jacobson C, Cornell RC, Savin RC: A comparison of Clobetasol propionate 0.05 percent ointment and an optimized betamethasone dipropionate 0.05 percent ointment in the treatment of psoriasis. Cutis 37:213–220, 1986.

A multicenter, double-blind paired control study of 130 patients found Temovate ointment to be significantly superior to Diprolene ointment after two weeks of application twice daily.

Roenigk HH Jr, Maibach HI (eds): Psoriasis. New York, Marcel Dekker Inc., 1985, 667 pp.

Our bible: written by 73 world-class scholars of this worldwide disease.

Lowe NJ: Practical psoriasis therapy. Chicago, Year Book Medical Publishers, Inc., 1986, 201 pp.

Twelve patient-caring clinicians detail exactly how to care for psoriatic patients.

Humenir D: Pet-associated illness. N Engl J Med 314:1046, 1986.

A houshold dog or cat may be the source of recurrent or persistent attacks of group A streptococcal pharyngitis in children or other family members. (This "pet-strep" vector deserves attention in psoriasis).

Rosenberg EW, Noah PW, Zanolli MD, et al. Use of rifampin with penicillin and erythromycin in the treatment of psoriasis. Preliminary report. J Am Acad Derm 14:761–764, 1986.

Nine patients were judged to have streptococcal-associated psoriasis on the basis of positive throat or skin fold cultures for beta-hemolytic streptococci or on the finding of elevated levels of antistreptococcal antibodies. None showed clinical improvement following two weeks of either **penicillin V** or **erythromycin** (250 mg qid). However, five of the nine patients had 95 to 100 per cent disappearance of their lesions when **rifampin** (300 mg bid) was given as a supplement on the final five days of a second course of penicillin or erythromycin (250 mg qid, 10 to 14 days). The remaining four had a good response (better than 80 per cent improvement).

Patients want the name of the treatment much more than the name of the disease.

Pustular Psoriasis, Generalized

Methotrexate	Dapsone
Hydroxyurea	Calcium
Retinoids	Vitamin D
PUVA	Rocephin

Although most examples of generalized pustular psoriasis are as idiopathic as psoriasis itself, it is imperative to stop prior drugs. We have had under our care a patient who had three attacks, each induced by butazolidine, before she and her internist would believe that it was the cause. It is always well to take a direct and indirect history repetitively, since patients frequently take medicines without recollection. We enlist the aid of relatives in this area also, and extend the net of questioning to include eyedrops, laxatives, mouthwashes, douches, vitamins, and tonics. A careful sympathetic review of problems such as tension, headache, and fatigue will also aid the patient in recall. Sometimes the list comes out piecemeal over a period of days.

We search for antecedent infections with equal zeal, since appropriate antibiotic therapy can be of tremendous value. Latent or apparent candidiasis, trichomoniasis, cystitis, or colitis deserves attention and consideration of therapy with ketoconazole or dapsone. Likewise, blood cultures may reveal a pathogen, and intravenous use of some of the newer aminoglycosides and cephalosporins (Rocephin) may be indicated. In all instances, secondary skin surface colonization with bacteria makes the oral administration of erythromycin advisable.

Hospitalization is usually necessary for these patients. They need intensive nursing care and careful monitoring of their toxic febrile state. Water and protein loss through the skin call for high fluid and protein intake. Many patients are erythrodermic and hypothermic from the constant heat loss through their flushed skin. Regular laboratory monitoring of blood chemistry profiles is necessary so that corrective measures can be taken early.

Topically, strong antipsoriatic medications must be strictly avoided, as well as greasy preparations. We generally prescribe warm saline baths daily, followed by Eucerin inunction.

Internally, we avoid steroids. Since some cases of pustular psoriasis have been associated with the abrupt cessation of corticosteroid therapy, we slowly taper any steroids the patient may be receiving. Our favorite drug is hydroxyurea (Hydrea 0.5 gm bid to qid), which produces rapid involution of lesions in our experience. Within days it can be replaced by methotrexate (2.5 mg q12h for three doses once weekly).

No one approach has been uniformly successful, and hence one can combine retinoids, methotrexate, and ultraviolet light (UVA) according to one's skills and experience. Our limited experience with PUVA-treated patients indicates that it must be used cautiously and in low dose to avoid development of Koebner lesions.

For most of these patients, long-term maintenance therapy is necessary. In this regard, the prognosis is as variable as with psoriasis vulgaris. This is not too surprising, as the two forms really differ only in the size of their essential lesion, the pustule.

Baker H, Ryan TJ: Generalized pustular psoriasis. A clinical and epidemiological study of 104 cases. Br J Dermatol 80:771–793, 1968.

A superb clinical review of the course of disease in 104 patients. Two out of three cases evolved into erythroderma. The best prognosis was in the exanthematous form due to drug exposure or infection. Other forms included the von Zumbusch, annular, and localized patterns.

Ryan TJ, Baker H: Systemic corticosteroids and folic acid antagonists in the treatment of generalized pustular psoriasis. Evaluation and prognosis based on the study of 104 cases. Br J Dermatol 81:134–145, 1969.

Methotrexate cleared the pustules in 37 of 47 patients, but was associated with three of eight deaths in their series. Systemic steroids gave control in only 12 of 73 patients and are usually avoided because of side effects and ineffectiveness.

Baker H: Pustular psoriasis. Dermatol Clin 2:455–470, 1984.

The management of generalized pustular psoriasis includes bedrest, mild sedation, applications of bland creams or lotions or low-potency topical steroids, and elimination of trigger factors such as infections, drugs (e.g., **lithium**), and irritating (**tar** or **anthralin**) topical antipsoriatic preparations. Systemic steroids and potent topical steroids should be withdrawn slowly (many cases of the disease are precipitated by withdrawal of steroids). Attention must be paid to correction of special problems of heat, water, and protein loss in these patients. For active treatment, **methotrexate** (5 to 10 mg IM or IV weekly) is the drug of choice. Hydroxyurea (Hydrea 500 mg bid) and dapsone (100 to 200 mg daily) may also be helpful. Oral steroids should be avoided unless the disease is life threatening. **Etretinate** (Tigason 0.5 to 0.75 mg/kg/day is helpful in conjunction with PUVA, started 10 days later with 0.5 J/sq cm.

Hubler WR Jr: Familial juvenile generalized pustular psoriasis. Arch Dermatol 120:1174–1178, 1984.

Oral **methotrexate** (5 to 15 mg/week given in three divided doses q12h) controlled localized acral pustular psoriasis with episodic generalized pustular psoriasis in three siblings ages 18, 20, and 21 years (one female).

Stein KM, Shelley WB, Weinberg RA: Hydroxyurea in the treatment of pustular psoriasis. Br J Dermatol 85:81–85, 1971.

In four patients, **hydroxyurea** (Hydrea 1 to 2 gm PO each day) induced resolution of lesions and fever within three to seven days of initiating treatment.

MacMillan AL, Champion RH: Generalized pustular psoriasis treated with dapsone. Br J Dermatol 88:183–185, 1973.

Dapsone (125 to 200 mg/day) combined with **triamcinolone** (8 to 12 mg/day) gave long-term complete control of life-threatening generalized pustular psoriasis in a 50-year-old man. Prior treatment failures included **methotrexate, chloroquine, azathioprine**, and **erythromycin**.

Hönigsmann H, Gschnait F, Konrad K, Wolff K: Photochemotherapy for pustular psoriasis (von Zumbusch). Br J Dermatol 97:119–126, 1977.

Complete clearing of skin lesions and systemic symptoms occurred in all eight patients using 8-MOP (**methoxsalen** 0.6 mg/kg two hours prior to exposure, four times per week) and UVA (1.0 to 5.0 J/sq cm initially, increased gradually to an average total of 50 J/sq cm over a three-week period). Maintenance doses were given once or twice a week for up to 18 months.

Wolska H, Jablonska S, Bounameaux Y: Etretinate in severe psoriasis. Results of double-blind study and maintenance therapy in pustular psoriasis. J Am Acad Dermatol 9:883–889, 1983.

This aromatic retinoid (widely used in Europe) is the authors' first choice for treating pustular psoriasis (dose: 1 mg/kg/day for a maximum of four months). They demonstrated moderate to complete clearing of lesions in four patients with von Zumbusch pustular psoriasis. **Etretinate** is not nearly as effective in psoriasis vulgaris.

Rosenbaum MM, Roenigk HH Jr: Treatment of generalized pustular psoriasis with etretinate (Ro 10-9359) and methotrexate. J Am Acad Dermatol 10:357–361, 1984.

Combination therapy (**etretinate** 1.25 mg/kg/day + **methotrexate** 50 mg IM weekly) was effective in a 60-year-old man, whereas each given alone was not.

Shelley WB: Generalized pustular psoriasis induced by potassium iodide: A postulated role for dihydrofolic reductase. JAMA 201:1009–1014, 1967.

Potassium iodide (500 mg oral challenge) induced attacks in two patients with recurrent generalized pustular psoriasis of von Zumbusch (fever, leukocytosis, hypoproteinemia, hypocalcemia, hepatitis). Salicylates and progesterone also triggered attacks.

Stewart AF, Battaglini-Sabetta J, Millstone L: Hypocalcemia-induced pustular psoriasis of von Zumbusch. Ann Intern Med 100:677–680, 1984.

Hypocalcemia in a woman with surgical hypoparathyroidism precipitated generalized pustular psoriasis on several occasions. It cleared rapidly with oral **calcium** supplements and **vitamin D** (ergocalciferol 200,000 U/day). Intravenous calcium infusions would also clear the lesions, but only after normocalcemia was achieved.

Lowe NJ, Ridgway HB: Generalized pustular psoriasis precipitated by lithium carbonate. Arch Dermatol 114:1788–1789, 1978.

A 44-year-old woman with psoriasis vulgaris for 22 years developed generalized pustular psoriasis three weeks after starting **lithium carbonate** (300 mg tid) prescribed for manic-depressive psychosis. At this same time she had discontinued **methotrexate** (20 mg/week) because of the mania. Resumption of methotrexate (25 mg IV + 20 mg IV five days apart) in the hospital led to methotrexate toxicity. PUVA was the successful treatment (**methoxsalen** 40 mg + 3 J/sq cm initially, given every other day), both this time and in a second attack precipitated by lithium.

Reshad H, Hargreaves GK, Vickers CFH: Generalized pustular psoriasis precipitated by phenylbutazone and oxyphenbutazone. Br J Dermatol 109:111–113, 1983.

Two cases (in women, ages 39 and 78 years) in which the **phenylbutazone** (Butazolidin) family of nonsteroidal anti-inflammatory drugs was clearly responsible for attacks of generalized pustular psoriasis.

Moy RL, Kingston TP, Lowe NJ: Isotretinoin vs etretinate therapy in generalized pustular psoriasis and chronic psoriasis. Arch Dermatol 121:1297–1301, 1985.

Isotretinoin (13-cis-retinoic acid, 1.5 to 2.0 mg/kg/day) controlled pustulation and systemic symptoms in 10 of 11 patients with generalized pustular psoriasis. The response was seen within two to five days. Maintenance dosage was determined by the clinical response to tapering dose and continued for six weeks.

Etretinate (0.75 mg/kg/day) was found to be more effective than isotretinoin (1.5 mg/kg/day) for chronic plaque psoriasis. After eight weeks of treatment with etretinate, 18 of 19 patients had moderate to complete clearing in contrast to only 4 of 10 patients with similar response in the isotretinoin treatment group.

Patients like to think their EDC (Expected Date of Cure) is sometime later this week.

Pyoderma

Erythromycin
Tegopen
Keflex
Dapsone
Rocephin

The sovereign remedy for this purulent plebeian affliction is a modern antibiotic. Erythromycin has long been the favorite treatment for the nondescript pyodermas, since most invaders are erythromycin-sensitive staphylococci and streptococci.

Recall these principles:

Systemic therapy is more effective than topical.
The organism must be sensitive to the antibiotic.
Most pyodermas are due to group A beta-hemolytic streptococci and *Staphylococcus aureus*, which are sensitive to erythromycin, cloxacillin (Tegopen), and cephalexin (Keflex).
The less common gram-negative pathogens are sensitive to neomycin, polymyxin, and gentamicin, which may be used topically.
Resistant organisms may emerge, requiring treatment with Rocephin.

Specific sections elsewhere in this book describe approaches to some nongeneric categories of pyoderma (impetigo, ecthyma, furuncles, folliculitis). Here, references are given for the principles of treating pyodermas, along with some specific treatment of rare pyodermas.

Dillon HC Jr: Topical and systemic treatment for pyodermas. Int J Dermatol 19:443–451, 1980.

Complete review by a leading investigator. **Erythromycin** is the drug of choice for bullous impetigo. Oral penicillin is preferred for streptococcal infections. Topical antibiotics may be effective in mild cases, but healing is less prompt than with systemic antibiotics.

Sebben JE: Surgical antiseptics. J Am Acad Dermatol 9:759–765, 1983.

Hibiclens (**chlorhexidine gluconate**) is the best, with broad-spectrum persistent residue on the stratum corneum and no absorption. Should not be applied directly to the middle ear.

Disadvantages of other surgical antiseptics:

benzalkonium chloride (Zephiran)
- inactivated by soaps and detergents on skin
- prone to contamination by gram-negative bacteria (not active against *Pseudomonas aeruginosa*)

hexachlorophene (pHisoHex)
- inactivated by alcohol on skin (including perfume and aftershave)
- narrow spectrum (little activity against gram-negative bacteria)
- absorption through skin
  - central nervous system toxicity
  - teratogenicity (do not use in pregnancy)

povidone-iodine (Betadine)
  skin reactions
  tissue irritation may increase infection
  addition of detergent decreases effectiveness
  release of iodine from iodophors may not be continuous
alcohol
  not adequate if used alone (about same effectiveness as soap and water)

Leyden JJ, Kligman AM: Rationale for topical antibiotics. Cutis 22:515–528, 1978.

Data on experimental pyodermas provide evidence of effectiveness of over-the-counter **neomycin-bacitracin-polymyxin B** ointments.

Wilson WR, Cockerill FR III: Tetracyclines, chloramphenicol, erythromycin, and clindamycin. Mayo Clin Proc 58:92–98, 1983.

Erythromycin is powerful against both streptococci and staphylococci. Reserve **chloramphenicol** and **clindamycin** for anaerobic infections. Avoid **tetracyclines** because of resistant strains and bacteriostatic rather than bactericidal action against *Staphylococcus aureus* and group A beta-hemolytic streptococci.

Thompson RL, Wright AJ: Cephalosporin antibiotics. Mayo Clin Proc 58:79–87, 1983.

The oral cephalosporins (Keflex, Velosef, Duricef) are bactericidal against most gram-positive cocci and gram-negative bacilli, except *Pseudomonas aeruginosa*. Use is restricted by cost and emergence of resistance.

MacDonald RH, Beck M: Neomycin: A review with particular reference to dermatological usage. Clin Exp Dermatol 8:249–258, 1983.

This aminoglycoside, used topically, is effective against staphylococci and most gram-negative organisms, but is not effective against streptococci and *Pseudomonas aeruginosa*.

Edson RS, Keys TF: The aminoglycosides: Streptomycin, kanamycin, gentamicin, tobramycin, amikacin, netilmicin, sisomicin. Mayo Clin Proc 58:99–102, 1983.

Despite toxicity, **gentamicin** and **tobramycin** play major roles in treating serious gram-negative infections. **Amikacin** is the first choice with gentamicin-resistant organisms.

Kucers A, Bennett N McK: The Use of Antibiotics: A Comprehensive Review with Clinical Emphasis, 3rd ed. London, Heinemann Medical Books, 1979, 1014 pp.

A marvelous reference!

Tells you the things your "detail man" never told you.

Nobel WC: Skin microbiology: Coming of Age. J Med Microbiol 17:1–12, 1984.

An attempt to alter skin surface ecology and disrupt pathogen colonization by using *Staphylococcus epidermidis* inoculations on skin was not successful.

Marples CR, Kligman AM: Pyoderma due to resistant *Staphylococcus aureus* following topical applications of neomycin. J Invest Dermatol 53:11–13, 1969.

A hazard of long-term self-medication with over-the-counter salves.

Massa MC, Su WPD: Pyoderma faciale. A clinical study of twenty-nine patients. J Am Acad Dermatol 6:84–91, 1982.

For this subset of acne, multiple forms of therapy were used simultaneously: Vlem Dome compresses, oral antibiotics, incision and drainage, UVB, and intralesional steroids. (Accutane is now the treatment of choice.)

Brown CS, Kligman AM: Mycosis-like pyoderma. Arch Dermatol 75:123–125, 1957.

Vegetating hypertrophic lesions resembling blastomycosis were cleared with three weeks of **procaine penicillin** (600,000 U/day) in two debilitated men. Cultures showed *Staphylococcus aureus* and beta-hemolytic streptococci.

Su WPD, Duncan SC, Perry HO: Blastomycosis-like pyoderma. Arch Dermatol 115:170–173, 1979.

Multiple verrucoid plaques caused by *Staphylococcus aureus* in a woman with chronic granulocytic leukemia cleared with three weeks of **erythromycin** (500 mg qid). In seven other cases both gram-negative bacteria and *Staphylococcus aureus* were frequently found, usually in an immunocompromised host.

Williams HM, Stone OH: Blastomycosis-like pyoderma: Case report of unusual entity with response to curettage. Arch Dermatol 93:226–228, 1966.

Cure by **curettage** of a large granulomatous ulcerating lesion that had failed to respond to topical and systemic antibiotics, intralesional and systemic steroids, oral SSKI (saturated solution of potassium iodide), and superficial x-ray. Obesity was the only predisposing factor. Cultures showed *Staphylococcus aureus* consistently, with a multitude of other organisms.

Jacyk WK: Treatment of pyoderma vegetans of Hallopeau with dapsone. Arch Dermatol 115:1035–1036, 1979.

Moist verrucous, vegetating, malodorous lesions in the inguinal folds, perineum, and axillae cleared with six weeks of **dapsone** (100 mg/day). Remarkable before and after photographs of a case in Nigeria.

Person JR, Schwartz JH: Dapsone-responsive, noninfectious verrucous pyoderma. Its occurrence following cisplatin therapy. Arch Dermatol 118:336–338, 1982.

Firm, round, erythematous nodules with verrucous centers on the dorsal surfaces of the hands and fingers cleared with two weeks of **dapsone** (50 mg tid). Contributing factors included metastatic bladder carcinoma and treatment with **cisplatin II**.

Powell FC, Winkelmann RK: Malignant pyoderma. Br J Dermatol 109:597–603, 1983.

Rapidly enlarging ulcers on the face and neck in young adults responded to a combination of **cytoxan** (100 to 200 mg/day) and corticosteroids (60 to 90 mg/day). Cultures were negative for pathogens. Clinically different from pyoderma gangrenosum.

Magnussen CR: Skin and soft tissue infections. In Reese RE, Douglas RG (eds): A Practical Approach to Infectious Diseases. 2nd ed. Boston, Little, Brown and Company, 1986, pp 99–122.

A first rate resource:

- Fournier's gangrene of the scrotum: IV **gentamicin** (1.5 mg/kg every 8 hours) and IV **clindamycin** (600 mg every 6 hours). Surgical incision and drainage.
- Perineal area abscess: Oral **amoxicillin** (250 mg every 8 hours) and oral **clindamycin** (600 mg every 6 hours).

Keep your patient's hostility down with a smile.

Pyoderma Gangrenosum

Corticosteroids	Minocin
Topical	Chemotherapy
Systemic	Purinethol
Pulse	Imuran
Benzoyl peroxide	Alkeran
Cromoglycate	Cytarabine
Hyperbaric oxygen	Cytoxan
Periactin	Thalidomide
Sulfapyridine	Clofazimine
Azulfidine	Cyclosporin A
Dapsone	

These patients have ulcer-prone skin in which the slightest trauma can initiate progressive chronic ulcers in a manner not yet explained. They must protect themselves from bumps, bruises, and bites, and you must protect them from casual vena punctures, injections, skin tests, and biopsies. Iodides are particularly malevolent in inducing flares in some of these individuals.

Treatment centers on good topical care, systemic steroids, and therapy for possible underlying disease. We like silver nitrate compresses (0.5 per cent aqueous 20 minutes tid) followed by packing of the ulcers each time with 10 per cent benzoyl peroxide gel. We also prescribe dapsone (100 mg/day) in conjunction with Minocin (100 to 300 mg/day) and zinc sulfate (220 mg tid). Kenalog (40 mg IM) is given every three weeks. Progress is measured in weeks rather than days.

Always the patients deserve continuing careful screening for any of the possible 25 associated systemic diseases. These include inflammatory bowel disease, hepatitis, and myeloproliferative disorders. Appropriate treatment for these may be of great benefit.

Holt PJA: The current status of pyoderma gangrenosum. Clin Exp Dermatol 4:509–516, 1979.

Excellent review of this enigmatic disease that is most commonly treated by high-dosage systemic corticosteroids.

Jennings JL: Pyoderma gangrenosum: Successful treatment with intralesional steroids. J Am Acad Dermatol 9:575–580, 1983.

A horrendous ulcer covering the entire dorsum of one hand was cured in six weeks with intralesional injections of **triamcinolone acetonide** (Kenalog suspension 10 mg/ml). Initially, 6 ml was injected in 0.3-ml quantities via a 30-gauge one-inch needle around the entire ulcer. A similar follow-up injection of 1 ml was given after 16 days. No Xylocaine dilution. Silvadene cream was the only other therapy. This article includes a valuable table of 25 diseases that have occurred in association with pyoderma gangrenosum, including rheumatoid arthritis (seropositive and seronegative), Hodgkin's disease, carcinoid tumor, metastatic carcinoma of the colon, and Takayasu's arteritis.

Peachey RDG: Pyoderma gangrenosum of scalp. Br J Dermatol 90:106–108, 1974.

Betamethasone 17-valerate lotion 0.1 per cent (Valisone) applied under polyethylene occlusion each night produced complete healing of ulceration that had been indifferent to courses of **prednisone, erythromycin, cephalexin, carbenicillin**, and **gentamicin**.

Nguyen LQ, Weiner J: Treatment of pyoderma gangrenosum with benzoyl peroxide. Cutis 19:842–844, 1977.

Gauze dressings impregnated with **benzoyl peroxide** lotion 20 per cent (Benoxyl lotion) and cut to the exact size of the ulcer produced healing in six weeks of a large ulcer on buttocks. Protect normal skin with Lassar's paste, cover with Saran wrap, pressure dress with a Pamper pad, and change every 12 hours. Necrotic tissue was debrided after one week. After four weeks, Neosporin powder and Lassar's paste replaced the benzoyl peroxide.

De Cock KM, Thorne MG: The treatment of pyoderma gangrenosum with sodium cromoglycate. Br J Dermatol 102:231–233, 1980.

A local spray of 2 per cent **cromoglycate** solution (Rynacrom nasal spray tid) induced healing in three weeks in two cases. (Available in the United States as a 1 per cent solution—Intal nebulizer solution. Could improvise a 2 per cent solution by dissolving contents of a 20-mg Intal [**cromolyn sodium**] capsule in 1 ml water).

Thomas CY, Crouch JA, Guastello J: Hyperbaric oxygen therapy for pyoderma gangrenosum. Arch Dermatol 110:445–446, 1974.

Case showing dramatic relief of pain and healing in 10 days following 30 minutes/day in a hyperbaric (two atmospheres) oxygen chamber. Adjunct therapy: **oxacillin** (1 gm qid), **prednisone** (5 mg qod), and 0.1 per cent **neomycin** solution soaks.

Gelernt IM, Kreel I: Pyoderma gangrenosum in ulcerative colitis: Prevention of the gangrenous component. Mt Sinai J Med 43:467–470, 1976.

Cyproheptadine (Periactin 4 mg qid), presumably acting as a platelet deaggregator to prevent platelet thrombi, was remarkably helpful when given early in two cases.

Perry HO, Brunsting LA: Pyoderma gangrenosum: A clinical study of nineteen cases. Arch Dermatol 75:380–386, 1957.

Introduced Azulfidine (**sulfasalazine** 4 gm/day), which gut bacteria convert to sulfapyridine and 5-aminosalicylic acid. Good results were seen in 9 of 12 patients (with and without associated ulcerative colitis).

Lorincz AL, Pearson RW: Sulfapyradine and sulfone type drugs in dermatology. Arch Dermatol 85:2–16, 1962.

Six cases of pyoderma gangrenosum were treated successfully with **sulfapyridine** (2 to 4 gm/day). Today's analogue is dapsone (100 mg/day).

Lynch WS, Bergfeld WF: Pyoderma gangrenosum responsive to minocycline hydrochloride. Cutis 21:535–538, 1978.

Minocin (100 mg tid) gave complete healing within several months in three of four cases. Note large dosage of **minocycline**. Associated ulcerative colitis also improved in one patient.

Davies MG, Piper S: Pyoderma gangrenosum: Successful treatment with minocycline. Clin Exp Dermatol 6:219–223, 1981.

Minocin (100 mg tid) was similarly effective in a 39-year-old woman with polyarthritis, vitiligo, and pyoderma gangrenosum, but was needed for one year with slowly tapered dose. Since cultures of lesions showed no growth, the authors felt that **minocycline** acts as an anti-inflammatory agent, possibly through suppression of leukocyte chemotaxis.

Johnson RB, Lazarus GS: Pulse therapy: Therapeutic efficacy in the treatment of pyoderma gangrenosum. Arch Dermatol 118:76–84, 1982.

Methylprednisolone sodium succinate (1 gm in 150 ml 5 per cent dextrose) given IV (60 to 90 minutes) each morning for five days produced dramatic remission in three severe, resistant cases. Therapy should be carried out only in the hospital. Must watch out for sudden electrolyte shifts and cardiac arrhythmias, which may cause cardiac arrest. Model of case reporting of new high-potency pulse therapy. 95 references.

Holt PJA, Davies MG, Saunders KC, Nuki G: Pyoderma gangrenosum: Clinical and laboratory findings in 15 patients with special reference to polyarthritis. Medicine 59:114–133, 1980.

Comprehensive review. Of the 15 patients, 6 developed lesions at the site of skin trauma. Only 2 had colitis. No vasculitis or immunofluorescence was seen histologically. In 6 of 12, steroid complications developed, with 4 deaths.

Maldonado N, Torres VM, Méndez-Cashion D, et al: Pyoderma gangrenosum treated with 6-mercaptopurine and followed by acute leukemia. J Pediatr 72:409–414, 1968.

Complete healing was induced in six months with **6-mercaptopurine** (Purinethol 2.5 mg/kg/day) in a seven-year-old boy with hypergammaglobulinemia and plasmacytosis of the bone marrow. However, he died one year later of acute leukemia.

Schöpf E, Schulz HJ, Schulz KH: Azathioprin-Behandlung der Dermatitis ulcerosa (Pyoderma gangrenosum). Hautarzt 20:558–563, 1969.

Imuran (150 mg/day) produced healing in four weeks in a 79-year-old man.

Möller H, Waldenström JG, Zettervall O: Pyoderma gangrenosum (dermatitis ulcerosa) and monoclonal (IgA) globulin healed after melphalan treatment. Case report and review of the literature. Acta Med Scand 203:293–296, 1978.

Alkeran (**melphalan** 2 mg/day) healed extensive lesions in an elderly woman with myeloma in six months. Surgical removal of a carcinoma of the colon had not altered the pyoderma gangrenosum.

Crawford SE, Sherman R, Favara B: Pyoderma gangrenosum with response to cyclophosphamide therapy. J Pediatr 71:255–258, 1967.

Cytoxan (150 mg/sq m/day) and **prednisone** (30 mg/day) produced complete healing of ulcers within three months in a nine-year-old girl. The problem began as an ulcer of the buttock following a penicillin injection and was unresponsive to systemic and topical antibiotics. Excision had been followed by new ulcers around the sutures and on the legs and at venipuncture sites. No pathogenic organisms were found, and histologic findings were simply inflammatory. The ulcers had persisted despite **amphotericin B** therapy, transfusions, skin grafting, and steroid therapy.

Byrne JPH, Hewitt M, Summerly R: Pyoderma gangrenosum associated with active chronic hepatitis. Arch Dermatol 112:1297–1301, 1976.

Azathioprine (Imuran 150 to 300 mg/day) induced complete healing of ulcers in two cases in two to five months. In one case, however, the drug caused severe leukopenia, and the ulcers broke down after the Imuran was stopped.

Olson K: Pyoderma gangrenosum with systemic L.E. Acta Derm Venereol 51:233–234, 1971.

Imuran (100 mg/day) caused rapid improvement in ulcers present for two years despite therapy with **chloroquine, sulfasalazine**, and **prednisolone**.

Lewis SJ, Poh-Fitzpatrick MB, Walther RR: Atypical pyoderma gangrenosum with leukemia. JAMA 239:935–938, 1978.

In two patients chemotherapy of acute myeloblastic leukemia with **cytarabine** (Cytosar-U) and **daunorubicin** (Cerubidine) induced healing of all ulcers within three months. Pyoderma gangrenosum has also been associated with other forms of leukemia, monoclonal gammopathy, myeloma, myeloid metaplasia, and polycythemia.

Newell LM, Malkinson FD: Pyoderma gangrenosum: Response to cyclophosphamide therapy. Arch Dermatol 119:495–497, 1983.

Complete review of chemotherapy reserved for the most destructive and resistant cases of these ulcers (also known years ago as Meleney's ulcers). Although Imuran is a favorite, the authors obtained a splendid response with **cyclophosphamide** (Cytoxan 150 mg/day) in a 33-year-old woman with severe pyoderma gangrenosum but without associated systemic disease. Complete healing occurred in three months. There was a four-year follow-up of the disease, which had been present for 17 years.

Happle R, Schiffer H-P, Kovary PM: Ocular involvement in pyoderma gangrenosum. Arch Dermatol 113:1612, 1977.

In a 64-year-old man with asymmetric seronegative arthritis and pyoderma gangrenosum of the left temple, conjoint **azathioprine** and **prednisone** cleared the skin lesions, but relapse occurred on stopping. Maintenance azathioprine (50 mg) and prednisone (5 mg) twice weekly have kept the patient clear for three years. He also had unique ulcerative scleritis with corneal opacity in the left eye, which responded to cryotherapy and systemic steroids (12 mg/day).

Work BA Jr: Pyoderma gangrenosum of the perineum. Obstet Gynecol 55:126–128, 1980.

Although excision and grafting are generally avoided in pyoderma gangrenosum, here is an exception to the rule. Vulvectomy and two-stage split-thickness grafting gave a 10-year cure in a woman with underlying ulcerative colitis.

Michaëlsson G, Molin L, Öhman S, et al: Clofazimine: A new agent for the treatment of pyoderma gangrenosum. Arch Dermatol 112:344–349, 1976.

Clofazimine (100 mg tid), a mycobacterial antimicrobial, gave rapid complete healing of ulcers in eight patients within six weeks to four months. Side effects: reddish discoloration of skin and urine, ichthyosiform dryness on arms and legs.

Thomsen K, Rothenborg HW: Clofazimine in the treatment of pyoderma gangrenosum. Arch Dermatol 115:851–852, 1979.

Seven of ten cases healed completely in two to five months with **clofazimine** (100 mg tid). Partial healing occurred in other cases.

Kark EC, Davis BR, Pomeranz JR: Pyoderma gangrenosum treated with clofazimine. Report of 3 cases. J Am Acad Dermatol 4:152–159, 1981.

First cases treated in the United States with this fabulous new drug, which remains experimental (Lamprene [Ciba-Geigy] 100 mg tid).

Venencie PY, Saurat JH: Pyoderma gangrenosum chez un enfant traitement par la thalidomide. Ann Pediatr (Paris) 29:67–69, 1982.

Thalidomide therapy, the newest approach. Extensive pyoderma gangrenosum in a three-year-old girl, unresponsive to **prednisone, minocycline,** and **clofazimine**, showed a spectacular recovery following **thalidomide** (150 mg/day that was gradually tapered to 100 mg every five days). Keloidal scarring did remain.

Talansky AL, Meyers S, Greenstein AJ, Janowitz HD: Does intestinal resection heal the pyoderma gangrenosum of inflammatory bowel disease? J Clin Gastroenterol 5:207–210, 1983.

Yes, particularly if inflammatory bowel disease is severe. In a study of eight cases, five with severe bowel disease healed within two months, but three others with milder bowel disease required an additional year for healing. After lesions had healed, there were no recurrences.

Curley RK, MacFarlane AW, Vickers CFH: Pyoderma gangrenosum treated with cyclosporin A. Br J Dermatol 113:601–604, 1985.

Cyclosporin A (500 mg/day, orally) induced healing of pyoderma gangrenosum ulcers of the legs of 14 years' duration. The ulcer healing was evident by 3 weeks and has continued for the ensuing 12 months. Maintenance dose is 200 mg/day. New areas of ulceration appeared when the dose was reduced to 150 mg/day.

The ulcers had previously failed to heal despite the following treatments:

Occlusive bandaging
Antibiotics, multiple
ACTH
Prednisolone (150 mg/day)
Azathioprine (150 mg/day)
Methotrexate (IV, 45 mg/week)
Dapsone (400 mg/day)
Cyclophosphamide (100 mg/day)
Aspirin and dipyridamole (300 mg/day)
Clofazimine (100 mg/day)
Sodium cromoglycate (topical)
Methylprednisolone pulse (1 gram/day for three days)
Plasma exchanges (× 14)
Skin grafting (× 2)

If the first five patients of the day are "better," everyone will be better that day.

Quixote Syndrome

Characterized by an unrelenting quixotic itch to write something for each letter in the alphabet, the Quixote syndrome usually runs a benign course. In our experience, it does not respond to treatment and hence, once recognized, is best ignored.

By the thread one comes to the ball of yarn.

DON QUIXOTE

Something is better than nothing at all.

DON QUIXOTE

A diamond is not as valuable as one's own tooth.

DON QUIXOTE

That which costs little is valued less.

DON QUIXOTE

Never assume that crazy problems can appear only in crazy patients.

Diagnosis is in the mind of the beholder, but therapy is in the hands of the patient.

Treat every patient who comes to your office as a VIP (Very Important Patient).

Relapsing Polychondritis

Corticosteroids	Dapsone
Nonsteroidal anti-inflammatory drugs	Colchicine
Immunosuppressants	Cyclosporine A

McAdam LP, O'Hanlan MA, Bluestone R, Pearson CM: Relapsing polychondritis: Prospective study of 23 patients and a review of the literature. Medicine 55:193–215, 1976.

The best general reference.

This is a rare disease of unknown etiology with episodic yet generally progressive inflammation of cartilaginous structures throughout the body. Major clinical features include auricular, nasal, and respiratory tract chondritis, ocular inflammation, seronegative inflammatory polyarthritis, and audiovestibular damage.

It uniformly responds to **prednisone** (80 to 100 mg/day initially, with maintenance 25 mg/day), as seen in 18 of 23 patients. Six patients could be reasonably well controlled with nonsteroidal anti-inflammatory drugs (**aspirin, indomethacin**, and **phenylbutazone**). In four patients an immunosuppressive drug (**6-mercaptopurine, cyclophosphamide, azathioprine**, or **melphalan**) was needed in addition to corticosteroids.

Seven of the 23 patients (30.5 per cent) died as a result of the polychondritis after an average duration of 4.2 years, usually of respiratory tract involvement or cardiac valvular or vasculitic involvement.

Martin J, Roenigk HH Jr, Lynch W, Tingwald FR: Relapsing polychondritis treated with dapsone. Arch Dermatol 112:1272–1274, 1976.

A 51-year-old man with painful erythematous swelling of the ears showed no response to **dapsone** (100 mg/day for five days) but clearing occurred with dapsone (200 mg/day for three weeks). Within four days of doubling the dose the ears had improved noticeably, and by 10 days the skin had returned to normal. During a four-month follow-up after the drug was discontinued, there had been no recurrence.

Barranco VP, Minor DB, Solomon H: Treatment of relapsing polychondritis with dapsone. Arch Dermatol 112:1286–1288, 1976.

Three patients with relapsing polychondritis were treated successfully with **dapsone** (100 to 200 mg/day). The response was uniformly rapid within one week.

Espinoza LR, Richman A, Bocanegra T, et al: Immune complex–mediated renal involvement in relapsing polychondritis. Am J Med 71:181–183, 1981.

Prednisone (60 mg/day) and **dapsone** (100 mg bid) rapidly cleared symptoms in an 80-year-old woman with a two-week history of ocular redness, nasal tenderness, jaw pain, fever, and weakness. The prednisone dose was tapered to 25 mg/day and the dapsone discontinued without any exacerbation of her disease in the subsequent year.

Askari AD: Colchicine for treatment of relapsing polychondritis. J Am Acad Dermatol 10:507–510, 1984.

Colchicine (0.6 mg bid for two weeks) induced dramatic improvement in four days and complete resolution after seven days of chondritis of the pinnae of the ears in two men (ages 27 and 44 years).

Ruhlen JL, Huston KA, Wood WG: Relapsing polychondritis with glomerulonephritis: Improvement with prednisone and cyclophosphamide. JAMA 245:847–848, 1981.

In a 32-year-old man, tracheal and laryngeal tenderness as well as hoarseness improved with **prednisone** (60 mg/day). The renal problem persisted until **cyclophosphamide** (Cytoxan 150 mg/day) was added. Control was maintained for more than a year with the cyclophosphamide (150 mg/day) and low-dose prednisone (5 mg every other day).

Svenson KLG, Holmdahl R, Klareskog L, et al: Cyclosporin A treatment in a case of relapsing polychondritis. Scand J Rheumatol 13:329–333, 1984.

A 52-year-old woman with relapsing polychondritis and high titers of anti-collagen II antibodies responded rapidly to oral **cyclosporine** (15 mg/kg/day for one month, then 6 mg/kg/day maintenance to give therapeutic plasma levels [70 ng/ml]). The condition had affected her ears, nose, joints, and trachea, and prior treatment with corticosteroids, **dapsone, azathioprine**, and **cyclophosphamide** had failed to stop its progression. Within nine months of the start of treatment the anti-collagen II antibodies had virtually disappeared. After two years the patient is in good health, but noninflammatory residual deformities remain.

One drug tried is worth a score of lab tests ordered.

Rosacea

Tetracycline Flagyl Dapsone Accutane

Today the greatest therapeutic challenge is posed not by simple rosacea but rather by iatrogenic rosacea induced by topical steroids. While the powerful fluorinated steroids erase the disease with ease, they induce a self-perpetuating steroid rosacea. The result is a topical steroid "addict" who will do anything to obtain more of "the only salve that works."

Such patients (mainly women) may have been dependent on powerful topical steroids for years. They need to know that the "steroid-rosacea" cycle can and must be broken. Stopping the topical steroid habit "cold turkey" with reliance on oral tetracycline is most desirable but results initially in a dramatic flare. Alternatives include injection of triamcinolone acetonide (40 mg IM) or graduated reductions in topical steroid potency. Newer systemic treatments include Flagyl and Accutane. But stop the topical steroid addiction, we must.

Wilkin JK: Rosacea. Int J Dermatol 22:393–400, 1983.

Complete review. Avoid heat, cold, sunlight (use sun screen), alcohol, seafood, and pork. In **tetracycline**-resistant cases, try **dapsone**. Other helpful antibiotics include **erythromycin, ampicillin, chloramphenicol, metronidazole**, and other tetracyclines. **Clonidine** (Catapres) may help by suppressing menopausal flushing. 75 references.

The problem of rosacea. Br Med J 4:366, 1975.

The most "embarrassing" disease:

It affects those who blush easily, in an area that cannot be covered.

The nose grows to be red and clownlike, which popular myth associates with heavy drinking.

Fluorinated steroids that help today make the face worse in the long run.

Result: a seriously depressed patient, needing your help and concern.

Treatment: **tetracycline** (250 mg bid), which also helps rosaceous keratitis.

Wilkin JK: Vasodilator rosacea. Arch Dermatol 116:598, 1980.

When taking a history for rosacea, ask about vasodilator drugs. The following 22 drugs cause flushing and worsen rosacea:

aminophylline
amyl nitrite
cyclandelate (Cyclospasmol)
diazoxide (Proglycem)
dioxyline phosphate
dipyridamole (Persantine)
erythrityl tetranitrate (Cardilate)
ethaverine (Ethatab)
ethyl alcohol
hydralazine (Apresoline)
isoproterenol (Isoprel)

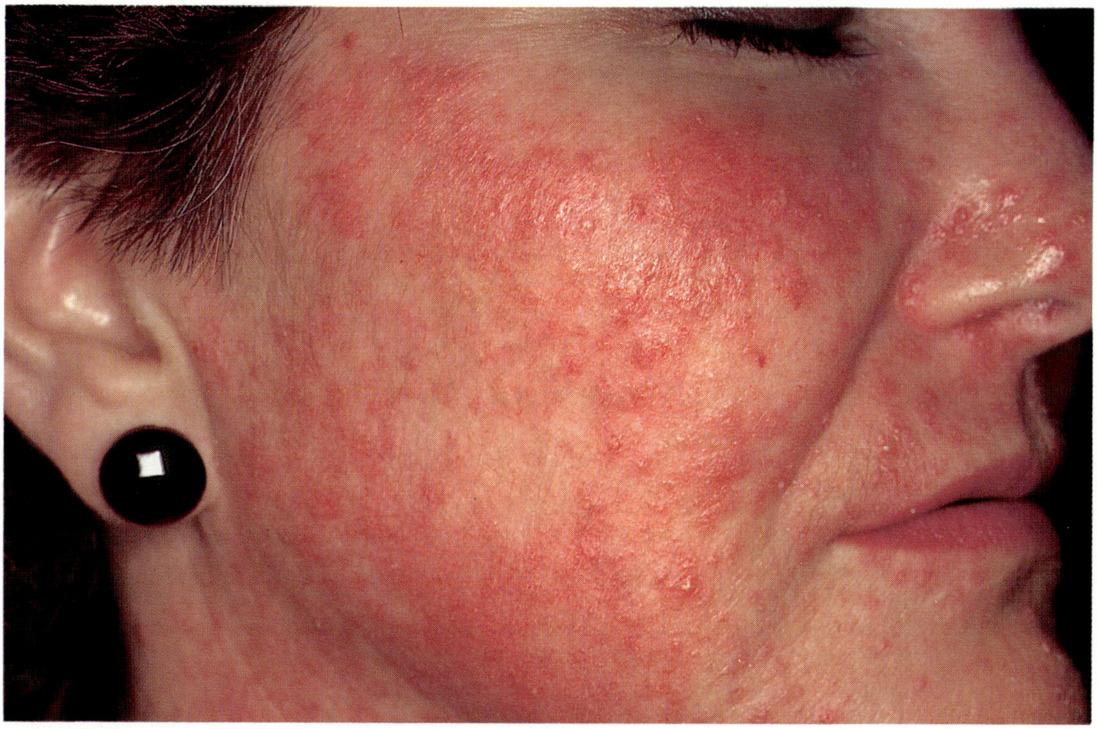

isosorbide dinitrate (Isordil)
isoxsuprine (Vasodilan)
niacin (nicotinic acid)
nicotinyl alcohol (Roniacol)
nitroglycerin
nylidrin
papaverine (Pavabid)
pentaerythritol tetranitrate (Pentritol, Peritrate)
reserpine (Serpasil)
theophylline
tolazoline (Priscoline)

Cites the case of a 74-year-old man who developed rosacea a few months after starting **pentaerythritol tetranitrate** prescribed for a myocardial infarction.

Wilkin JK: Oral thermal-induced flushing in erythematotelangiectatic rosacea. J Invest Dermatol 76:15–18, 1981.

Heat, not caffeine, in coffee favors the flush. Study of 24 patients showed that very hot fluids, including decaffeinated coffee, should be avoided to reduce flushing. Ingested heat in the oral cavity probably leads to flushing through countercurrent heat exchange at the level of the internal jugular vein and common carotid artery and a subsequent central thermoregulatory reflex.

Rosacea in hot water. Lancet 1:647, 1981.

Since the face does not sweat excessively in rosacea, the erythema is probably mediated by locally acting vasoactive substances rather than a neural mechanism.

Flushing in rosacea may be similar to that induced by alcohol in diabetics taking **chlorpropamide** (Diabinese). This can be blocked by both **indomethacin** and **aspirin**, which are prostaglandin inhibitors.

Topical **salicylic acid** may help rosacea through inhibiting prostaglandin synthesis.

Question: Would sucking on ice reduce facial blood flow and help rosacea?

Tan SG, Cunliffe WJ: Rosacea and migraine. Br Med J 1:21, 1976.

Of 137 patients with rosacea 60 (44%) also had migraine. Both have abnormal vascular reactivity and are aggravated by stress.

Rosacea may be related to:

facial migraine (episodic facial neuralgia, flushing, lacrimation, and reddening of the skin)

facial flushing and migraine at menopause

Questions:

Do oral contraceptives, chocolate, and cheese aggravate rosacea (as they do migraine)?

Could drugs used in migraine also help rosacea?

Cunliffe WJ, Dodman B, Binner JG: Clonidine and facial flushing in rosacea. Br Med J 1:105, 1977.

Since rosacea and migraine may be associated, a trial of **clonidine** (Catapres 0.05 mg bid), which helps migraine, was given to 17 patients with rosacea.

Results: In five flushing improved. Four had to stop the drug because of increased pustulation.

Topical clonidine (2 per cent in cream base applied qid for two weeks) was without effect in 20 patients with rosacea.

Sneddon I: Adverse effect of topical fluorinated corticosteroids in rosacea. Br Med J 1:671–673, 1969.

In 14 cases, telangiectasia and erythema were increased and aggravated by prolonged use (two to six months) of topical fluorinated steroids. A severe rebound of superficial edema, pustules, and inflammation developed within one week upon cessation of fluorinated steroids and required three months of **tetracycline** (250 mg bid) and **hydrocortisone** ointment (1 per cent) for clearing. Hydrocortisone topically did not produce the rebound phenomenon and helped to quiet the inflammation.

Go MJ Th H, Wuite J: Comparative study of triamcinolone acetonide and hydrocortisone 17-butyrate in rosacea with special regard to the rebound phenomenon. Dermatologica 152(Suppl 1):239–246, 1976.

No rebound flare developed with low-potency topical steroid therapy (Kenalog cream 0.1 per cent or Locoid cream bid).

Ellis CN, Stawiski MA: The treatment of perioral dermatitis, acne rosacea, and seborrheic dermatitis. Med Clin North Am 66:819–830, 1982.

Excellent review emphasizing topical therapy:

sulfur ppt (2 to 10 per cent in cream base bid); may add **hydrocortisone** (1.0 per cent)

salicylic acid (1 to 3 per cent in 70 per cent isopropyl alcohol bid)

resorcinol (3 to 5 per cent in 70 per cent isopropyl alcohol bid)

Kwell lotion (to face and scalp at bedtime for two treatments in one week) to eliminate large *Demodex* population.

Residual telangiectatic vessels may be eradicated by electrodesiccation.

Russell BF: Some aspects on the biology of the epidermis. Br Med J 1:815–820, 1962.

Patients with follicular papular rosacea often have a heavy infestation of *Demodex folliculorum*, which thrive in the environment of vascular dilatation and seborrhea. The use of facial cleansing creams instead of soap may be responsible. Topical sarcopticides (**sulfur, benzyl benzoate**, or **crotamiton**) often help rosacea patients.

Mills OH Jr, Kligman AM: Topically applied erythromycin in rosacea. Arch Dermatol 112:553–554, 1976.

Erythromycin (2 per cent in equal parts of ethanol and water) bid for two months gave good to excellent results in 13 of 15 patients.

Montes LF, Cordero AA, Kriner J, et al: Topical treatment of acne rosacea with benzoyl peroxide acetone gel. Cutis 32:185–190, 1983.

Enthusiasm for 5 per cent Persa-Gel (applied one or two times daily) following a four-month double-blind controlled study.

Sneddon IB: The treatment of steroid-induced rosacea and perioral dermatitis. Dermatologica 152(Suppl 1):231–237, 1976.

Recommends **tetracycline** (250 mg bid) and **hydrocortisone** (1 per cent) cream, but should use the mild topical steroids as little as possible because of relapses when they are discontinued. Alert patient to rebound, which will be severe for two weeks after fluorinated steroid is stopped. Do not give tetracycline to pregnant patients. **Ampicillin** is good alternative to tetracycline, whereas **clindamycin** is not effective.

Sneddon IB: A clinical trial of tetracycline in rosacea. Br J Dermatol 78:649–652, 1966.

In 78 cases, patients were given **tetracycline** (250 mg bid) but no local treatment: 78 per cent improved within one month, but relapse occurred unless they were given a small maintenance dose (100 mg daily).

Jenkins MS, Brown SI, Lempert SL, Weinberg RJ: Ocular rosacea. Am J Ophthalmol 88:618–622, 1979.

Tetracycline (250 mg qid) greatly helped 37 patients in 4 to 17 days. Most patients could gradually taper the dose, but prolonged therapy was needed for symptoms of burning, pain, and foreign body sensation. Other common findings included conjunctival hyperemia, superficial punctate erosions of the cornea, chalazia, and blepharitis.

Bartholomew RS, Reid BJ, Cheesbrough MJ, et al: Oxytetracycline in the treatment of ocular rosacea: A double-blind trial. Br J Ophthalmol 66:386–388, 1982.

Of 35 patients with ocular rosacea who received **oxytetracycline** (Terramycin 200 mg bid for 6 weeks), 19 had sustained remission for more than eight months with improvement beginning after the first two weeks. Nonspecific inflammatory changes (lid swelling, redness, blepharitis, chalazia, and conjunctival hyperemia) responded well, as did corneal infiltrates, marginal ulcers, and superficial punctate erosions. No permanent improvement was seen in conjunctival or corneal vascularization. Relapses occurred two to three weeks after stopping tetracycline. Progressive keratitis occurs in 5 per cent of rosacea patients.

Marks R, Ellis J: Comparative effectiveness of tetracycline and ampicillin in rosacea: A controlled trial. Lancet 2:1049–1052, 1971.

In a double-blind study of 56 patients for six weeks, **ampicillin** (250 mg tid for one week, then bid) was of value in rosacea, but was somewhat less effective than **tetracycline** (identical dosage).

Bajdekoff B: Die Behandlung der Rosacea mit Breitspectrum-Antibiotika. Z Haut-Geschlkrkh 43:933, 1968.

Chloromycetin (**chloramphenicol** 1 gm/day for one month) coupled with topical Chloromycetin cream (1 per cent) was helpful in 26 cases.

Pye RJ, Burton JL: Treatment of rosacea by metronidazole. Lancet 1:1211–1212, 1976.

Serendipitous discovery that Flagyl (200 mg bid) prescribed for another condition cleared rosacea. It vanquishes pustules and papules but not erythema. Double-blind study of 29 patients demonstrated significant benefit after six weeks, with further clearing when drug was continued up to three months. The only side effect was headache (not related to alcohol ingestion).

Saihan EM, Burton JL: A double-blind trial of metronidazole versus oxytetracycline therapy for rosacea. Br J Dermatol 102:443–445, 1980.

There was no difference in a three-month trial with 40 patients taking either **tetracycline** (250 mg bid) or Flagyl (200 mg bid). Mechanism of action is not known, but possibly antibacterial. The authors feel that **metronidazole** can be used safely during pregnancy.

Burton JL, Saihan EM: Rosacea, metronidazole, and pregnancy. Br J Dermatol 103:585–586, 1980.

Metronidazole has been used safely for 20 years to treat trichomoniasis in pregnancy with no evidence of teratogenicity. There is no evidence of carcinogenicity in humans with short- or long-term treatment. Should limit course of metronidazole to three months to avoid risk of sensory peripheral neuropathy (which is usually, but not always, reversible).

Braun-Falco O, Korting HC: Metronidazoltherapie der Rosazea: Medikament und Indikation. Hautarzt 34:261–265, 1983.

Summary of good responses to Flagyl in 218 patients reported in the world literature. The authors feel it should *not* be used in pregnancy. Avoid use for longer than three months.

Molavi A, LeFrock, JL, Prince RA: Metronidazole. Med Clin North Am 66:121–133, 1982.

Comprehensive review with 152 references.

Note: Adverse effects—all have low incidence

Urine possibly turning dark red-brown because of azometabolite of drug
Anorexia, nausea, vomiting
Unpleasant metallic taste
Furring of tongue due to *Candida* glossitis
Colitis—one case—*Clostridium difficile*
Disulfiram-like reaction to alcohol (rare)
Increases hypoprothrombinemic effect of warfarin (Coumadin)
No evidence of carcinogenicity or teratogenicity in humans (but numbers studied are small—avoid use in first trimester of pregnancy)

Dolezal R, Schultz RC: Early treatment of rhinophyma—A neglected entity? Ann Plast Surg 11:393–396, 1983.

Recommends early surgical treatment for minimal rhinophyma using subsection with scalpel blade and dermabrasion sculpturing. Nine patients were all pleased: better airway, better appearance.

Strempel H: A new dermatome for surgical treatment of rhinophyma. J Dermatol Surg Oncol 7:153–156, 1981.

Good review of surgical techniques used in rhinophyma. Introduces use of an electrically driven "mucotome" (used in palate surgery) which cuts to a constant depth of 1.0 mm as blade moves to and fro. It permits delicate sculpturing in narrow spaces around alar margins. Operations were done under general anesthesia. Keep tip of index finger in each nostril to estimate depth of shaving and avoid damage to nasal cartilages.

Shapshay SM, Strong MS, Anastasi GW, Vaughan CW: Removal of rhinophyma with the carbon dioxide laser. Arch Otolaryngol 106:257–259, 1980.

Four cases with good to excellent results.

Advantages are bloodless field and better sculpturing.
Eschar lasts about 10 days.
Healing is complete in three to four weeks.

Nikolowski J, Plewig G: Orale Behandlung der Rosazea mit 13-cis-Retinsäure. Hautarzt 32:575–584, 1981.

In 13 severe cases not responsive to **tetracycline, metronidazole**, and dermabrasion, 95 per cent were cleared within 8 weeks by using a small to modest dose of Accutane (0.05 to 1.0 mg/kg/day), although treatment continued 12 to 28 weeks. Seborrhea disappeared as sebaceous glands became markedly reduced in size. Fabulous before-and-after color pictures. (English version: J Am Acad Dermatol 6:766–785, 1982).

A rosacea is a rosacea is a rosacea—if treated with topical steroids.

Sarcoidosis

Chloroquine	Ketoconazole
Allopurinol	Accutane
Methotrexate	Thalidomide
Chlorambucil	

The mysterious immune granulomas of sarcoidosis represent a markedly delayed (four to six weeks) type of hypersensitivity response involving monocytes and an unidentified antigen. We consider it a reaction pattern to multiple antigens, prototypically related to the zirconium, beryllium, or mycobacterial sarcoid reactions. Eventually the offending allergen may be degraded by the monocytes and eliminated by the body, producing a "spontaneous remission" of all lesions.

Our initial therapy centers on elimination of possible causal antigens, using a variety of antimicrobial agents. Although it is rarely achieved, we have accomplished this with streptomycin, ketoconazole, and dapsone, respectively, in three patients whose lesions cleared within six weeks of initiation of therapy.

The nonspecific attack against this perplexing indolent noninflammatory reaction uses immunosuppressants such as steroids, chlorambucil, and methotrexate. The results are temporary. In our minds, intralesional steroids are most consistently effective in causing prolonged paralysis of the monocyte response, but risk atrophy. We find that topical steroids are disappointing, and systemic steroids provide relief only while being given. The therapeutic net can be further widened using chloroquine and allopurinol. Even Accutane, the wonder drug of the 80s, offers promise.

Sharma OP: Sarcoidosis: Clinical Management. London, Butterworths, 1984, 186 pp.

A masterpiece monograph, covering every aspect of this disease.

Hanno R, Needelman A, Eiferman RA, Callen JP: Cutaneous sarcoidal granulomas and the development of systemic sarcoidosis. Arch Dermatol 117:203–207, 1981.

Eleven patients with sarcoidosis limited to the skin were treated with intralesional or topical steroids with fair success. Involvement of other organs was found in half of the patients who sought dermatologic help.

All such patients with skin lesions deserve:

- ophthalmologic examination to rule out uveitis (precursor of glaucoma and cataracts)
- search for systemic sarcoidosis:
  - chest roentgenogram and pulmonary function tests
  - liver function tests
  - serum angiotensin-converting enzyme (ACE) (increased in systemic sarcoidosis)
  - urinary calcium excretion (more sensitive than serum calcium)
  - lymph node biopsy

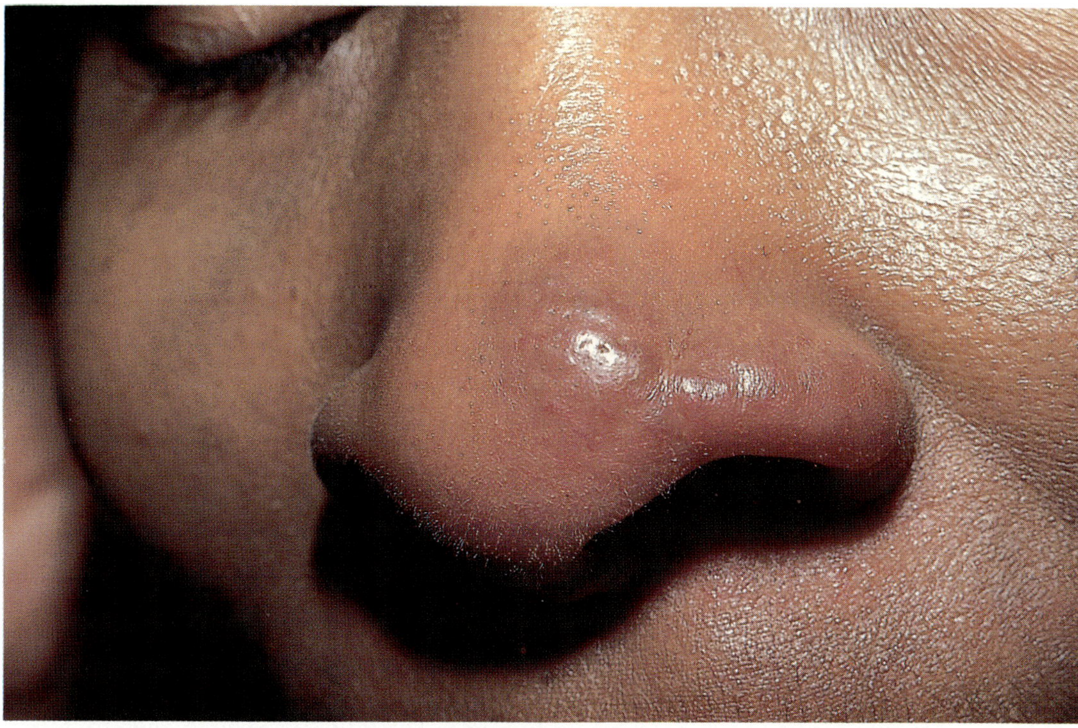

intradermal skin tests—PPD, *Candida*, mumps (we would also include bacterial and trichophytin skin tests)

Shaffer B, Cahn MM, Levy EJ: Sarcoidosis apparently cured by quinacrine (Atabrine) hydrochloride. Arch Dermatol 67:640–641, 1953.

First report of an antimalarial drug (Atabrine 100 mg tid) clearing cutaneous sarcoidosis within two months.

Soderström N: Two cases of sarcoidosis treated with mepacrine. Lancet 2:947–948, 1960.

Similar account of two cases with spectacular complete involution of all sarcoid lesions within one month of starting Atabrine (100 mg tid for two weeks, bid for two weeks, and then daily for two months). **Chloroquine** (Aralen 250 mg daily) was eventually substituted for **mepacrine** in one patient. All skin lesions resolved with atrophic brown scars.

Morse SI, Cohen ZA, Hirsch JG, Schaedler RW: The treatment of sarcoidosis with chloroquine. Am J Med 30:779–784, 1961.

Chloroquine (500 mg/day) resulted in significant or complete involution of skin lesions in seven patients. Therapy continued for six months. Reversible relapse occurred within three months of stopping chloroquine. Mechanism of action is unknown.

Siltzbach LE, Teirstein AS: Chloroquine therapy in 43 patients with intrathoracic and cutaneous sarcoidosis. Acta Med Scand Suppl 425:302–306, 1964.

Chloroquine (250 mg bid) was regularly effective in suppressing cutaneous sarcoidosis, but *not* pulmonary lesions in 14 cases. Relapse on stopping drug. Treatment should be limited to six months, followed by a rest period, to reduce risk of eye problems.

Rosof BM: Allopurinol for sarcoid? N Engl J Med 294:447, 1976.

Serendipitous discovery that **allopurinol** (Zyloprim 100 mg tid) given for gout cleared steroid-resistant sarcoidosis of 17 years' standing in a 60-year-old man. The finding was confirmed in a second patient, with relapse on stopping allopurinol.

Pollock JL: Sarcoidosis responding to allopurinol. Arch Dermatol 116:273–274, 1980.

Two more cases responded brilliantly to **allopurinol** (100 mg/day and 100 mg tid respectively) within four to eight weeks. Therapy was continued for six months.

Veien NK, Brodthagen H: Cutaneous sarcoidosis treated with methotrexate. Br J Dermatol 97:213–216, 1977.

Methotrexate (25 mg PO once a week) caused involution of skin lesions within two months in 12 of 16 patients. Uveitis also cleared in 3 of 4 patients. Average treatment period was two years. More than half of the patients showed relapse two to four weeks after stopping methotrexate.

Kataria YP: Chlorambucil in sarcoidosis. Chest 78:36–43, 1980.

Chlorambucil (4 to 6 mg/day) cleared sarcoid erythema nodosum in three months in a 55-year-old diabetic white woman. Lesions relapsed twice when the drug was stopped, but always responded when it was restarted.

Franck WA, Fossum DR, Katz RI: Candidiasis and sarcoidosis. NY State J Med 77:122–124, 1977.

Amphotericin B (750 mg IV given over three months) eliminated *Candida albicans* from sputum and dramatically ameliorated pulmonary sarcoidosis. (**Ketoconazole** would be prescribed today.)

Waldinger TP, Ellis CN, Quint K, Voorhees JJ: Treatment of cutaneous sarcoidosis with isotretinoin. Arch Dermatol 119:1003–1005, 1983.

In one patient Accutane (40 to 80 mg/day) cleared 75 per cent of nodules within three months. Erythematous and erosive changes developed in many lesions after two weeks. By the end of the 7½ month course 75 per cent of the peripheral lymphadenopathy had also cleared. Pulmonary function tests remained unchanged after four months of treatment.

Patterson JW, Fitzwater JE: Treatment of hypopigmented sarcoidosis with 8-methoxypsoralen and long wave ultraviolet light. Int J Dermatol 21:476–480, 1982.

A single case (in a 43-year-old black woman) required eight months of home black light therapy (GE F15 T8 BLB) coupled with 1 per cent **methoxypsoralen** lotion pretreatment for good response; 80 treatments were given three times a week with maximum exposure of 60 minutes at 25 cm. First help was noted at four months.

Barriere H: Sarcoïdes cutanées: Traitement par la thalidomide. Presse Med 12:963, 1983.

Four cases were helped within two months with **thalidomide** therapy. Treatment continued for six to twelve months.

Prigent F, Ouazzani W: Sarcoïdose cutanée: Traitement par la thalidomide. Presse Med 12:3007, 1983.

Confirmation of **thalidomide** report. Thalidomide (300 mg/day) gave rapid clearing in one case of ulcerative sarcoid lesions.

Barnhill RL, McDougall AC: Thalidomide: Use and possible mode of action in reactional lepromatous leprosy and in various other conditions. J Am Acad Dermatol 7:317–323, 1982.

Thalidomide probably acts as an immunosuppressant by inhibiting neutrophil chemotaxis in inflammatory conditions similar to erythema nodosum leprosum. Sarcoid is not mentioned. Hazards of polyneuritis and teratogenicity preclude the use of thalidomide in the United States except on a research basis.

James DG, Williams WJ: Sarcoidosis and Other Granulomatous Disorders. Philadelphia, WB Saunders Co, 1985, 254 pp.

Comprehensive monograph on every aspect of this disease and present-day therapy:

Prednisolone	First line of treatment and consistently most successful
Indomethacin	Helpful in erythema nodosum
Immunosuppressives	Permit dose of steroid to be cut in half
Chloroquine	Helpful in fibrotic form (250 mg q.o.d., maximum, nine months)
Methotrexate	Very helpful (5 mg once/week for three months)
Cyclosporin A	Under study

Knowing how a drug works isn't knowing that it will work.

Scabies

Lindane	Nitrofurazone
Sulfur	Malathion
Benzyl benzoate	Crotamiton
Thiabendazole	Methotrexate

The treatment of scabies fulfills the therapist's dream and the patient's fantasy: absolute cure with thorough application of a simple chemical that is nonirritating, nonsensitizing, and nonexpensive.

The chemical, which sat on the laboratory shelf for over a century before it was discovered to be a magic bullet for killing mites, is gamma benzene hexachloride (lindane). Its 1 per cent formulation in lotion or cream (Kwell) has swept the field because of unquestioned effectiveness. Alternate effective measures need rarely be employed.

The skill in using Kwell hinges on careful patient instruction and compliance and in treating all of the skins with which the patient comes in contact. We prefer Kwell lotion with simultaneous treatment of the entire family and household help. Treatment should also be given to the extended family of a commune, nursing home, or primitive village. The *Scarcoptes scabiei* mite travels widely, but its passage is nearly always one of skin to skin.

Estes SA: Diagnosis and management of scabies. Med Clin North Am 66:955–963, 1983.

Superb concise reference. Stresses insidious onset of pruritus and rash four to six weeks after infestation as the immune system starts to react to the increasing mite population. Intense nocturnal pruritus leads to hemorrhagic excoriations. Apply Kwell lotion over every square inch of skin from neck down, including nails, umbilicus, perineum, and soles. Will need help for back area. No prior bath! For Norwegian scabies, must also treat face and scalp.

Shower off in morning and launder bedding.

Two-ounce trade package suffices for retreatment the following night, if desired.

No further Kwell. Use topical steroids for residual eczematization, antibiotics for secondary pyoderma, and intralesional steroids for persistent pruritic nodules that develop in intertriginous areas.

Ways to identify burrows:

1. Cover hyperkeratotic areas with mineral oil and examine closely.
2. Apply Topicycline (liquid **tetracycline**), dry for a few minutes, wipe vigorously with isopropyl alcohol, illuminate with Wood's light to reveal yellow green linear lesions.
3. Burrow ink test: Cover lesions with black or blue ink from a fountain pen, wipe with alcohol pad to remove surface ink, look for burrows penetrated by ink.

Woodley D, Saurat JH: The burrow ink test and the scabies mite. J Am Acad Dermatol 4:715–722, 1981.

Details of the diagnostic test used routinely at Hôpital Saint-Louis in Paris, with helpful photographs showing zigzagged lines of burrows

Best yield: papules (not vesicles or excoriations)

Best location: medial wrists and medial hypothenar area of hands (where skin is taut and thick)

Hurwitz S: Scabies in babies. Am J Dis Child 126:226–228, 1973.

Must treat babies from neck up as well as neck down, since head is not a mite-free site in children.

Taplin D, Rivera A, Walker JG, et al: A comparative trial of three treatment schedules for the eradication of scabies. J Am Acad Dermatol 9:550–554, 1983.

Timed applications of Kwell lotion, including the scalp:

2 hours: cured 82 per cent
6 hours: cured 96 per cent
12 hours: cured 98 per cent

This study took place on an island off Panama where 70 per cent of the population of 2076 persons were infested with scabies. The entire population at risk was treated at the same time to prevent reinfestation. There were no adverse reactions.

Taplin D: Resistance to antiscabietic drugs. J Am Acad Dermatol 8:121–123, 1983.

Treatment failures are never due to mites developing resistance to Kwell. They are likely to be due to concomitant bacterial infection with crusted lesions or to failure of the patient to apply the scabicide behind the ears, in the intergluteal cleft, or between the toes.

Taplin D, Arrue C, Walker JG: Eradication of scabies with a single treatment schedule. J Am Acad Dermatol 9:546–550, 1983.

One application of Kwell lotion for 16 to 20 hours will stop an epidemic if everybody at risk is treated simultaneously. Patients with pyoderma should have a second treatment after the infection has been treated, as crusts prevent adequate penetration of gamma benzene hexachloride lotion.

One family physician in the San Blas Islands, treating approximately 30 new scabies patients per week for almost two years, did not reduce the incidence of scabies (which was over 50 per cent in the island population of 2000).

Moral: Treating only the patient in your office is a good practice-builder, but not a good public health measure.

Church RE, Knowelden J: Scabies in Sheffield: A family infestation. Br Med J 1:761–763, 1978.

New epidemics of scabies appear approximately every 30 years, with each cycle consisting of 15 years of widespread infestation followed by 15 years of only rare cases. A possible explanation is the development of herd resistance and a resistant generation, succeeded by a nonsensitized generation.

How to control a scabies epidemic:

Ensure adequate treatment of affected households.

Follow up contacts.

Lessons from this epidemic:

Schoolchildren and teenagers, especially girls, brought scabies into the household.

Schools were not a major source of infestation (cases were few and sporadic).

Friends and relatives living outside the household were the initial contact source in 90 per cent.

If a young child was the first affected member of a household, relatives were the source.

Thirty-eight per cent of family contacts within a household became infested.

Kanaaneh HAK, Rabi SA, Badarneh SM: The eradication of a large scabies outbreak using community-wide health education. Am J Public Health 66:564–567, 1976.

Success in an underdeveloped Arabic village by examining and treating the entire population at risk. **Benzyl benzoate** emulsion (25 per cent) was used to treat all household members whenever a case of scabies was found. Exterminators then visited houses and sprayed all bedding, clothing, and fomites with **lindane** (0.5 per cent in kerosene).

Lerche NW, Currier RW, Juranek DD, et al: Atypical crusted "Norwegian" scabies: Report of nosocomial transmission in a community hospital and an approach to control. Cutis 31:637–642, 668, 684, 1983.

Elderly debilitated and immunosuppressed patients are likely to harbor large numbers of mites (100 to 1000) without a lot of itching and be highly contagious. Failure to recognize scabies in a pruritic diabetic led to infestation of 54 per cent of the hospital staff. **Crotamiton** (Eurax 10 per cent lotion) applied for 24 hours on three occasions cleared the condition after Kwell lotion had failed. All contacts were also treated with Eurax (applied every 24 hours for 2 days) with repeat treatment in seven days for persons in close contact.

Parish LC, Millikan LE, Witkowski JA, Schwartzman R: Scabies in the extended care facility. Int J Dermatol 22:380–382, 1983.

Nursing homes become loci of endemic scabies unless *all* residents, nursing staff employees, and families of patients and employees are treated (without exception) at the same time. Very instructive article on how to "quell" scabies epidemics in nursing homes. Watch out for overuse of scabicides leading to irritant dermatitis.

Aforismo JF: Infection control procedure for scabies in the long-term care facility. Hosp Pharm 17:200–201, 1982.

Exquisitely detailed directions your hospital administrator will appreciate.

One ounce of Kwell lotion or cream is sufficient for one treatment of an adult.

Seal personal articles (shoes, books, knitting, purse) in a plastic bag for 10 days.

(We also suggest "retiring" the mattresses temporarily, as 10 days without a host spells death for the mite.)

Elmros T, Hornqvist R: Infestation of scabies in the scalp area. Acta Derm Venereol 61:360–362, 1981.

Scabies simulating dandruff in the scalp of a 25-year-old woman was not cured until both head *and* body were treated with **benzyl benzoate** (available in the United States as a 28 per cent lotion USP and a 50 per cent emulsion). She had previously been treated for scabies on the body. Application of a topical steroid to the scalp for treatment of seborrheic dermatitis probably worsened the eruption.

Scher RK: Subungual scabies. Am J Dermatopathol 5:187–189, 1983.

A subungual biopsy revealed an adult mite under the distal nail plate. Failure to cut nails short and brush fingertips and free edges of nails with a scabicide on several consecutive days can also lead to treatment failure. Treatment should be given on several consecutive days. This procedure stopped long-lasting epidemics in two nursing homes.

Mellanby K: Human guinea pigs. London, Merlin Press, 1973.

It's not the bedding but what's in the bed that spreads scabies.

Millard LG: Norwegian scabies developing during treatment with fluorinated steroid therapy. Acta Derm Venereol 57:86–88, 1977.

Avoid topical steroids until after the mites are dead.

Macmillan AL: Unusual features of scabies associated with topical fluorinated steroids. Br J Dermatol 87:496–497, 1972.

A massive mite invasion with crisscrossing burrows developed in a seven-month-old boy treated for over half his life with topical steroids. Iatrogenically depressed immunity plus the universal inability of infants to scratch allowed the mites to thrive while the baby wriggled up a storm.

Charlesworth EN, Johnson JL: An epidemic of canine scabies in man. Arch Dermatol 110:572–574, 1974.

Fifteen patients developed a pruritic eruption from contact with a litter of five puppies infested with *Sarcoptes scabiei* var. *canis.* Lesions in dogs usually involve the external ear margins, legs, and ventral abdomen, but may become generalized with large areas of alopecia and crusting. Sometimes it is the dog, not the patient, that needs treatment.

Chakrabarti A, Chatterjee A, Chakrabarti K, Sengupta DN: Human scabies from contact with water buffaloes infested with *Sarcoptes scabiei* var. *bubalis.* Ann Trop Med Parasitol 75:353–357, 1981.

The story of 35 individuals in India who acquired scabies from scabietic water buffaloes. Protect your patient from *Sarcoptes*-infested dogs, cats, pigs, sheep, goats, horses, mules, cows, and water buffaloes (and people)!

Rasmussen JE: The problem of lindane. J Am Acad Dermatol 5:507–516, 1981.

Complete review of hazards of the toxic active ingredient of Kwell (**gamma benzene hexachloride**). Adverse reactions are essentially due to misuse (repeated daily application or oral ingestion). Patients should never re-treat within 1 week—warning them about possible convulsions helps insure compliance. Over 50 million treatments in the last five years attest to safety.

Solomon LM, Fahrner L, West DP: Gamma benzene hexachloride toxicity: A review. Arch Dermatol 113:353–357, 1977.

Presents the chemistry and pharmacology of this neurologic poison used so successfully in curing scabies.

Special alert: hazard to infants and pregnant women. 88 references.

Lange M, Nitzsche K, Zesch A: Percutaneous absorption of lindane in healthy volunteers and scabies patients. Arch Dermatol Res 271:387–399, 1981.

Avoid bathing before application to reduce percutaneous absorption. The authors recommend showering with lukewarm water and soap 10 hours after applying Kwell lotion to minimize absorption.

Davies JE, Dedhia HV, Morgade C, et al: Lindane poisonings. Arch Dermatol 119:142–144, 1983.

Oral **cholestyramine** resin (Questran 4 gm q8h) was used as an adjunctive absorptive measure to save a comatose convulsing 16-year-old boy who had ingested **lindane** shampoo (1 per cent).

Pramanik AK, Hansen RC: Transcutaneous gamma benzene hexachloride absorption and toxicity in infants and children. Arch Dermatol 115:1224–1225, 1979.

A four-month-old marasmic baby boy developed seizures and abnormal neurologic function two days after receiving one total-body treatment with 1 per cent **lindane** lotion left on 24 hours. His blood level was 17 times greater than that of normal children treated with lindane, probably because of malnourishment.

Orkin M, Maibach HI: Scabies in children. Pediatr Clin North Am 25:371–386, 1978.

The authors favor **sulfur** (6 per cent finely precipitated in petrolatum) applied nightly to the entire body for three days as alternative to **lindane**.

Mellanby K: Scabies. London, Oxford University Press, 1943.

Some treatments of yesteryear and a scoreboard of cure rates:

Treatment	***% Cures***
Benzyl benzoate 20 per cent emulsion in water	99.9
Sulfur 10 per cent ointment	97–100
Marcussen's ointment (polysulfides)	100
Dimethyl diphenylene disulfide	100
Sulfur soap	17
Sulfur orally 10 gm/day	0

Hernandez-Perez E: Topically applied thiabendazole in the treatment of scabies. Arch Dermatol 112:1400–1401, 1976.

A **thiabendazole** 10 per cent suspension (Mintezol applied bid for five days) cleared the condition in 80 per cent of 40 patients after one course and in an additional 15 per cent after two courses. Persistent violaceous periumbilical nodules resolved after a single intralesional steroid injection.

Chowdhury SPR: Nitrofurazone in scabies. Lancet 1:152, 1977.

Sixteen of twenty cases cleared with Furacin ointment (**nitrofurazone** 0.2 per cent) when supplies of **benzyl benzoate** ran short in Bangladesh.

Hanna NF, Clay JC, Harris JRW: *Sarcoptes scabiei* infestation treated with malathion liquid. Br J Vener Dis 54:354, 1978.

Malathion liquid (0.5 per cent) topically gave an 83 per cent cure rate in 30 cases.

Cubela V, Yawalkar SJ: Clinical experience with crotamiton cream and lotion in treatment of infants with scabies. Br J Clin Pract 32:229–231, 1978.

Crotamiton 10 per cent (Eurax cream or lotion) applied on three to five consecutive days resulted in cure in only 26 of 50 patients. Results were best (69 per cent cured) with Eurax cream applied on five consecutive days.

Ward WH: Scabies norvegica: Treatment with methotrexate. Australas J Dermatol 12:44–51, 1971.

Report of nine cases with mongolism. Suppression of thick psoriasiform scale by **methotrexate** (2.5 mg daily for six days, then rest six days, then repeat, etc.) was the key to success. Apparently the thick scale physically protected mites from the scabicide before methotrexate therapy.

Shelley WB, Shelley ED: Common causes of treatment failure in scabies. Ill Med J 163:112–114, 1983.

Four major failures:

unrecognized scabies (The well-washed should stop bathing for one week.)
not treating the entire skin surface
close contacts not simultaneously treated (Infestation in bedfellows, playmates, babysitters, grandparents, etc., may precede itching by weeks.)
continuing use of a scabicide for hyperalgesic postscabetic skin (instead of topical steroids and systemic antibiotics)

To itch is human, to scratch divine.

Scleredema

Chloroquine

Scleredema, whether it be "adultorum or juvenilis," is still beyond our regular therapeutic grasp. We have no way of curbing the wayward fibrocyte that fills the dermis of these patients with polysaccharide polymers (glycosaminoglycans, especially hyaluronic acid). We can look for predisposing factors such as diabetes mellitus or a febrile illness, but identification and correction of such factors are still without effect on this skin problem.

We have steroids to modulate lymphocyte function, dapsone to affect the neutrophil, and tretinoin to control the keratinocyte. Yet nothing comparable has been discovered to affect the fibrocyte, as witness our struggle with the cognate problems of keloids and scleroderma.

But these patients need more than sympathy. We explain that the swelling is due to avidity of the abnormal polysaccharides for binding water. We explain that the disease is not a sign of cancer and that it will not affect the hands or feet. We stress that most cases undergo resolution in a year or two without heroic treatment. We point out that both surgery and pregnancy are well tolerated.

For the severe example we prescribe new or previously untried drugs for short therapeutic trials. Recently in one of our patients nodular scleredema on the shoulders cleared rapidly with chloroquine (Aralen 300 mg daily). If this fails in the next patient, we will prescribe ketoconazole (200 mg bid), cimetidine (300 mg qid), or phenytoin sodium (100 mg tid). Remember, serendipitous therapeutic success comes only to those who try, try, and try again.

Venencie PY, Powell FC, Su WPD, Perry HO: Scleredema: A review of thirty-three cases. J Am Acad Dermatol 11:128–134, 1984.

Systemic corticosteroids, methotrexate, or D-penicillamine had no effect on this insidious disease. Patients should be checked for diabetes mellitus as well as for involvement of the heart (ECG) and esophagus (swallowing function). The cutaneous process may be so mild as to actually escape the patient's notice.

Curtis AC, Shulak BM: Scleredema adultorum: Not always a benign self-limited disease. Arch Dermatol 92:526–541, 1965.

A review of 223 cases showed that 1 in 4 had the disease longer than two years. Note the therapeutic failures of 20 years ago:

calcium gluconate	para-amino benzoate
estradiol	penicillin
fever	pituitary extract
hot baths	steroids
hyaluronidase	thyroid
nicotinic acid	vitamin D
ovarian extract	

Christy WC, Buckingham RB, Barnes EL, Prince RK: Scleredema adultorum of Buschke: A clinical, pathologic, and cell culture study of two patients. J Rheumatol 10:595–601, 1983.

The authors postulate that a chemical mediator from injury, drug, or infection activates fibroblasts to synthesize increased amounts of glycosaminoglycans (particularly hyaluronic acid) that avidly bind water with resultant "hard edema."

Rees R, Moore A, Nanney L, King L: Scleredema adultorum: The surgical implications of a rare dermatologic disorder. Plast Reconstr Surg 72:90–93, 1983.

In a 44-year-old black man with previously unrecognized diabetes mellitus, a large indurated hyperpigmented plaque developed over the right scapula following an insect bite and secondary pustule and abscess formation due to *Staphylococcus aureus*. Drainage of a large abscess was followed by poor wound healing, which necessitated skin grafting.

The disease usually remits spontaneously in 6 to 24 months.

Verghese A, Noble J, Diamond RD: Scleredema adultorum: A case of the recurrent cellulitis syndrome. Arch Dermatol 120:1518–1519, 1984.

Recurrent attacks of cellulitis ("pseudoerysipelas") in areas of scleredema in a 52-year-old diabetic woman were readily controlled with oral **penicillin V potassium**. One attack, however, required hospitalization for **cephapirin** (Cefadyl 2 gm IV q6h). No organisms could be found in either skin aspirates or skin biopsy. Note: The onset of the scleredema had followed an attack of acute pharyngitis.

Kovary PM, Vakilzadeh F, Macher E, et al: Monoclonal gammopathy in scleredema: Observations in three cases. Arch Dermatol 117:536–539, 1981.

Paraproteinemia was found in three of the authors' six patients with widespread scleredema (Buschke's disease). Attention is directed to one case in the literature associated with multiple myeloma. The authors advise that immunoelectrophoresis be performed at regular intervals.

Carrington PR, Sanusi ID, Winder PR, et al: Scleredema adultorum. Int J Dermatol 23:514–522, 1984.

To date, no therapy has been shown to be efficacious in this disease.

No machine can replace the searching eye *linked to the discriminating brain.*

J. M. Ziman

Scleroderma

Nitroglycerin ointment	Azathioprine
Emollients	Stanozolol
Prazosin	D-Penicillamine
Nifedipine	Estriol
Captopril	Dilantin
Ketanserine	Physiotherapy

This disease is more than skin deep. In its progressive systemic form, it slowly sentences the patient to death by constriction. As the patient's skin becomes a sclerotic shroud, the internal organs become similarly fibrotic. Death comes as fibrosis. Hence the therapeutic attack should be on the fibroblast. As of yet, however, there is no specific drug that blocks this insidious lethal fibroplasia.

But we *can* interfere with the collagen bonding itself. After making certain that the sclerosis is not the result of drugs, chemicals, toxins, or internal malignant disease, we can prescribe D-penicillamine (Cuprimine 1 gm/day), which inhibits cross-linkages within the collagen molecule. Used indefinitely, it can halt and indeed slowly reverse some of the fibrosis. It is not a risk-free drug, but it offers hope to the patient experiencing cardiac and renal failure or facing starvation due to a fibrotic gut that will neither move nor absorb food. In addition to penicillamine, these patients need long-term medical management by a sympathetic internist versed in hypertension, heart failure, and renal failure. Some patients may even need dialysis or a renal transplant.

Management of the skin changes largely centers on problems caused by acrosclerosis, as it is in the extremities that the reduced blood flow in constricted arterioles becomes most evident. Raynaud's phenomenon, pain, ulceration, contractures, and calcinosis all may ensue. Here the focus is on prevention and symptomatic relief.

We emphasize the need for warmth. Air conditioning is dangerous. Even entering an air conditioned store to shop may precipitate painful vasospasm. Conversely, hand warmers in the winter are necessary. We emphasize the need for avoiding trauma. Patients should not be engaged in manual labor. Even forcing a key or removing a bottle cap poses a serious risk to be avoided. Their taut, glossy, atrophic skin does best with frequent use of a lubricant such as Eucerin.

Once an ulcer forms, we prescribe nitroglycerin ointment for local use. Silver sulfadiazine cream (Silvadene) topically and erythromycin (250 mg qid) will clear secondary infection. The critical prescription, however, is a vasodilator to improve the arterial circulation. Our favorite is prazosin (Minipress 4 mg tid), but the calcium channel blocker nifedipine (Procardia) also has proven to be very effective. Another alternative is captopril (Capoten), an enzyme inhibitor that reduces formation of the vasoconstrictor angiotensin. Everything possible is

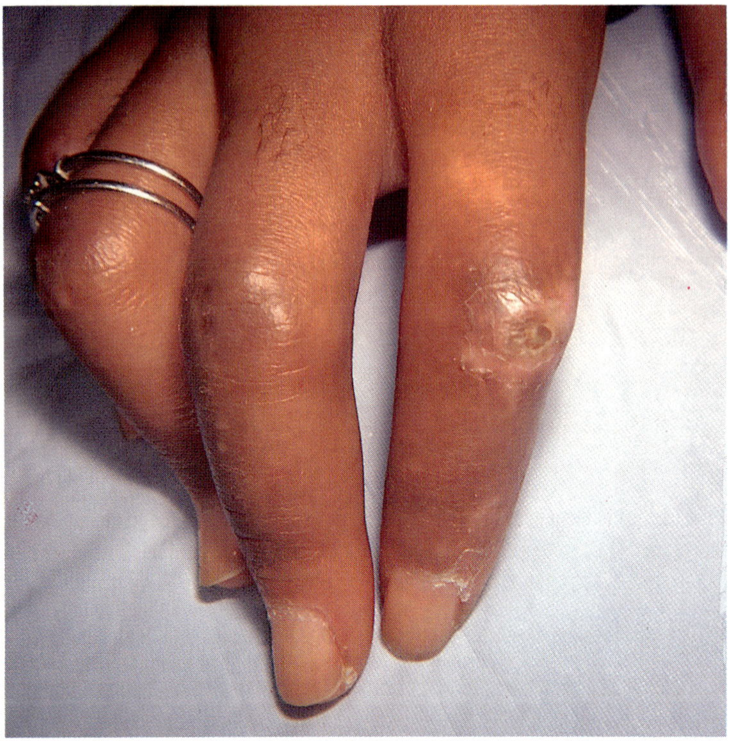

done to improve the cutaneous blood flow. For this reason, use no corticosteroids locally because of their vasoconstrictive action. Xylocaine ointment, however, is valuable in providing analgesia.

Scleroderma remains a strange, terrible disease with no evidence of its true cause. It does not respond to the classic nonspecific measures such as corticosteroids, immunosuppressants, or antibiotics. It has ignored waves of enthusiasm for such drugs as chelators, dimethylsulfoxide (DMSO), and para-aminobenzoate. Its cure must await the serendipitous or programmed finding of a drug that can master the fibroblast. Until then, we must give our patients symptomatic relief, judicious trials of new drugs, and real hope for a remission.

Jablonska S, Szczepanski A: Drugs used in the treatment of systemic and localized scleroderma. *In* Jablonska S (ed.): Scleroderma and Pseudoscleroderma, 2nd ed. Warsaw, Polish Medical Publishers, 1975, pp 610–631.

In this definitive book about scleroderma, the authors review 22 classes of drugs that have been used with limited success. Still there is no specific effective treatment despite the 177 references cited.

Some of the remedies include:

procaine penicillin (600,000 U/day to total of 24 million U, repeat every 6 to 8 weeks for several courses)

procaine (2 per cent solution 4 cc IM two to three times weekly for 10 to 12 weeks)—for morphea: inject around lesions

vitamin E (300 mg daily PO or IM for 8 to 10 weeks, repeat every 2 to 3 months)

piascledine (soya + avocado oils—6 × 50 mg daily for six months or more)
EDTA (**disodium EDTA** 2.5 to 3.0 gm in 500 ml 5 per cent dextrose slow IV drip over four to six hours daily for 15 days, to a total dose of 35 to 50 gm. Repeat after several months.) Supplement treatment with **pyridoxine** (50 mg/day) and **nicotinamide** (200 mg/day).
EACA (**epsilon-aminocaproic acid,** Amicar 1.0 to 4.0 gm/day orally for 25 months)
low-molecular-weight **dextran** (400 ml daily IV to a total dose of 10,000 ml; or 2 liters IV over 48 to 72 hours every five to eight weeks)
penicillamine (Cuprimine 1.0 to 2.0 gm/day for several months)—Supplement treatment with **vitamin B_6** (150 to 200 mg daily)
β-aminopropionitrile (1.0 to 3.0 gm daily for six weeks)
colchicine (1 mg daily for six months)
madecassol (three to six 10-mg tablets daily for several months or 2 per cent [20 mg/ml] IM every other day for several months, then twice weekly)
hyaluronidase (Wydase 1500 units IV three times weekly for five months to a total of 90,000 units)
PABA (**para-aminobenzoic acid** 12 gm/day for several months)
norlestrin (15 mg daily from days 16 to 19 of cycle, to total of 110 gm in 18 months). May give 10 to 15 mg weekly to men
relaxin (20 mg daily IM for several weeks)
indomethacin (Indocin 50 to 75 mg/day for one to six months)
chloroquine (Aralen 500 mg daily for two weeks, then 250 mg daily for 10 months)
prednisone (30 to 40 mg/day for a few months)
immunosuppressors (not recommended)—**azathioprine** (Imuran 100 to 200 mg daily for one to five months); **chlorambucil** (Leukeran 0.1 mg/kg/day for one to five months)
phenoxybenzamine (Dibenzyline 30 to 60 mg daily) or **phentolamine** (Regitine mesylate 5 mg IM or IV daily or 40 mg PO bid or tid)
reserpine (Serpasil, Sandril intra-arterial)
alpha-methyldopa (Aldomet)
nicotinic acid
griseofulvin (500 mg daily)
tetracycline (250 mg qid) or **erythromycin** (250 mg qid) to stop diarrhea

Local treatment:

warm paraffin baths for hands

DMSO (**dimethylsulfoxide**) gel (873 mg/ml) or solution (890 mg/ml)

fluocinolone ointment (Synalar-HP 0.2 per cent under occlusion)

triamcinolone intralesional injections—not recommended

Black CM, Myers AR (eds): Systemic Sclerosis (Scleroderma). Current Topics in Rheumatology, Vol 2. New York, Gower Medical Publishing, 1985, 480 pp.

The latest: 78 papers from the International Conference on Progressive Systemic Sclerosis (ICPSS). Includes state-of-the-art therapy.

Barnett AJ: Scleroderma (progressive systemic sclerosis): Progress and course based on a personal series of 118 cases. Med J Aust 2:129–134, 1978.

Scleroderma is subject to remissions and relapses, but one in five will not survive five years. Data are based on 118 cases personally treated over a 25-year period.

Cunningham PH, Andrews BS, Davis JS IV: Scleroderma: Developments from Osler to the present. South Med J 73:770–774, 1980.

A complete review, pointing out the need in some patients for vigorous antihypertensive therapy, nephrectomy, dialysis, or renal transplant.

Rush PJ, Bell MJ, Fam AG: Toxic oil syndrome (Spanish oil disease) and chemically induced scleroderma-like conditions. J Rheumatol 11:262–264, 1984.

Specific causes that if eliminated may result in regression of both cutaneous and other lesions of scleroderma:

Plastics
- polyvinylchloride
- epoxy resins

solvents
- trichloroethylene
- perchloroethylene
- trichloroethane
- benzene
- toluene
- xylene

drugs
- bleomycin
- L-5-hydroxytryptophan-carbidopa (oxitriptan + carbidopa)
- pentazocine (Talwin)

other
- paraffin or silicone implants
- cocaine abuse
- contaminated rapeseed oil

Winkelmann RK: Pathogenesis and staging of scleroderma. Acta Derm Venereol 56:83–92, 1976.

Examine and think about your patient in respect to sclerodermoid changes that may be seen with these factors:

metabolic
- porphyria
- amyloid
- biliary cirrhosis

immunologic
- lupus erythematosus
- dermatomyositis
- Sjögren's syndrome
- scleromyxedema

environmental
- vibratory tools
- silicosis
- polyvinylchloride

neoplastic
- carcinoid
- malignancy

genetic
- Werner's syndrome
- phenylketonuria

Connolly SM: Scleroderma: Therapeutic options. Cutis 34:274–276, 1984.

General measures:

Avoid vasospasm due to cold, nicotine, ergot alkaloids, epinephrine.
Avoid cutaneous trauma.
Undertake physical therapy to preserve function.
Provide nutritional support.

Winkelmann RK, Kierland RR, Perry HO, et al: Management of scleroderma. Mayo Clin Proc 46:128–134, 1971.

Valuable advice:

frequent use of skin emollients
room temperature 78°F
high-protein, high-calorie snacks or meals six times a day
sleep with head of bed on six-inch blocks to prevent gastric reflux esophagitis
tetracycline (250 mg tid) to reduce overgrowth of bacteria in aperistaltic intestines
hot paraffin baths, massage, exercise
pregnancy and surgery tolerated
vocational rehabilitation to avoid manual trauma

Vasoactive drugs (vasodilators) helpful in scleroderma:

phenoxybenzamine (Dibenzyline 30 to 60 mg/day)
tolazoline (Priscoline 30 to 60 mg/day)
alpha-methyldopa (Aldomet 1.0 to 2.0 gm/day)
reserpine (intra-arterial)
nicotinic acid
procaine (IV)

Franks AG Jr: Topical glyceryl trinitrate as adjunctive treatment in Raynaud's disease. Lancet 1:76–77, 1982.

A double-blind cross-over study of 17 patients with Raynaud's disease using topical **nitroglycerin** ointment (1 per cent tid and during attacks for six weeks), applied to the fingers on one hand only, showed:

13 had fewer attacks
11 had less severe attacks
7 of 9 had ulcers decrease in size

Nitroglycerin is available as a 2 per cent ointment (Nitro-Bid), which could not be used because of a high incidence of nitrite headaches. It was diluted to 1 per cent with petrolatum.

Scherbel AL: The effect of percutaneous dimethyl sulfoxide on cutaneous manifestations of systemic sclerosis. Ann NY Acad Sci 411:120–130, 1983.

Topical DMSO (46 per cent aqueous, immersion of affected areas 30 minutes qid for three months) healed 22 of 30 ulcers in 15 patients with scleroderma. In the control group, only 5 of 31 ulcers healed. The treatment is only palliative, since the underlying scleroderma was unchanged.

Williams HJ, Furst DE, Dahl SL, et al: Double-blind, multicenter controlled trial comparing topical dimethyl sulfoxide and normal saline for treatment of hand ulcers in patients with systemic sclerosis. Arthritis Rheum 28:308–314, 1985.

In a double-blind study in 13 centers of 84 patients with scleroderma, DMSO (70 per cent soaks, 15 minutes tid for three months) proved to be of no value for treating digital ulcers. Severe skin reactions (cracking, blistering, sloughing, and burning) from DMSO caused withdrawal of nine patients from the study.

Surwit RS, Gilgor RS, Allen LM, Duvic M: A double-blind study of prazosin in the treatment of Raynaud's phenomenon in scleroderma. Arch Dermatol 120:329–331, 1984.

By blocking the alpha-adrenergic receptors in the vascular smooth muscle, **prazosin hydrochloride** (Minipress 1 mg tid for two months) was effective in reducing both the frequency and severity of vasospasm in 19 patients with scleroderma and Raynaud's phenomenon. There was a 50 per cent reduction within one week, and this persisted even after the drug was stopped. Because of postural hypotension and syncope, treatment with Minipress should be started slowly with 1 mg at bedtime. The drug may also induce a positive ANA test result.

Rodeheffer RJ, Rommer JA, Wigley F, Smith CR: Controlled double-blind trial of nifedipine in the treatment of Raynaud's phenomenon. N Engl J Med 308:880–883, 1983.

The calcium channel blocker **nifedipine** (Procardia 20 mg tid for one month) produced subjective symptomatic relief in 21 of 32 (66 per cent) patients with Raynaud's phenomenon by inducing vascular smooth muscle relaxation.

Woo TY, Wong RC, Campbell JP, et al: Nifedipine in scleroderma ulcerations. Int J Dermatol 23:678–680, 1984.

Nifedipine (Procardia 40 mg tid, later 10 mg tid for four months), daily whirlpool, and Op-Site dressings produced impressive resolution of a 3- by 3-cm ischemic ulcer on the medial area of the left foot of a 68-year-old woman with scleroderma. Prior treatment with high-dose **erythromycin** (500 mg qid) and Bactrim (2 tablets qid) had failed to heal this ulcer of three years' duration.

Nifedipine, by lowering intracellular calcium in smooth muscle, is the most powerful cutaneous vasodilator available. Nifedipine (30 to 120 mg daily) is also reportedly effective for treating Raynaud's phenomenon.

Lopez-Ovejero JA, Saal SD, D'Angelo WA, et al: Reversal of vascular and renal crisis of scleroderma by oral angiotensin-converting enzyme blockade. N Engl J Med 300:1417–1419, 1979.

Captopril (Capoten 150 mg q6h for six weeks) healed chronic sclerodermatous ulcers of the hands in two patients. As an angiotensin-converting enzyme inhibitor, it acts by reducing formation of the vasoconstrictor angiotensin.

Katayama H, Ohsawa K, Yaoita H: Improvement of progressive systemic sclerosis (PSS) with estriol treatment. Acta Derm Venereol 64:168–171, 1984.

Estriol (Estriel Depot 10 mg subcutaneously once a week for 10 months), a natural steroidal estrogen, induced significant clinical and histologic improvement in the skin lesions of two Japanese women with scleroderma. The skin became palpably softer, and the biopsy no longer showed homogenization of connective tissue.

Martin MFR, Dowd PM, Ring FJ, et al: Prostaglandin E_1 infusions for vascular insufficiency in progressive systemic sclerosis. Ann Rheum Dis 40:350–354, 1981.

In a double-blind cross-over study of 12 patients with systemic sclerosis and severe Raynaud's phenomenon, the potent vasodilator and inhibitor of platelet aggregation **prostaglandin E_1** (PGE_1 6 to 10 ng/kg/min IV in saline or 5 per cent dextrose for 72 hours) resulted in:

Two patients noted healing of ischemic ulcers.

All patients noted (1) less pain, (2) improved cold tolerance, (3) that the attacks of Raynaud's phenomenon were less prolonged, less frequent, and less severe for several weeks after treatment. However, there was no objective change in hand function.

Kang B, Veres-Thorner C, Heredia R, et al: Successful treatment of far-advanced progressive systemic sclerosis by D-penicillamine. J Allergy Clin Immunol 69:297–305, 1982.

Penicillamine (1.0 to 1.5 gm/day for 12 to 30 months) induced good to excellent improvement in eight patients with scleroderma. It acts by blocking critical cross-linkages in collagen synthesis. The most common side effect was transient hypogeusia.

Steen VD, Medsger TA, Rodnan GP: D-Penicillamine therapy in progressive systemic sclerosis (scleroderma): A retrospective analysis. Ann Intern Med 97:652–659, 1982.

D-Penicillamine (500 to 1500 mg/day, median 750 mg, for two years) was the only drug found helpful in the treatment of scleroderma. Skin thickness was reduced in 73 patients as compared with 45 controls. Furthermore, during treatment new visceral involvement was not seen, and the five-year survival rate climbed from 66 per cent (control group) to 88 per cent (treatment group). This Pittsburgh center has studied 530 patients with scleroderma and found corticosteroids, potassium para-aminobenzoate, vasodilators, colchicine, cyclophosphamide, azathioprine, and chlorambucil to be ineffective.

Jarrett PEM, Morland M, Browse NL: Treatment of Raynaud's phenomenon by fibrinolytic enhancement. Br Med J 2:523–525, 1978.

An anabolic steroid, **stanozolol** (Winstrol 5 mg bid for three months), relieved symptoms of vasospasm and improved grip strength in 14 patients with scleroderma. Each had had prior cervical sympathectomy without help. Stanozolol enhances natural blood fibrinolysis by reducing plasma fibrinogen. Clinical improvement lasted two to three months. Further three-month courses of stanozolol were given intermittently with rest periods of one to two months.

Greer KE: Newer therapies for the sclerodermas. Dermatol Clin 1:505–515, 1983.

Azathioprine (Imuran 50 to 200 mg/day) or **cyclophosphamide** (Cytoxan 100 to 150 mg/day) completely cleared two patients of debilitating generalized morphea within 12 months.

Seibold JR, Jageneau AHM: Treatment of Raynaud's phenomenon with ketanserin, a selective antagonist of the serotonin$_2$ (5-HT$_2$) receptor. Arthritis Rheum 27:139–146, 1984.

Of 18 patients with systemic sclerosis 15 reported moderate or marked relief from **ketanserin** therapy (20 mg tid for one week, then 40 mg tid for three weeks). This treatment also reduced hand edema and facilitated healing of ischemic digital ulcerations.

Dau PC, Kahaleh MB, Sagebiel RW: Plasmapheresis and immunosuppressive drug therapy in scleroderma. Arthritis Rheum 24:1128–1136, 1981.

Conjoint plasmapheresis (5 to 6 per cent of body weight, once weekly for 10 weeks, then every one to four weeks) and **cyclophosphamide** (2.5 mg/kg/day) induced clinical improvement in 14 of 15 scleroderma patients, as seen by gradual loosening of hidebound skin, relaxation of contractures, and healing of cutaneous ulcers. In addition, the ANA titer and endothelial cell cytotoxic factor levels fell.

Talpos G, Horrocks M, White JM, Cotton LT: Plasmapheresis in Raynaud's disease. Lancet 1:416–417, 1978.

By reducing viscosity and thereby favoring better blood flow, plasmapheresis per se (2.5 liters of plasma removed once a week for five weeks) gave striking improvement that lasted at least six months in five patients with Raynaud's disease. Most of the digital ulcerations healed, and the frequency and intensity of attacks of Raynaud's symptoms were reduced.

Coffman JD: β-blocking agents and Raynaud's phenomenon. JAMA 254:116, 1985.

If possible, avoid beta-blockers in patients with Raynaud's phenomenon and peripheral vascular disease, since these drugs may induce vasospastic phenomena, even to the point of gangrene. Although approximately 3 per cent of patients require withdrawal of drug treatment for these reasons, the beta-blockers still are not contraindicated when needed for treatment of ischemic heart disease.

Morgan RJ: Scleroderma: Treatment with diphenylhydantoin. Cutis 8:278–282, 1971.

Of 29 patients with scleroderma treated with **diphenylhydantoin** (phenytoin—Dilantin 100 mg daily qid) 15 had complete clearing of sclerosis, in contrast to only 6 of 36 given other treatments. The length of treatment with Dilantin was not specified, but the original case that cleared was treated for two years.

Hazen PG, Walker AE, Carney JF, Stewart JJ: Cutaneous calcinosis of scleroderma: Successful treatment with intralesional adrenal steroids. Arch Dermatol 118:366–367, 1982.

Triamcinolone acetonide (20 mg/ml, 1 to 2 ml intralesionally every four to eight weeks for one year) healed large preauricular ulcers in an 83-year-old woman with scleroderma. A total dose of approximately 200 mg of triamcinolone acetonide per area treated was required for healing.

Gahhos F, Ariyan S, Frazier WH, Cuono CB: Management of sclerodermal finger ulcers. J Hand Surg 9:320–327, 1984.

A splendid reprise of management of the major dermatologic problems in scleroderma. In a study of 59 patients with sclerodactyly, digital phalangeal resorption, calcinosis cutis, and digital contractures, the authors found medical management with systemic vasodilators (e.g., reserpine) to be unsatisfactory. The best treatment for pain was intra-arterial (radial) injection of **reserpine** (1.25 mg), which depleted the arterial wall of catecholamine. It gave three weeks of relief. In those patients with persistent crippling ulcers and arteriographic evidence of luminal constriction, conservative finger amputation was the best way to eradicate the ulcer and pain, as well as restore the hand to useful function.

Noncompliant patients are usually fully "complaintive."

Seborrheic Dermatitis

Shampoo
Ketoconazole
UVL

The enemy was sighted in 1904, but the right bullet was not found until recently. Such is the story of seborrheic dermatitis. Only now do we have the "magic bullet," ketoconazole, so needed in the war against the pathogenic yeast *Pityrosporon ovale*. It has proven to be remarkably effective and is our treatment of choice for severe seborrheic dermatitis.

Prior to ketoconazole our favorite approach was wash, wash, wash. Failure to remove the yeast-loaded oil regularly led to seborrheic dermatitis. This is seen every day in hospitals where seriously ill patients receive minimal washing of the face and soon become the object of dermatologic consultation. It is seen in the parkinsonian patients whose muscular rigidity regularly leads to inadequate washing and consequent seborrheic dermatitis. But the most dramatic example of the need for frequent washing comes from observing the ipsilateral dermatitis that evolves in 10 days when washing is interdicted on one side of the face of anyone with the seborrheic diathesis. In an infant, seborrheic dermatitis can usually be simply washed away, whereas atopic dermatitis becomes worse with frequent bathing. It is evident to us that the pathogen can be scrubbed off, washed away, or shampooed out. Indeed, much of the simplest, mildest form of seborrheic dermatitis, namely, dandruff, responds to a daily shampoo with almost any over-the-counter preparation. DHS and Sebulex shampoos are popular examples.

If the dandruff persists we prescribe Selsun shampoo, since its 20 per cent surfactant formulation, plus the selenium sulfide, attacks the yeast problem in a twofold manner. Alernates include a host of coal tar products. We favor Sebutone or Zetar shampoo. It is important to instruct the patient that treatment of dandruff is somewhat like dental care, requiring daily, lifelong attention. There is no true cure. As one observer put it, "The only doctor who ever cured dandruff was Dr. Guillotine." Accordingly, the patient must be aided in his search for a pleasant, safe, and acceptable shampoo. More than 200 are available, since in the United States the defense budget against dandruff and dirty hair now runs to $1.4 billion a year.

These hundreds of different shampoos, containing multiple antigens such as parabens, formaldehyde, and proteins, at times are the cause of mild contact dermatitis which, with its sequential scaling, masquerades as seborrheic dandruff. It is important to recognize that this may happen, as cure comes with the substitution of a wash without the allergens. When such a contact reaction is suspected we recommend washing the hair with an unperfumed soap such as Neutrogena.

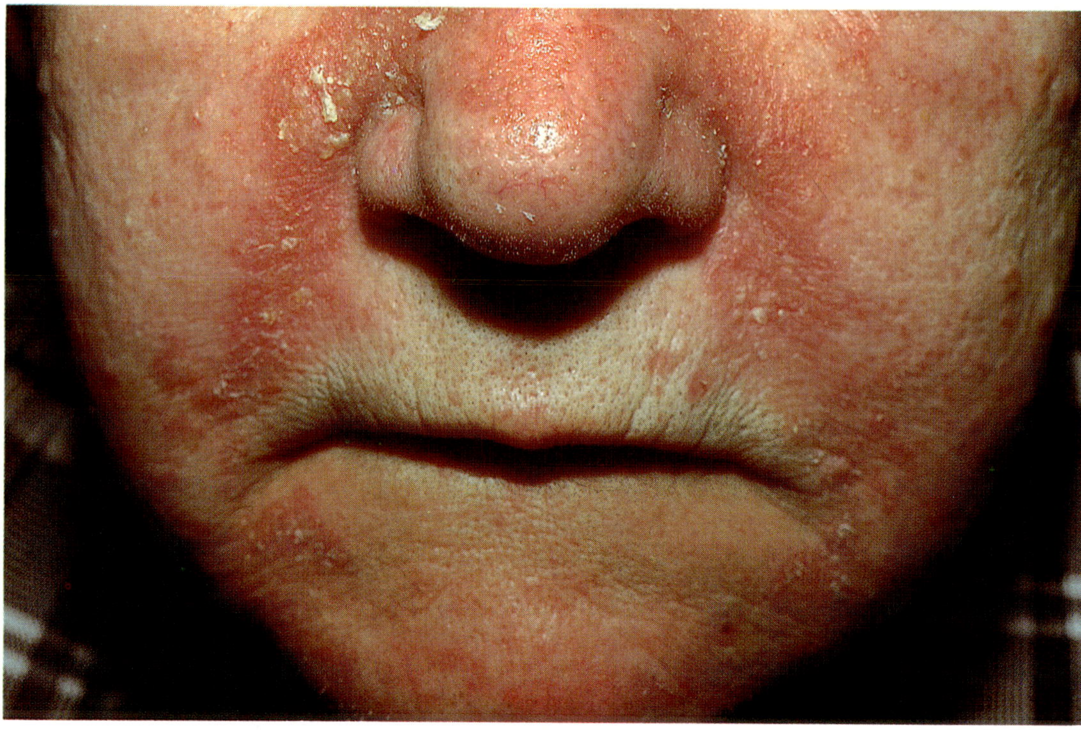

Another pitfall in the treatment of dandruff is the failure to recognize the atopic form. It is important to remain alert to this form that requires the specific measures appropriate for the control of atopic dermatitis. An even more insidious example of nonseborrheic dandruff is tinea capitis due to *Trichophyton tonsurans*. It occurs in adults as well as children and reveals its presence only to one who will do fungal cultures. It does not produce fluorescence under the Wood light. One cannot sit back diagnostically and therapeutically relaxed when a patient complains of a "dry scalp" or dandruff. White scales on the shoulders of the blue serge suit are not always the hallmark of seborrheic dermatitis, but may be those of psoriasis. It is wise to take a history and look the patient over carefully before leaping to the prescription pad.

As the yeast makes its descent down from the scalp onto the face, and still later to the oily ramparts of the chest, treatment can be mild topical corticosteroids coupled with washing. We like sunlight or ultraviolet light therapy as well. For severe examples, particularly if the patient fails to actually wash the areas, ketoconazole remains our most powerful weapon with short courses of 200 mg/day giving rapid help.

The effectiveness of topical steroids, in particular the fluorinated forms, has led to virtual addiction in some patients. We always stop the long-term use of fluorinated steroids because of the inevitable transformation of seborrheic dermatitis into rosacea. This is particularly important in the facial area.

Another aid in management is to be aware of the possibility that drugs may induce a seborrheic-like dermatitis. We recently had a particularly vivid example due to Lopressor. The antipsychotic drugs that induce parkinsonian side effects (e.g., haloperidol) are well-known offenders in this regard. Strangely and paradoxically, a few patients develop a seborrhea-like eruption from exposure to sunlight. A careful history is always one of your best guides.

Seborrheic dermatitis is now a disease in which we can take new effective measures against its immediate cause, the *Pityrosporon* yeasts. **Ketoconazole** has given us new firepower.

Shuster S: The aetiology of dandruff and the mode of action of therapeutic agents. Br J Dermatol 111:235–242, 1984.

Clever, convincing evidence that the pathogen in seborrheic dermatitis is *Pityrosporon ovale.*

Ford GP, Farr PM, Ive FA, Shuster S: The response of seborrhoeic dermatitis to ketoconazole. Br J Dermatol 111:603–607, 1984.

Of 17 patients with scalp scaling and 15 patients with widespread seborrheic dermatitis, 12 and 10, respectively, showed regression of their lesions over a one-month period of oral **ketoconazole** therapy (200 mg/day). In this double-blind randomized study, three of the four failures responded well to an increased dose of ketoconazole (400 mg/day for one month). Relapse occurred rapidly after the drug was stopped.

Farr PM, Shuster S: Treatment of seborrhoeic dermatitis with topical ketoconazole. Lancet 2:1271–1272, 1984.

Eight of nine cases of seborrheic dermatitis of the face and trunk cleared following daily application of topical **ketoconazole** (Nizoral 2 per cent cream for one to four weeks). One month after stopping of the cream, relapse occurred in two of the four original patients studied. The cream was not suitable for scalp application.

Skinner RB, Noah PW, Taylor RM, et al: Double-blind treatment of seborrheic dermatitis with 2% ketoconazole cream. J Am Acad Dermatol 12:852–856, 1985.

Of 20 seborrheic dermatitis patients 18 showed 75 to 95 per cent improvement with the application of **ketoconazole** cream (2 per cent bid). Ketoconazole has a low rate of percutaneous absorption and should not produce side effects.

Cram DL: How I treat seborrheic dermatitis. Med Times 108(3):74–76, 1980.

Mild

face:

- 1 per cent **hydrocortisone** cream tid

scalp:

- Sebulex shampoo (sulfur, salicylic acid) used two or three times a week

Recalcitrant

face:

- Tridesilon (**desonide** cream 0.05 per cent tid)
- Westcort (**hydrocortisone valerate** cream 0.2 per cent)

scalp:

- Baker's P&S liquid (liquid paraffin oil, sodium chloride, phenol less than 1 per cent)
- Capitrol (**chloroxine**) shampoo daily
- 10 per cent liquor carbonis detergens (LCD 10 per cent) in Nivea oil
- **anthralin** pomade (0.6 per cent hs)

steroid lotions and sprays
Barseb Thera-Spray (**hydrocortisone** 0.6 per cent, **salicylic acid** 0.48 per cent)
Aeroseb-HC (**hydrocortisone** 0.5 per cent)

Wheatley D: Topical corticosteroids in seborrhoeic dermatitis. Practitioner 226:1178–1179, 1982.

Ten physicians in a multicenter double-blind study were unable to see any therapeutic difference between a mild topical steroid (Locoid lotion—**hydrocortisone 17-butyrate** 0.1 per cent) and a potent topical steroid (Betnovate lotion) after a three-week treatment period. Both were highly effective.

Olansky S: Old drug—in a new system—revisited. Cutis 19:852–854, 1977.

Recommends Sulfacet-HC lotion (**sodium sulfacetamide** 10 per cent, **sulfur** 5 per cent, and **hydrocortisone** 0.5 per cent) for treating seborrheic dermatitis. (No longer available in the United States, but can make it using Sulfacet-R lotion and hydrocortisone 0.5 per cent).

Christodoulou GN, Vareltzides AG: Positive side effects of lithium? Am J Psychiatry 135:1249, 1978.

Two cases of seborrheic dermatitis showed dramatic clearing after one month of lithium (300 mg/day) therapy.

Oliver R: The dandruff story. Cent Afr J Med 28:22–23, 1982.

Advises use of a cream with 1 per cent **hydrocortisone**, 2 per cent **sulfur**, and 3 per cent Vioform. For the scalp apply Pragmatar ointment (sulfur 3 per cent, **salicylic acid** 3 per cent, **cetyl alcohol–coal tar** distillate 4 per cent) one or two times a day and shampoo the following day with Polytar shampoo. Avoid topical steroids on the scalp because of rebound exacerbation upon stopping treatment.

Treatment of dandruff. Med Lett Drugs Ther 19:63–64, 1978.

Simple dandruff can be treated effectively by washing the hair every one to three days with any shampoo. If stronger therapy is required, use a shampoo containing **zinc pyrithione**, **selenium sulfide**, or a **coal tar** product.

Ellis CN, Stawiski MA: The treatment of perioral dermatitis, acne rosacea, and seborrheic dermatitis. Med Clin North Am 66:819–830, 1982.

Capitrol (**chloroxine** 2 per cent) shampoo is especially valuable for institutionalized patients who cannot shampoo frequently. However, it may discolor gray or light-colored hair.

Seborrheic blepharitis responds well to ophthalmic ointments such as Blephamide (**prednisolone** 0.2 per cent and **sulfacetamide** 10 per cent).

Veien NK, Pilgaard CE, Gade M: Seborrheic dermatitis of the scalp treated with a tar/zinc pyrithione shampoo. Clin Exp Dermatol 5:53–56, 1980.

Using a shampoo containing 2.5 per cent tar and 2 per cent **zinc pyrithione** (5 ml left on scalp for 5 minutes twice weekly) 17 of 27 patients had complete remission of itch and scale during a six-week double-blind study.

Sheth RA: A comparison of miconazole nitrate and selenium disulfide as antidandruff agents. Int J Dermatol 22:123–125, 1983.

Both of these agents, known to be effective against *Pityrosporon ovale*, induced temporary remission of dandruff. The study compared two shampoos: **miconazole nitrate** 2 per cent (9 of 15 patients improved) and **selenium disulfide** 2.5 per cent (4 of 8 patients improved). Making cytologic smears of scales from the scalp and staining with Giemsa and Gram stains was helpful in guiding therapy. A preponderance of bacteria or yeast cells led to use of an antibacterial or antifungal agent, while clumps of nucleated parakeratotic keratinocytes suggested seborrheic dermatitis, psoriasis, or ichthyosis.

Garcia RL, Miller JD, Miller WN: Occlusive tar extract therapy for recalcitrant psoriasis and seborrheic dermatitis of the scalp. Cutis 22:90–91, 1978.

Four of six patients with seborrheic dermatitis had good results when they massaged an 8.75 per cent tar shampoo (Pentrax) into the scalp, covered it with a shower cap, and allowed it to remain for two hours before shampooing. The treatment period was three weeks. Similar results were seen in seven of ten patients with scalp psoriasis.

Fox C: Shampoo components—1985. Cosmet Toiletr 100(3):31–46, 1985.

Complete listing of the hundreds of compounds actually present in 200 shampoos. These include a variety of surfactants, lather boosters, conditioners, thickeners, opacifiers, preservatives, and Madison Avenue pacifiers. (Do not forget, shampoo may cause contact dermatitis simulating seborrheic dermatitis. Switch shampoos.)

Krestin D: The seborrhoeic facies as a manifestation of post-encephalitic parkinsonism and allied disorders. Q J Med 21:177–186, 1927.

Think of Parkinson's disease with the unexpained onset of seborrheic dermatitis of the face.

Binder RL, Jonelis FJ: Seborrheic dermatitis in neuroleptic-induced parkinsonism. Arch Dermatol 119:473–475, 1983.

Three antipsychotic drugs were associated with the onset of seborrheic dermatitis and drug-induced parkinsonism in many patients receiving them:

haloperidol (Haldol): 11 of 22 patients had seborrheic dermatitis and 16 of 22 had parkinsonism.

chlorpromazine (Thorazine): 4 of 21 patients had seborrheic dermatitis and 2 had parkinsonism.

thiothixene (Navane): 6 of 16 patients had seborrheic dermatitis and 10 had parkinsonism.

Honig PJ, Smith LR: Tinea capitis masquerading as atopic or seborrheic dermatitis. J Pediatr 94:604–605, 1979.

Trichophyton tonsurans infection was present in 10 of 30 children referred for treatment of diffuse scaling of the scalp without hair loss. The "dandruff" was not cleared until two months of **griseofulvin** (10 to 12 mg/kg/day) therapy was given. This diagnosis should be suspected if scattered broken "black dot" hairs are present or if the scaling increased after application of topical steroid solutions.

Sudan BJL, Brouillard C, Sterboul J, Sainte-Laudy J: Nicotine as a hapten in seborrhoiec dermatitis. Contact Dermatitis 11:196–197, 1984.

Avoidance of tobacco smoke was curative in at least three patients with seborrheic dermatitis who had demonstrable hypersensitivity to nicotine.

Salo VO, Lassus A, Juvakoski T, et al: Behandlung der Dermatitis atopica und der Dermatitis seborrhoica mit selektiver UV-Phototherapie und PUVA. Dermatol Monatsschr 169:371–375, 1983.

Broad-spectrum ultraviolet light therapy (UVA-UVB, 3 m W/sq cm four times a week for two months) was as effective as PUVA in controlling seborrheic dermatitis. It was favored because of the fewer side effects noted in the 48 patients studied. This therapy induced symptom-free remissions in 63 per cent of the group.

Dahl KB, Reymann F: Photochemotherapy in erythrodermic seborrhoeic dermatitis. Arch Dermatol 113:1295–1296, 1977.

PUVA provides an excellent therapeutic alternative to systemic steroids in the treatment of erythrodermas of seborrheic origin. In this study of three patients, clearing was achieved in 1 to 7 months, in which 9 to 32 treatments were given.

Storrs LA: Management of the ear canal seborrhea with cerumen. Laryngoscope 91:1231–1233, 1981.

Normal cerumen is not produced in patients with chronic ear canal seborrheic dermatitis, and the inner two thirds of the ear canal often appear shiny and polished. Replacement of cerumen (collected from healthy children and young adults, dispensed in 50 per cent glycerin*) helps control the problem.

℞: Cerumen in 50 per cent glycerin—two drops placed in the external ear canal once weekly

Other helpful local measures include:

Avoid soap and water.
Avoid scratching with hairpins, pencils, etc.
Wear gloves at night to avoid fingernail reinfection.
Avoid hair spray and cosmetics.
Remove water and sweat with 70 per cent alcohol.
Physician must periodically cleanse the ear.

Flandermeyer KL, Brauner GJ: Surgical management of an uncommon complication of seborrheic dermatitis. J Dermatol Surg Oncol 4:768–769, 1978.

Excise and close fissured areas with superficial ulcerations occurring in intertriginous areas. Example illustrated: cure of a postauricular fissure.

---

* Suspend cerumen in 50 per cent glycerin; leave for several weeks to sterilize, heat, and strain through a fine filter.

If you'd like to see more patients, do more for the patients you're seeing.

Sézary Syndrome

Chlorambucil Steroids Electron beam

This is basically a rare chronic leukemia with exfoliative dermatitis that deserves conjoint attention from the dermatologist, oncologist, and radiation therapist. Although electron beam therapy may be necessary, we favor the steroid-chlorambucil treatment program used at the Mayo Clinic. This consists of chlorambucil (2 to 4 mg/day) coupled with prednisone (20 to 40 mg/day). It may have to be given for several years.

Always, symptomatic relief of the erythroderma can be achieved with bedrest, hospitalization, topical Synalar ointment, and saline compresses.

As the special leukemic variant of mycosis fungoides, Sézary syndrome has proven less responsive to measures that mainly affect the skin, such as PUVA or topical nitrogen mustard. On the other hand, intensive chemotherapy is neither necessary nor effective. Both the patient and the disease seem to respond best to the gentle arm of long-term, low-dose chlorambucil and prednisone.

Winkelmann RK, Caro WA: Current problems in mycosis fungoides and Sézary syndrome. Ann Rev Med 28:251–269, 1977.

Sézary syndrome (erythroderma with circulating atypical mononuclear cells) can develop from drug reactions, contact dermatitis, and atopic dermatitis. Patients often have multiple positive patch tests, indicating active cutaneous delayed hypersensitivity. Chronic contact dermatitis may be the most common cause of the erythroderma.

Winkelmann RK, Perry HO, Muller SA, et al: Treatment of Sézary syndrome. Mayo Clin Proc 49:590–592, 1974.

Chlorambucil (2 to 4 mg/day) coupled with **prednisone** (20 to 40 mg/day) produced long-term remission in eight patients. Previous aggressive chemotherapy with nitrogen mustard, cyclophosphamide, chlorambucil, triethylenemelamine, methotrexate, and vinblastine was not effective.

Winkelmann RK, Perry HO, Muller SA, et al: The pre-Sézary erythroderma syndrome. Mayo Clinic Proc 49:588–589, 1974.

Seven of these patients with severe pruritus and chronic erythroderma were treated with **chlorambucil** (2 to 4 mg/day) and **prednisone** (20 to 40 mg/day) for more than a year. Three are completely clear and need no treatment.

Dawkins RL, Zilko PJ, Harper JM, et al: Atypical Sézary syndrome: "T-cell leukemia" associated with reversible clubbing, acrolysis and infiltration of skin and liver. Australas J Dermatol 16:9–12, 1975.

Chlorambucil (10 mg/day) produced a dramatic response in a 63-year-old woman. The rash, leukocytosis, hepatomegaly, and clubbing regressed within six weeks.

Lutzner M, Edelson R, Schein P, et al: Cutaneous T-cell lymphomas: The Sézary syndrome, mycosis fungoides, and related disorders. Ann Intern Med 83:534–552, 1975.

Treatment with **cyclophosphamide**, **methotrexate**, **actinomycin D**, or **vincristine** produces partial response for only a few months in 25 to 80 per cent of patients with Sézary syndrome.

Spittle M: Treatment of skin reticuloses. Clin Exp Dermatol 7:93–97, 1982.

Sézary syndrome, the leukemic phase of mycosis fungoides, does not respond well to topical nitrogen mustard, PUVA, cyclosporin A, or intravenous chemotherapy. Whole-skin or whole-body irradiation as well as leukophoresis gives only temporary benefit. Recommends **chlorambucil-prednisone** therapy.

Holmes RC, McGibbon DH, Black MM: Mycosis fungoides: Progression towards Sézary syndrome reversed with chlorambucil. Clin Exp Dermatol 8:429–435, 1983.

A 74-year-old man showed good clinical response to **chlorambucil** (4 mg/day) and **prednisone** (20 mg/day). There was a concomitant decrease in pruritus, erythema, and the number of circulating Sézary cells.

Herbst M, Muller R: Ganz-Haut-Elektronentherapie der Mycosis fungoides und des Sézary-Syndroms. Hautarzt 35:16–21, 1984.

Review of details of the technique and results in the world literature concerning the 1078 patients with mycosis fungoides and Sézary syndrome treated with electron beam irradiation. At Stanford University Medical Center 84 per cent of patients achieved complete remission by aggressive total skin irradiation (more than 3000 rads), but the overall survival rate at 10 years was 46 per cent, with the initial extent of skin involvement being the major prognostic factor.

Patients like lotions (and physicians) that are creamy and smooth.

Stomatitis

Decadron elixir
Clotrimazole troches
Metronidazole
Eliminate cause

Effective management of stomatitis is a "search and eradicate mission." In most instances of acute stomatitis the cause is a primary irritant the patient has recognized and already eliminated. Occasionally the irritant may be of an occult nature. We recall vividly a patient with severe erosive stomatitis that followed eating a pretzel. She had never been bothered by pretzels previously. Investigation revealed that during manufacture the pretzels had been inadvertently coated with crystals of lye rather than salt.

Chronic stomatitis may be due to an irritant of a more subtle nature. The cause may also be a food or chemical acting as a true allergen. Since testing for irritability and allergenicity on the oral mucosa is not ordinarily practicable, we have our patients rigorously monitor and reduce their oral contactants.

We instruct them as to the hazard of anything held in the mouth. Lozenges, candy drops, Lifesavers, cough drops, mouthwashes, and toothpaste are all strictly forbidden. Teeth and dentures are to be cleaned only with saline or sodium bicarbonate. Aerosol breath fresheners must be interdicted. The patient must be aware that the inflamed mucosa cannot tolerate that which was previously harmless. The patient must not smoke, chew tobacco, chew gum, or drink coffee.

Time spent reviewing and reviewing the patient's habits can be rewarding. We have seen stomatitis due to chewing on rubber binders, from eating Philadelphia scrapple, and from allowing aspirin tablets to dissolve in the mouth. Food can act as an allergen as well as an irritant. Given the innumerable potential causes, and our limited diagnostic skills, we stress keeping a complete 24-hour-a-day diary of all that enters the mouth. This focuses attention on possible causes and better acquaints the physician with the patient's habits. At the same time we encourage a sharp reduction in the variety of foods ingested. Saline brushing of the teeth after each meal is advised, followed by copious flushing with water to minimize contact time.

If the stomatitis persists, we routinely do scout tray patch tests for identification of specific allergens. We eliminate all possible medications, since drug-induced stomatitis is always a distinct possibility.

For immediate symptomatic relief we prescribe Decadron elixir (dexamethasone 0.5 mg/ml)—hold one teaspoonful in mouth for 3 minutes tid but do not swallow. Note that this elixir is red, so dye-sensitive individuals may have to avoid it. We tend not to use viscous lidocaine since the pain in most cases of stomatitis is not major.

Any candidiasis is treated with clotrimazole troches, Mycostatin oral suspension, or systemic ketoconazole. Denture wearers need particular help in this regard, but usually the cure of their stomatitis lies in new dentures that are free of the "barnacles" of microbial plaques.

With prolonged attention to detail, with continued patient instruction, and with a dash of serendipity, you can solve many of these strange stomatitides. "Elementary, my dear Watson, it was the onion."

Nally FF: The sore mouth: A review. J R Soc Med 77:50–55, 1984.

Physical or chemical trauma is the most common cause. Be alert to stomatitis artefacta. Favors **metronidazole** (Flagyl) for treating acute ulcerative gingivostomatitis. Suspect depression in the patient complaining of soreness when the mouth looks normal. A biopsy may be lifesaving, but must be correctly done, particularly to diagnose pemphigus vulgaris.

Glenert U: Drug stomatitis due to gold therapy. Oral Surg 58:51–56, 1984.

Eighteen patients had nonspecific ulcerations, mainly of the buccal mucosa, associated with intramuscular **gold** therapy for rheumatoid arthritis. All cases cleared when the drug was stopped. Other signs included reticular lichen-planus-like changes, diffuse erythema of the oral mucosa, and atrophy of the filiform papillae of the tongue.

Bergendal T: Treatment of Denture Stomatitis. A clinical, microbiological and histological evaluation. Linköping, Sweden, Tryck-Center AB, 1982, 116 pp.

A monographic investigation of this multifactorial disease concludes:

1. The presence of microbial plaque and crusts on the fitting surface of the denture base is of critical importance in the development and maintenance of denture stomatitis.
2. **Nystatin** powder (thin layer on the maxillary denture three times a day) reduced yeast colonization, but had no long-term effect on the stomatitis.
3. Reduction of denture contact time is beneficial. Avoid wearing dentures at night.
4. Good denture hygiene heals not only the stomatitis, but also associated glossitis and angular cheilitis.

Stohler C: Etiology and occurrence of denture stomatitis. A review of the literature. Schweiz Monatsschr Zahnmed 94:187–194, 1984.

Allergic reactions are rarely the cause. Look for candidiasis, dental plaque, and trauma.

White IR, Smith BGN: Dental amalgam dermatitis. Br Dent J 156:259–260, 1984.

A 36-year-old man who recurrently developed widespread dermatitis after having dental fillings was found to be allergic to mercury. Treatment was to remove the existing amalgams and use only composite glass-ionomer, gold, or porcelain restorations.

The dental series of allergens used at St. John's Hospital for diseases of the skin includes:

amethocaine 1 per cent
procaine 1 per cent
cetavlon 0.25 per cent
hexachlorophene 1 per cent
mercury ammonium chloride 1 per cent
methyl methacrylate 5 per cent
hydroquinone 1 per cent

oil of cloves 1 per cent
benzoyl peroxide 5 per cent
impregum 5 per cent
impregum catalyst 5 per cent

Watson CJ, Walker DM, Bates JF, Newcombe RG: The efficacy of topical miconazole in the treatment of denture stomatitis. Br Dent J 152:403–406, 1982.

Miconazole gel 2 per cent (applied tid for 14 days to the fitting surface of the maxillary denture) helped reduce candidal populations in a double-blind controlled study of 45 patients. However, no cures were achieved until the patients painstakingly brushed their dentures to remove plaque.

Ayres S: Sore mouth caused by electrogalvanic current. J R Soc Med 77:708–709, 1984.

Burning, irritation, and ulceration may be due to an electrogalvanic current that develops between dissimilar metals (gold and amalgam fillings), with saliva acting as an electrolyte. Advises replacement of amalgam with gold if more than 75 μA of current is demonstrated by placing electrodes of a microammeter on adjacent fillings.

If you make one or two ridiculous assumptions, any therapy becomes logical.

Subcutaneous Fat Necrosis

Primum non nocere

This nonspecific disorder, possibly due to obstetric or birth trauma, requires more in the way of diagnosis than treatment.

Moreno-Gimenez JC, Hernández-Aguado I, Arguisjuela MT, Camacho-Martinez F: Subcutaneous-fat necrosis of the newborn. J Cutan Pathol 10:277–280, 1983.

Multiple hard, painless, slowly growing, subcutaneous nodules on the cheeks, arms, and buttocks of a two-month-old infant completely regressed slowly and spontaneously over a five-month period.

Dont's for Diagnosticians

1. *Don't be too clever.*
2. *Don't diagnose rarities.*
3. *Don't be in a hurry.*
4. *Don't be faddy.*
5. *Don't mistake a label for a diagnosis.*
6. *Don't diagnose two diseases simultaneously in the same patient.*
7. *Don't be too cock-sure.*
8. *Don't be biassed.*
9. *Don't hesitate to revise your diagnosis from time to time in a chronic case.*

Sir Robert Hutchison

Do you rush back from vacation because your patients need you or because you need your patients?

Syphilis & STD

Penicillin
Erythromycin
Tetracycline
Doxycycline

Forty years of experience with spirocheticidal penicillin has codified the therapy of syphilis.

Rein MF, Caine V, Grossman JH, et al.: 1985 STD treatment guidelines. J Am Acad Dermatol 14:707–726, 1986.

The Centers for Disease Control (CDC) suggest the following treatment for these sexually transmitted diseases (STD):

- AIDS: None known
- Chancroid:
  - **Erythromycin** (500 mg qid for seven days)
- *Chlamydia trachomatis* infection:
  - **Tetracycline** (500 mg qid for seven days)
- Enteric infections:
  - Campylobacter jejuni:
    - **Erythromycin** (500 mg qid for seven days)
  - Shigella species:
    - **Trimethoprim/sulfamethoxazole** (160/800 mg bid for seven days)
  - Amebiasis:
    - **Metronidazole** (750 mg tid for 10 days) plus
    - **Iodoquinol** (650 mg tid for 20 days)
  - Giardiasis:
    - **Quinacrine** (100 mg tid for seven days)
- Epididymo-orchitis:
  - **Amoxicillin** (3.0 gm, single oral dose)
- Gonococcal infection:
  - **Amoxacillin** (3.0 gm, single oral dose)
- Genital herpes simplex virus infection:
  - **Acyclovir** (200 mg 5 times a day for 10 days) or continuously for recurrent attacks.
- Lymphogranuloma venereum:
  - **Tetracycline** (500 mg qid for two weeks)
- Nongonoccal urethritis:
  - **Tetracycline** (500 mg qid for seven days)
- Pediculosis pubis and scabies:
  - **Lindane** (1 per cent lotion for eight hours)
- Pelvic inflammatory disease:
  - **Doxycycline** (100 mg IV bid) plus **cefoxitin** (2.0 gm IV qid) for four days, followed by doxycycline (100 mg by mouth bid for two weeks)
- Syphilis:
  - Early—**Benzathine penicillin G** (2 to 4 million units IM once)
  - More than one year duration—same dose once a week for three successive weeks
- Trichomoniasis:
  - **Metronidazole** (2.0 gm, single oral dose)

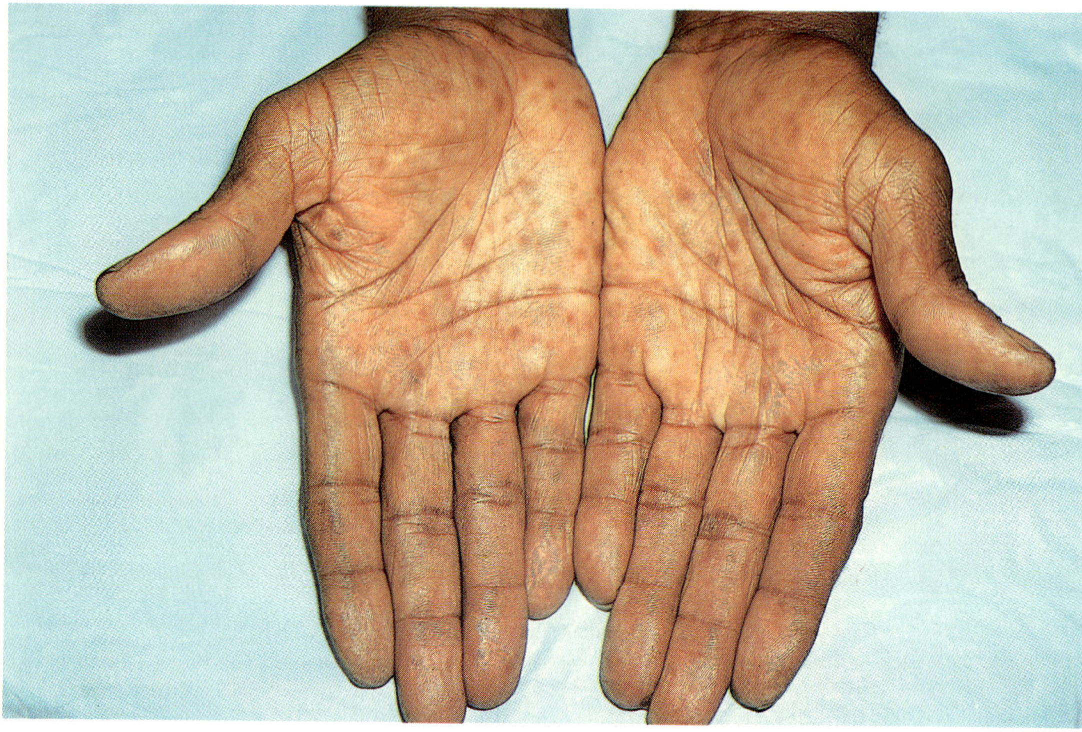

Vaginosis, bacterial:
Metronidazole (500 mg bid for seven days)
Warts:
Cryotherapy or **podophyllin** (10 per cent in compound tincture of benzoin)

Crissey JT, Denenholz DA: Syphilis. Clin Dermatol 2(1):1–166, 1984.

The definitive monograph with all the answers in its 166 pages.

Treatment schedules:

Type	***Treatment***	***Alternate***
Early syphilis		
Primary Secondary Early latent	Benzathine penicillin G (Bicillin L-A 2.4 million U IM one-time dose)	Erythromycin or tetracycline (500 mg qid for 15 days)
Late syphilis		
Late latent (>1 year)	Benzathine penicillin G (Bicillin L-A 2.4 million U IM once a week for three weeks)	Erythromycin or tetracycline (500 mg qid for 30 days)
Benign tertiary Cardiovascular		
Neurosyphilis* or if spinal tap is not done	Aqueous penicillin G (2.4 million U IM daily for 10 days) plus probenecid (Benemid 500 mg qid for 10 days), then benzathine penicillin G (2.4 million U IM weekly for 3 weeks)	Doxycycline (Vibramycin 100 mg tid for 30 days)

* Give Tegretol and Dilantin for lightning pains of tabes dorsalis.

A drug is worth trying if the chance of its helping is greater than the chance the disease will go away without help.

Tinea

Lotrimin cream	Tinactin
Spectazole cream	Castellani's Paint
Loprox cream	Griseofulvin
Monistat-Derm cream	Ketoconazole
Nizoral cream	

The treatment of fungal infections is a proud moment in clinical practice. Not only do we have systemic therapy in the form of griseofulvin and its new alternate, ketoconazole, but we have a rich variety of topical imidazole agents that attack all the pathogenic fungi and many gram-positive bacteria. They do this safely and with remarkable effectiveness. With one of these "universal" antifungal agents also available in combination with a corticosteroid (Lotrisone), it would seem that treating fungal infections should be a most elementary undertaking. Indeed, one of our most effective antifungal prescriptions (MicaTin cream) has defected to "over-the-counter land." Nonetheless, certain fungal infections of the feet and toenails and invasive lesions in immunocompromised patients remain a first-class challenge to the clinician.

For simple uncomplicated tinea corporis or tinea cruris our primary choices are creams: Lotrimin, Spectazole, and Loprox (not an imidazole, but a pyridone derivative), as alternates for the patient who says "Oh, I've used that and it's no help." Lotrimin contains the first imidazole, clotrimazole, to be introduced in this field, and Spectazole contains econazole, a second generation imidazole antifungal. And now ketoconazole is in a topical formulation (Nizoral). These three imidazoles and miconazole (Monistat-Derm, MicaTin) belong to a family of drugs long known to us by its other members: thiabendazole (anthelmintic), metronidazole (trichomonacide), and levamisole (parasiticide). Selective laboratory testing of more than 1000 imidazole analogues led to clotrimazole and these newer antimicrobials. They all act by disrupting the cell membrane. More significantly, clotrimazole, miconazole, econazole, and ketoconazole act against dermatophytes, yeasts, and gram-positive bacteria. Thus, their use in the groin practically erases the need for distinguishing tinea cruris, candidiasis, and erythrasma.

In extensive cases of tinea corporis or cruris or invasive forms (tinea profunda, Majocchi's granuloma) we turn to systemic therapy with griseofulvin (micronized, 500 mg bid with food) or to ketoconazole (Nizoral 200 mg once a day). For a view of other specific forms see tinea capitis, tinea pedis, tinea versicolor, and onychomycosis.

Jones HE: Therapy of superficial fungal infection. Med Clin North Am 66:873–893, 1982.

Excellent review filled with good advice, e.g., Majocchi's granuloma requires three to five months of **griseofulvin**. Lists 14 topical, 3 oral, and 2 intravenous antifungal agents, along with major side effects.

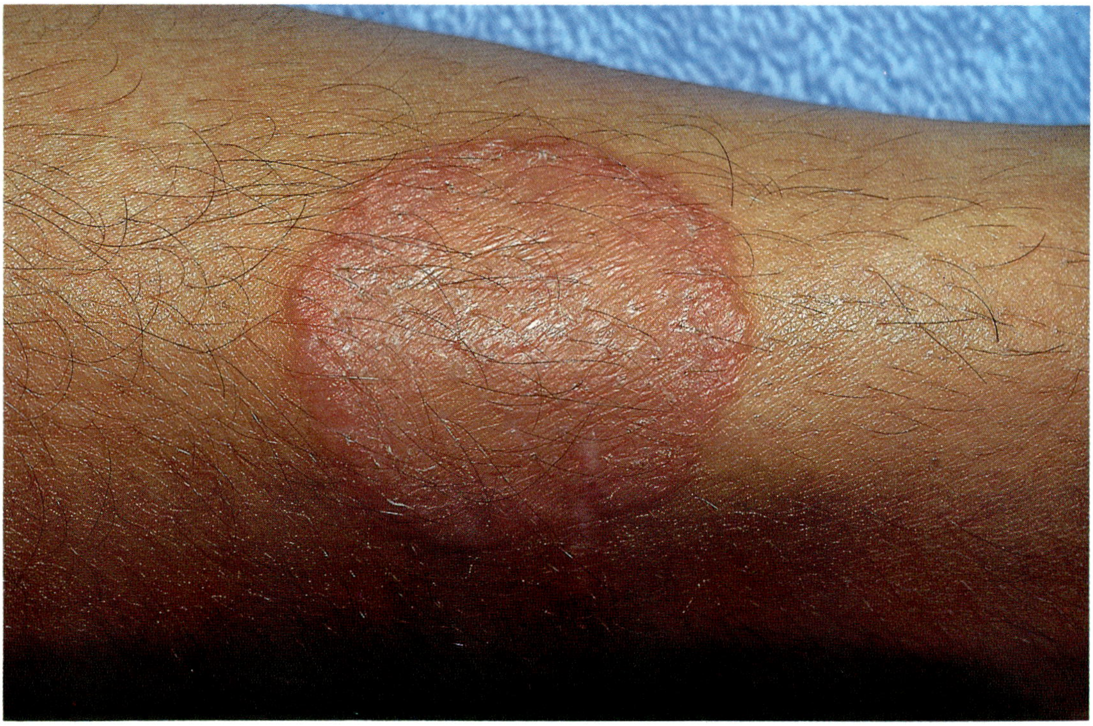

Griseofulvin

can use up to 2 gm/day

watch drug interactions:

sodium warfarin (Coumadin): must increase dose of anticoagulant

barbiturates: must increase dose of griseofulvin

monitor CBC and chemistry profile periodically

Raab WPE: The Treatment of Mycosis with Imidazole Derivatives. New York, Springer-Verlag, 1980, 157 pp.

The imidazoles (**clotrimazole, miconazole, econazole, ketoconazole**) are active against all fungi and yeasts and many gram-positive bacteria pathogenic for man. Superb practical handbook on a new group of drugs as revolutionary in antifungal therapy as the penicillins were in the antibacterial field.

Hall-Smith P: Dermatomycoses: A brief history of therapy and initial results with clotrimazole. Postgrad Med J 50(Suppl 1):70–72, 1974.

Castellani's fuchsin paint is the best all-purpose topical treatment for crural and toe web fungal infections. A double-blind trial of **clotrimazole** cream 1 per cent and **tolnaftate** cream 1 per cent showed comparable results in treating assorted tineas of glabrous skin.

Clayton YM, Connor BL: Comparison of clotrimazole cream, Whitfield's ointment and Nystatin ointment for the topical treatment of ringworm infections, pityriasis versicolor, erythrasma and candidiasis. Br J Dermatol 89:297–303, 1973.

Whitfield's ointment (3 per cent **salicylic acid**, 6 per cent **benzoic acid** in an emulsifying ointment) was shown to be the equal of **clotrimazole** cream in a double-blind study of 32 tinea patients. Approximately 50 per cent still had a (+) KOH preparation after eight weeks of treatment.

VanDersarl JV, Sheppard RH: Clotrimazole vs haloprogin treatment of tinea cruris. Arch Dermatol 113:1233–1235, 1977.

Four weeks after stopping treatment, 63 per cent of cases treated with **clotrimazole** (Lotrimin 1 per cent solution bid for 14 days) were clear, but only 34 per cent of those treated with **haloprogin** (Halotex 1 per cent solution bid for 14 days) were clear. Haloprogin caused stinging, burning, or an unpleasant odor in 37 per cent of patients, while clotrimazole caused no adverse effects.

Mandy SJ, Garrott TC: Miconazole treatment for severe dermatophytoses. JAMA 230:72–75, 1974.

A cure rate of greater than 90 per cent in men with tinea cruris using **miconazole** cream (2 per cent bid for four weeks). Follow-up: four weeks after treatment was stopped, one of 20 had relapse.

Clayton YM, Gange RW, MacDonald DM, Carruthers JA: A clinical double-blind trial of topical haloprogin and miconazole against superficial fungal infections. Clin Exp Dermatol 4:65–73, 1979.

In fungal infections of the groin, the cure rate was 89 per cent with either **miconazole** cream (2 per cent bid) (a phenethyl imidazole derivative) or **haloprogin** ointment (1 per cent bid) (halophenyl-γ-iodo propargyl ether) after four weeks of treatment. For tinea pedis, cure rates were 93 per cent with miconazole and 70 per cent with haloprogin. Final assessment four weeks after stopping treatment.

Katz HI, Bard J, Cole GW, et al: SCH 370 (clotrimazole-betamethasone dipropionate) cream in patients with tinea cruris or tinea corporis. Cutis 34:183–188, 1984.

The incorporation of 0.05 per cent **betamethasone dipropionate** into a 1 per cent **clotrimazole** cream resulted in a product (Lotrisone cream) that relieved inflammatory symptoms more rapidly than either ingredient alone. Report of 331 patients in a double-blind multicenter study who applied the creams twice a day for two weeks. Follow-up: two weeks post-treatment.

Grigoriu D, Grigoriu A: Double-blind comparison of the efficacy, toleration and safety of tioconazole base 1% and econazole nitrate 1% creams in the treatment of patients with fungal infections of the skin or erythrasma. Dermatologica 166(Suppl 1):8–13, 1983.

Spectazole (**econazole nitrate** cream 1 per cent bid for six weeks) achieved a 93.5 per cent clinical and mycologic cure rate in 31 patients. All remained clear of infection six weeks after the end of treatment. No statistical difference between cure rates of the two products (**tioconazole** not available in the United States).

Heel RC, Brogdeu RN, Speight TM, Avery GS: Econazole: A review of its antifungal activity and therapeutic efficacy. Drugs 16:177–201, 1978.

Details on this topical **imidazole** antifungal agent (Spectazole cream) reveal it to be impressive. 78 references.

Battistini F, Zaias N, Sierra R, Rebell G: Clinical antifungal activity of thiabendazole. Arch Dermatol 109:695–699, 1974.

Used as a broad-spectrum antihelminthic since 1961, this early **imidazole** will clear tinea corporis if applied daily as a 0.25 per cent solution in 70 per cent alcohol or three times a day as a 10 per cent cream. Not available as such. Ineffective in propylene glycol. Also useful in tinea capitis and tinea cruris.

Cox FW, Stiller RL, South DA, Stevens DA: Oral ketoconazole for dermatophyte infections. J Am Acad Dermatol 6:455–462, 1982.

Overall cure rate of 63 per cent in 19 patients; 75 per cent of patients with chronic dermatophyte infections that had failed to respond to **griseofulvin** were cured or improved by **ketoconazole** (200 to 400 mg daily for 2½ months). Overall relapse rate 38 per cent. Relapse occurred in three patients with *Trichophyton rubrum* infection one month after stopping ketoconazole, despite treatment longer than nine months in two of the patients. Adverse reactions included nausea (3), increased appetite (1), and generalized erythematous eruption after the first dose (1).

Laurberg G: Ketoconazole in *Trichophyton rubrum*. Acta Derm Venereol 62:273–274, 1982.

Ketoconazole (200 mg/day for two months, but if no change after one month, 400 mg/day for second month) cleared 6 of 10 *Trichophyton rubrum* skin infections previously resistant to **griseofulvin** and topical antifungal agents. Three patients had recurrence two months after stopping ketoconazole, indicating that eight weeks of treatment was too short.

Baker RL, Para MF: Successful use of ketoconazole for invasive cutaneous *Trichophyton rubrum* infection. Arch Intern Med 144:615–617, 1984.

A 56-year-old man receiving chemotherapy for acute lymphocytic leukemia developed generalized tender hemorrhagic papules caused by invasive *Trichophyton rubrum*. The lesions cleared after three months of oral **ketoconazole** (400 mg/day). Recurrence three months later required maintenance ketoconazole.

Artis WM, Odle BM, Jones HE: Griseofulvin-resistant dermatophytosis correlates with in vitro resistance. Arch Dermatol 117:16–19, 1981.

Failure to respond to **griseofulvin** (or other regimens) may reflect:

inadequate dosage
poor patient compliance
malabsorption
diminished capacity to reach site (thicker stratum corneum or harder keratin of nails or hair)
drug resistance of dermatophyte (minimal inhibitory concentration level above 3 μg/ml)

Antimycotic sensitivity testing may become useful in the future for selection of antimycotic therapy.

Carr JF, Lewis CW: Tinea nigra palmaris: Treatment with thiabendazole topically. Arch Dermatol 111:904–905, 1975.

A case not responsive to **tolnaftate** (Tinactin) or **salicylic acid** ointment cleared in two weeks with **thiabendazole** suspension 10 per cent (Mintezole 100 mg/ml) applied bid. Follow-up: three months.

Pradinaud R: The treatment of two cases of tinea nigra by miconazole. Mykosen 21:99–102, 1978.

Tinea nigra palmaris cleared after 7 to 10 days of **miconazole** gel therapy. Cites failure of **griseofulvin** (500 mg/day for one month) and **5-fluorocytosine** cream 10 per cent and poor response to **amphotericin B** cream.

Marks JG Jr, King RD, Davis BM: Treatment of tinea nigra palmaris with miconazole. Arch Dermatol 116:321–322, 1980.

Another case cleared in three weeks with **miconazole** cream 2 per cent (MicaTin) applied twice a day. No recurrence in six months.

Mattar J, Solbach W: Tinea imbricata in Papua-New Guinea. Treatment with griseofulvin and haloprogin in a population of the Gogol-Valley, Madang Province. Mykosen 25:355–367, 1981.

This picturesque tropical tinea responded beautifully to either oral **griseofulvin** or topical **haloprogin** over a four-week course, but relapsed within a week of stopping therapy. 39 cases.

Levine HB, Cobb JM, Friedman RH: Griseofulvin in dimethylsulfoxide: Penetration into guinea-pig skin and clinical findings in feline ringworm. Sabouraudia 9:43–49, 1971.

A paste made by grinding in a mortar **griseofulvin** 500-mg tablets with anhydrous DMSO (result 250 mg/ml) was applied once daily for 5 to 10 days to 11 cats infected with *Microsporum canis*. (Before treatment, hair was removed with a surgical clipper.) All cats were cured.

Meinhof W, Girardi RM, Stracke A: Patient noncompliance in dermatomycosis: Results of a survey among dermatologists and general practitioners and patients. Dermatologica 169(Suppl 1):57–66, 1984.

Personal interviews of 35 physicians and 230 dermatomycosis patients revealed:

48 per cent neglected proper daily dosage schedule (44 per cent reduced the number of applications, especially young, well-educated patients)
25 per cent stopped treatment after symptoms disappeared (especially elderly patients)

Recommendations:

more thorough doctor-patient communication
aim for a single daily dose treatment
aim for reduced length of therapy

Knight AG: The activity of various topical griseofulvin preparations and the appearance of oral griseofulvin in the stratum corneum. Br J Dermatol 91:49–55, 1974.

Griseofulvin 1 per cent in dimethylacetamide (DMAC) was still detectable in the stratum corneum 96 hours after application. One application for 15 minutes (prior to washing) prevented experimental *Trichophyton mentagrophytes* infections in humans.

Hay RJ, Clayton YM: Treatment of chronic dermatophyte infections. The use of ketoconazole in griseofulvin treatment failures. Clin Exp Dermatol 7:611–617, 1982.

Ketoconazole (200 mg/day for three to six months) cleared 72 per cent of unresponsive infections on the trunk, groin, or proximal limbs.

Barson WJ: Granuloma and pseudogranuloma of the skin due to *Microsporum canis*: Successful management with local injections of miconazole. Arch Dermatol 121:895–897, 1985.

Injection of **miconazole nitrate** (Monistat 20 mg/ml) into granulomatous nodules, one at a time on an every-other-day basis for one month, produced striking regression of nodules due to intradermal growth of *Microsporum canis*. The patient was an immunosuppressed (cyclophosphamide and prednisone) 25-year-old woman with systemic lupus erythematosus. Although courses of griseofulvin and ketoconazole of over four months' duration had produced improvement, relapses occurred promptly when these drugs were stopped. After the month of intralesional miconazole therapy, cultures of the nodules were negative and there was no relapse in the subsequent three years.

Do unto patients as you would have doctors do unto you.

Tinea Capitis

Griseofulvin
Ketoconazole
Selsun shampoo
Corticosteroids

Detection of tinea capitis masquerading as folliculitis in a child or dandruff in the adult is far more difficult than prescribing the necessary griseofulvin. We take it as a rule that any child with unexplained scaling or hair loss should be given a therapeutic course of griseofulvin. We are not convinced that topical antifungals have the capacity to cure either ectothrix or endothrix infections.

Griseofulvin is prescribed in a high dose until all evidence of fungal infection is gone. This means a dose of 2 teaspoonsful bid of the griseofulvin oral suspension (125 mg/teaspoonful) for young children. Very young children should be given griseofulvin 5 mg/pound daily for at least two weeks. The usual cause of failure is too little griseofulvin for too short a time. We treat for a minimum of three weeks and often continue for several months. Careful shampooing of the scalp with Selsun shampoo or Ionil shampoo reduces the scaling, and the former appears to be sporicidal. Often there is concurrent pyoderma or bacterial folliculitis of the scalp, so that oral erythromycin is an important adjunctive measure. In these instances topical Spectazole cream twice a day affords both antifungal and antibacterial action. The presence of a kerion may call for systemic steroids and indicates need of more prolonged griseofulvin therapy. The prognosis for complete hair regrowth must be guarded in these instances.

Although we have not had failures with systemic griseofulvin, the possibility exists of a griseofulvin-resistant tinea capitis. In such an instance, ketoconazole therapy must be considered.

To avert recurrence, siblings, playmates, and pet cats must all be checked for tinea (clinically and under Wood's light) and appropriately treated.

Allen HB, Honig PJ, Leyden JJ, McGinley KJ: Selenium sulfide: Adjunctive therapy for tinea capitis. Pediatrics 69:81–83, 1982.

In children with *Trichophyton tonsurans* scalp infections who were also taking **griseofulvin** (10 mg/kg/day), the addition of Selsun shampooing twice a week rendered hair cultures negative at two weeks. In contrast, cultures remained positive up to eight weeks with griseofulvin alone or griseofulvin plus daily **clotrimazole** (Lotrimin) lotion. All groups receiving griseofulvin showed clinical improvement within two to four weeks. **Selenium sulfide** remains on the scalp surface and is sporicidal to *Trichophyton tonsurans.*

Weston WL, Thorne EG: Two cases of tinea in the neonate treated successfully with griseofulvin. Clin Pediatr 16:601–602, 1977.

In month-old baby boys, tinea capitis due to *Microsporum audouini* (Wood's light–negative) and *Microsporum canis* (Wood's light–positive) infection, respectively, cleared with two weeks of oral **griseofulvin** (10 mg/kg/day).

Barriér H, Litoux P: Intéret et justification de la corticothérapie générale des trichophyties suppurées (Kérions). Ann Dermatol Venereol 104:294–297, 1977.

A kerion is a clarion call for systemic corticosteroids. Observations of six cases, including four in children with tinea capitis and two in men with tinea barbae.

Dosage: **Prednisone**—10 to 20 mg/day in children
—50 to 80 mg/day in adults

Additional treatment: **griseofulvin** and antibiotic (**erythromycin** or **doxycycline**).

Foged EK, Jepsen LV: Hair loss following kerion celsi. A follow-up examination. Mykosen 27:411–414, 1984.

Two-year follow-up of hair regrowth at site of kerions caused by *Trichophyton verrucosum* in 18 patients treated with **griseofulvin**. No patients had entirely normal regrowth:

Four had nearly normal regrowth.
Eleven had marked reduction in hair counts (103/sq cm vs 302/sq cm).
Three had severe scarring alopecia.

The authors suggest the addition of corticosteroids to rapidly decrease inflammation and subsequent scarring.

Rasmussen JE, Ahmed AR: Trichophytin reactions in children with tinea capitis. Arch Dermatol 114:371–372, 1978.

Skin tests with trichophytin antigen (0.1 ml intradermal into skin of arm) showed strongly positive reactions after 48 hours in 15 of 16 patients with kerions, in contrast to little or no reaction in 37 patients with noninflammatory tinea capitis. All patients had *Trichophyton tonsurans* infections. The probable role of cell-mediated immunity suggests therapeutic benefit from systemic or intralesional steroids.

Warin RP: Persistent *Trichophyton tonsurans* infection. Br J Dermatol 97(Suppl 15):48–49, 1977.

A 57-year-old woman had tinea capitis for 14 years, unresponsive to **griseofulvin** (500 to 2000 mg/day), oral **clotrimazole**, and topical **miconazole** and **tolnaftate**. Serum assays showed a negligible amount of griseofulvin, presumably as a result of interference from long-term (20 years) barbiturates given for petit mal and anxiety.

Herbet AA, Head ES, MacDonald EM: Tinea capitis caused by *Trichophyton tonsurans*. Pediatr Dermatol 2:219–223, 1985.

A family epidemic revealed positive cultures from the couch, rug, floor, vinyl chair, beds, toys, baby blanket, telephone receivers, combs, and brushes.

Recommendations for control of *Trichophyton tonsurans*:

Examine and culture the scalp in any case of tinea corporis due to *T. tonsurans*.
Obtain scalp cultures (with moistened sterile cotton swab) from all immediate family members.
Watch for spread to the newborn baby from a mother who is a subclinical chronic carrier on the scalp.
Clean the environment.
Treat with **griseofulvin** for four to six weeks, then repeat cultures.
To prevent the carrier state, you must keep treating until you obtain a negative culture.

For a physician, the deadliest sin of all is the sin of indifference.

Tinea Pedis

Spectazole cream	Griseofulvin
Lotrimin cream	Ketoconazole
Loprox cream	Drysol
Nizoral cream	

In this commonplace skin affliction, therapy is firmly entrenched in the public domain. Numerous OTC preparations are offered in every pharmacy and supermarket. They include the truly powerful and helpful imidazole, miconazole (MicaTin). Thus the physician's prescription must offer something better.

The "something better" for severe recalcitrant cases is systemic therapy. Marked amelioration can be best achieved with griseofulvin (500 to 1000 mg/day) or ketoconazole (200 mg/day). Each should be given for at least the epidermal turnover time of one month, and each should be followed by a regimen of long-term topical antifungal therapy with such agents as Loprox, Lotrimin, Spectazole, or Nizoral creams.

The intertriginous form is often best attacked by applying Castellani's paint between the toes every few weeks and using Drysol each night on the sole to counteract hyperhidrosis. Many cases seen in the physician's office are compounded by bacterial infection requiring appropriate systemic antibiotics such as erythromycin.

The most difficult type of tinea pedis to treat is the chronic, noninflammatory, scaling "tinea plantaris," which is due to *Trichophyton rubrum*. Very large doses of griseofulvin or ketoconazole over a period of months are indicated, and relapse is common.

Prevention is aided by aeration, achieved through wearing light or open shoes, and having the shoes off whenever possible. Drysol application nightly to the soles under Saran wrap greatly reduces hyperhidrosis, as well as both fungal and bacterial reinfection. Many find dusting of the feet with Desenex (zinc undecylenate) powder or MicaTin powder also very helpful.

Jones HE: Therapy of superficial fungal infection. Med Clin North Am 66:873–893, 1982.

An important practical survey by a grand master. Divides tinea pedis into three types:

web space: use topical **imidazole**
vesicular: use **griseofulvin** and compresses
hyperkeratotic and erythrodermic moccasin: use topical imidazole, peeling agent (Whitfield's ointment, 40 per cent **urea**, or 5 per cent **salicylic acid** [Keralyt]), and oral antifungal agent (griseofulvin or **ketoconazole** 200 to 400 mg/day for eight weeks)

Smith EB, Graham JL, Ulrich JA: Topical clotrimazole in tinea pedis. South Med J 70:47–48, 1977.

Clotrimazole solution 1 per cent cleared 19 of 33 cases of tinea pedis. The chronic dry scaling type was the most difficult type to treat.

Gentles JC, Jones GR, Roberts DT: Efficacy of miconazole in the topical treatment of tinea pedis in sportsmen. Br J Dermatol 93:79–84, 1975.

Four weeks of **miconazole** cream 2 per cent gave a mycologic and clinical cure rate of 60 per cent in 45 university athletes who used gymnasium showers. Approximately one of three shower users in an unselected sample had tinea pedis.

Ongley RC: Efficacy of topical miconazole treatment of tinea pedis. Can Med Assoc J 119:353–354, 1978.

Miconazole nitrate cream 2 per cent (MicaTin, Monistat-Derm applied bid for 28 days) was effective in 95 per cent of 20 patients with tinea pedis in an extended-care hospital at the six-week follow-up. **Tolnaftate** cream 1.0 per cent cleared 65 per cent of 20 cases in the same study.

Fuerst JF, Cox GF, Weaver SM, Duncan WC: Comparison between undecylenic acid and tolnaftate in the treatment of tinea pedis. Cutis 25:544–549, 1980.

Desenex ointment and Tinactin cream applied twice a day for four weeks in double-blind study of 103 patients gave effective cure rates of 66 and 47 per cent respectively.

Guess W, Engley FB Jr, Blaylock WK, Shelley ED, et al: Topical antifungal drug products for over-the-counter human use: Establishment of a monograph. Fed Reg 47:12480–12566 (Mar 23) 1982.

"Safe and effective" ingredients for OTC use in athlete's foot and "jock itch" are discussed in detail, including:

haloprogin
iodochlorhydroxyquin
miconazole nitrate
nystatin
tolnaftate
undecylenic acid and its salts (calcium, copper, and zinc)

Also, comprehensively discussed by the OTC panel were the following ingredients, felt to be safe but incompletely evaluated for effectiveness:

aluminum salts
basic fuchsin
benzethonium chloride
benzoic acid
borates
caprylates
chlorothymol
chloroxylenol
cresols
dichlorophen
oxyquinolines
parabens
phenyl salicylate
povidone-iodine
propionic acid and its salts (sodium, zinc)
salicylic acid
sulfur
triacetin

Prazak G, Ferguson JS, Comer JE, McNeil BS: Treatment of tinea pedis with griseofulvin. Arch Dermatol 81:821–826, 1960.

Good control in 12 patients taking **griseofulvin** (1 gm/day) for five weeks, but prompt relapse in three patients upon stopping the drug. Better results were seen in a group of 13 who also used Whitfield's ointment at bedtime and hexachlorophene (pHisoHex) wash of feet in the morning in addition to taking griseofulvin.

Zaias N, Battistini F, Gomez-Urcuyo F, Rojas RF, Ricart R: Treatment of "tinea pedis" with griseofulvin and topical antifungal cream. Cutis 22:196–199, 1978.

Griseofulvin alone was much more effective than Lotrimin cream alone in treating all types of tinea pedis. Griseofulvin plus Lotrimin cream was much better than either alone for the intertriginous type (84 per cent cure rate three months after stopping treatment), but was no better than griseofulvin alone for the plantar scaling type (64 per cent cure rate three months post-treatment).

Leyden JJ, Kligman AM: Aluminum chloride in the treatment of symptomatic athlete's foot. Arch Dermatol 111:1004–1010, 1975.

Aqueous **aluminum chloride** ($AlCl_3 \cdot 6H_2O$) 30 per cent solution applied with a cotton-tipped applicator bid for seven days was as effective as Castellani's paint in the treatment of interdigital athlete's foot in 10 patients.

Chretien JH, Esswein JG, Sharpe LM, Kiely JJ, Lyddon FE: Efficacy of undecylenic acid–zinc undecylenic powder in culture-positive tinea pedis. Int J Dermatol 19:51–54, 1980.

A foot powder (Desenex, Cruex, Ting) containing **undecylenic acid** 2 per cent and **zinc undecylenate** 20 per cent used bid for four weeks cleared 88 per cent of culture-positive cases, compared to 17 per cent in controls using placebo powder. Two weeks post-treatment, KOH preparations were still negative in 77 per cent of the active group (compared to 48 per cent of the placebo group).

Williams DI: Griseofulvin and *Trichophyton rubrum* infections. Arch Dermatol 81:769–771, 1960.

The "lively pocket of enemy resistance" between the fourth and fifth toes failed to clear in 38 patients despite **griseofulvin** 1 gm/day (KOH preparations and cultures remained positive). Could griseofulvin be washed away by sweat? (To counteract this, we apply Xerac AC [**aluminum chloride hexahydrate** 6.25 per cent] to toe webs at bedtime).

Hay RJ, Clayton YM: Treatment of chronic dermatophyte infections. The use of ketoconazole in griseofulvin treatment failures. Clin Exp Dermatol 7:611–617, 1982.

Of infections of the soles and toenails unresponsive to **griseofulvin**, 82 per cent remained unresponsive to ketoconazole (200 mg/day for nine months) or relapsed within six months of stopping the drug.

Kligman AM, Bogaert H, Cordero C, et al: Evaluation of ciclopirox olamine cream for the treatment of tinea pedis: Multicenter double-blind comparative studies. Clin Therap 7:409–417, 1985.

One per cent **ciclopirox olamine cream** (Loprox) applied twice daily for one month gave a clinical cure rate of 60 per cent in a study of 43 patients with tinea pedis. By contrast, 1 per cent **clotrimazole** cream (Lotrimin) induced cure in only 41 per cent of a comparable group of 44 patients.

Diseases that harm call for drugs that harm less.

Tinea Versicolor

Selsun shampoo Clotrimazole Loprox Ketoconazole

The treatment of this superficial *Pityrosporon* infection is a pleasant exercise. There is a small pharmacopeia of effective remedies. The problem is not one of treatment, but of prevention. These patients frequently become reinfected, and repeated courses of treatment become the rule.

Selsun shampoo applied to the entire trunk and arms as well as the scalp for five minutes each day for one month eradicates the hyphae and spores as well as the scaling. Subsequently the hypopigmentation or hyperpigmentation generally disappears slowly over a period of months. If one does not wish to use Selsun shampoo, other shampoos containing zinc pyrithione may be equally effective. Topical creams or lotions with the imidazole antifungals (clotrimazole, miconazole, econazole, or ketoconazole) are very satisfactory, but cannot be applied as simply as a shampoo five minutes before showering.

For extensive cases, those present many years, or cases involving the face or producing severe dyschromia, systemic therapy is our favorite. We use Nizoral (200 mg/day for 15 days) followed by one tablet each day on the first three days of every month. It is the ultimate "magic bullet" and requires no adjuvant topical measures. The advantage of such internal treatment is that it attacks all sites of infection, not simply those recognized and treated topically by the patient.

Clothes must be freshly laundered or cleaned once treatment is begun, and the patient should be cautioned against the future wearing of communal sweat shirts, sweaters, or T-shirts. Other family members or individuals in close contact should be checked for the presence of the disease. Many individuals serve as carriers, never showing more than minimal signs of infection. Husband and wife "Ping-Pong" tinea versicolor can occur. Moreover, we have personally treated two deep-sea divers who acquired the disease from diving suits shared with divers who had the disease.

Once the infection is cleared, topical corticosteroids may aid in hastening correction of the dyschromic changes.

Faergemann J, Djärv L: Tinea versicolor: Treatment and prophylaxis with ketoconazole. Cutis 30:542–545, 1982.

Ketoconazole (200 mg/day) cured 26 of 32 patients in three weeks, and the remainder in five weeks. Among 30 of these patients subsequent doses of ketoconazole (200 mg/day) for three consecutive days every month for at least six months prevented recurrence in all but one patient, compared with seven relapses in patients taking a placebo.

Symoens J, Moens M, Dom J, et al: An evaluation of two years of clinical experience with ketoconazole. Rev Infect Dis 2:674–687, 1980.

Of 99 patients with tinea versicolor 94 per cent were clinically and mycologically cured in three to six weeks with **ketoconazole** (200 mg daily). Long-term follow-up not available.

Savin RC: Systemic ketoconazole in tinea versicolor: A double blind evaluation and a 1 year follow-up. J Am Acad Dermatol 10:824–830, 1984.

Ketoconazole (200 mg/day for one month) healed each of the author's 33 patients. One year after treatment 66 per cent were still clear. For first-time patients he favors **selenium sulfide** lotion (USP) applied from ear lobes to knees 20 minutes before showering, followed by a shampoo with selenium sulfide. Miconazole cream is then applied over the same area. Repeat daily for two weeks.

Fredrikssen T, Faergemann J: Double-blind comparison of a zinc pyrithione shampoo and its shampoo base in the treatment of versicolor. Cutis 31:436–437, 1981.

After two weeks all 20 patients were completely cleared of infection with a daily five-minute application (prior to showering) of **zinc pyrithione** 1 per cent shampoo (Danex) to the trunk, arms, and thighs. Use bathrub brush to apply to back. Follow-up: four weeks post-treatment.

Bamford JTM: Treatment of tinea versicolor with sulfur-salicylic shampoo. J Am Acad Dermatol 8:211–213, 1983.

Nightly application for one week of a shampoo lotion containing 2 per cent **sulfur** and 2 per cent **salicylic acid** (Sebulex shampoo) cleared 21 cases. Reexamination at six months showed 16 of 20 still clear.

Faergemann J, Fredriksson T: Propylene glycol in the treatment of tinea versicolor. Acta Derm Venereol 60:92–93, 1980.

A 100 per cent cure rate in 20 patients using **propylene glycol** (50 per cent in water) applied with a gauze pad to the trunk and arms twice a day for two weeks. No side effects except slight burning in two patients. Follow-up: two weeks after stopping treatment.

Prestia AE: Topical benzoyl peroxide for the treatment of tinea versicolor. J Am Acad Dermatol 9:277–278, 1983.

Nine cases cleared following nightly application of 5 per cent Persa-Gel (**benzoyl peroxide**, acetone-based **propylene glycol** gel) for one month. Avoid the axillae, but treat from the hairline to the waist area and down the arms to the elbows. Shower each morning.

Mills OH, Kligman AM: Tretinoin in tinea versicolor. Arch Dermatol 110:638, 1974.

Stresses the lifelong nature of this affliction. Retin-A cream (0.1 per cent twice a day for two weeks) gives temporary cure. Treats hypopigmentation with sunlight.

El-Gothamy Z, Abdel-Fattah A, Ghaly AF: Tinea versicolor hypopigmentation: Histochemical and therapeutic studies. Int J Dermatol 14:510–515, 1975.

The classic old treatment, **sodium thiosulfate** (30 per cent solution applied twice a day for six weeks) cleared every one of 79 cases. (Available in the United States in 25 per cent concentration [Tinver lotion].)

Vicik GJ, Mendiones M, Quinones CA, Thorne EG: A new treatment for tinea versicolor using econazole nitrate 1.0 percent cream once a day. Cutis 33:570–571, 1984.

Spectazole cream applied once a day for three weeks gave an excellent response in 76 per cent of 67 patients with tinea versicolor, compared with 55 per cent of 59 patients using placebo cream. On day 21, positive KOH preparations were still present in 20 per cent of patients using **econazole nitrate** cream. No follow-up after stopping treatment.

Cullen SI, Frost P, Jacobson C, et al: Treatment of tinea versicolor with a new antifungal agent ciclopirox olamine cream 1%. Clin Therapeut 9:574–583, 1985.

Application of 1 per cent **ciclopirox** cream (Loprox) twice a day for two weeks to 65 patients with tinea versicolor gave a clinical and mycologic cure rate of 77 per cent. Using randomized, double-blind, parallel group studies, the cure rate for 1 per cent **clotrimazole** cream applied similarly was 45 per cent. Fourteen days post treatment the cure rate was 86 per cent for Loprox cream and 73 per cent in the clotrimazole group.

Consultants commonly see patients who are more difficult than their problems.

WALTER C. LOBITZ, JR.

A good therapeutic eye looks at the patient's problem from both inside and out.

Trichotillomania

TLC

Actions speak louder than words. And the act of pulling hair out of the scalp or eyelids is a loud nonverbalized cry of the child for something. Treatment centers on hearing the call, deciphering it, and then doing your best to have the parents answer it.

We generally do not confront the parents with the exact nature of the hair loss, since, in our experience, very few will accept the diagnosis. We try to learn the child's wish and orient the parent to help. Sometimes the task is easy. One child simply did not want to go to special religious instruction classes. Once the requirement was lifted, no further hair loss occurred. On other occasions it is more difficult. One of our patients, age 8 years, was being driven by a perfectionist father to superperform in school. It took more than a year to reduce the pressures and thereby the call for help. Sometimes the cry goes unheeded even when deciphered and recognized. We have seen many instances in which the hair loss was signaling an impending divorce.

All this takes time. During this period we have reassured the parents that the child is healthy (CBC, urinalysis), the skin and hair normal (microscopic examination of the hair). We have offered an excellent prognosis. We make it evident to the child that we know the true cause by pointing out that their hair roots are fragile and that they must not comb vigorously or pull or tug on the hair at any time. We suggest the wearing of a night cap so that no hairs will be pulled out "accidentally" when the patient is asleep.

At each visit we explore the child's wishes as much as possible. We encourage the parents to reduce stress, "spoil the child a little," get a pet or a special toy to watch the hair grow back. All of this spells TLC (tender loving care) by everyone concerned.

We prescribe a special shampoo (DHS with zinc), and oral biotin (0.3 mg tid). We examine the scalp for hair growth at each visit. We praise the child for progress, and we praise the parents when we see the child emerge into the sunlight of having their wish come true. Happiness for all is a full head of hair.

Jillson OF: Alopecia. II. Trichotillomania (trichotillohabitus). Cutis 31:383–389, 1983.

Some cogent observations:

Many examples are a minor tic, analogous to thumb-sucking or nail biting.

Seven times more common in children than in adults.

Tell, and if necessary, prove to the parent that the hair is being pulled out, and even possibly being eaten so that no evidence of hair loss is present in the bed in the morning.

Be certain that the patient has a teddy bear or security blanket to fondle and pull at.

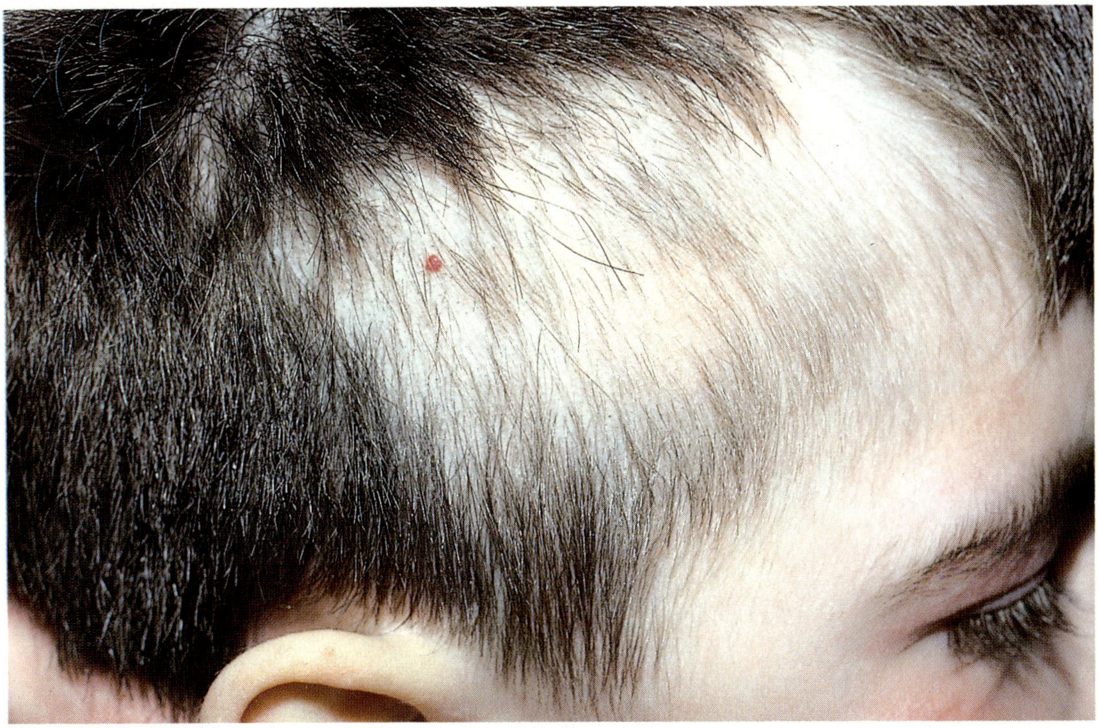

Do not recommend psychiatric help if this is a solitary problem.

Enlist the parents' gentle concern and provision of full security for the child.

Watch out for malingering in adults ("My hair won't grow since that beautician burned me.")

Brown AC: Alopecia. *In* Rakel RE: Conn's Current Therapy. Philadelphia, WB Saunders Co, 1985, pp 615–618.

Trichotillomania:

This may be nothing more than a minor transient neurotic habit comparable to nail biting. Each child or patient must be evaluated for the need for psychiatric consultation.

Reassurance and a kind, understanding attitude by the physician are frequently all that is necessary.

Clearly understand the stresses and anxiety that cause a patient to pull the hair out.

For some, use of **chromotherapy** (1 per cent **gentian violet** applied to the involved areas) is helpful, since the fingers pulling the hair become stained and the area is an eyesore. This probably draws more attention to the patient than was desired!

Meiers HG, Rechenberger H-G, Rechenberger I: Trichotillomanie: untersuchungen zur Ätiologie, Diagnostik und Therapie. Hautarzt 24:248–252, 1973.

An exquisite study of 17 cases of diffuse, focal, and patterned hair loss, each demonstrating a need for psychotherapy to reduce tensions. In one case, the doll of a patient also developed patterned hair loss.

Hamann K: Onychotillomania treated with pimozide (Orap). Acta Derm Venereol 62:364–366, 1982.

A 70-year-old woman had a $5\frac{1}{2}$ year history of a nail dystrophy due to use of nail scissors, rough sponges, and chlorine to remove "nail disease" consisting of "hardness" of the nail plate and skin surrounding the nail. All of her fingernails had been plucked away, and the great toenails were partially affected. A sister had the same problem. **Pimozide** (Orap 2 to 4 mg/day for seven months) resulted in perfect nails, but a maintenance dose (2 mg/day) was continued to counteract her prolonged tendency to manipulate the nails. The sister responded equally well.

To the patient complaining about the fee: "You were expecting a Cadillac for the price of a Ford?"

WALTER C. LOBITZ, JR.

Using the right drug for the wrong reason is better than using the wrong drug for the right reason.

Uncombable Hair

Biotin

Congenital anomalies usually receive more diagnostic than therapeutic attention. But in the uncombable hair syndrome, exhibiting nonpliable grooved trihedron-shaped hairs (pili trianguli et canaliculi), there is at least one therapeutic approach, i.e., biotin. The administration of biotin in modest dosage rapidly reversed the uncombability of the hair in one of our patients.

Thus the usefulness of biotin supplementation now extends from the treatment of noncompliant to nonexistent hair. Some babies with congenital failure of hair growth or retarded hair growth have benefited from biotin given orally in a dose of 3 to 10 mg a day. Like zinc, which is so essential to the activity of many enzymes, biotin has proved helpful also in the treatment of unexplained dermatitides and candidiasis in infants. It is evident that biotin-dependent carboxylases are of importance in the integrity and growth of hair and epidermis. Thus, low levels of biotin, biotinidase, or multiple carboxylases in the serum clearly indicate a need for biotin therapy.

Interestingly, the common localized patch of scalp hair that will not comb down, i.e., the cowlick, is not a forme fruste of the uncombable hair syndrome. Scanning electron microscopy of hair samples from 10 "cowlicks" failed to reveal any significant number of trihedron hair shafts.

Shelley WB, Shelley ED: Uncombable hair syndrome: Observations on response to biotin and occurrence in siblings with ectodermal dysplasia. J Am Acad Dermatol 13:97–102, 1985.

Biotin (0.3 mg tid) reversed scaling, hair loss, hair fragility, and uncombability of hair within four months in a two-year-old boy with the pili trianguli syndrome. It did not alter the trihedron form of the hair, however. (Follow-up: After one year of biotin therapy the hair remains combable and scanning electron microscopy revealed that the number of triangular hairs present has dropped from 90 per cent to 10 per cent).

A great therapist is the sum of all he has seen, heard, read, and thought.

Urticaria

Chlor-Trimeton	Epinephrine
Periactin	Corticosteroids
Cimetidine	Dapsone
Hydroxyzine	Indomethacin

Among the most interesting patients we see are those with urticaria. Each comes with the challenging question not of "What?" but of "Why?" Each is an adventure in detection that calls for a confident, knowledgeable physician and a faithful, helpful patient.

The easy answers come in cases of acute drug sensitivity or food intolerance. A simple history often suffices for the detection of a penicillin or seafood reaction. Antihistamines to the point of suppression or tolerance will aid the patient through the week or two of antigen degradation and elimination. In severe reactions immediate relief is available with epinephrine injections and powerful suppression by systemic steroids.

The hard answers come in the case of chronic recurrent urticaria. Again, the history is the simple most valuable area of help. It must be carefully recorded and enlarged and reviewed on each subsequent visit. No observation of the patient or family is too insignificant to be ignored. The patient must be encouraged to watch for immediate antecedents of each major attack. He must be informed that virtually any ingestant, inhalant, or contactant may be responsible. The search need not extend beyond the 12-hour period just prior to the sudden flare.

We enlist the total cooperation of the patient in this pursuit. He is not to take antihistamines in a dose that will eradicate all evidence of hives. The idea is to subdue but not submerge the eruption. The patient must look for triggering relationships with work, hobbies, diurnal cycles, menses, or unusual events and must understand that the search is for a specific antigen. He must fully recognize that the "antigen" for which he is searching is innocuous to his family and friends and indeed was innocuous to him prior to the onset of his hives. Urticaria is never due to "nerves" alone, but only to some external or internal chemical to which he has become sensitized. This approach is particularly valuable in urticarial attacks that are episodic.

We regularly reduce the potential antigen exposure in every way possible. A monastic life style is necessary until the problem is solved: no candies, toothpaste, eyedrops, cigarettes, hair tonic, perfume, perfumed soap, or cosmetics. Furthermore, we eliminate all aspirin, drugs, medicines, cough drops, laxatives, vitamins, minerals, and antacids. We ask that the patient minimize dust, pollen, and vapor (aerosol) exposures; especially stressed is avoidance of contact with wool. We immediately start him on a diet in which all beer, chocolate, corn, eggs, fish, milk, nuts, pork, seafood, and tomatoes are eliminated for two weeks.

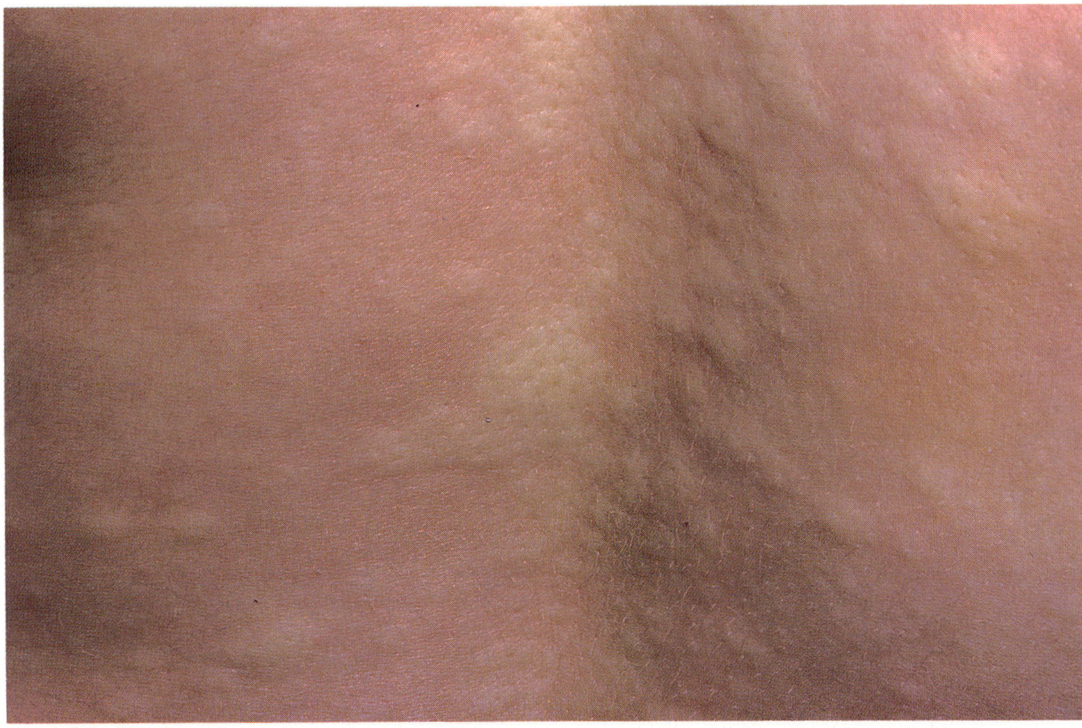

We teach the patient to expect and anticipate rapid success. If there is no change in two weeks we begin a program of short therapeutic trials. Our favorite drug is Nizoral (200 mg/day) or its alternate, Mycostatin, to reduce the yeast antigen load. When there is no response in two weeks, we try seriatim, an antibacterial regimen with erythromycin (250 mg qid), tetracycline (250 mg qid), and Flagyl (250 mg tid). This is particularly relevant in examples of urticaria in which the single lesions persist for more than 24 hours. Biopsy will usually show vasculitis in these cases, and bacterial sensitivity is often present.

In all instances, if there is symptomatic or physical evidence of infection or disease, this aspect is addressed. If a biopsy of the urticarial lesion shows vasculitis, we redouble our effort to locate and treat occult infection, such as cystitis or prostatitis. Blood studies revealing hepatitis call for conservative measures until resolution occurs. The presence of a positive ANA may necessitate dapsone or chloroquine therapy. In the physical urticarias with obvious causes, induction of tolerance by gradually ascending exposures to light, heat, cold, water, or vibrating trauma is undertaken if the causal agent cannot be avoided.

Whenever intensive outpatient management fails, hospitalization is indicated. Here, the environmental control of the patient can be idealized. In this setting a 48-hour fast allows one to determine whether the cause of the recurrent urticaria is from the outside or inside. Later challenges with the food colorant tartrazine (10 mg or a glass of Tang), the common preservative sodium benzoate

(50 mg), or specific foods or drugs in the hospital under controlled conditions are always valuable. It is also a time for an in-depth search for occult systemic disease and focal infection.

No disease requires a more cooperative effort on the part of physician and patient. The greatest success comes to the physicians and patients who have the drive and courage to continue to look for and eradicate the cause. Despite the pessimism of those who merely write a prescription for Atarax and thereby write off the cause, the real answers come to those who work the hardest. Do not give up until the hives do.

Warin RP, Champion RH: Urticaria. Philadelphia, WB Saunders Co, 1974, 173 pp.

Reviews over 150 specific documented causes of chronic urticaria. Also gives details of how to find which one caused your patient's problem.

Marks R: Chronic idiopathic urticaria: The dilemma of treatment. Int J Dermatol 21:19–20, 1982.

In 1876, treatment centered on **bichloride of mercury**, acid solution of **iron, chloride of arsenic**, and total avoidance of beer. Only the latter remains of proven value today.

Mathews KP: Management of urticaria and angioedema. J Allergy Clin Immunol 66:347–357, 1980.

In 1950, 35 drugs were considered useful. Today, all of those have been abandoned except the H_1 blockers.
Most useful drugs:

hydroxyzine
- low dose at first, titering upward to minimize drowsiness

cyproheptadine
- drug of choice for cold urticaria
- may produce weight gain
- suppresses ACTH and growth hormone; must avoid prolonged use in children

cimetidine
- not to be used alone—add to an H_1 blocker

epinephrine

ephedrine

steroids
- drug of choice for serum sickness and delayed pressure urticaria

Champion RH, Highet AS: Investigation and management of chronic urticaria and angio-oedema. Clin Exp Dermatol 7:291–300, 1982.

Do not blame hives solely on emotional factors.

Eliminate aspirin in all forms, since it aggravates urticaria in 50 per cent of the patients. Aspirin modulates prostaglandin synthetase, as does **indomethacin**. Also eliminate tartrazine. Test for *Candida* sensitivity with intradermal skin test read at 15 minutes and four to six hours. Treat with oral **nystatin, amphotericin** lozenges, and vaginal **nystatin** tablets.

Guin JD: Treatment of urticaria. Med Clin North Am 66:831–849, 1982.

Excellent review. 172 references.

Must avoid **aspirin**, wintergreen flavoring, balsam of Peru, **cinnamic aldehyde** and **acid, benzaldehyde**, and **benzoic acid**. Must avoid the yellow dye **tartrazine** (FD&C yellow No. 5), including antihistamines with this coloring. (Atarax and Periactin are okay.) Also avoid seafood (lobster, scallops), which contains tyramine, a histamine liberator.

Tyramine also occurs in foods altered by yeast or mold, which may explain why a "low-yeast" diet combined with anti-*Candida* treatment helps many urticaria patients, especially if they have an immediate positive scratch or intradermal test to *Candida*. Also avoid vasodilating influences:

heat
exercise
sunburn
drugs (including **thiamine, quinine**, and **chlortetracycline**)
fever
alcohol

Helpful hints:

scratch tests
- Molds are the most common inhalant in urticaria, especially in farmers, hunters, and construction workers.
- Pollens, house dust, animal epidermals, and common foods should also be checked.

diet diary
- This consists of four vertical columns, seven horizontal lines (for days of week). List meals and snacks in first three columns and time of flare in last column.

elimination of aspirin (give list)
elimination of foods

milk	peanuts
citrus	peas
chocolate	beans
cola	eggs
cinnamon	pork
tomato	nuts
fish	wheat
strawberries	artificial food colors

if inhalant sensitivity is established, give two months of hyposensitization.
checking of OTC medications

cold tablets	rectal medications
cough medicine	reducing pills
decongestants	sleeping pills
douches	tonic (quinine)
laxatives	vaginal medications
lozenges	vitamins
mouthwashes	

other drugs to consider for therapy
- tricyclic antidepressants (**doxepin** + **amitriptyline**): strong antihistaminic effect
- acute urticaria: epinephrine (temporary effect—induces refractory state following mast cell degranulation)
- chronic urticaria: terbutaline (beta$_2$-agonist) + ketotifen—both increase cAMP levels within mast cells
- drug urticaria: systemic steroids
- pressure urticaria: systemic steroids

drugs that help asthma and might help urticaria
- **theophylline** (inhibits breakdown of cAMP by phosphodiesterases)
- **cromolyn sodium**, **doxantrazole** } stabilize mast cell (mechanism unknown)

A careful history with a search for psychosomatic influences may not solve the problem, but helps cooperation, communication, and confidence. Drug history should include:

laxatives	headache remedies
vitamins	artificial sweeteners
OTC medications	topical medications

Speer F, Carrasco LC, Kimura CC: The management of urticaria. Ann Allergy 40:387–392, 1978.

Very practical approach to urticaria—need optimism, patience, and an open mind. **Penicillin**, sulfa, and **aspirin** are the drugs that most commonly cause urticaria. Eggs, strawberries, citrus, fish, and chocolate are the foods most commonly responsible. Gives valuable table of 83 common odors and fumes that may cause urticaria, including chlorine and moth balls.

Twarog FJ: Urticaria in childhood: Pathogenesis and management. Pediatr Clin North Am 30:887–898, 1983. 51 references.

Tests of value in directing treatment include biopsy, challenges, ANA, hepatitis screen, IgE, and immune complex assay.

Harvey RP, Wegs J, Schocket AL: A controlled trial of therapy in chronic urticaria. J Allergy Clin Immunol 68:262–266, 1981.

Hydroxyzine (25 mg qid) and **cimetidine** (300 mg qid) used conjointly gave best results in 19 patients. "Nonresponders" to antihistamine therapy may be noncompliant—an important factor to remember in the management of all patients with chronic urticaria.

Commens CA, Greavens MW: Cimetidine in chronic idiopathic urticaria: A randomized double-blind study. Br J Dermatol 99:675–679, 1978.

In 19 patients, **chlorpheniramine** (Chlor-Trimeton 4 mg qid) alone was as effective as chlorpheniramine (4 mg qid) in conjunction with **cimetidine** (400 mg qid). Since only one third of patients have a good response to H_1-blockers, mediators other than histamine, such as kinins or prostaglandins, may be important in these refractory cases.

Farnam J, Grant JA, Guernsey BG, et al: Successful treatment of chronic idiopathic urticaria and angioedema with cimetidine alone. J Allergy Clin Immunol 73:842–845, 1984.

Be alert to the exceptional patient: A 50-year-old man had too much sedation and too little relief from **diphenhydramine, hydroxyzine**, and **chlorpheniramine**. Three years of successful therapy with nonsedating **cimetidine** (300 mg qid) suggested that his urticaria was uniquely mediated by H_2 histamine receptors.

Coutts A, Greaves MW: Evaluation of six antihistamines in vitro and in patients with urticaria. Clin Exp Dermatol 7:529–536, 1982.

The winner: Periactin (**cyproheptadine**) for effectiveness against pruritus and for fewer side effects.

Millns JL, Randle HW, Solley GO, Dicken CH: The therapeutic response of urticarial vasculitis to indomethacin. J Am Acad Dermatol 3:349–355, 1980.

Indomethacin (25 to 50 mg qid) cleared all lesions in 6 of 10 patients within three weeks. These patients had painful hives, angioedema, arthralgias, abdominal pain, low-grade fever, and leukocytoclastic vasculitis with positive direct immunofluorescence.

Thormann J, Laurberg G, Zachariae H: Oral sodium cromoglycate in chronic urticaria. Allergy 35:139–141, 1980.

Cromolyn (200 mg qid) for four weeks was no help in preventing symptoms in 15 patients with food allergies when challenged with the known precipitating oral agents.

Sullivan TJ: Pharmacologic modulation of the whealing response to histamine in human skin: Identification of doxepin as a potent in vivo inhibitor. J Allergy Clin Immunol 69:260–267, 1982.

Doxepin (Sinequan 5, 10, or 25 mg q12h for five doses) was a very effective inhibitor of histamine-induced whealing. Drowsiness may occur in nondepressed individuals at 10 to 25 mg bid. The tricyclic antidepressants were originally developed as H_1 antihistamines.

Kennes B, De Maubeuge J, Delespesse G: Treatment of chronic urticaria with a beta-adrenergic stimulant. Clin Allergy 7:35–39, 1977.

The antiasthmatic drug **terbutaline** (Brethine 1.25 mg tid for two months) greatly helped 24 patients with chronic urticaria resistant to antihistamines. Maximum therapeutic effect was seen after one month.

Only one patient had palpitations. Probable mechanism: $beta_2$-receptor stimulation, which inhibits mast cell degranulation.

Saihan EM: Ketotifen and terbutaline in urticaria. Br J Dermatol 104:205–206, 1981.

Ten of 14 patients unresponsive to antihistamines were helped by **ketotifen** (1 mg tid—not available in the United States) plus **terbutaline** (5 mg tid) taken separately with one hour between drugs.

Side effects of fine tremor and palpitations caused discontinuation of treatment in three patients.

Metcalfe DD: Food hypersensitivity. J Allergy Clin Immunol 73:749–762, 1984.

Details of exactly how to test scientifically for food allergy, with data on food groupings by chemical composition.

Illig L, Paul E: Foodborne allergic and pseudoallergic reactions on skin and mucous membranes under special consideration of foodborne urticaria and RAST. Z Hautkr 59:793–813, 1983.

Best to eliminate any food that gives prodromal mucosal symptoms.

Verschave A, Stevens E, Degreef H: Pseudo-allergen-free diet in chronic urticaria. Dermatologica 167:256–259, 1983.

Elimination of food additives (coloring, flavoring, preservatives) and shellfish, bread, peas, tomatoes, oranges, bananas, pineapple, strawberries, cheese, and nuts as well as alcohol gave favorable results in more than half of the 67 patients under study. Responders were usually atopic with associated gastrointestinal disturbances.

Michaëlsson G, Juhlin L: Urticaria induced by preservatives and dye additives in food and drugs. Br J Dermatol 88:525–532, 1973.

Recurrence could be prevented by strict elimination of preservatives (benzoates) and azo coloring dyes (tartrazine) in half of the 52 patients. Includes helpful list of foods likely to contain these chemicals.

Noid HE, Schulze TW, Winkelmann RK: Diet plan for patients with salicylate-induced urticaria. Arch Dermatol 109:866–869, 1974.

Very helpful lists of do's and don'ts for a salicylate-free diet. Since tartrazine is a "salicylate-related" compound, patients are often allergic to it also. The diet is very limited in fruits, so that a vitamin C supplement (devoid of tartrazine dye) is advisable.

Lee M, Gentry AF, Schwartz R, Bauman J: Tartrazine-containing drugs. Drug Intel Clin Pharm 15:782–788, 1981.

Includes tabulated lists of manufacturers of tartrazine-free products, as well as 366 tartrazine-containing drugs from 60 other drug companies. A few surprises with tartrazine—Mycostatin oral tablets, Cleocin capsules, Bicillin tablets, Ortho-Novum 1/50 tablets, **ferrous sulfate**, Librium, and Synthroid.

Effective June 26, 1980, The Food and Drug Administration required package labeling of FD&C yellow No. 5 dye on all prescription and over-the-counter oral, rectal, vaginal, and nasal products.

Note:
incidence of tartrazine intolerance: approximately 1 in 10,000
particular risk: asthmatic patients with aspirin sensitivity
symptoms: asthma, urticaria, angioedema, rhinorrhea
sensitivity mechanism unknown: tartrazine structure similar to aminopyrine, an analgesic that adversely affects patients allergic to aspirin

Must warn patients that tartrazine appears in color blends such as turquoise, green, and maroon—not only in bright yellow products.

Settipane GA: Adverse reactions to sulfites in drugs and foods. J Acad Dermatol 10:1077–1080, 1984.

The antioxidant potassium metabisulfite, used as a preservative in foods (e.g., restaurant salads) and drugs (e.g., Gantrisin), can initiate urticaria within minutes. **Vitamin B_{12}** (a sulfite oxidant), if taken in an oral dose of 1 to 5 mg, can prevent this reaction, as can **atropine, cromolyn**, and **doxepin**. Includes lists of 56 drugs and 19 foods that contain sulfites.

Thomas DR, Pursley TV, Jorizzo JL: Chronic urticaria secondary to aminobenzoic acid. Arch Dermatol 120:961–962, 1984.

A strange case of urticaria of six months' duration not solved until the offending multivitamin tablet containing **aminobenzoic acid** (a quasivitamin) was stopped. A positive challenge was observed within 20 minutes after an oral dose of 50 mg aminobenzoic acid, a denouement that required months of cross-examining the patient.

Dewdney JM, Edwards RG: Penicillin hypersensitivity—Is milk a significant hazard?: A review. J R Soc Med 77:866–877, 1984.

No! (Probably due to extreme dilution of the antigen through pooling of milk sources.)

Papa CM, Shelley WB: Menthol hypersensitivity: Diagnostic basophil response in a patient with chronic urticaria, flushing, and headaches. JAMA 189:546–548, 1964.

Attacks of urticaria in a 31-year-old woman following use of toothpastes, Life Savers, cigarettes, or Noxzema were traced to a single allergen, menthol. She was thus at risk with prescribed or over-the-counter medications, mouthwashes, toothpastes, cosmetic creams, nose drops and sprays, chest rubs, dusting powder, douches, cough drops, candy, analgesic balm, massaging lotions, shaving creams, chewing gum, aerosols, food, ice cream, cigarettes, liquors, mixed drinks, and mint gardens. The common "antigen" thread was always menthol.

James J, Warin RP: An assessment of the role of *Candida albicans* and food yeasts in chronic urticaria. Br J Dermatol 84:227–237, 1971.

C. albicans sensitivity was an important factor in 26 per cent of 100 consecutive patients with chronic urticaria.

Evaluation
- prick test with *C. albicans* antigen (5000 PNU/ml); read at 15 minutes and four to eight hours
- diet challenge with bakers' yeast (0.4 gm) or brewers' yeast (*Saccharomyces cerevisiae*)

Treatment
- **nystatin**: oral (1 million U tid for two weeks, then 500,000 units tid for two weeks); vaginal pessaries (bid for one week)
- **amphotericin B** troches (10 mg bid for one week—suck on)
- remove and clean dentures at bedtime
- low-yeast diet—eliminate:
  - bread
  - buns

sausage
wines
beer
cider
grapes
sultanas
cheese
vinegar
tomato ketchup
pickles
yeast tablets
canned foods with yeast (must read label)

Juhlin L: Clinical studies on the diagnosis and treatment of urticaria. Ann Allergy 39:356–361, 1977.

Ask where the patient has traveled, since amebiasis, ascariasis, trichinosis, and hookworm disease are common causes of urticaria in certain areas.

Van Dellen RG, Ottesen EA, Gocke TM, Neafie RC: Loa loa: An unusual case of chronic urticaria and angioedema in the United States. JAMA 253:1924–1925, 1985.

A 49-year-old woman developed urticaria nine months after hunting big game in Africa. Serologic tests for parasites revealed high titers for filariasis, but blood sera were negative. She had eosinophilia (27 per cent) and elevated levels of IgE. Initial treatment with **diethylcarbamazine citrate** (100 mg tid) led to malaise, arthralgias, migratory myalgias, and subcutaneous swelling. Skin biopsy revealed a gravid *Loa loa* worm. After three days, the reaction subsided, and the dosage was slowly increased (to 400 mg/day) for three weeks. Recurrence three months later was due to a second adult worm and required a second course of treatment.

Veronesi S, Palmerio B, Negosanti M, Tosti A: Urticaria and giardiasis. Dermatologica 166:42–43, 1983.

Giardia lamblia was isolated in 6 of 50 (12 per cent) patients with chronic urticaria. None had eosinophilia, and only 3 of 6 had periodic mushy foul stools and abdominal distention. Treatment with **metronidazole** (Flagyl 125 to 250 mg tid for 10 days) was curative.

Nizami RM, Baboo MT: Office management of patients with urticaria: An analysis of 215 patients. Ann Allergy 33:78–85, 1974.

No psychogenic factors were found, even with the help of a psychiatrist, and the use of tranquilizers or sedatives is discouraged. Five cases cleared after patients received definitive therapy for sinusitis. One patient had allergy to silver contained in a metal compound, Nobilium, used in a dental plate.

Bushkell LL: Chronic urticaria and gallbladder disease: Clearing after cholecystectomy. Arch Dermatol 115:638, 1979.

This 30-year-old woman noted permanent disappearance of her hives 48 hours after surgery.

Tanphaichitr K: Chronic urticaria associated with bacterial infection. Cutis 27:653–656, 1981.

Urticaria of 5 years' duration in a 35-year-old man was cured by extraction of abscessed carious teeth and treatment of periodontal disease.

Bretag AH, Archer RS, Atkinson HM, Woods WH: Circadian urticaria: Another *Campylobacter* association. Lancet 1:954, 1984.

Urticaria that developed every evening for 10 days was associated with proven *Campylobacter jejuni* enteritis.

von Krogh G, Maibach HI: The contact urticaria syndrome—An updated review. J Am Acad Dermatol 5:328–342, 1981.

Handy list of agents producing contact urticaria, including many chemicals present in standard patch test screening trays. For open tests: 0.03 ml of substance to ventral forearm or back; observe 30 to 60 minutes for follicular erythema evolving into a wheal or wheal-and-flare response. Animal danders, foods, cosmetics, plants, textiles, and woods may be similarly tested. If no response, apply test to previously affected or presently involved areas. Lastly, try leaving closed patches on for 15 to 20 minutes.

Werman BS, Rietschel RL: Chronic urticaria from tantalum staples. Arch Dermatol 117:438–439, 1981.

Removal of tantalum staples from the legs was necessary to cure this 39-year-old woman with peculiar localization of hives in the surgical scars on her legs. Prior to this, the diagnostic use of the powerful metal chelator **disulfiram** (Antabuse 250 mg bid) gave marked temporary relief. Intradermal testing with tantalum reproduced the lesions.

Shelley WB, Rawnsley HM: Aquagenic urticaria: Contact sensitivity reaction to water. JAMA 189:895–898, 1964.

In three patients, contact with water or sweat elicited small follicular hives in areas rich in sebaceous glands. In one patient, Chlor-Trimeton (**chlorpheniramine maleate**) controlled the attacks, and use of a bath oil containing lanolin, mineral oil, and a nonionic emulsifier (Alpha Keri, 1 teaspoonful to the tub) greatly reduced the number of hives. (Now we favor showering every hour to induce tolerance. This can be done once weekly, with each shower being only long enough to provoke hives. Tolerance can then be maintained with a once-daily shower.)

Sibbald RG, Black AK, Eady RAJ, et al: Aquagenic urticaria: Evidence of cholinergic and histaminergic basis. Br J Dermatol 105:297–302, 1981.

In two patients with lesions indistinguishable from cholinergic urticaria, **cyproheptadine** (Periactin 4 mg qid) or **promethazine** HCl (Phenergan 50 mg hs) were more effective than **hydroxyzine** (10 mg qid) or **chlorpheniramine** (4 mg qid). Both hot and cold water evoked lesions. Pretreatment of the skin with petrolatum ointment prevented lesions.

Tkach JR: Aquagenic urticaria. Cutis 28:454–463, 1981.

Cyproheptadine HCl (Periactin 4 mg) taken one hour before bathing prevented hives in a 30-year-old woman sensitive to tap water, snow, and sweat. She could drink water and swim in the ocean without difficulty.

Ramsay CA: Solar urticaria treatment by inducing tolerance to artificial radiation and natural light. Arch Dermatol 113:1222–1225, 1977.

Induction of tolerance requires a highly motivated patient, an appropriate fluorescent light source (based on determination of action spectrum for urticaria), and a daily maintenance dose (approximately 10 minutes' exposure using four to six lamps). Alternatives of **chloroquine**, sunscreens, or staying indoors seemed more attractive to some patients.

Parrish JA, Jaenicke KF, Morison WL, et al: Solar urticaria: Treatment with PUVA and mediator inhibitors. Br J Dermatol 106:575–580, 1982.

Incremental suburticarial UVA dosage three times a week for four to eight weeks, given two hours after oral **methoxsalen** (0.6 mg/kg), induced a tolerance that could be maintained by one-hour sun exposure three times a week during the summer.

Bernhard JD, Jaenicke K, Momtaz-T K, Parrish JA: Ultraviolet A phototherapy in the prophylaxis of solar urticaria. J Am Acad Dermatol 10:29–33, 1984.

Three of five patients experienced marked increase in sunlight tolerance treated with only UVA (three days a week for six weeks). Maintenance was achieved with summer sun exposure (one hour three times a week).

Keahey TM, Lavker RM, Kaidbey KH, et al: Studies on the mechanism of clinical tolerance in solar urticaria. Br J Dermatol 110:327–338, 1984.

Tolerance to ultraviolet radiation was induced in three patients by administering graded whole-body exposures to long-wave ultraviolet radiation in a UVA phototherapy cabinet. Tolerance may be due to an increase in mast cell degranulation threshold.

Tatnall FM, Gaylarde PM, Sarkany I: Localised heat urticaria and its management. Clin Exp Dermatol 9:367–374, 1984.

Hospitalize the patient. Induce heat intolerance with hourly immersion in water at 38 to 40.5°C, starting with the legs and working up to the total body after four days. Then gradually increase the time between baths to eight hours over the next two weeks, followed by daily baths for one month. The patient was eventually kept symptom free for six months with a hot bath every third day.

Black AK, Sibbald RG, Greaves MW: Cold urticaria treated by induction of tolerance. Lancet 2:964, 1979.

Although induction of cold tolerance is possible, it is not a routine treatment. A study of 19 patients hospitalized for induction of cold tolerance through hourly five-minute immersion in cold water (15°C), starting with one arm and moving sequentially to other body areas.

Results: Three patients stopped because of unpleasantness, four received no help, and the rest found it hard to maintain tolerance after induction during one to three weeks in the hospital.

Highet AS, Titterington M: Treatment of cold urticaria. Br J Dermatol 101:51–55, 1979.

Hydroxyzine (Atarax) proved to be superior to **diphenhydramine** (Benadryl), **cyproheptadine** (Periactin), and **cimetidine** (Tagamet) in a very carefully studied patient with essential acquired cold urticaria.

Sigler RW, Evans R, Horakova Z, et al: The role of cyproheptadine in the treatment of cold urticaria. J Allergy Clin Immunol 65:309–312, 1980.

Six patients were completely cleared of cold urticarial responses to ice cube challenge after two weeks of **cyproheptadine** (Periactin 4 to 8 mg qid). Mechanism: H_1 receptor antagonist (blocks effects of histamine).

Illig L: Physical urticaria: Its diagnosis and treatment. Curr Probl Dermatol 5:79–116, 1973.

Cold urticaria—50 per cent of cases cleared with 1 million U **penicillin** IM twice weekly for a total of 10 million units. Unique to cold urticaria. No help from oral penicillin.

Kaplan AP, Garofalo J: Identification of a new physically induced urticaria: Cold-induced cholinergic urticaria. J Allergy Clin Immunol 68:438–441, 1981.

Report of four patients who developed tiny hives only after exposure of the entire body to cold for 5 to 15 minutes. Ice cube tests, cold immersion tests, and exercise in a warm environment failed to produce lesions. Histamine levels were increased by cold exposure. Successful treatment consisted of **hydroxyzine** (100 mg/day) plus **cyproheptadine** (16 mg/day). Moral: "Challenge patients in a cold environment when the history suggests cold or cholinergic urticaria and the usual confirmatory tests are negative."

Bentley-Phillips CB, Eady RAJ, Greaves MW: Cold urticaria: Inhibition of cold-induced histamine release by doxantrazole. J Invest Dermatol 71:266–268, 1978.

Doxantrazole (400 mg tid—not available in the United States) given for periods of up to four weeks suppressed cold-evoked histamine release in 8 of 13 patients, with clinical improvement in 6 patients. Its mechanism of action is similar to **disodium cromoglycate** (which is active only when inhaled).

Asad SI, Kemeny DM, Youlten LJF, et al: Effect of aspirin in "aspirin sensitive" patients. Br Med J 288:745–748, 1984.

Aspirin-induced urticaria is usually a pharmacologic phenomenon to which tolerance can be achieved by repeated administration of the drug (up to 650 mg daily).

Mathews KP: Management of urticaria and angioedema. J Allergy Clin Immunol 66:347–357, 1980.

If no cause can be found, avoid alcoholic drinks, heat, exertion, emotional stress, aspirin.

Shelley WB: Case report: An analysis of a case of chronic urticaria. Ann Allergy 24:421–425, 1966.

Success demands physician confidence, an informed helpful patient, hospitalization, imagination, and persistence. Urticaria is "antigenic," not psychogenic. In this case, urticaria was caused by sensitivity to Pantopaque, an iodized fatty acid dye used in myelography, which was slowly released from the lumbar canal over several years.

Akers WA, Naversen DN: Diagnosis of chronic urticaria. Int J Dermatol 17:616–627, 1978.

No patient should be considered to have chronic idiopathic urticaria until after the following therapeutic trials for occult infections:

yeast

nystatin (500,000 U tid) for 10 days

yeast-free diet, avoid:

- bread
- beer
- grapes
- raisins
- cheeses
- sausages
- vinegar
- pickles
- ketchup
- mushrooms
- yeast tablets

in women: nystatin vaginal tablet (100,000 U tid). (Today, Nizoral 200 mg/day is an excellent alternative.)

bacterial cystitis

Tetracycline (250 mg qid) for five days

Ampicillin (250 mg qid) for five days or **methenamine mandelate** (Mandelamine 1 gm qid) for five days—must acidify urine with ascorbic acid (1 gm daily for five days)

enteritis

Azulfidine (**sulfasalazine** 500 mg qid) for five days

amebic

Diiodohydroxyquin (Amebaquin 650 mg tid) for 1 week

trichomonas
Metronidazole (Flagyl 250 mg tid) for one week
helminth
Thiabendazole (Mintezol 25 mg/kg bid) for four days
fungal
Griseofulvin (500 mg/day) for three weeks
dermatitis herpetiformis
Dapsone (100 mg bid) for five days or **sulfapyridine** (500 mg bid) for five days
scabies
Kwell lotion (topically, leave on for 12 hours)

Kulczycki A: Aspartame-induced urticaria. Ann Intern Med 104:207–208, 1986.

The common artificial sweetener, **aspartame** (NutraSweet, dipeptide of aspartic acid and the methyl ester of phenylalamine) was proven by challenge to be the cause of chronic urticaria and angioedema in two women. The author cites 11 other cases of hives circumstantially linked to the use of aspartame. Its presence in diet soft drinks, chewing gums, cereals, desserts, and sugar substitutes may account for more hives than now realized. Challenge can be done with a single oral dose of 50 mg aspartame (Equal) or even a half can of Tab or Diet Pepsi. The sensitive patient will develop obvious hives within a few hours.

Shelley WB, Shelley ED: Adrenergic urticaria: A new form of stress-induced hives. Lancet 2:1031–1033, 1985.

A new form of pharmacologic allergy in which stress triggers autonomic norepinephrine release and in turn hives. The beta-blocker **propranolol** (Inderal 20 mg tid) afforded specific therapy for two patients with this analogue of cholinergic urticaria. Lesions are tiny red wheals with white halos.

Moneret-Vautrin DA, Bene MC, Faure G: She should not have chewed. Lancet 1:617, 1986.

Butylate hydroxytoluene (BHT) proved to be the cause of a puzzling generalized urticaria in a gum-chewing young woman. The answer came from provocation tests at four-day intervals with the chewing gum ingredients (chlorophyll, menthol, and BHT). Other sources of BHT, which is used as an antioxidant in foods, include potato chips, salted peanuts, and cake mixes.

Champion RH, Greaves MW, Kobza Black A, Pye RJ: The urticarias. Edinburgh, Churchill Livingstone, 1985, 237 pp.

This records the proceedings of a 1984 symposium on the chronic urticarias. Although only 20 per cent of these challenges are solved etiologically, food allergy can be eliminated as a cause if the patient does not improve after seven days of a diet limited to green tea, cane sugar, lamb, rice, sea salt, and water.

Never underestimate the power of a case report to help you with your case.

Urticaria Pigmentosa

Antihistaminics	Systemic Steroids
Aspirin	PUVA
Cromolyn	

Parental reassurance with a correct diagnosis is often sufficient therapy for an infant with one or more asymptomatic lesions. However, the patient with pruritus, flushing, urticaria, or bullae deserves much more. This is even more apparent in the individual with diarrhea, headaches, or the bone pain of systemic mastocytosis.

Antihistamines are the cornerstone therapy, since the symptoms and signs result from the histamine released by mast cell infiltrates. Both H_1 and H_2 receptor blockers are valuable, particularly when used in conjunction with each other. Since prostaglandins are also mediators in this disease, aspirin merits consideration as a prostaglandin synthetase inhibitor. Aspirin initially must be given carefully, with physician guidance, in low dosage since it is a powerful histamine liberator. Patients must be alerted to the potential hazard of other histamine liberators like codeine, polymyxin B, and bee sting venom, which may result in anaphylaxis or a generalized bullous eruption.

An alternate approach is the use of cromolyn sodium (100 mg bid), an inhibitor of mast cell degranulation. This drug can dramatically inhibit bullae formation in infants and eliminate gastrointestinal symptoms. It has a remarkable effect for a drug absorbed to the extent of only 1 per cent.

Systemic corticosteroids are indicated occasionally, since they do suppress the reaction. Topical steroids are helpful only on denuded skin, when soothing compresses and systemic antibiotics also may be required.

James MP: The treatment of urticaria pigmentosa. Clin Exp Dermatol 7:311–320, 1982.

Careful modern review of pathogenesis and treatment. Check for leukemia. Try reserpine (1 mg/day) in patients not responding to more conventional therapy, but watch out for depression.

Caplan RM: The natural course of urticaria pigmentosa. Arch Dermatol 87:146–157, 1963.

A study of 112 cases showed slow spontaneous remission of lesions of infancy over a period of years, whereas lesions of adult onset do not disappear.

Muller UR, Horat W, Wuthrich CM, Reisman RE: Anaphylaxis after *Hymenoptera* stings in three patients with urticaria pigmentosa. J Allergy Clin Immunol 72:685–689, 1983.

In three adult patients with urticaria pigmentosa, anaphylaxis after honeybee and yellow jacket stings was not an IgE-mediated sensitivity reaction, but was due to pharmacologic liberation of histamine by components of the

Hymenoptera venoms. Skin tests to various venoms were not helpful. Alert patients or parents to this danger as well as that of other histamine liberators, such as aspirin and codeine.

Gerrard JW, Ko C: Urticaria pigmentosa: Treatment with cimetidine and chlorpheniramine. J Pediatr 94:843–844, 1979.

Chlorpheniramine (2.5 mg q8h) and **cimetidine** (60 mg q6h) each helped, and together they were excellent in treating a three-year-old boy with bullous mastocytosis.

Johnson GJ, Silvis SE, Roitman B, Blumenthal M, Gilbert HS: Long-term treatment of systemic mastocytosis with histamine H_2 receptor antagonists. Am J Gastroenterol 74:485–489, 1980.

Cimetidine (300 mg qid) used daily for four years alleviated gastric hypersecretion, healed a duodenal ulcer, and ameliorated the marked pruritus and erythema experienced by a man after bathing. Skin test reactivity to histamine was also demonstrably reduced.

Achord JL, Langford H: The effects of cimetidine and propantheline on the symptoms of a patient with systemic mastocytosis. Am J Med 69:610–614, 1980.

Nearly two years of treatment with **cimetidine** (300 mg qid) failed to reduce lesional skin pigmentation in a 24-year-old woman with lifelong systemic mastocytosis. However, her episodic flushing, headaches, palpitations, and profuse diarrhea were greatly helped. Addition of an anticholinergic, **propantheline bromide** (Pro-Banthine 15 mg qid), kept her asymptomatic.

Roberts LJ, Sweetman BJ, Lewis RA, Folarin VF, Austen KF, Oates JA: Markedly increased synthesis of prostaglandin D_2 in systemic mastocytosis. Trans Assoc Am Physicians 93:141–147, 1980.

Overproduction of PGD_2 accounts for flushing and hypotension unresponsive to H_1, H_2 blockers. The authors recommend a therapeutic cocktail of histamine blockers and the prostaglandin synthetase blocker, **aspirin.**

Chlorpheniramine 12 mg qid
Cimetidine 300 mg qid
Aspirin 15 grains qid

Fabulous results in one adult with life-threatening attacks of flushing, dyspnea, hypotension, diarrhea, and chest pain. Symptoms were not controlled with **chlorpheniramine** (Chlor-Trimeton 12 mg qid) plus **cimetidine** (300 mg tid) until aspirin (3.9 gm/day) was added. Must start with small aspirin dosage (40 mg/day or less) and increase slowly to avoid massive histamine liberation.

Soter NA, Austen KF, Wasserman SI: Oral disodium cromoglycate in the treatment of systemic mastocytosis. N Engl J Med 301:465–469, 1979.

Cromolyn sodium (100 mg qid) produced marked amelioration of all symptoms in five adult patients, but did not reduce histaminuria or eosinophilia. Double-blind study for up to 2½ years.

Czarnetzki BM, Behrendt H: Urticaria pigmentosa: Clinical picture and response to oral disodium cromoglycate. Br J Dermatol 105:563–567, 1981.

Good response in 9 of 13 patients. Disadvantages: Costly large dose (up to 800 mg/day), side effects (headaches, insomnia), and recurrence on stopping.

Evans S, Vickers CFH: Bullous urticaria pigmentosa (cutaneous mastocytosis) and sodium cromoglycate. Acta Derma Venereol 61:572–575, 1981.

Sodium cromoglycate (20 to 100 mg tid) was effective in two infants with the severe bullous form. Dosage was increased to 300 mg daily for control in one child age three years.

Welch EA, Alper JC, Bogaars H, Farrell DS: Treatment of bullous mastocytosis with disodium cromoglycate. J Am Acad Dermatol 9:349–353, 1983.

Convincing color photos show complete involution of bullae in two infants taking **disodium cromoglycate** (cromolyn sodium in the United States). In a 19-month-old boy an initial dose of 20 mg bid was increased to 100 mg/day, then decreased to 60 mg/day maintenance. A 9-month-old girl received 5 to 10 mg bid with good control, followed by a larger maintenance dosage of 160 to 200 mg daily for 12 months.

Christophers E, Honigsmann H, Wolff K, Langner A: PUVA—Treatment of urticaria pigmentosa. Br J Dermatol 98:701–702, 1978.

Ten cases (nine adults, one child) responded to PUVA, given four times a week until no dermographism or whealing could be produced with physical trauma (loss of Darier's sign). All patients noted relief of itching, and two patients had relief of migraine. Shielded areas did not clear. Relapse occurred in three to six months without treatment. Dosage: 8-MOP (0.5 to 0.8 mg/kg) + total UVA (12 to 417 J/sq cm) over 3 weeks to 10 months.

Vella Briffa D, Eady RAJ, James MP, Gatti S, Bleehen SS: Photochemotherapy (PUVA) in the treatment of urticaria pigmentosa. Br J Dermatol 109:67–75, 1983.

Eight adult patients responded to oral **8-methoxypsoralen** (0.6 mg/kg) followed by UVA exposure (1.5 to 2.5 J/sq cm) two hours later. An average of 27 exposures (range 15 to 69) given twice weekly (2 to 12 J/sq cm total) was required to fade the lesions and decrease pruritus and whealing. Disadvantages: Slow, partial response and relapse on stopping.

Vaatainen N, Hannuksela M, Karvonen J: Trioxsalen baths plus UV-A in the treatment of lichen planus and urticaria pigmentosa. Clin Exp Dermatol 6:133–138, 1981.

To avoid the systemic effects of oral psoralens use **trioxsalen** (50 mg dissolved in 20 ml alcohol) in 150 L warm bath water for 10 minutes prior to UVA. Five adult cases improved. Total UVA dose 3 to 36 J/sq cm. Starting dose 0.12 to 0.24 J/sq cm, increased by 25 to 50 per cent every third treatment. Maintenance dose at two- to four-week intervals.

Czarnetzki BM: A double-blind cross-over study of the effect of ketotifen in urticaria pigmentosa. Dermatologica 166:44–47, 1983.

Ketotifen (2 mg daily), the newest mast cell degranulation inhibitor (not yet available), was effective in 10 adults with urticaria pigmentosa. It should replace **cromolyn**, as it is easily absorbed from the gastrointestinal tract and was much more effective.

Lewis RA: Mastocytosis. J Allergy Clin Immunol 74:755–765, 1984.

Complete review of current status. 58 references. Note that in episodes of shock, if **dopamine** fails to act, intravenous **epinephrine** is effective therapy for these patients. Albumin-based plasma volume expanders are always a valuable adjunct. H_1 receptor antagonists must also be given until the released mediators are cleared by the body.

Barton J, Lavker RM, Schechter NM, et al: Treatment of urticaria pigmentosa with corticosteroids. Arch Dermatol 121:1516–1523, 1985.

Betamethasone dipropionate ointment (Diprolone) applied under occlusion eight hours daily for six weeks induced almost complete clearing of adult-onset urticaria pigmentosa lesions in six patients. The areas treated remained clinically clear for the following year.

Patients know more than you think, and think more than you know.

Vasculitis

Bedrest	Colchicine
Antihistamines	Chloroquine
Antibiotics	KI
Corticosteroids	Cytoxan
Dapsone	

Our therapy for vasculitis centers on the elimination of "bugs and drugs." Most of the vasculitis we see is an immune complex–mediated inflammatory reaction within the microvasculature of the skin. As such, it has numerous different causes and an enormously broad spectrum of clinical lesions. This ranges from a few petechiae to frighteningly deep ulcers. Accordingly, therapy can range from antihistamines to intravenous pulse steroids, long-term immunosuppressants, and even reparative plastic surgery.

Vasculitis is a disease that tries the patience of victim and physician alike. Aside from the trivial transitory forms, it is a problem that requires months, even years, of thoughtful treatment. Therefore the patient-doctor relationship must be good. The patient must understand the nature of this ordeal, and the doctor must not expect rapid cures or be unduly discouraged by relapses. But always the patient should be on an incline of recovery, no matter how slight the slope. We do not persist in therapy that shows no promise.

The only specific curative therapy we have for vasculitis is the detection and elimination of antigens (bacterial, viral, or chemical). These combine with circulating antibodies and then deposit in vessel walls where blood flow is slow (lower legs, cold extremities) or the vessel wall has been damaged (trauma, folliculitis). Once deposition has occurred, inflammation is initiated and can only be stopped with nonsteroidal or steroidal anti-inflammatory agents.

The search for possible antigens must be ongoing. Although a careful temporal history may reveal an offending drug, we use the all-out approach of stopping all drugs (except those immediately essential to the patient's life). It is surprisingly hard to do this, as often the patient fails to acknowledge his vitamins, laxative, eye drops, medicated lozenges, or aspirin. We repeatedly question the patient and family to be certain that this supposedly simple interdiction is being followed.

If there is no improvement we expand the elimination program to include toothpaste, candies, gums, mouthwash, sprays, cigarettes, perfumes, insecticides, flowers, turpentine, and specific inhalants or ingestants with antigenic potential. We encourage and elicit help from the patient to seek out hidden antigen sources. It is a serious search, for if occult antigen remains, the vasculitis remains. The story is no different from that of contact dermatitis persisting when the allergen remains unidentified in the patient's environment.

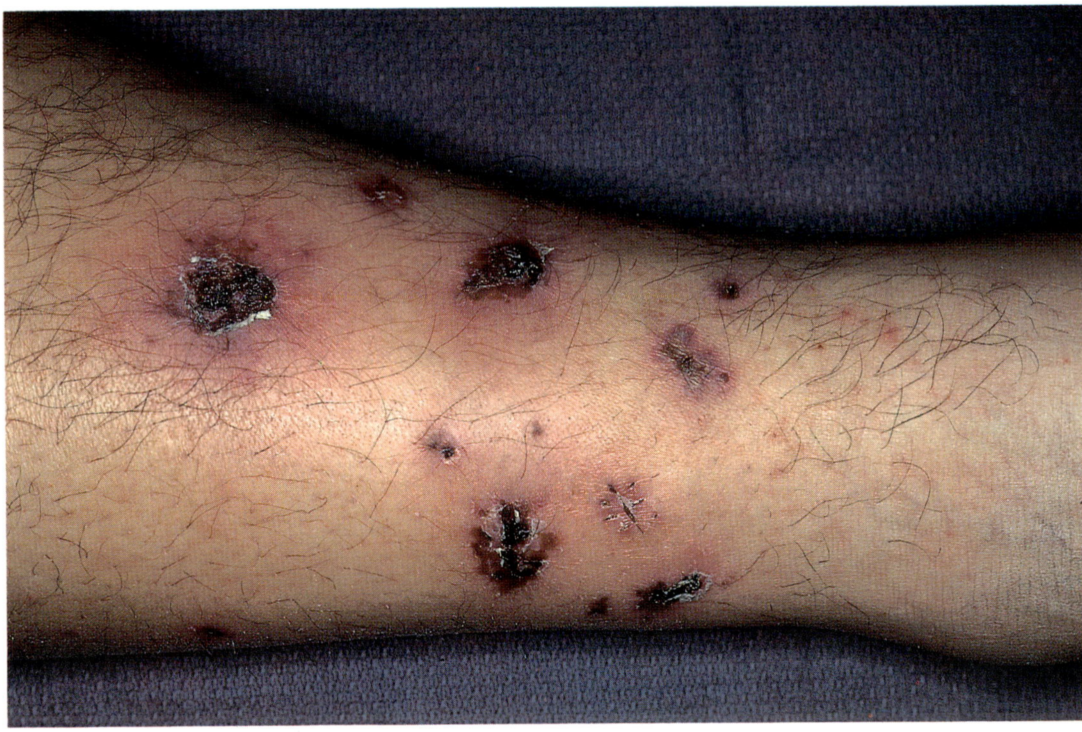

From the microbial side, we look for recurrent pharyngitis, sinusitis, bronchitis, dental abscesses, cystitis, and cholecystitis. If there is no specific organism identifiable, we treat first with erythromycin (250 mg qid). If this fails we use alternatives such as amoxicillin (Augmentin 500 mg tid). We also check for tinea pedis as an antigen source, treating it with griseofulvin (500 mg bid) or ketoconazole (200 mg/day).

Hepatitis screening, careful histories, and knowledge of current contagions are helpful. The most valuable blood test, however, is the immune complex assay, which assesses the potential hazard present and helps monitor the course. We regularly secure a health profile, ANA, and CEA, since underlying disease such as autoimmunity or a tumor may be responsible. In that regard, lymphomas are likely candidates. It is also advisable to screen for cryoglobulins and macroglobulins, which may be present in such quantities as to occlude small vessels and give a clinical picture similar to vasculitis.

For the patient who has passed all of these gates, we prescribe dapsone (100 mg/day), which has given us the greatest help in treating cutaneous vasculitis. We tend to avoid systemic steroids although a test injection of Kenalog (40 mg IM) will quickly assess whether or not the vasculitis is steroid responsive. It has the added advantage that you, not the pharmacist, are in control of the drug and its dosage. Colchicine and potassium iodide remain alternatives. For a few rare patients the powerful immunosuppressants (particularly, Cytoxan 50 mg tid) are useful, as they block the formation of antibodies and hence reduce the noxious immune complex level.

Local treatment is very useful in the care of necrotizing vasculitis wherein the reaction is so severe and massive that the skin becomes necrotic, sloughs, and ulcerates. Such an ulcer becomes a crusted purulent nidus for organisms of all shapes and sizes. The first law of therapy here is compresses-debridement. We favor 0.5 per cent aqueous silver nitrate (one hour qid) compresses using white cotton cloth (rather than gauze) applied eight layers thick. A topical antibiotic such as Silvadene cream (silver sulfadiazine 1 per cent) is then applied to the ulcer base. At night the ulcer is packed with a 10 per cent benzoyl peroxide gel (e.g., Persa-Gel W 10 per cent) to kill residual organisms, especially anaerobes.

The therapy of vasculitis can be a long, long road. Throughout it all the patient must take every precaution to avoid trauma. A bruise on the skin may spell a new lesion for anyone with such an immune complex load. The patient must take every precaution to prevent stasis, as the immune complexes will surely deposit in vessels filled with slow-moving sludged blood. The patient should wear Supphose and avoid long periods of immobility, sitting on a bus, or standing at work. Chilling and cyanosis of the extremities should be prevented, as cryoglobulins and possibly the immune complexes are precipitable in the chilled blood of cold skin. The uniqueness of the skin in regard to these three factors of trauma, stasis, and low temperature accounts in part for the fact that vasculitis of the skin is generally not associated with vasculitis of the internal organs.

Likewise, the skin is unique in having a pain sensory system not found in the internal organs. As a result the pain of cutaneous vasculitis of the necrotizing type is a major burden for the patient. Indeed, the ulcers can be covered and hidden, but never the pain. These patients need analgesics and, at times, steroid therapy to reduce the pain. Intralesional xylocaine and triamcinolone suspension may also be considered.

In the weeks and months to come the patient must do everything possible to maintain good health and avoid intercurrent infections. A good diet, supplemental zinc, adequate rest, and avoidance of crowds are well acknowledged aids that merit special attention by these patients.

The master clinician, Eugene Stead, often said on rounds, "What this patient needs is a good doctor." For these patients we would add, "and for a good long time!"

Cupps TR, Fauci AS: The vasculitides. Philadelphia, WB Saunders Co, 1981, 211 pp.

The master review of therapy stresses the need to:

1. Eliminate the antigen if identifiable
2. Treat any underlying disease
3. Treat the vasculitis directly with corticosteroids, immunosuppressants (especially **cyclophosphamide**), and nonsteroidal anti-inflammatory agents (**aspirin**, **indomethacin**, **colchicine**).

Fauci AS: Vasculitis. J Allergy Clin Immunol 72:211–223, 1983.

An updated summary of N.I.H. experience:

1. Most cases have an immunologic basis, often immune complex mediated.
2. Individualized therapy is based on the extent and scope of vasculitis. Less aggressive measures are indicated if the process is limited to the skin.

3. If nonsteroidal anti-inflammatory drugs fail, use corticosteroids (**prednisone** 1 mg/kg/day in three divided doses, gradually tapered to a single alternate-day dose for three to six months).
4. If steroids fail, use a cytotoxic drug. The best is **cyclophosphamide** (2 mg/kg/day in a single dose, or 4 mg/kg IV for three to four days initially if critically ill). Treatment must be continued for at least one year.
5. Alternate cytotoxic drugs that are useful: **chlorambucil**, **azathioprine**, **6-mercaptopurine**, and **methotrexate**.
6. Plasmapheresis may be considered to prevent deposition of immune complexes (especially cryoglobulinemic complexes) in the vascular bed.

Wolff K, Winkelmann RK: Vasculitis. Philadelphia, WB Saunders Co, 1980, 338 pp.

A classic reference source on all aspects of this disease pattern that features inflammation and damage to vessels of all sizes.

Sams WM Jr: Necrotizing vasculitis. J Am Acad Dermatol 3:1–13, 1980.

The clinical spectrum of vasculitis includes leukocytoclastic, rheumatic, and granulomatous types (with diseases such as dermatomyositis and granuloma annulare), and giant cell arteritis, polyarteritis nodosa, and infarcts.

The search is for antigenic antecedents:

- microbial (streptococci, mycobacteria, hepatitis virus, influenza virus)
- drugs
- serum proteins (vaccines, hyposensitization, antigens)
- chemicals (insecticides, petroleum products)
- autoimmune diseases
- malignant tumors

Mackel SE: Treatment of vasculitis. Med Clin North Am 66:941–954, 1982.

Laboratory evaluation recommended:

- chest roentgenogram
- urinalysis
- complete blood count
- sedimentation rate
- SGOT
- BUN or creatinine
- complement
- ANA
- rheumatoid factor
- serum protein electrophoresis and immunoelectrophoresis
- hepatitis B–associated antigen
- cryoglobulins

Callen JP: Cutaneous vasculitis and its relationship to systemic disease. DM 27:1–48, 1981.

Alteration of predisposing factors such as dependency and cool environment by simple measures may be beneficial. In mild cases, antihistamines, salicylates, or nonsteroidal anti-inflammatory agents (NSAID) are enough.

Cupps TR, Springer RM, Fauci AS: Chronic recurrent small-vessel cutaneous vasculitis: Clinical experience in 13 patients. JAMA 247:1994–1998, 1982.

This form of vasculitis, limited to the skin, is relatively unresponsive to steroid and immunosuppressant therapy. Only 4 of 13 patients were helped by steroid therapy, and only 2 of 6 were helped with Cytoxan. Strangely, anticoagulants, **phenformin**, **ethylestrenol**, and plasmapheresis were also ineffective. In a few instances, **colchicine** or **dapsone** gave real relief. Pain is a serious problem in the cutaneous form and requires analgesics. The value of bedrest is also noted.

Callen JP, Kalbfleisch S: Urticarial vasculitis: A report of nine cases and review of the literature. Br J Dermatol 107:87–93, 1982.

The vasculitis in seven of nine patients could not be controlled without systemic steroid therapy. In one instance, **azathioprine** allowed reduction in steroid dosage. Antihistamines, **indomethacin**, and **hydroxychloroquine** were also ineffective.

Millns JL, Randle HW, Solley GO, Dicken CH: The therapeutic response of urticarial vasculitis to indomethacin. J Am Acad Dermatol 3:349–355, 1980.

In 6 of 10 patients clearing occurred within three weeks when they were given indomethacin (Indocin 25 to 50 mg qid), but the vasculitis reappeared within 48 hours of stopping indomethacin.

Hazen PG, Michel B: Management of necrotizing vasculitis with colchicine: Improvement in patients with cutaneous lesions and Behçet's syndrome. Arch Dermatol 115:1303–1306, 1979.

Four patients with cutaneous vasculitis of two to nine years' duration responded well to three months of **colchicine** therapy (0.6 mg bid or tid with food). In three of these, improvement was sustained on stopping colchicine.

Ledermann JA, Hoffbrand BI: Dapsone in allergic vasculitis: Its use in Henoch-Schönlein disease following vaccination. J R Soc Med 76:613–614, 1983.

Henoch-Schönlein purpuric vasculitis appeared in a 33-year-old male following cholera, yellow fever, and typhoid-paratyphoid vaccination. **Prednisolone** (30 mg/day) was ineffectual. **Dapsone** (50 mg bid) induced clearing in 48 hours, but nine months of therapy was necessary before the dapsone could be stopped. Interestingly, an upper respiratory infection induced a new attack of purpura, which subsided when dapsone therapy (75 mg/day) was reinstituted.

van der Horst JC, Bronsveld W: Urticarial vasculitis in a patient with systemic lupus erythematosus: A case report. Clin Exp Dermatol 6:489–494, 1981.

A 56-year-old man with SLE developed annular erythematous wheal-like lesions with central vesicles, which proved on biopsy to be leukocytoclastic vasculitis. Specific therapy: Plaquenil (**hydroxychloroquine** sulfate 200 mg tid) coupled with **prednisone** (40 mg/day). Skin lesions involuted within a few days and did not recur after slow tapering and discontinuation of both drugs.

Horio T, Danno K, Okamoto H, et al: Potassium iodide in erythema nodosum and other erythematous dermatoses. J Am Acad Dermatol 9:77–81, 1983.

Seven of 11 patients with nodular vasculitis showed complete remission of lesions within two weeks after taking oral KI (300 mg tid).

Valbonesi M, Garelli S, Mosconi L, et al: Plasma exchange in the management of a patient with diffuse necrotizing cutaneous vasculitis. Vox Sang 39:241–245, 1980.

Extensive palpable purpura and focal necrosis developed in a 36-year-old woman starting 10 days after an acute febrile illness. The lesions rapidly responded to two sessions of discontinuous-flow centrifugal plasmapheresis exchange. After 9 liters of plasma exchanged in six sessions over nine days, therapy was stopped. Reappearance of the lesions four days later necessitated further plasmapheresis and Cytoxan (**cyclophosphamide** 2 mg/kg/day) therapy. Five days later the plasmapheresis was discontinued, and control was maintained with Cytoxan. Plastic surgery was necessary to heal the necrotic areas.

Do not use plasmapheresis unless the immune complex level is high. It acts only by physically removing these complexes that otherwise deposit and cause vasculitis.

Parish WE: Microbial antigens in vasculitis. *In* Wolff K, Winkelmann RK (eds): Vasculitis. Philadelphia, WB Saunders Co, 1980, pp 129–150.

Immune complexes are likely to form during or after every instance of bacteremia, e.g., following tooth extraction, sigmoidoscopy, or barium enema. Streptococcal group A antigen was the most frequent of the six microbial antigens detected in the skin vessels of these patients.

Lucas SB, Moxham J: Recurrent vasculitis associated with beta-haemolytic streptococcal infections. Br Med J 1:1323, 1978.

A 17-year-old girl developed biopsy-proven—vasculitic lesions in the skin associated with polyarthritis, beginning while she had a sore throat of four weeks' duration, unresponsive to **penicillin** and **tetracycline**. A throat culture showed *Streptococcus pyogenes* and the ASO titer was 230. There was no clinical improvement with further courses of **erythromycin**, **ampicillin**, and tetracycline. However, she received dramatic help following **hydrocortisone** and **azathioprine**. She remained clear of the disease for nine years, until the same sequence developed following a sore throat, with an ASO titer of 1600. The same therapeutic response was observed, but cortisone (70 mg/day) was necessary as maintenance to suppress the disease.

Hilton AM, Hasleton PS, Bradlow A, et al: Cutaneous vasculitis and immune complexes in severe bronchiectasis. Thorax 39:185–191, 1984.

Three bronchiectasis patients with purpuric vasculitis (C3, IgG, and IgA in their cutaneous vessels) were found to have *Hemophilus influenzae* in their sputa and circulating immune complexes. The treatment of choice was antibiotics, e.g., clearing occurred in one patient within six weeks when **amoxicillin** (500 mg qid) was prescribed in conjunction with **prednisone** (80 mg/day). Interestingly, 80 per cent of all bronchiectasis patients have circulating immune complexes.

Popp JW, Harrist TJ, Dienstag JL, et al: Cutaneous vasculitis associated with acute and chronic hepatitis. Arch Intern Med 141:623–629, 1981.

A report of 11 patients, most of whom also had arthralgias and cryoglobulins, but no overt liver disease. Palpable purpura was seen only with chronic hepatitis, while urticaria and maculopapular lesions were seen in acute hepatitis. Do not forget to do a panel screen for hepatitis.

Hoffman GS, Franck WA: Infectious mononucleosis, autoimmunity, and vasculitis: A case report. JAMA 241:2735–2736, 1979.

A 31-year-old man with fever, sore throat, myalgias, arthralgias, and petechial lesions on the feet and ankles was found to have antibodies to Epstein-Barr virus in high titer, microscopic hematuria, increased liver enzymes, cryoglobulins, and cutaneous vasculitis. Clearing was gradual over 10 weeks, with treatment centered on pain relief using:

acetaminophen (Tylenol)
propoxyphene HCl (Darvon)
codeine
salicylates to reduce fever

Newton JA, McGibbon DH, Marsden RA: Leukocytoclastic vasculitis and angiooedema associated with inflammatory bowel disease. Clin Exp Dermatol 9:618–623, 1984.

Purpuric skin plaques and angioedema of the arms were the presenting signs of inflammatory bowel disease in two instructive cases:

male, 68 years: cleared with Azulfidine (**sulfasalazine** 1 gm tid)
male, 61 years: **dapsone** gave control, but was discontinued because of anemia induced by it. Subsequently **colchicine** (0.25 mg tid) gave excellent control, but relapse occurred whenever it was stopped.

Sandbank M, Weltfriend S, Wolf R: Bowel bypass arthritis dermatitis syndrome: A histological and electron microscopical study. Acta Derm Venereol 64:79–82, 1984.

This syndrome develops in 20 per cent of those who have bowel bypass surgery for control of morbid obesity, and virtually all patients have circulating immune complexes. A 36-year-old woman developed abdominal pain, joint pains, and large vesiculopustules with red haloes (sterile on culture) one year after having ileojejunal bypass surgery. Treatment with Achromycin (**tetracycline** 500 mg qid) and topical **zinc** lotion and Terramycin (**oxytetracycline**) powder resulted in gradual disappearance of lesions after 10 days of treatment.

Marks CR, Willkens RF, Wilske KR, Brown PB: Small vessel vasculitis and methotrexate. Ann Intern Med 100:916, 1984.

This vasculitis was observed in eight patients receiving **methotrexate** (15 mg/week or less) for treatment of rheumatoid and psoriatic arthritis. In two patients, rechallenge with methotrexate confirmed the etiologic diagnosis. All of the patients had previously had reactions to **gold**, **penicillamine**, or other medications.

Mitchell GG, Magnusson AR, Weiler JM: Cimetidine-induced cutaneous vasculitis. Am J Med 75:875–876, 1983.

Biopsy-proven vasculitis was reproduced with a **cimetidine** challenge in a 63-year-old man with generalized urticaria. The rash began four days after starting cimetidine (300 mg qid). Treatment consisted of **prednisone** (40 mg/day for seven days), **hydroxyzine** (100 mg qid), and discontinuance of cimetidine.

Ruzicka T, Ring J, Braun-Falco O: Vasculitis allergica durch vitamin B_6. Hautarzt 35:197–199, 1984.

Bullous hemorrhagic lesions on the lower legs of a 68-year-old patient rapidly cleared on elimination of vitamin B_6.

Lambert WC, Kolber LR, Proper SA: Leukocytoclastic angiitis induced by clindamycin. Cutis 30:615–619, 1982.

A 56-year-old diabetic man with osteomyelitis developed a palpable purpuric rash on the sixth day after starting IV **tobramycin** (70 mg q8h) and **clindamycin** (600 mg q6h). The rash was preceded by generalized arthralgias. Allergy to clindamycin was proven by challenge, with new skin lesions developing within 24 hours of restarting IV clindamycin.

Kerdel FA, Fraker DL, Haynes HA: Necrotizing vasculitis from radiographic contrast media. J Am Acad Dermatol 10:25–29, 1985.

Radiocontrast material resulted in generalized cutaneous vasculitis and nephritis in two patients within 12 to 22 hours of being given intravenously. These agents or their metabolic products act as haptens to which antibodies attach, forming soluble immune complexes. If not removed by reticuloendothelial cells, these complexes lodge in blood vessel walls, activate complement, and induce a surge of neutrophils with consequent vessel damage.

Note: The site of an **epinephrine** injection given four hours before the contrast material was devoid of any change, probably because vasoconstriction prevented deposition of immune complexes. In contrast, intradermal **histamine** localizes deposits of immune complexes through vasodilatation.

Other drugs to suspect of causing necrotizing vasculitis:

aspirin
allopurinol
gold
iodides
penicillin

phenacetin
sulfonamides
thiazides
thiouracils
phenothiazines

Tanay A, Yust I, Brenner S, et al: Dermal vasculitis due to coumadin hypersensitivity. Dermatologica 165:178–185, 1982.

Rechallenge confirmed that **coumadin** induced a purpuric eruption with vasculitis in a 65-year-old man following only 10 days of coumadin treatment. The challenge dose of one tablet of coumadin caused a temperature of 39°C within six hours and purpuric lesions on the legs that lasted one week.

Vasily DB, Tyler WB: Propylthiouracil-induced cutaneous vasculitis. Case presentation and review of the literature. JAMA 243:458–461, 1980.

A 31-year-old woman with Graves' disease, controlled with **propylthiouracil** (200 mg bid), developed polyarthralgias and indurated, dusky, violaceous lesions on the malar area, thighs, and buttocks. Skin biopsy showed necrotizing vasculitis. Splenomegaly and leukopenia were also present. The condition cleared after propylthiouracil was eliminated and **methimazole** (Tapazole) was substituted.

Note: The face and ear lobes are frequently involved with this type of vasculitis.

Curd JG, Milgrom H, Stevenson DD, et al: Potassium iodide sensitivity in four patients with hypocomplementemic vasculitis. Ann Intern Med 91:853–857, 1979.

Four patients are reported in whom KI induced urticarial vasculitis. Oral challenge in two of these reproduced lesions within two hours, with severe symptoms in one patient resembling periarteritis nodosa.

Houston TP: Small vessel vasculitis following simultaneous influenza and pneumococcal vaccination. NY State J Med 83:1182–1183, 1983.

Conjoint injections of trivalent influenza virus vaccine and polyvalent pneumococcal vaccine were associated eight days later with biopsy-proven cutaneous vasculitis. **Prednisone** (60 mg/day for two days, then tapered by 5 mg/day for two weeks) cleared the eruption in five days.

Menne T, Christophersen J, Gram N, Bjerrehus T: Scabietic leukocytoclastic vasculitis with focal glomerulonephritis. Acta Derm Venereol 64:445–447, 1984.

Palpable purpura was intermixed with scabies burrows in two middle-aged patients (one with Parkinson's disease, the other with diabetes mellitus and a large abscess). Treatment with a scabicide (**gamma benzene hexachloride** lotion 1 per cent) was curative.

Bruynzeel DP, van den Hoogenband HM, Koedijk F: Purpuric vasculitis-like eruption in a patient sensitive to balsam of Peru. Contact Dermatitis 11:207–209, 1984.

In an 80-year-old woman contact dermatitis on the face, due to the application of an ointment containing balsam of Peru, was followed shortly by the development of purpuric vasculitis lesions on the lower legs. The vasculitis was thought to be an unusual manifestation of allergic contact dermatitis, presumably through endogenous spread of the allergen.

Harper JI, Copeman PWM: Dermatitis artefacta presenting as a "vasculitis." J R Soc Med 76:970–971, 1983.

A 22-year-old woman novice in a closed religious order was hospitalized for a month with a vasculitis-like eruption (C3 deposits but no immunoglobulin in the vessel walls). Denouement: Removal of lye crystals found in the patient's possession was associated with rapid healing. Sequel: long-term warm sympathetic understanding, psychiatric counseling and release from commitments. Even with these necessary steps, the prognosis remains poor.

To get the best clues, examine and cross-examine your patient the day after a flare.

When instructing patients, make the implicit explicit.

Verrucae

Curettage	Cantharone
Liquid nitrogen	Bleomycin
Duofilm	Contact sensitization
Podophyllin	Laser
Formaldehyde	

Bertrand Russell said that "all human knowledge is uncertain, inexact and partial." This would seem to be a particularly accurate description of our knowledge of how to treat warts. Nonetheless, the majority of patients with warts who seek help can be cured. With no virucidal agent available, a variety of techniques may have to be employed. The approach always should be nonscarring, destroying or removing the epidermal growth only. This eliminates techniques such as excision and electrosurgery. Recall that most warts in children clear spontaneously within several years, without medicine and without scarring.

Our favorite technique of treating warts is simple surgical removal by curettement. For filiform or digitate warts of the bearded region this is done without anesthesia, but with Monsel's solution (ferric subsulfate) hemostasis. Wart bases must be wiped and kept bloodless with the skin taut before application, since Monsel's solution does not stop capillary bleeding, only prevents it.

In the case of other warts, large or small, curettage is always preceded by removal of the keratinous bulk of the wart (down to bleeding points), using subsection with a Gillette Super Blue Blade half. On the palm and sole such curettage must be complete and deep. The most common cause of recurrence is timid, incomplete curettage. To prevent scarring, electrosurgery should not be used in the wart removal or control of bleeding. The latter is achieved with pressure dressings.

Liquid N_2 cryotherapy is equally effective in many patients. Using a cotton-tipped swab, we apply the nitrogen for a full minute. Generally a single treatment is sufficient to induce complete involution in three weeks, with or without antecedent blistering. If one treatment is not dramatically effective we turn to chemoexfoliation of the wart.

Our choice is the use of Duofilm (16.7 per cent salicylic acid, 16.7 per cent lactic acid in collodion base). It is applied by toothpick precisely to the wart surface after the maceration of a 10-minute soak. The area is covered with Cordran tape, the tape removed, and the procedure repeated every 24 hours. Again, we expect involution or significant clearing in three weeks.

For moist warts in the vulvar or penile areas we use 20 to 25 per cent podophyllin in tincture of benzoin. It is applied only by us and at weekly intervals. Talcum powder dusted over the treated warts helps to prevent smearing of the podo-

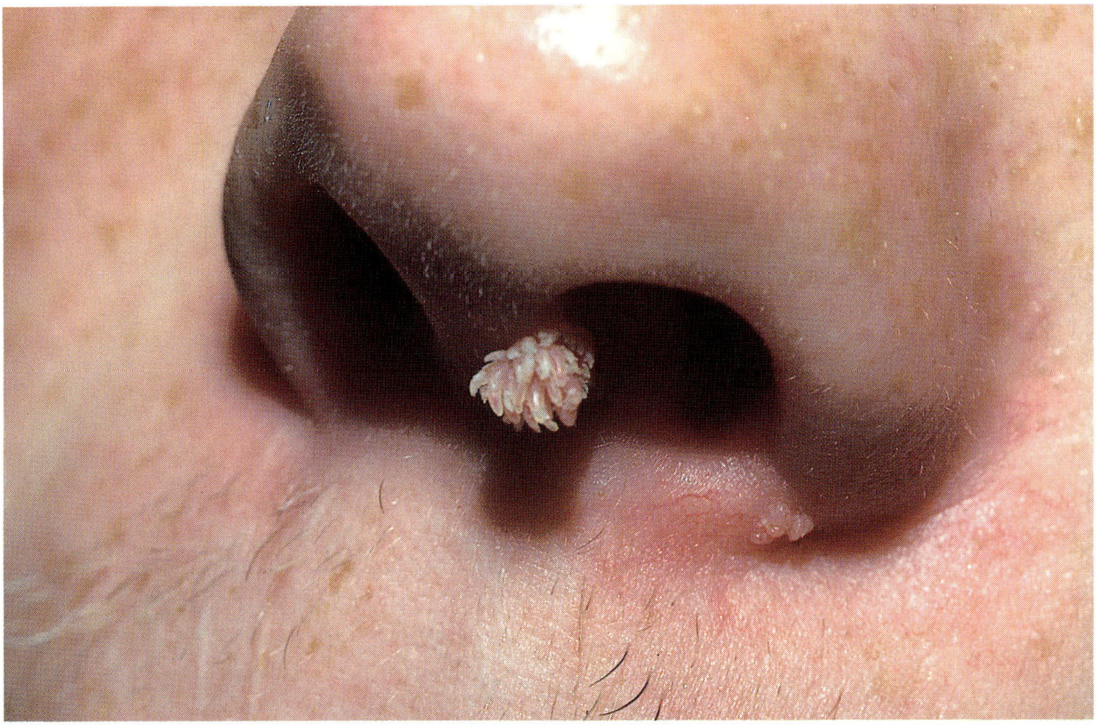

phyllin onto normal skin. It is washed off in a tub bath five hours after the first treatment, and at lengthening intervals up to 18 hours if no primary irritation develops. Some warts in these areas of loose skin can best be removed by simple excision with iris scissors. No sutures are required, and the scarring is minor.

Extremely recalcitrant warts, especially around the fingernails, may require the current darling of wart therapy, intralesional bleomycin. Again, the wart should be pared and the area anesthetized prior to injection. No more than three injections should be required over a six-week period.

On the sole where massive extensive warts abound, "sole soaks" in 4 per cent formaldehyde (formalin, diluted 1 to 10 in water) for 10 minutes each day, coupled with wart parings every two weeks, are highly effective, but require patience, since the warts are deep and epidermal turnover is slow. Plantar warts in children often respond well to the painless daily application of salicylic acid plaster (40 per cent), with paring of the warts every one to two weeks. Children are always warned of the hazard of bare feet.

The fearsome invasion and resistance of warts in the immunocompromised patient has taught us the importance of cell-mediated immunity in clearing warts, no matter what method is used. We use oral zinc (zinc sulfate 220 mg tid) in an effort to enhance immunity. We also use Aquasol A (50,000 IU tid) to alter the host keratinocytes and thereby help dislodge the unwelcome virus. In all instances we expect results within three weeks. We also warn patients that they must return if they see any sign of recurrence during the 90 days after treatment.

When all is said and done, there are still warts that defy every rational therapeutic approach. We recall vividly a patient with her entire sole covered by a mosaic wart. After a year of intensive treatment the wart remained in full bloom. We did not see her during a 3-month summer vacation, but when she returned the warts had vanished without a trace. "What ever did you do?" was our immediate inquiry. "Nothing at all, but my 12-year-old son prayed that they would go away, and they did!"

Bunney MH: Viral warts: Their biology and treatment. New York, Oxford University Press, 1982.

Ninety-nine pages by a master therapist giving detailed help in converting a frequently frustrating dermatologic challenge into a welcome adventure.

Mahrle G, Alexander W: Surgical treatment of recalcitrant warts. J Dermatol Surg Oncol 9:445–450, 1983.

A helpful list of current methods with more detailed discussion of cryosurgery (with and without blister formation) and electrosurgery.

Conservative treatment

- keratolytic agent: **salicylic acid**
- cytotoxic agents: podophyllin, cantharidin, **colchicine**
- chemotherapy: **fluorouracil**, **bleomycin**, **tretinoin**, **etretinate**, **interferon**
- photochemotherapy: light and dyes, PUVA
- immunotherapy: DNCB, bacille Calmette-Guérin vaccine, **gamma globulin**

Surgical treatment

- stepwise debridement
- blunt dissection
- curettage
- cryosurgery
- electrosurgery
- laser

Jillson OF: Warts. Cutis 27:32–37, 1981.

Facial warts: if digitate, use curettage without anesthesia; if flat, use an effective placebo.

Pringle WM, Helms DC: Treatment of plantar warts by blunt dissection. Arch Dermatol 108:79–82, 1973.

Of 58 plantar warts 49 (85 per cent) were cured with one treatment consisting of encirclement of wart with blunt dissection followed by curettage.

Gibbs RC: Conservative management of plantar warts by gentle chemocautery. J Dermatol Surg Oncol 4:915, 1978.

Apply 60 per cent **salicylic acid** in petrolatum; curet off dead wart once a week.

Thomson S: The treatment of plantar warts by formalin. Br J Dermatol 55:267–269, 1943.

Soak sole in 3 per cent aqueous formalin for 10 minutes each night. After three weeks, most warts are easily removed by curettage; 31 of 33 cases were cured.

Allenby CF: The treatment of viral warts with glutaraldehyde. Br J Clin Pract 31:12–13, 1977.

Soak soles in **glutaraldehyde** (2 per cent aqueous) for 15 minutes a day. There was clearing in 60 days in three out of every four patients in this study of 178 patients. Brown stain is excellent evidence of patient compliance. An alternative treatment with glutaraldehyde (10 per cent in an aqueous ethanol solution applied twice a day) resulted in clearing in 6 weeks in 15 of 21 patients with plantar warts.

Rosenberg EW, Amonette RA, Gardner JH: Cantharidin treatment of warts at home. Arch Dermatol 113:1134, 1977.

Cantharone (0.7 per cent **cantharidin** solution in acetone-flexible collodion) containing green food dye was applied daily at home until a blister formed or the wart disappeared. Result: 215 of 336 warts on the hands were cured. Only one patient developed a "fairy ring" of tiny satellite warts.

Thomas JR, Su WPD: The treatment of plane warts. Arch Dermatol 118:626, 1982.

Transact (2 per cent **sulfur** gel applied twice a day) cleared three of four resistant cases in two to three months.

de Bersaques J: Vitamin A acid in the topic treatment of plantar warts. Dermatologica 150:369–371, 1975.

Vitamin A acid (2 per cent in petrolatum) applied once daily under occlusion cured only 17 of 50 cases after 2 to 10 weeks of treatment.

Cajee YD: Household cleaners in the treatment of warts. S Afr Med J 62:1016, 1982.

Proprietary household cleaners containing liquid ammonia (Handy Andy, Ajax) were diluted with three parts of water and applied every four to seven days to warts for 10 minutes with cotton wool soaked in the solution. Within five weeks, 21 cases of warts were cured, including vulgaris, filiform, and acuminata varieties.

Warszawer-Schvarcz L: Treatment of plantar warts with banana skin. Plast Reconstr Surg 226:1342–1343, 1981.

Daily occlusive dressing with the innerside of fresh banana skin cured one case of very impressive large plantar warts within six weeks. The hyperkeratotic material was removed once a week.

Dunagin WG, Millikan LE: Dinitrochlorobenzene immunotherapy for verrucae resistant to standard treatment modalities. J Am Acad Dermatol 6:40–45, 1982.

Dinitrochlorobenzene (DNCB) 400 μg (20 μg/μl in acetone) was applied every two weeks to warts in patients previously sensitized to DNCB with 400 μg applied in two to three sites on the forearm. A phenomenal 87 per cent cure rate resulted in 24 patients after five to six treatments. Pruritus and mild inflammation occurred routinely at treatment sites, and two patients developed dyshidrosiform dermatitis of the palms and soles.

Claudy AL, Roche H: Traitement Des Verrues Multiples et Récidivantes par induction d'une hypersensibilité retardée. II. Etude critique de l'utilisation du dibutylester de l'acide squarique. Ann Dermatol Venereol 108:765–767, 1981.

Since DNCB is mutagenic in the Ames test, the authors used a nonmutagenic compound, squaric acid dibutyl ester (SADBE). In patients previously sensitized to SADBE with multiple recurring warts, only 2 of 18 were cured after three months.

Lahti A, Hannuksela M: Topical immunotherapy with tuberculin jelly for common warts. Arch Dermatol Res 273:153–154, 1982.

Three months of nightly application of tuberculin jelly preparation led to disappearance of recalcitrant warts in 8 of 14 (60 per cent) tuberculin-sensitive patients after three to four months. (In Finland, immunity to tuberculosis is high, since 95 per cent of babies are vaccinated against tuberculosis.)

Bunney MH, Nolan MW, Buxton PK, Going SM, Prescott RJ: The treatment of resistant warts with intralesional bleomycin: A controlled clinical trial. Br J Dermatol 111:197–207, 1984.

Fresh **bleomycin sulfate** (0.1 per cent in normal saline, 5 mg/5 ml) injected intralesionally every three weeks (up to 0.2 ml, one to three treatments) gave a cure rate of 76 per cent in a double-blind controlled study with matched pairs of hand warts. The authors preferred a tuberculin syringe with a 25-gauge Luer needle. Injection should blanch the wart. Expect moderate pain, usually well tolerated, for 48 hours. The solution is stable in glass (but not plastic) at 4°C for 60 days, but watch out for contamination.

Shumer SM, O'Keefe EJ: Bleomycin in the treatment of recalcitrant warts. J Am Acad Dermatol 9:91–96, 1983.

Details on clearing 123 of 151 (81 per cent) warts in 40 patients by one or two biweekly intralesional injections of **bleomycin** (1 U/ml in normal saline, 0.2 to 1.0 ml per wart). Careful intralesional injection necessary to avoid local necrosis. Very painful for large plantar warts. Long-term safety not known.

Cure rates: periungual 94 per cent, plantar 60 per cent, others 95 per cent.

Munkvad M, Genner J, Staberg B, Kongsholm H: Locally injected bleomycin in the treatment of warts. Dermatologica 167:86–89, 1983.

With the jet injection technique, **bleomycin** was absolutely without effect.

Bauer DJ: Treatment of plantar warts with acyclovir. Am J Med 73(Suppl):313–314, 1982.

Case report of an 18-year-old woman with painful plantar warts of seven years' duration, indifferent to curettage, **salicylic acid**, formalin, cryotherapy, cauterization, excision, and reexcision. The warts cleared within a few months with **acyclovir** ointment 2.5 per cent (Zovirax) applied under cellophane occlusion every 48 hours.

Lockshin NA: Flat facial warts treated with fluorouracil. Arch Dermatol 115:929–930, 1979.

Dramatic example of a 28-year-old woman with an eight-year history of 300 asymptomatic flat facial warts that all disappeared after 21 days of 5 per cent **fluorouracil** cream twice a day. They had not recurred after six months. Four more patients had the same result.

LoCricchio J Jr, Haserick JR: Hot-water treatment for warts. Cleve Clin Q 29:156–161, 1962.

Convincing photos of the cure of warts on the feet, hands, and face in 9 of 15 patients by using water of 45°C (113 to 118°F) in a foot bath or wash basin for one hour twice a week for up to three months. Hyperemia occurred, but no blistering at this temperature (which is about as hot as can be tolerated).

Wyre HW, Stolar R: Extirpation of warts by a loop electrode and cutting current. J Dermatol Surg Oncol 3:520–522, 1977.

An even hotter treatment. They use a tungsten wire loop 0.25-inch (6.35 mm) in diameter, which may be used on any electrosurgical unit with cutting-current capability.

Hughes E, Marshall H, Mehlmauer M, Koch M, Whitaker K, Weinstein R: Human warts permanently removed by static electricity. Cutis 31:319–325, 1983.

Static electricity via spark discharge (tesla coil) moved over the entire wart surface for 15 seconds to 20 minutes once a week resulted in clearing in 13 of 16 (81 per cent) patients treated for two months.

Kent H: Warts and ultrasound. Arch Dermatol 100:79–81, 1969.

Only a 35 per cent cure rate in 1000 patients treated once a week for three months with a Burdick ultrasonic unit (1.5 w/sq cm for 15 minutes each time).

McBurney EI, Rosen DA: Carbon dioxide laser treatment of verrucae vulgares. J Dermatol Surg Oncol 10:45–48, 1984.

The 1984 bloodless eradication of warts: Cure rate of 81 per cent of recalcitrant warts on the hands and feet in 27 patients with a single laser treatment. Cure achieved in all others following one or two additional treatments. While no scarring was seen on the feet, atrophic scars occurred on the hands in 50 per cent of patients.

Stahl D, Veien NK, Wulf HC: Photodynamic inactivation of virus warts: A controlled clinical trial. Clin Exp Dermatol 4:81–85, 1979.

Not recommended: Only 5 of 65 cases cleared after eight weekly treatments consisting of UVA exposure following application of methylene blue (0.1 per cent in 80 per cent DMSO-20 per cent alcohol).

Macht SH, Cordero JM: Superficial radiotherapy of warts: Results of treating 531 warts. Radiology 122:231–232, 1977.

A retrospective questionnaire study of 360 patients who received a classic therapy now rarely used because of the hazards of radiation. The cure rate was 97 per cent in children under 12 and 79 per cent in patients over 25 years of age.

Moncada B, Rodriguez ML: Levamisole therapy for multiple warts. Br J Dermatol 101:327–330, 1979.

Levamisole (5 mg/kg given as 50-mg tablets on three consecutive days every two weeks) cured 17 of 22 patients (77 per cent) in a period of one to four months. Most patients had 12 cycles of therapy. Levamisole is a wide-spectrum antiparasitic drug that increases cellular immunity (not available in the United States).

Gross G, Pfister H, Hagedorn M, Stahn R: Effect of oral aromatic retinoid (Ro 10-9359) on human papilloma virus-2–induced common warts. Dermatologica 166:48–53, 1983.

The new retinoid (Tigason 1 mg/kg [not available in the United States]) induced rapid dramatic involution within 10 days of numerous large warts on the hands in an 81-year-old man with chronic lymphatic leukemia, treated for three months. On stopping of the drug, the warts returned full force within the following week. The drug appears to be more keratinocidal than virucidal and does not eliminate HPV-2 DNA.

Boyle J, Dick DC, Mackie RM: Treatment of extensive virus warts with etretinate (Tigason) in a patient with sarcoidosis. Clin Exp Dermatol 8:33–36, 1983.

Similar example in which massive warts on the hands could be eliminated with Tigason (100 mg/day for 1 month) only to recur with a maintenance dose of less than 30 mg/day. **Etretinate** may be of value in treating multiple warts associated with immunosuppression.

Sinclair-Gieben AHC, Chalmers D: Evaluation of treatment of warts by hypnosis. Lancet 2:480–482, 1959.

Suggestion during truly deep hypnosis that the warts on one side of the body would disappear was followed by unilateral cure in 9 of 10 patients. The "control" side showed no change.

Litt JZ: Don't excise—exorcise: Treatment for subungual and periungual warts. Cutis 22:673–676, 1978.

Apply specially labeled "wart tape" (Zonas adhesive tape) lengthwise to the finger. Draw a face on the tape, then wrap the finger with more tape. Remove in 6½ days. Reapply exactly the same way 12 hours later. See patient every 2 weeks for liquid phenol–nitric acid (1 drop phenol and 1 drop nitric acid) "cloud" treatment, which turns warts brown. Wart will be gone by the second or third visit. (No need for potatoes or a cemetery).

Smith EL: The occult removal of warts: A continuing practice. Int J Dermatol 18:89–91, 1979.

The common denominator in folklore therapy is faith, but the neurologic or hormonal mechanism remains completely unknown.

Howard WR, Garcia RL: Complications of wart therapy. J Assoc Mil Dermatol 9:12–13, 1983.

Rogues' gallery (in color) of adverse effects of overzealous treatment: Chemical burns, erosions, ulcers, scars, keloids, ectropion, permanent nail dystrophy.

Bunney MH, Nolan MW, Willians DA: An assessment of methods of treating viral warts by comparative treatment trials based on a standard design. Br J Dermatol 94:667–680, 1976.

Warts on the hand should be treated with **liquid N_2** every 2 to 3 weeks for a cure rate of 75 per cent. Treatment every 4 weeks dropped the cure rate to 40 per cent.

Nightly application of a **salicylic acid** paint (salicylic acid 1 part : **lactic acid** 1 part : flexible collodion 4 parts) was a satisfactory treatment for hand warts and plantar warts. The keratolytic acids remove infected cells and wart virus and provoke mild inflammation. (Duofilm = salicylic acid 16.7 per cent + lactic acid 16.7 per cent in flexible collodion.)

Hard core of resistant warts: common warts 30 per cent, simple plantar warts 20 per cent, mosaic plantar warts 50 per cent.

de Bersaques J: Vitamin A acid in the topical treatment of warts. Acta Derm Venereol 55(Suppl 74):169–170, 1975.

Concise review of the literature. **Vitamin A acid** ointment (0.1 to 0.3 per cent) for four to six weeks was good for seborrheic keratoses.

Verruca plana cleared in 1 to 11 weeks with these vitamin A acid preparations applied twice a day: 0.2 to 0.5 per cent in cold cream, 0.05 to 0.3 per cent solution.

Gollock JM, Slatford K, Hunter JM: Scissor excision of anogenital warts. Br J Vener Dis 58:400–401, 1982.

A 71 per cent success rate in 28 cases. Patients were hospitalized and treated while under general anesthesia in the lithotomy position. The affected areas were infiltrated with a saline-**adrenaline** solution (1 : 300,000) to separate the warts and control bleeding.

Gabriel G, Thin RNT: Treatment of anogenital warts: Comparison of trichloracetic acid and podophyllin versus podophyllin alone. Br J Vener Dis 59:124–126, 1983.

Weekly treatment in a double-blind study of 60 men with either a **trichloroacetic acid** (50 per cent)—**podophyllin** (25 per cent) mixture or podophyllin (25 per cent) alone showed no difference after 3 months. In both series, two of three were clear after six weeks, but only one of three was clear after three months. Warts persisting after six weeks were treated with either cryocautery or trichloroacetic acid (100 per cent).

von Krogh G: 5-Fluoro-uracil cream in the successful treatment of therapeutically refractory condylomata acuminata of the urinary meatus. Acta Derm Venereol 56:297–301, 1976.

Mucosal warts at the urinary meatus were cleared within three weeks in 13 of 14 cases by daily application of 5 per cent **5-FU** cream (Efudex). Dysuria (tolerable) occurred in 33 per cent. Perianal warts cleared in 43 per cent, but treatment was painful because of fissures and sores at the mucocutaneous junction.

Simmons PD, Langlet F, Thin RNT: Cryotherapy versus electrocautery in the treatment of genital warts. Br J Vener Dis 57:273–274, 1981.

No difference in 42 male patients after three months. Cryotherapy was more acceptable to patients.

Dodi G, Infantino A, Moretti R, Scalco G, Lise M: Cryotherapy of anorectal warts and condylomata. Cryobiology 19:287–288, 1982.

Freezing for 30 to 120 seconds (Frigitonics CM 73, nitrous oxide) cured 19 of 21 patients after an average of three treatments.

Abcarian H, Sharon N: Long-term effectiveness of the immunotherapy of anal condyloma acuminatum. Dis Colon Rectum 25:648–651, 1982.

A cure rate of 84 per cent in 200 patients (mainly male homosexuals) after use of autogenous vaccine made from 5 gm of wart. Subcutaneous injections of vaccine, 0.5 ml each, were given weekly for six weeks.

Vance JC, Bart BJ, Hansen RC, et al: Intralesional recombinant alpha-2 interferon for the treatment of patients with condyloma acuminatum or verruca plantaris. Arch Dermatol 122:272–277, 1986.

Although of no value in treatment of 100 patients with plantar warts. **alpha-2 interferon** (0.2 ml containing 10 IU intralesional injection, three times a week for three weeks) did produce complete clearing of condyloma acuminatum lesions in 16 of 30 patients.

Khawaja HT: Treatment of condyloma acuminatum. Lancet 1:208–209, 1986.

Comparative cure rates in 29 patients with first episode of condyloma acuminatum:

	at 6 weeks	***at 42 weeks***
Surgical excision	100%	81%
Podophyllin	77%	30%

Eighty-eight per cent of patients were satisfied with surgical treatment, while only 23% were satisfied with **podophyllin treatments.**

Silva PD, Micha JP, Silva DG: Management of condyloma acuminatum. J Am Acad Dermatol 13:457–463, 1985.

Podophyllin (10 to 25 per cent in tincture of benzoin applied by physician only, at weekly intervals up to three times, always washed off one to four hours after application) is an effective first-line therapy for external genital and perianal condyloma acuminatum. Do not use in vagina or on cervix, nor on infants or pregnant women.

Second-line therapy is trichloroaetic acid (50 per cent, one to three weekly applications).

Alternate approaches with cure rates of 90 per cent are:

1. Cryosurgery. (Nitrous oxide cryosurgical probe, moisten lesion with saline, freeze until entire lesion and 2 mm of surrounding skin is in ice ball.) If necessary, can retreat at one or two weeks for one or two more times.
2. Carbon dioxide laser photocoagulation (local or general anesthesia, with photocoagulation of several centimeters of surrounding normal-appearing skin). This laser method is the one of choice for extensive or giant lesions.

Article further details the specialized therapy for those who venture to treat condylomata of vagina, cervix, anorectal area, urethra, and mouth.

Jablonska S (ed): Warts/human papilloma viruses. Clin Dermatol 3(4):1–220, 1985

The last word!

Enter into your patient's delusion, but only as a visitor, not as a permanent resident.

Vitiligo

Fluorinated corticosteroids
Psoralen-sunlight
PUVA

There are few triumphs in the therapy of vitiligo, for the problem is a daunting one: completely mysterious, total destruction of all the pigment cells in the affected epidermis. Today's treatment centers on summoning functioning melanocytes from the unaffected hair bulbs in the dermis up into the epidermis. It is not successful if the hair bulb melanocytes have also been destroyed, as evidenced by the presence of white hair. Nor is it successful if there are no hair bulbs in the area, as in vitiligo of the vermilion border of the lips or the ends of the fingers.

Given pigmented hair bulbs, what is the signal that calls forth the long migration of melanocytes from the deep dermis into the epidermis? It is ultraviolet light, amplified by psoralens. The newly mobilized colonizers will not reach the epidermis and elaborate melanin in grossly visible amounts for several months. And initially, the pigment will only be punctate, that is, perifollicular. The patient expects uniformly gradually darkening repigmentation, but this does not occur. He must be instructed to take heart with the dotted color. These spots in turn will widen as the melanocytes migrate laterally. And all this will take several years of steady treatment. And in many it will never happen. Vitiligo is indeed a "bete blanche."

Despite all this, there is much that can be done. Our first effort is to rule out "chemical" vitiligo, i.e., destruction of the melanocyte by a contactant or inhalant. We explore exposure to rubber, plastics, and germicidal agents that contain a variety of depigmenting phenol derivatives. Elimination of these hazardous exposures is imperative.

Once certain that the problem is true idiopathic vitiligo, confirmed on occasion by biopsy and an epidermal dopa stain, we check for the presence of associated diseases, such as diabetes mellitus, thyroid disease, and pernicious anemia. We are then prepared to reassure and instruct the patient:

1. It is a cosmetic problem, not a sign of cancer or disease.
2. It is common; several million other Americans have it.
3. It is of unknown cause, but often is seen as a family trait.
4. It will not spontaneously go away, and medical treatment is not always effective.

We review with the patient the cosmetic options:
Covermark opaque makeup
Vitadye stain
Quick-tan preparations containing dihydroxyacetone

We stress the importance of staying out of the sun. Sunburn will induce new lesions as a Köbner's response (and so will scratches and abrasions). If avoiding the sun is not acceptable, we recommend the use of a sun screen, with a sun-protective factor (S.P.F.) of 15 (such as Solbar), to reduce tanning of the surrounding skin, which accentuates the whiteness of the vitiliginous sites.

For most pale-skinned individuals this is sufficient. For those who wish greater help, we prescribe Lidex cream (fluocinonide 0.05 per cent twice a day) to be applied precisely to the areas of vitiligo of most concern. This is done for two months. If no follicular dots of pigment are seen at that time, it is discontinued.

For the rare patient who has the drive and dedication to do everything possible, we prescribe 8-methoxypsoralen (20 to 30 mg to be taken orally two hours before graded high-noon sun exposure, three times a week). If this is not possible, we prescribe graded UVA exposures in our office or appropriate tanning centers. We explain:

1. UVA protective eyeglasses must be worn each day of psoralen therapy.
2. At least 40 treatments will be needed before any sign of response will be evident—and then only as dots.
3. Ultraviolet light exposure should keep the vitiligo areas pink, but not burned. The program must be kept up for about two years, and even then repigmentation will never be completely uniform and cosmetically perfect.
4. The possibility of no response is real.
5. Aspirin (5 grains tid) enhances repigmentation in some patients.

In the instance in which psoralen and sunlight or psoralen and UVA produce no pigment in four months, the patient is advised that if we cannot repigment, what we can do is depigment. In a few instances the cosmetic disfigurement is so marked that permanent removal of the melanocytes in the normal skin is acceptable. Again, here it takes months of topical Benoquin (20 per cent monomethyl ether of hydroquinone applied twice a day) to destroy the normal melanocyte and thereby produce an indistinguishable blend of idiopathic and "chemical" vitiligo. For this, it is well to have informed consent forms signed, since the MMEH, unlike hydroquinone, produces an irreversible lifetime loss of color.

It is evident that the intensive treatment of serious examples of vitiligo cannot be casual. Both the doctor and the patient need motivation to an uncommon degree. But few things are more gratifying to see than the light in these patient's eyes as the light disappears from their skin.

Klaus S, Lerner AB: Vitiligo. J Am Acad Dermatol 11:997–1000, 1984.

due to loss or destruction of melanocytes by an unknown factor
vitiligo present in 1 per cent of U.S. inhabitants
develops before the age of 20 years in half of the patients
no spontaneous remissions
no entirely safe or effective treatment available
therapy centers on:

- cosmetic cover
- steroid creams
- bleaching creams to reduce contrast with adjacent skin
- PUVA—but results partial and require several years

Naughton GK, Elsinger M, Bystryn J-C: Antibodies to normal human melanocytes in vitiligo. J Exp Med 158:246–251, 1983.

Most patients with active vitiligo, 82 per cent of 61, had circulating antibodies directed to a common antigen on normal human melanocytes. These antibodies were not found in 35 controls and were present in only 3 (12 per cent) of 24 patients with melanoma.

Nordlund JJ, Lerner AB: Vitiligo: It is important. Arch Dermatol 118:5–8, 1982.

These patients may have:

- antithyroid antibodies
- anti–smooth muscle antibodies
- anti–parietal cell antibodies
- antinuclear antibodies

These patients may have:

- multiple myeloma
- Hodgkin's disease
- thymomas
- mycosis fungoides
- dysgammaglobulinemia

Lerner AB: Vitiligo. J Invest Dermatol 32:285–310, 1959.

Familial incidence: 4 of 10.

Ortonne J-P, Mosher DB, Fitzpatrick TB: Vitiligo and Other Hypomelanoses of Hair and Skin. New York, Plenum Medical Book Co., 1983, 683 pp.

The ultimate reference source with more than 20 pages of treatment for vitiligo.

Before making a diagnosis of vitiligo, rule out chemically induced leukoderma from contact with:

- wire disk trays
- adhesive tape
- hat bands
- contraceptive diaphragms
- rubber finger cots
- rubber clothing
- rubber condoms
- rubber dolls
- neoprene (a synthetic rubber)
- fabric-lined rubber gloves
- shoes (rubber cement)
- insecticides
- deodorants
- detergents
- germicidal disinfectants
- writing ink
- latex adhesives
- fumigants

Mathias CGT, Maibach HI, Conant MA: Perioral leukoderma simulating vitiligo: From use of a toothpaste containing cinnamic aldehyde. Arch Dermatol 116:1172–1173, 1980.

Cinnamic aldehyde in a toothpaste used for two years proved to be the cause of loss of perioral pigment in a 25-year-old Oriental woman. The patch test site still showed depigmentation after three months. Elimination of the toothpaste was curative, with total return of pigment in six months.

Stevenson CJ: Occupational vitiligo: Clinical and epidemiological aspects. Br J Dermatol 105(Suppl 21):51–56, 1981.

Phenolic compounds are the major cause. These include:

- para-tertiary butyl catechol (TBC)
- para-tertiary butyl phenol (PTPB)
- para-tertiary amyl phenol (PTAP)
- monobenzyl ether of hydroquinone (MHQ)
- monomethyl ether of hydroquinone (MMEH)
- hydroquinone (HQ)

James O, Mayes RW, Stevenson CJ: Occupational vitiligo induced by p-tert-butylphenol, a systemic disease? Lancet 2:1217–1219, 1977.

Loss of pigment identical to vitiligo was seen in 54 of 198 men exposed to *p*-tert-butylphenol (PTBP) in the air in concentrations above 1 ppm. The occurrence of vitiligo was related to the duration and intensity of exposure to PTBP, which was probably absorbed through inhalation. This chemical is used in the production of resins for adhesives used in the car industry. There was no evidence of an autoimmune disturbance, but reversible liver damage occurred in six workers.

Kersey P, Stevenson CJ: Vitiligo and occupational exposure to hydroquinone from servicing self-photographing machines. Contact Dermatitis 7:285–287, 1981.

The contactant here was 7 per cent hydroquinone solution. A 54-year-old man who serviced black-and-white photography machines had no place to wash the material off his skin and "chemical" vitiligo of his hands, wrists, and mouth became evident after one year.

El Mofty AM, El Mofty ME: Vitiligo: A symptom complex. Int J Dermatol 19:237–244, 1980.

Vitiligo, which may begin simultaneously with metastasis of the tumor, develops in 20 per cent of all patients with malignant melanoma. (Be sure to check the entire skin of vitiligo patients.)

Todes-Taylor N, Abel EA, Cox AJ: The occurrence of vitiligo after psoralens and ultraviolet A therapy. J Am Acad Dermatol 9:526–532, 1983.

PUVA is a double-edged sword capable of both inducing and reducing vitiligo.

Zackheim HS, Epstein EH Jr, Grekin DA, McNutt NS: Mycosis fungoides presenting as areas of hypopigmentation: A report of three cases. J Am Acad Dermatol 6:340–345, 1982.

In a 30-year-old black man, an unsuspected microscopic focus of mycosis fungoides was found in a purely macular hypopigmented area previously treated as vitiligo.

Repigmentation was slowly achieved following daily applications of **carmustine** (BCNU 0.05 per cent in 95 per cent ethanol) for one month.

Rampertaap MP: Vitiligo-like syndrome following the use of fluphenazine enanthate. Mo Med 82:24–26, 1985.

The phenothiazine neuroleptic drug, **fluphenazine enanthate** (Prolixin 50 mg IM every two weeks + 10 mg orally tid), produced depigmented patches on the breasts, pubic area, and hands of a 44-year-old schizophrenic black woman. After stopping of the drug and switching to **thiothixene hydrochloride** (Navane), the skin repigmented in 2½ months.

Lane AT, Rasmussen JE, Stein DH: Meeting report: Society for Pediatric Dermatology, 1984. J Am Acad Dermatol 12:1115–1123, 1985.

Vitiligo treatment: Method of James J. Nordlund, M.D.

Trimethylpsoralen (Trisoralen 20 to 30 mg three times a week) followed in one to two hours by sunlight outdoors; must wear UVA-blocking glasses.

Rarely uses topical psoralen because of the hazard of blistering. If necessary, advises **methoxsalen** lotion (Oxsoralen lotion 0.01 per cent).

If no response, may permanently destroy melanocytes in the surrounding skin by months of topical **monobenzyl ether of hydroquinone** (Benoquin 20 per cent cream), which, unlike hydroquinone, is melanocidal.

Grimes PE, Minus HR, Chakrabarti SG, et al: Determination of optimal topical photochemotherapy for vitiligo. J Am Acad Dermatol 7:771–778, 1982.

Topical **8-methoxypsoralen** (8-MOP 0.1 to 1 per cent in Acid Mantle creme; or Oxsoralen 1 per cent 8-MOP lotion) coupled one hour later with UVA (0.25 joule/sq cm with increments, once a week for six months) resulted in total repigmentation in only 9 per cent of 69 black patients studied; 15 per cent had no repigmentation, and the rest showed varying degrees. A broad-spectrum **benzophenone** sun screen was used between UVA treatments. A phototoxic response preceded repigmentation in each instance.

Mosher DB, Parrish JA, Fitzpatrick TB: Monobenzylether of hydroquinone: A retrospective study of treatment of 18 vitiligo patients and a review of the literature. Br J Dermatol 97:669–679, 1977.

Among 8 of 18 severely affected vitiligo patients, complete permanent depigmentation was achieved with application of **monobenzyl ether of hydroquinone** (Benoquin 20 per cent twice a day for 10 months). For use only in persons over 40 years of age with disfiguring vitiligo involving more than half of the body.

Urbanek RW: Tar vitiligo therapy. J Am Acad Dermatol 8:755–756, 1983.

Topical **crude coal tar** (300 mg/ml, Zetar bath oil emulsion) applied by the physician every week, coupled with topical applications of **betamethasone 17-valerate** cream (Valisone 0.1 per cent cream twice a day) induced 50 per cent repigmentation in five months in all five subjects studied.

The literature shows that repigmentation may be induced also by UVL, x-ray, topical **nitrogen mustard**, **cyclophosphamide**, **clofazimine**, quinolines, **ACTH**, PUVA, topical steroids in DMSO, and intralesional injection of steroids.

Kumari J: Vitiligo treated with topical clobetasol propionate. Arch Dermatol 120:631–635, 1984.

Intermittent topical applications of the steroid **clobetasol propionate** (0.05 per cent in 50 per cent isopropyl alcohol applied twice a day for two months, maximum of four courses over a 3-year period) achieved 90 to 100 per cent repigmentation in 80 per cent of patients with vitiligo of the face. Only 40 per cent of patients with vitiligo elsewhere attained this degree of repigmentation. A total of 75 patients was studied, with each course of treatment being two months only. Repigmentation was not seen until one to four months after starting treatment. Eyelids were treated with clobetasol propionate (0.05 per cent in a paraffin base twice a day) which is not irritating to the eyes.

Tsuji T, Hamada T: Topically administered fluorouracil in vitiligo. Arch Dermatol 119:722–727, 1983.

In 28 patients, vitiligo lesions were lightly epidermally abraded with either sandpaper or an electric rotary grinder following local anesthesia. They were then treated with 5 per cent **fluorouracil** cream (Efudex applied once daily under continuous polyethylene-occlusive dressing, for seven to nine days). Treatment was stopped when the sites were completely eroded. The treatment spots in 18 patients showed nearly complete repigmentation, while in 5 patients there was no response. The hyperpigmentation induced initially usually lightened to normal with time, although uneven repigmentation remained in some patients, particularly near the joints.

Imamura S, Tagami H: Treatment of vitiligo with oral corticosteroids. Dermatologica 153:179–185, 1976.

Of 17 patients with generalized vitiligo 6 showed more than 75 per cent repigmentation in at least one patch following **prednisolone** (5 mg, three to five times daily for three months, then 2.5 to 5 mg/day for three months). Repigmentation became evident in one month and was most striking in exposed areas.

Hernández-Pérez E: Vitiligo treated with ACTH. Int J Dermatol 18:578–579, 1979.

Of 20 patients with extensive vitiligo 6 had repigmentation after 15 weeks of **ACTH** gel (40 mg IM twice weekly for five weeks, rest five weeks, then repeat for five weeks), but depigmentation recurred when treatment was stopped.

Koga M: Vitiligo: A new classification and therapy. Br J Dermatol 97:255–261, 1977.

In 16 of 28 patients with dermatomally distributed vitiligo, the use of a monoamine oxidase inhibitor (**nialamide** 50 mg tid) to suppress catecholamine metabolism at autonomic nerve endings resulted in 50 per cent repigmentation. No improvement was seen in patients with nondermatomally distributed vitiligo. (Not available in the United States, but perhaps other monamine oxidase inhibitors can be considered: **isocarboxazid** [Marplan], **phenelzine sulfate** [Nardil], **tranylcypromine sulfate** [Parnate], and **pargyline hydrochloride** [Eutonyl Filmtab].)

Falabella R: Repigmentation of segmental vitiligo by autologous minigrafting. J Am Acad Dermatol 9:514–521, 1983.

Cosmetic success was achieved in three adolescent patients with segmental vitiligo by placing hundreds of 1-mm punch grafts 5 mm apart in areas of vitiligo. Best results were seen after one to two years. Approximately 50 to 100 minigrafts were harvested at each session from donor sites in the gluteal or inner arm areas. After transplantation, firm pressure was applied with Telfa and gauze dressings covered with micropore tape, left in place for 15 days.

Gopinathan T: A study of the lesion of vitiligo. Arch Dermatol 91:397–404, 1965.

Epidermodermal trauma via linear scarification of totally uninvolved skin resulted in local depigmentation in 5 of 13 subjects with vitiligo. Epidermal trauma alone via tape stripping did not cause depigmentation.

Porter J, Beuf A, Nordlund JJ, Lerner AB: Personal responses of patients to vitiligo. The importance of the patient-physician interaction. Arch Dermatol 114:1384–1385, 1978.

Patients clearly need emotional support from physicians, since they may feel shame, embarrassment, depression, and anxiety about their disease.

The art of dermatologic therapy is in the restoration of the original cutaneous masterpiece.

White Sponge Nevus et al.

Penicillin

We have never seen a white sponge nevus or a golden tongue, but we would rather see than be one.

Alinovi A, Benoldi D, Pezzarossa E: White sponge nevus: Successful treatment with penicillin. Acta Derm Venereol 63:83–85, 1983.

Penicillin (1.2 million U IM every third day for one month) induced dramatic involution of a white sponge nevus in the oral mucosa of a 23-year-old medical student. The lesions had been present since infancy, and his mother and grandmother had similar growths. Prior treatment with **vitamin A** (one year), **nystatin** (two months), and **liquid nitrogen** had been unsuccessful. This report confirms the effectiveness of penicillin as previously recorded in two other patients with white sponge nevi.

"This treatment is based on practical experience without reference to scientific principles, but it seems to be the only available remedy." (And we sure will use it, if we ever see one!)

Rippon JW, Arnow PM, Larson RA, Zang MS: 'Golden Tongue' syndrome caused by *Ramichloridium schulzeri*. Arch Dermatol 121:892–894, 1985.

A patient with acute lymphocytic leukemia under chemotherapy developed a golden orange erosion on the tip of her tongue. Rapidly extending over the dorsum of the tongue, it was shown to be due to *R. schulzeri*, a fungus that grows on Sabouraud's agar as a golden orange colony.

The lesion healed in response to oral ketoconazole (200 mg bid for six days), although an additional course of intravenous amphotericin was given (0.5 mg/kg/day) for eight days.

Medical Care:
The better half is letting the patient know you care.
The other half is prescribing with care!

Xerosis

Superfatted soap	Aquasol A
Bath oil	Synalar ointment
Emollients	Lac-Hydrin

Dry skin is the bane of the atopic person and the aged. Industry has spawned scores of emollients, cold creams, lotions, bath oils, and soaps to respond to their needs, but still many patients need your dermatologic help.

For the atopic patient we prescribe Synalar ointment (0.025 per cent) to be applied to the worst areas after each shower. For the aged we recommend Eucerin, Complex 15, or Nutraderm (lanolin free) lotion applied sparingly each night over the entire skin. Other favorites are Acid Mantle creme, Curél, Mi Fine skin cream, and Moisturel. For dry, chapped hands, the best treatment we have found is Neutrogena hand cream. Keeping a humidifier in the bedroom in the winter is of proven worth as well. Both groups should bathe as infrequently as possible, sponging only the intertriginous areas on a daily basis. Indeed, we ask for a seven-day moratorium on bathing at the time of the first visit. We encourage "the Saturday night bath" only. Many will follow this advice once they feel the normal texture of their stratum corneum returning. We begrudgingly allow soap only sparingly, using Neutrogena dry skin soap or Oilatum soap. We do not recommend the use of bath oils for the elderly because of the hazard of slippery tubs. We do suggest Alpha Keri bath oil on a trial basis for others. Only once have we seen allergic contact dermatitis due to the dye in this product.

We often prescribe **vitamin A** (Aquasol A 50,000 U tid for two to three months), as it can have a profound effect on reversing the dryness. In the elderly, restoration of night vision and olfaction are pleasing dividends for these patients. In summary, we teach our xerotic patients that for the skin they'll love to touch, it's "an emollient and Aquasol A, but never a bath every day."

Pascher F: Cosmetic products for people with dry or oily skin. *In* Frost P, Horwitz SN (eds.): Principles of Cosmetics for the Dermatologist. St. Louis, C. V. Mosby Co., 1982, pp 297–301.

Dry skin may be due to a genetic trait, excessive cleansing, climate, or aging.

Treatment centers on:

controlling exposure to:
- hot water, detergents, soaps, lipid solvents

using superfatted soaps:
- Neutrogena dry skin soap, Cold Cream soap, Basis soap, Oilatum soap, or Dove bar.

possibly using cleansing lotion or cream in lieu of soap for dry facial skin:
- Deep Mist, combination skin cleanser (Allercreme), cold cream (USP)

using dispersible bath oils:
- Alpha Keri bath oil (soak for 20 minutes)

Idson B: Moisturizers, emollients, and bath oil. *In* Frost P, Horwitz SN (eds.): Principles of Cosmetics for the Dermatologist. St. Louis, C. V. Mosby Co., 1982, pp 37–40.

Low humidity in ambient air, household detergents, and mechanical abrasion all conspire to cause chapped, cracked, rough, reddened hands. The benefits derived from hand lotions are transient, but easily renewable by simply applying more.

Bath oils useful for lubricant effects come in three versions:

1. Dispersible oils:
   Mineral oil with emulsifiers give milky cloudiness to the bath water (Alpha Keri).
2. Floating or spreading oils:
   Mineral oil floats on the surface of the water in the tub, coating the patient's skin on emerging. These have low amounts of emulsifier.
3. Bath oil beads:
   Sodium hexametaphosphate (Calgon) beads are coated with oil that separates in the bath and rises to the surface. Milk solids are added to yield a "milk bath oil."

Frosch PJ: Irritancy of soaps and detergent bars. *In* Frost P, Horwitz SN (eds.): Principles of Cosmetics for the Dermatologist. St. Louis, C. V. Mosby Co., 1982, pp 5–12.

Using a chamber exposure test for erythema, scaling, and fissures on 10 subjects to test 12 soaps, the author found that the mildest soaps were Dove, Aveenobar, and Neutrogena, while the most irritating soaps were Zest, Lava, and Irish Spring.

Marks R: Methods to evaluate effects of skin surface texture modifiers. *In* Frost P, Horwitz SN (eds.): Principles of Cosmetics for the Dermatologist. St. Louis, C. V. Mosby Co., 1982, pp 50–58.

Products that cause "smoothing" and "softening" of the skin include:

Emollients, which act simply by hydrating the stratum corneum, and should be known as hydrating or moisturizing agents. Their effects are transient, rapidly altered, and reversible.

Keratolytics, which enhance desquamation of abnormal stratum corneum, probably through specific effects on intercellular cement substance within the stratum corneum. Their effects are slow and irreversible.

Wehr R, Krochmal L, Baqatell F, et al: A controlled two-center study of lactate 12 percent lotion and a petrolatum-based creme in patients with xerosis. Cutis 37:205–209, 1986.

Lac-Hydrin (**lactate 12 per cent** lotion) proved to be significantly better in relieving dry skin than a popular petrolatum-based creme. Seventy-three subjects participated in the study which involved twice daily applications for three weeks. The significant difference between products was seen at two weeks, and persisted for two weeks after therapy was discontinued.

Therapy is not what you do, but what you accomplish.

Yellow Nail Syndrome

Biotin	Corticosteroid injection
Vitamin E	Antibiotics
Stilbestrol	

A wonderful area for new therapeutic approaches from Aquasol A to zinc!

Venencie PY, Dicken CH: Yellow nail syndrome: Report of five cases. J Am Acad Dermatol 10:187–192, 1984.

All five men had yellow nails, primary lymphedema, and respiratory tract involvement, and four of the five had noted the onset after pneumonia. Two had bronchiectasis, two had chronic sinusitis, and one had chronic pleural effusion. Two experienced spontaneous improvement of their yellow nails.

Defective lymph drainage is thought to be the cause of the nail changes, consisting of slow growth, yellow or yellow green discoloration, overcurvature, thickening, cross-ridging, plate separation, shedding, and loss of lunulae and cuticles.

Maisels DO, Korachi AOA: Lymphoedema of the eyelids in the yellow nail syndrome. Br J Plast Surg 38:93–96, 1985.

Yellowing, hardening, and onychomadesis of the fingernails and toenails developed in a 27-year-old woman three months following a flulike illness that was accompanied by facial swelling. The swelling spread to the limbs and trunk and had persisted for more than 11 years. The eyelid lymphedema was severe enough to require excision and grafting.

Pavlidakey GP, Hashimoto K, Blum D: Yellow nail syndrome. J Am Acad Dermatol 11:509–512, 1984.

Yellow nail syndrome in a 61-year-old man cleared in nine months following treatment of *Proteus mirabilis* pulmonary infection with intensive long-term intravenous and oral antibiotic therapy. The authors completely review the literature, pointing out that the yellow nail syndrome usually occurs in relation to pulmonary problems, although it has been reported also with rheumatoid arthritis, nephrotic syndrome, thyroiditis, underlying malignant disease, mental retardation, Raynaud's disease, diabetes mellitus, penicillamine therapy, tuberculosis, and lichen planus.

Nelson LM: Yellow nail syndrome. Arch Dermatol 100:499–500, 1969.

Initiation of therapy for diabetes in a 36-year-old woman was associated with rapid improvement of her problem with slow-growing thick yellow nails.

Guin JD, Elleman JH: Yellow nail syndrome: Possible association with malignancy. Arch Dermatol 115:734–735, 1979.

Removal of a laryngeal carcinoma in a 65-year-old man was associated with clearing of his 20 yellow nails, beginning four to six weeks postoperatively.

Solal-Celigny P, Cormier Y, Fournier M: The yellow nail syndrome: Light and electron microscopic aspects of the pleura. Arch Pathol Lab Med 107:183–185, 1983.

In a 55-year-old man with recurrent pleural effusions, leg edema, and yellow dystrophic fingernails and toenails, a left parietal pleurectomy done to control the effusions led to clearing the fingernail changes.

Ayres S Jr, Mihan R: Yellow nail syndrome: Response to vitamin E. Arch Dermatol 108:267–268, 1973.

Vitamin E (d, alpha-tocopheryl acetate 400 IU bid) led to normal nails within 6½ months in a 65-year-old woman who had had thick yellow fingernails and toenails for 11 months. Noteworthy was the concomitant improvement in chronic bronchitis and chronic sinusitis.

Meiers HG, Greuel H, Perschmann U, et al: Skleronychie-syndrom (yellow nail syndrome): Skleronychie-lymphödem-atemwegsaffektionen. Dtsch Med Wochenschr 98:1829–1834, 1973.

The thick dystrophic and yellow nail changes in a 30-year-old woman totally disappeared after treatment with **biotin** (100 mg/day). Previous treatment with antifungal agents, radiation therapy, nail removal, **vitamin A**, and **L-cysteine** had had no effect.

The authors recommend treatment of underlying lymphedema with compressive support and diuretics, as well as treatment for respiratory tract infections.

Spontaneous remission after a course of many years has been observed in only 2 of 33 cases recorded in the literature.

Lebioda J, Budzanowska E: Zespol zoltych paznokci (The yellow nail syndrome). Przegl Dermatol 59:523–526, 1972.

A case is described in which edema of the face, legs, and knuckles developed simultaneously with yellow nails. Two series of treatments with **stilbestrol** (0.25 mg IM weekly for five weeks) produced a complete and permanent cure.

Abell E, Samman PD: Intradermal triamcinolone acetonide injection in the yellow nail syndrome. Trans St. John Hosp Dermatol 59:114–117, 1973.

Triamcinolone acetonide (5 mg/ml) injections of the posterior fingernail fold induced complete recovery in some or all yellow nails in 5 of 10 patients after five to nine months. Port-O-Jet injections delivered 0.1 ml, with two to four injections per nail given every two to four weeks for three times, then every six to eight weeks.

Baran R: Pigmentation of the nails (chromonychia). J Dermatol Surg Oncol 4:250–254, 1978.

Yellow nails may be the result of external contact with:

- dinitrotoluene
- fluorescein
- picric acid
- resorcin
- dinobuton
- insecticides
- weed killers
- red varnish

or internal "contact" with:

- quinacrine
- tetracycline

or:

- aging
- jaundice

Cohen SR: Yellow staining caused by 4,4′-methylenedianiline exposure: Occurrence among molded plastic workers. Arch Dermatol 121:1022–1027, 1985.

Nails, as well as hair and skin, became stained yellow by direct and airborne contact with this aromatic amine, also known as 4,4′-diaminodiphenylmethane, used as a curing agent in the manufacture of an expoxy-plastic. It is a potent contact allergen and possible photosensitizer and is available for routine patch testing. The cure lies in avoidance. It is a known hepatotoxin in man and a carcinogen in mice.

Norton L: Further observations on the yellow nail syndrome with therapeutic effects of oral alpha-tocopherol. Cutis 36:457–462, 1985.

Vitamin E (800 to 1200 IU/day for six months) therapy was associated with complete clearing of yellowing of nails in four of six patients.

The more tests you do on patients, the more patients you'll have to test.

A double-blind study finds out if a drug works in other *patients. Keeping your eyes wide open lets you see if it works in* your *patient.*

Z Last Notes

Alphabetized annotated references on additional diseases.

Acrokeratosis Paraneoplastica

Jacobsen FK, Abildtrup N, Laursen SO, et al: Acrokeratosis paraneoplastica (Bazex syndrome). Arch Dermatol 120:502–504, 1984.

This violaceous psoriasiform eruption of the ears, nose, and fingers heralded a lung tumor for over a year before it was detected in a 63-year-old man.

Bazex A, Griffiths A: Acrokeratosis paraneoplastica: A new cutaneous marker of malignancy. Br J Dermatol 102:301–306, 1980.

Classically, this eruption shows no response to antibiotics and topical steroids. The underlying neoplasm must be found and removed to cure the skin lesions.

Amyloidosis

Breathnach SM: The cutaneous amyloidoses: Pathogenesis and therapy. Arch Dermatol 121:470–473, 1985.

Treatment of primary systemic amyloidosis has included conjoint **melphalan-prednisone, colchicine, DMSO,** and peritoneal dialysis, but these do not halt the inexorable progression to cardiac and renal failure.

Atypical Mycobacterial Infection

Arai H, Nakajima H, Nagai R: *Mycobacterium marinum* infection of the skin in Japan. J Dermatol (Tokyo) 11:37–42, 1984.

Minocycline (Minocin) was the drug of choice in a study of 75 patients who acquired atypical mycobacterial infections from trauma associated with occupational fish handling or home aquaria. The average healing time was six weeks. **Rifampin, tetracycline,** and **doxycycline** (Vibramycin) are alternate drug choices. In some instances, thermotherapy or surgical excision was employed with success. This classic study points out that although *Mycobacterium marinum* was responsible for 82 per cent of the lesions, eight other species of mycobacteria accounted for the remainder.

Song M, Vincke G, Vanachter H, Benekens J, Achten G: Treatment of cutaneous infection due to *Mycobacterium ulcerans.* Dermatologica 171:197–199, 1985.

A large chronic ulcer of the foot, present for two years, healed only after unrelenting systemic antibiotic therapy for over one year. Topical treatment was limited to the dextran polymer Debrisan. Internal treatment was initiated with **co-trimoxazole** (Bactrim 80/400 mg bid). After three months **rifampin** (Rifadin 600 mg/day) was prescribed, and six months later **minocycline** (Minocin 100 mg/day) was given with the other two drugs for the final six months.

Basal Cell Nevus Syndrome

Cristofolini M, Zumiani G, Scappini P, et al: Aromatic retinoid in the chemoprevention of the progression of nevoid basal-cell carcinoma syndrome. J Dermatol Surg Oncol 10:778–781, 1984.

Tigason (1 mg/kg/day for five months) caused regression of 85 basal cell carcinomas in a 53-year-old woman. Persistent lesions were treated successfully with cryotherapy. The dose was gradually reduced to 0.25 mg/kg every other day over a four-month period.

New recurrences were first noted three months after the Tigason was discontinued, but these were less aggressive and easily cured with cryotherapy.

Bites and Stings

Ginsburg CM: Fire ant envenomation in children. Pediatrics 73:689–692, 1984.

Recommends local treatment: ice, compresses, and frequent cleansing to prevent secondary infection.

Rhoades RB, Schafer, WL, Schmid WH, et al: Hypersensitivity to the imported fire ant. J Allergy Clin Immunol 56:84–93, 1975.

In 49 patients, immediate angioedema and generalized urticaria followed stings of two South American species of fire ants, which now occupy 150 million acres in 13 southern states. A sterile pustule develops at the sting site within 24 hours (unique sting reaction in the United States). Immediate treatment included antihistamines, steroids, catecholamines, and general supportive measures. Hyposensitization with aqueous extracts (Greer Laboratory, Inc., Lenoir, NC) prevented systemic reactions in 9 of 10 patients who were subsequently stung.

Shelley WB, Shelley ED, Welbourn WC: Polypodium fern wreaths (Hagnaya): A new source of occupational mite dermatitis. JAMA 253:3137–3138, 1985.

Success in treating mite dermatitis rests on detecting and eliminating the cause. Call on both veterinarian and acarologist for help in surveying possible hideouts:

cheese	dogs	grain
dried fruit	cats	straw
oatmeal	rats	hay
bean paste	rabbits	feather pillows
	chickens	bird nests
	animals	dried vegetation
	birds	

Don't forget to check cerumen for ear mites in pets.

King LE, Rees RS: Treatment of brown recluse spider bites. J Am Acad Dermatol 14:691–692, 1986.

Based on observations in 31 patients with severe brown recluse spider bites (necrotic within 72 hours), they recommend:

Ice bags and elevation of the bite site
Erythromycin or cephalosporins to prevent secondary infection
Aspirin
Testing for hemolytic anemia and thrombocytopenia
Avoiding immediate surgical excision
Avoiding intralesional steroids

King LE Jr, Rees RS: Dapsone treatment of a brown recluse bite. JAMA 250:648, 1983.

A 27-year-old man with a large (32 × 14 cm) *Loxosceles reclusa* bite on the leg required hospitalization 48 hours after the bite. Treatment with **dapsone** (100 mg bid for 14 days), ice packs, and leg elevation rapidly reduced the pain, erythema, and induration and prevented cutaneous necrosis. For outpatient treatment of spider bites, they have successfully used lower doses of dapsone (50 to 100 mg daily) to prevent necrotic skin ulcers.

Powell RF, Palmer SM, Palmer CH, Smith EB: *Cheyletiella* dermatitis. Int J Dermatol 16:679–682, 1977.

The best treatment for an infested dog is daily 1 per cent **gamma benzene hexachloride shampoo** (Kwell) for one week.

Lockey RF: Management of anaphylactic reaction to bee sting. JAMA 251:2862, 1984.

An injection of **epinephrine** immediately following a bee sting is the preferred self-treatment for any patient with anaphylactic sensitivity to bee stings. Aerosol preparations, while convenient, provide a far lower dosage.

Any individual who experiences systemic reactions after Hymenoptera stings (bees, hornets, wasps, or yellow jackets) are candidates for venom extract immunotherapy. It is an extremely protective, life-saving measure.

Medleau L, Miller WH Jr: Flea infestation and its control. Int J Dermatol 22:378–379, 1983.

Fleas remain on the animal only at meal time, so that for every flea seen on the pet, there are 10 to 100 fleas in the environment.

To break the flea life-cycle, one must treat the homes, the pets, and the yard. Because the eggs are very resistant, and some stages of the life-cycle are months in length, treatment should be residual in effect and repeated periodically.

The use of foggers (insect bombs) is popular, since they are convenient and inexpensive. However, they fail to deliver adequate amounts of insecticide under baseboards and furniture. Professional help or a careful attack on all sites with a hand-held spray tank is the best.

The yard should be treated three times a week at two-week intervals (**carbonyl, malathion, diazesion**). *All* pets must be treated, since if one has fleas, all of them do. Flea collars are ineffective against high-density flea infestations, and flea shampoos remove fleas but have no residual effect. The correct approach is to use aerosol sprays every other day, or flea powder twice a week, or mists or dips once a week. Avoid strong insecticides on very young pets, since they can easily be poisoned.

The classic example of a quick-kill insecticide is **pyrethrin**. The best known residual insecticides are micro-encapsulated synergized pyrethrins, carbonyl, and malathion.

Bites—Animal

Tunnessen WW Jr: Practical aspects of bacterial skin infections in children. Pediatr Dermatol 2:255–265, 1985.

For dog and cat bites, administer the following prophylactic therapy for wounds to face, deep wounds of hands, or contaminated wounds:

Penicillin V to cover anaerobes, streptococci, and *Pasteurella multocida*.

Cephalosporin to eliminate *Staphylococcus aureus* and *Staph. epidermidis*.

Jaffu AC: Animal bites. Pediatr Clin North Am 30:405–413, 1983.

Meticulous wound toilet with copious irrigation.

Debride devitalized tissue.

No sutures if a hand wound.

No antibiotic until clinical signs of infection.

Dog bite: (*P. multocida* responsible for 50 per cent of infections)

℞: **Penicillin**

Human bite:

℞: **Erythromycin** or Keflex

Consider the possibility of tetanus and rabies.

Burdge DR, Scheifele D, Speert DP: Serious *Pasteurella multocida* infections from lion and tiger bites. JAMA 253:3296–3297, 1985.

Penicillin G, cloxacillin sodium, and **gentamicin sodium** were given intravenously for three weeks to a young Masai warrior bitten by a lion. This was followed by oral penicillin G for an additional two weeks. Because he was unimmunized, both tetanus antitoxin and tetanus toxoid were given.

A second patient was an 11-year-old girl bitten on the neck by a children's zoo Bengal tiger. Within hours purulent meningitis developed, which responded to intravenous **penicillin G potassium, chloramphenicol sodium succinate,** and **gentamicin.** This was given for two weeks, since *P. multocida* was the only organism found in the blood and CSF cultures.

Bite wounds from any of the great cats must be considered to be deep and to be contaminated by *P. multocida,* since this is the most common pathogen found in cultures of the upper respiratory tracts of lions, tigers, panthers, leopards, and the small house pet cats.

Sensitivity tests reveal that penicillin G is the antibiotic of choice for treating infected wounds following scratch or bite wounds inflicted not only by the great cats but by the domestic cat at home.

Blastomycosis

Van Tyle JH: Ketoconazole: Mechanism of action, spectrum of activity, pharmacokinetics, drug interactions, adverse reactions, and therapeutic use. Pharmacotherapy 4:343–373, 1984.

Cites report of *Blastomyces dermatitidis* infection following a dog bite that was successfully treated with **ketoconazole** (at least 400 mg/day for six months).

Ketoconazole is now the treatment of choice for blastomycosis.

Bromoderma

Millns JL, Rogers RS III: Furosemide as an adjunct in the therapy of bromism and bromoderma. Dermatologica 156:111–119, 1978.

In a woman with pyoderma gangrenosum–like skin lesions, **furosemide** (Lasix 40 mg bid for 10 days) facilitated renal excretion of bromides she had taken for three years in the form of Miles Nervine tablets. Lactated Ringer's solution (4 to 6 liters/day) was also administered while she was in the hospital to mobilize the bromides. **Prednisone** (80 mg/day for 10 days) also aided in completely clearing the eruption in three weeks.

Carpet Beetle Dermatitis

Ahmed AR, Moy R, Bark R, Price Z: Carpet beetle dermatitis. J Am Acad Dermatol 5:428–432, 1981.

A 22-year-old man with a five-year history of recurrent urticarial and papulovesicular lesions was cured by fumigations of the house with **sulfuryl fluoride** (Vikane). He was proven, by intradermal testing, to be exquisitely sensitive to the carpet beetle larvae (*Anthrenus verbasci*) that had colonized the wool rug in his bedroom.

Cellulitis

Hurwitz RM, Tisserand ME: Streptococcal cellulitis proved by skin biopsy in a coronary artery bypass graft patient. Arch Dermatol 121:908–909, 1985.

Bed rest, **erythromycin** (333 mg tid), and 1 per cent **econazole nitrate** (Spectazole cream) gave complete clearing in 72 hours of a cellulitis that developed in the left leg two years after surgical removal of the saphenous vein. Significantly, the patient had tinea pedis, and the infected toe web most likely provided the portal of entry for streptococci into the skin with compromised venous circulation.

Tunnessen WW Jr: Practical aspects of bacterial skin infections in children. Pediatr Dermatol 2:255–265, 1985.

Chloramphenicol is suggested as the drug of choice for the initial treatment of facial cellulitis, since *Haemophilus influenzae* type b is often the cause. Penicillinase-resistant **penicillin** should be added to cover staphylococci and streptococci. In view of the high risk of meningitis or systemic infection, these children should be hospitalized for parenteral antibiotic therapy. Cultures of blood and CSF should be obtained along with cultures of an aspirate from the leading edge of the cellulitis.

The portal of entry gives clues for therapy.

1. Tooth abscess: anaerobic organisms responsive to penicillin.
2. Insect bites, laceration: *Staphylococcus aureus* and *Streptococcus pyogenes* responsive to semisynthetic penicillinase-resistant penicillin.
3. None evident: *H. influenzae* type b responsive to chloramphenicol (blood cultures positive in 15 of 38; edge aspirates positive in 7 of 17).

Chondrodermatitis Nodularis Helicis

Beck MH: Treatment of chondrodermatitis nodularis helicis and conventional wisdom? Br J Dermatol 113:504–505, 1985.

Betamethasone valerate 0.1 per cent (Valisone) and 3 per cent **clioquinol** proprietary cream applied twice daily completely cleared five patients of chondrodermatitis nodularis helicis within two to six weeks. It is suggested that first-line treatment should not be surgical, but topical.

Chromomycosis

Van Tyle JH: Ketoconazole: Mechanism of action, spectrum of activity, pharmacokinetics, drug interactions, adverse reactions, and therapeutic use. Pharmacotherapy 4:343–373, 1984.

Of 31 patients with chromomycosis (chromoblastomycosis), 77 per cent experienced moderate to marked improvement or clinical cure when given oral **ketoconazole** (Nizoral 200 to 800 mg daily for one to four months). In case of failure, conjoint therapy with **5-flucytosine** (Ancobon) is indicated.

Tagami H, Ginoza M, Imaizumi S, et al: Successful treatment of chromoblastomycosis with topical heat therapy. J Am Acad Dermatol 10:615–619, 1984.

Five patients with localized chromoblastomycosis were completely cured solely by prolonged topical application of tolerable heat from pocket warmers. The lesions involuted in a median time of three months and did not recur.

Coccidioidomycosis

Van Tyle JH: Ketoconazole: Mechanism of action, spectrum of activity, pharmacokinetics, drug interactions, adverse reactions, and therapeutic use. Pharmacotherapy 4:343–373, 1984.

Of 307 patients with coccidioidomycosis, 266 (87 per cent) reported in the literature were either cured or markedly improved with **ketoconazole** therapy. Oral ketoconazole (400 to 800 mg/day for three months to two years) has replaced **amphotericin B** as the treatment of choice for coccidioidomycosis.

Cold Agglutinin Acrocyanosis

Shelley WB, Shelley ED: Acrocyanosis of cold agglutinin disease successfully treated with antibiotics. Cutis 33:556–557, 1984.

Penicillin V potassium (Pen Vee K 500 mg qid) in one case and **cephradine** (Velosef 250 mg qid) in another resulted in complete clearing of tender red to bluish toes. Both patients had low-titer cold agglutinins.

Confluent and Reticulated Papillomatosis (Gougerot-Carteaud)

Friedman SJ, Albert HL: Confluent and reticulated papillomatosis of Gougerot and Carteaud: Treatment with selenium sulfide lotion. J Am Acad Dermatol 14:280–281, 1986.

Selenium sulfide lotion (Selsun, Exsel 2.5 per cent at bedtime for five weeks) cleared skin lesions on the neck, trunk, and axillae of a 22-year-old black male. Recurrence of lesions three months after stopping treatment was again controlled by focal application of the selenium sulfide lotion.

Bruynzeel-Koomen CAFM, de Wit RFE: Confluent and reticulated papillomatosis successfully treated with the aromatic etretinate. Arch Dermatol 120:1236–1237, 1984.

Oral **etretinate** (50 mg/day) produced marked improvement within one month in a 25-year-old man with Gougerot-Carteaud papillomatosis of one year's duration. It was not possible to reduce the dose below 35 mg/day without exacerbation. **Tretinoin** ointment (0.1 per cent daily) had failed to produce any change.

Nagy R, Fairfield JC: Confluent and reticulated papillomatosis. Cutis 29:48–50, 1982.

Tretinoin gel (Retin-A 0.01 per cent) and **urea cream** (10 per cent) were two topical agents of value in treating the papillomatosis of Gougerot and Carteaud in two patients.

Cowden's Syndrome

Lazar AP, Lazar P: Cowden's disease (multiple hamartoma and neoplasia syndrome) treated with isotretinoin. J Am Acad Dermatol 14:142–144, 1986.

Isotretinoin (Accutane 40 mg daily for 152 days) produced "remarkable improvement" in the papillomatous growths on the face and oral mucosa of a 55-year-old woman. Discontinuation of treatment was followed by the return of all skin lesions three months later.

Cryptococcosis

Baes H, Van Cutsem J: Primary cutaneous cryptococcosis. Dermatologica 171:357–361, 1985.

Ketoconazole (200 mg bid for three months) cured a severe *Cryptococcus neoformans* infection of the wrist in a 53-year-old corticosteroid-immunosuppressed patient. Previously, therapy for this disease was limited to IV **amphotericin B,** IV **miconazole,** or massive oral doses of **flucytosine** (Ancobon).

Delusions of Dermatosis

Koblenzer CS: The dysmorphic syndrome. Arch Dermatol 121:780–784, 1985.

Haloperidol (Haldol 1 mg bid indefinitely) is valuable treatment for patients with the dysmorphic syndrome (delusions of offensive odors, facial distortions, "holes" in the skin, intense burning sensations of the tongue, scalp, or vulva, or all-consuming attention to changes in the skin perceived by them alone). Alternately, the tricyclic antidepressant **amitryptyline hydrochloride** (Elavil ascending dose to 100 mg/day) is valuable, but all of these patients need symptomatic treatment. None can imagine that their problems are imaginary!

The patient reported in this detailed review of 18 examples was a 49-year-old woman who complained of pain and facial contour changes. During 4½ years she had seen 60 physicians representing 12 different specialties, and had spent over $12,000 on a dozen classes of drugs in a fruitless search for relief. Haloperidol resulted in slow, steady improvement within six weeks, but the drug had to be taken indefinitely to prevent relapse.

(We call this condition delusions of dermatosis (the DOD syndrome) and prescribe **pimozide** (Orap 2 mg tid), but patient compliance is poor. These individuals are generally reluctant to relinquish the delusion. They dread the drug more than the disease!)

Dermatitis

ORDER OF POTENCY OF TOPICAL STEROID PREPARATIONS

Group*	Brand Name		Generic Name
I	Diprolene cream	0.05%	Betamethasone dipropionate
	Diprolene ointment	0.05%	Betamethasone dipropionate
	Temovate cream	0.05%	Clobetasol propionate
	Temovate ointment	0.05%	Clobetasol propionate
II	Cyclocort ointment	0.1%	Amcinonide
	Diprosone ointment	0.05%	Betamethasone dipropionate
	Florone ointment	0.05%	Diflorasone diacetate
	Halog cream	0.1%	Halcinonide
	Lidex cream	0.05%	Fluocinonide
	Lidex gel	0.05%	Fluocinonide
	Lidex ointment	0.05%	Fluocinonide
	Maxiflor ointment	0.05%	Diflorasone diacetate
	Topicort cream	0.25%	Desoximetasone
	Topicort ointment	0.25%	Desoximetasone
III	Aristocort cream	0.5%	Triamcinolone acetonide
	Diprosone cream	0.05%	Betamethasone dipropionate
	Florone cream	0.05%	Diflorasone diacetate
	Kenalog ointment	0.5%	Triamcinolone acetonide
	Maxiflor cream	0.05%	Diflorasone diacetate
	Valisone ointment	0.1%	Betamethasone valerate
IV	Aristocort ointment	0.1%	Triamcinolone acetonide
	Benisone gel	0.025%	Betamethasone benzoate
	Cordran ointment	0.05%	Flurandrenolide
	Cyclocort cream	0.1%	Amcinonide
	Fluonid ointment	0.025%	Fluocinolone acetonide
	Kenalog ointment	0.1%	Triamcinolone acetonide
	Synalar ointment	0.025%	Fluocinolone acetonide
	Topicort LP cream	0.05%	Desoximetasone
	Uticort gel	0.025%	Betamethasone benzoate
V	Aristocort A cream	0.1%	Triamcinolone acetonide
	Cloderm cream	0.1%	Flurandrenolide
	Cordran cream	0.05%	Clocortolone pivalate
	Diprosone lotion	0.05%	Betamethasone dipropionate
	Fluonid cream	0.025%	Fluocinolone acetonide
	Kenalog cream	0.1%	Triamcinolone acetonide
	Kenalog lotion	0.1%	Triamcinolone acetonide
	Locoid cream	0.1%	Hydrocortisone butyrate
	Synalar cream	0.025%	Fluocinolone acetonide
	Synemol cream	0.025%	Fluocinolone acetonide
	Topicort LP	0.05%	Desoximetasone
	Tridesilon ointment	0.05%	Desonide
	Valisone cream	0.1%	Betamethasone valerate
	Valisone lotion	0.1%	Betamethasone valerate
	Westcort cream	0.2%	Hydrocortisone valerate
VI	Locorten cream	0.03%	Flumethasone pivalate
	Synalar solution	0.01%	Fluocinolone acetonide
	Tridesilon cream	0.05%	Desonide
VII	Hytone cream	1%	Hydrocortisone
	Hytone cream	2½%	Hydrocortisone

Courtesy of Richard B. Stoughton, M.D.

* Group I is the most potent; Group VII is the least potent. Preparations within each group have similar potency.

Diaper Dermatitis

Zimmerer RE, Lawson KD, Calvert CJ: The effect of wearing diapers on skin. Pediatr Dermatol 3:95–101, 1986.

Wet diapers induce skin wetness, which leads to undesirable skin property changes: increased coefficient of skin friction (thus abrasions are more damaging), and reduced barrier friction (more permeable to irritants). Skin wetness also promotes bacterial (and yeast) overgrowth. Cloth diapers produce wetter skin than disposable diaper material at equivalent loadings.

Jordan WE, Blaney TL: Factors influencing infant diaper dermatitis. In Maibach H, Boisits EK (eds): Neonatal Skin: Structure and Function. New York, Marcel Dekker, Inc., 1982, pp 205–221.

Since maceration leads to irritation, an infant's diaper ideally should be changed promptly once there has been passage of urine or feces. This challenge is not met, since mothers on an average make only five diaper changes a day. Newborns urinate more than 20 times a day, and one-year-olds average six to seven times a day.

In a study of 400 infants, increased bathing frequency and the use of a **zinc oxide**–based ointment significantly reduced the incidence and severity of diaper rash.

Boisits EK, McCormack JJ: Diaper dermatitis and the role of predisposition. In Maibach H, Boisits EK (eds): Neonatal Skin: Structure and Function. New York, Marcel Dekker, Inc., 1982, pp 191–204.

Zinc oxide paste prevents virtually all occlusion-induced hydration and irritation.

Dafforn-Ierodiaconou E: Greek babies bottoms. Br Med J 287:764, 1983.

Greek babies don't get diaper dermatitis because these infants are regularly cleansed by their mother who cradles them in her left arm while her right hand washes away dry urine, feces, and bacteria with a stream of warm tap water.

(With the experience of three babies born since this book was conceived, we can vouch for the Greek method.)

Dry Mouth

Tetrault GA, Weintraub M: How to handle drug related dry mouth. Drug Therapy 14:(Feb):159–166, 1984.

Increase fluid intake.

Use saliva substitute (**carboxymethyl cellulose** preparations):

Xero-Lube artificial saliva
Moi-Stir artificial saliva
Salivart synthetic saliva (aerosol, with no parabens)

Rule out: emotional disturbance, neurologic disease, aging, sarcoidosis, Sjögren's syndrome, and drugs, e.g., antidepressants, anticholinergics.

Xerostomia leads to gingivitis, periodontitis, caries, parotitis, and dysphagia.

Shearn MA: Sjögren's syndrome. Philadelphia, WB Saunders Co, 1971, pp 201–202.

To minimize the pain, dysphagia, and difficulty in speaking that comes with xerostomia:

1. Avoid dehydration:
   Drink large amounts of water with meal.
   Sip water all day.

2. Suck on hard candy.
3. Maintain immaculate dental hygiene: Treat any infections.
4. Remove calculi of major salivary ducts.
5. Avoid drugs that dry the mouth (decongestants, antihistamines, atropine).
6. Sialogogues are of no real benefit.

Ehlers-Danlos Syndrome

Brighton P: The Ehlers-Danlos syndrome. London, William Heinemann Medical Books, Ltd., 1970.

Avoid trauma.

Wounds: Best treated by strapping rather than suturing.
Hematomas: Compression pad; may need aspiration.
Surgery: Meticulous, carefully layered suture closure.

Enterostomy Dermatitis

Rodriquez JT, Huang TL, Ferry GD, et al: Treatment of skin irritation around enterostomies with cholestyramine ointment. J Pediatr 88:659–661, 1976.

Cholestyramine ointment (Questran 20 per cent in aquaphor) gave rapid relief in eight patients with inflammation of the skin around the stoma.

Cola B, Farella S, Bacalini GC, et al: Le dermatiti peristomali: Considerazioni eziopatogenetiche, cliniche e terapeutiche a prosposito di 102 casi. Minerva Chir 36:1565–1570, 1984.

The three causes of enterostomy dermatitis in 102 patients were fecal contamination of the skin, trauma from the prosthesis, and sensitization to the prosthesis or its glue. Secondary bacterial and yeast infections also required attention.

Erythema Dyschromicum Perstans

Novick NL, Phelps R: Erythema dyschromicum perstans. Int J Dermatol 24:630–633, 1985.

Reassure the patient as to benign nature of the problem, but make no therapeutic promises. Treatment has been uniformly unsuccessful in halting progress or in reversing hyperpigmentation. The modalities that have failed include avoidance of sun exposure, sun blocking agents, chemical peels, antibiotics, oral and topical corticosteroids, vitamins, chloroquine, griseofulvin, and DMSO.

Erythema Elevatum Diutinum

Kohler IK, Lorincz AL: Erythema elevatum diutinum treated with niacinamide and tetracycline. Arch Dermatol 116:693–695, 1980.

Niacinamide (Nicotinamide 100 mg tid) and **tetracycline hydrochloride** (250 mg qid) for four weeks healed the painful papules in a 60-year-old woman who had failed to respond to dexamethasone and erythromycin.

Katz SI, Gallin JI, Hertz KC, et al: Erythema elevatum diutinum: Skin and systemic manifestations, immunologic studies, and successful treatment with dapsone. Medicine 56:443–455, 1977.

A detailed study of four patients who responded dramatically within two days of starting **dapsone** (50 to 300 mg daily). However, the skin lesions and systemic complaints recurred within 12 to 48 hours after discontinuing the dapsone. Long-term maintenance dosage schedules were established by trial.

Erythrasma

Habif TP: Clinical Dermatology: A Color Guide to Diagnosis and Therapy. St. Louis, CV Mosby Company, 1985, pp 214–215.

Erythrasma responds equally well to either oral **erythromycin** (250 mg qid for two weeks) or topical erythromycin (A/T/S, EryDerm, Staticin bid for two weeks). (An alternate is Achromycin ointment.)

Raab WPE: The treatment of mycosis with imidazole derivatives. New York, Springer-Verlag, 1980, p 122.

Erythrasma responds well to **econazole**. In one series 23 of 25 cases were cured by the topical application of econazole nitrate cream (Spectazole 1 per cent cream).

Erythroplasia of Queyrat

Sonnex TS, Ralfs IG, DeLanza MP, Dawber RPR: Treatment of erythroplasia of Queyrat with liquid nitrogen cryosurgery. Br J Dermatol 106:581–584, 1982.

Owing to its location and its nature, erythroplasia of Queyrat (Bowen's disease of the glans penis) calls for a treatment that is destructive of all tumor tissue yet cosmetically reasonable. Prior mutilating procedures (phallectomy, curettage and electrosurgery, wide local excision) have been replaced by local applications of 5 per cent **5-fluorouracil** cream (Efudex). The current report is a cure in two patients following cryosurgery (two freeze cycles with a five-minute thaw interval).

Fatty Acid Deficiency Dermatitis

Press M, Hartop PJ, Prottey C: Correction of essential fatty acid deficiency in man by the cutaneous application of sun-flower seed oil. Lancet 1:597–599, 1974.

Cutaneous application of sunflower seed oil (230 mg of oil daily for 12 weeks, containing 120 mg of the essential fatty acid linoleic acid), restored normal skin and serum fatty acid levels in three patients. They had developed a dry, scaly rash and drop in serum essential fatty acids from malnutrition associated with a low-fat diet, prescribed to prevent postoperative diarrhea.

Follicular Dermographism

Shelley WB, Shelley ED: Follicular dermographism. Cutis 32:244–245, 1983.

Follicular dermographism, reproducible by rubbing the skin with a tongue blade, showed an excellent immediate response to **hydroxyzine hydrochloride** (Atarax 25 mg at bedtime) in four patients.

Frostbite

McCauley RL, Hing DN, Robsen MC, et al: Frostbite injuries: A rational approach based on the pathophysiology. J Trauma 23:143–147, 1983.

1. Rapid rewarming in warm water (104 to 108°F) for 15 to 30 minutes. Not done if frostbite is over 24 hours old.
2. Debride bullae unless hemorrhagic and apply aloe vera (Dermaide Aloe) every six hours.
3. Elevate affected parts with splinting as indicated.
4. Tetanus prophylaxis.
5. **Morphine** or Demerol IV or IM, as indicated.
6. **Aspirin** (5 grains every six hours for three days.)
7. **Penicillin** (500,000 U q6h IV) until edema resolves.
8. Daily hydrotherapy.

Christenson C, Stewart C: Frostbite. Am Fam Physician 30:111–122, 1984.

1. No smoking, to prevent nicotine vasospasm.
2. High-calorie, high-protein diet.
3. If lower extremity injury, use wheelchair or litter. Shower in sitting position.
4. Whirlpool bid with **povidone-iodine** (Betadine) solution.
5. Wound care:

   Lower extremity:
   Feet to air under sheet cradle
   Cotton between digits
   Stockinette cover
   Elevate foot of bed
   Buerger's exercises (20 minutes qid)

   Upper extremity:
   Elevate hands with pillow
   Stockinette covering
   Constant digital exercises while awake
   Plastic mitten or bag for bowel care, oral hygiene, and shaving
6. Medication
   Phenoxybenzamine (Dibenzyline 10 mg daily for 10 days)
   Tetanus booster as indicated
   Propoxyphene napsylate (Darvocet-N 100 q4h prn) for pain
   Diazepam (Valium 5 mg q6h for three days) for anxiety
   Temazepam (Restoril 15 to 30 mg at bedtime prn) for sleep

Glossitis

Perry HO, Deffner NF, Sheridan PJ: Atypical gingivostomatitis: Nineteen cases. Arch Dermatol 107:872–878, 1973.

Discontinuance of both gum chewing and dentifrices resulted in resolution of glossitis in 12 of 19 patients. The glossitis was reproduced in each of the 12 by chewing gum challenges, with Doublemint accounting for 8 of the reactions. Patch tests did not prove to be a reliable method of identifying the cause.

Gooseflesh

Green JB: Pilomotor seizures. Neurology 34:837–839, 1984.

Two cases of episodic widespread gooseflesh were shown to be due to a glioblastoma of the right hemisphere. Palliative surgery was followed by a reduction in severity of attacks.

Green Hair

Person JR: Green hair: Treatment with a penicillamine shampoo. Arch Dermatol 121:717–718, 1985.

Green hair from exposure to copper salts in tap water or copper algicides in swimming pools can be restored to its normal color by shampooing a few times with **penicillamine shampoo** (penicillamine 250 mg in 5 ml water and 5 ml shampoo).

Alternatively, one could use a shampoo to which **EDTA** has been added. The patient described had shown no change in her green hair following H_2O_2 rinses and hot vegetable oil treatments.

Grover's Disease

Helfman RJ: Grover's disease treated with isotretinoin. J Am Acad Dermatol 12:981–984, 1985.

Isotretinoin (13-cis-retinoic acid, Accutane 40 mg/day) induced dramatic remission within two to four weeks in four patients. In three of the four treated for two to four months, there was no relapse in ten months after stopping the therapy.

Harlequin Fetus

Lawlor F, Peiris S: Harlequin fetus successfully treated with etretinate. Br J Dermatol 112:585–590, 1985.

Etretinate (1 mg bid) plus careful control of fluid balance, caloric intake, and ambient temperature and humidity proved lifesaving for this infant who was five months of age at the time of reporting.

Henoch-Schöenlein Purpura

Heng MCY: Henoch-Schöenlein purpura. Br J Dermatol 112:235–240, 1985.

The treatment of choice in severe cases is plasmapheresis, which removes the IgA immune complexes causing vascular blockade and infarcts.

For less threatening cases **dapsone** and **corticosteroids** may be helpful. Cytotoxic drugs are indicated if there is an underlying lymphoma.

In all instances, there must be an intense continuing search for any causal antigen or underlying disease which can be eliminated.

Look for the following:

Streptococcal infection
Bacterial infections, e.g., yersiniosis
Viral infections, e.g., varicella
Food sensitivity
Drug sensitivity, e.g., ampicillin, penicillin, erythromycin, quinidine
Lymphomas
Cancer of the colon, bronchi, prostate

This unique IgA vasculitis is not always a simple palpable purpura. It may strike the kidney (accounts for as many as 15 per cent of children in renal dialysis for end-stage kidney failure), the gastrointestinal tract (intestinal infarction and perforation), the nervous system (Guillain-Barré syndrome, mononeuropathies), or even the heart (coronary infarct). Sixty-nine references add to the value of this excellent précis of our current knowledge.

Histiocytosis

Monk BE, McKee PH, du Vivier A: Histiocytosis X of the scalp and face responding to topical nitrogen mustard. J R Soc Med 78(Suppl 11):6–7, 1985.

In a 23-year-old man, **topical nitrogen mustard** (20 per cent in aqueous solution, applied daily for six months) resulted in complete clinical clearing of localized histiocytosis of the scalp and face of five years' duration. The treatment has continued for over 1.5 years, since relapse invariably occurs when treatment is stopped.

Roper SS, Spraker MK: Cutaneous histiocytosis syndromes. Pediatr Dermatol 3:19–30, 1985.

A review with 88 references.

Although immunosuppressive drugs currently offer the greatest hope of survival, **prednisone** alone may result in complete clearing or a temporary remission.

Consider using **nitrogen mustard, chlorambucil, cyclophosphamide, methotrexate, 6-mercaptopurine, vinblastine,** or **vincristine**.

Histoplasmosis

Hawkins SS, Gregory DW, Alford RH: Progressive disseminated histoplasmosis: Favorable response to ketoconazole. Ann Intern Med 95:446–449, 1981.

Ketoconazole (200 to 400 mg daily for one year) produced improvement in four patients with disseminate histoplasmosis, two of whom had late relapses after treatment with **amphotericin B**. Particularly noteworthy was the resolution of oral ulcers observed in two patients.

Van Tyle JH: Ketoconazole: Mechanism of action, spectrum of activity, pharmacokinetics, drug interactions, adverse reactions and therapeutic use. Pharmacotherapy 4:343–373, 1984.

In 53 cases of disseminated histoplasmosis reported in the literature, **ketoconazole** (200 to 400 mg for 6 to 12 months) was 80 to 90 per cent efficacious.

Hypereosinophilic Syndrome

Shelley WB, Shelley ED: Erythema annulare centrifugum as the presenting sign of the hypereosinophilic syndrome: Observations on therapy. Cutis 35:53–55, 1985.

Therapy for the hypereosinophilic syndrome centers on **prednisone** and **hydroxyurea,** always with an attempt to find an underlying tumor or other cause.

In the patient reported here, the urticarial presentation of the hypereosinophilic syndrome cleared after one month of conjoint **dapsone** (100 mg/day), **ketoconazole** (Nizoral 200 mg/day), and **trimethoprim-sulfamethoxazole** (Bactrim DS 1 tablet at bedtime).

Nir MA, Westfried M: Hypereosinophilic dermatitis: A distant manifestation of the hypereosinophilic syndrome with response to dapsone. Dermatologica 162:444–450, 1981.

Dapsone (100 mg/day) rapidly cleared the pruritic papules of a 24-year-old Puerto Rican with an 18 per cent blood eosinophilia.

Hyperkeratosis

Kuokkanen K, Alavaikko M, Pitkanen R: Hyperkeratosis lenticularis perstans (Flegel's disease). Acta Derm Venereol 63:357–360, 1983.

The aromatic retinoid **Ro 10-9359** (Tigason 0.4 mg/kg/day) had to be taken indefinitely to maintain the excellent response seen with 0.8 mg/kg/day in one patient with these small horny papules of the legs.

Kuhlman DS, Hodge SJ, Owen LG: Hyperkeratosis of the nipple and areola. J Am Acad Dermatol 13:596–598, 1985.

Salicylic acid gel 6 per cent (Keralyt gel applied daily) induced resolution in one week and in two months, respectively, in two elderly men who had suffered from progressive thickening of the nipples and areolae.

Gibbs RC, Boxer MC: Abnormal biomechanics of feet and their cause of hyperkeratosis. J Am Acad Dermatol 6:1061–1069, 1982.

For those who fail to respond to a pad under the medial aspect of the sole, osteotomy may be helpful in restoration of an asymptomatic foot, free of hyperkeratoses.

Ingrown Toenails

Fishman, HC: Practical therapy for ingrown toenails. Cutis 32:159–160, 1983.

Insert a cotton wick saturated with **tincture of iodine** into the affected sulcus, separating the nail plate from the skin. Any granulation tissue is treated with a cotton applicator saturated with 50 per cent silver nitrate solution.

Prior treatments listed include a dozen surgical variations on removal of the nail plate, nail bed, or matrix.

Kaposi's Sarcoma of AIDS

Cooper JS, Fried PR, Laubenstein LJ: Initial observations of the effect of radiotherapy on epidemic Kaposi's sarcoma. JAMA 252:934–935, 1984.

Radiotherapy (total dose 1800 to 3000 cGy) induced complete involution in 12 of 17 lesions of Kaposi's sarcoma in 15 patients with acquired immune deficiency syndrome (AIDS). The other five lesions showed partial regression. This response, similar to that long known to occur in the classic form of the disease, occurred during or within weeks to months after the modest doses of radiation.

Keratoacanthomas

Haydey RP, Reed ML, Dzubow LM, et al.: Treatment of keratoacanthomas with oral 13-cis-retinoic acid. N Engl J Med 303:560–562, 1980.

13-cis-retinoic acid (Accutane 2 mg/kg/day) completely prevented the appearance of new keratoacanthomas in a 43-year-old man who had been developing them since he was seven years old. Nothing used previously had blocked this neoplastic cascade of new tumors which eventually confined him to a wheelchair. After the retinoid therapy and surgery of the remaining lesions, the patient returned to a normal life, which included soccer playing.

Other reported successful treatments are **methotrexate IM,** systemic **etretinate, podophyllin,** intralesional **bleomycin,** intralesional or topical **fluorouracil,** radiation, curettage and desiccation, laser treatment, and wide excision.

Keratoderma

Tan OT, Sarkany I: Severe palmar keratoderma in myxoedema. Clin Exp Dermatol 2:287–288, 1977.

Fissured bilateral palmar hyperkeratosis in a patient with hypothyroidism cleared dramatically within 10 days of starting thyroxine.

Machino H, Miki Y, Kawatsu T, et al: Successful control of tyrosinemia II. J Am Acad Dermatol 9:533–539, 1983.

A low phenylalanine-tyrosine (300 mg/day) diet completely cleared a painful localized palmoplantar hyperkeratosis within one month in a three-year-old child. The lesions recurred within a few weeks of provocation with a non-restricted diet. They disappeared on resuming the low-phenylalanine and tyrosine diet and have not recurred in three years.

Larva Currens

Orecchia G, Pazzaglia A, Scaglia M, Rabbiosi G: Larva currens following systemic steroid therapy in a case of strongyloidiasis. Dermatologica 171:366–367, 1985.

An analogue of thiabendazole (**mebendazole** 300 mg bid for 10 days) eliminated larvae from the skin and gut in a 73-year-old farmer.

Larva Migrans

Edelglass JW, Douglass MC, Stiefler R, et al: Cutaneous larva migrans in northern climates: A souvenir of your dream vacation. J Am Acad Dermatol 7:353–358, 1982.

In two young women just back from the Caribbean, oral **thiabendazole** (Mintezol 750 mg bid) combined with topical application of the same thiabendazole 10 per cent oral suspension (applied qid) induced complete resolution of serpiginous tracks in one week. Topical application (four times a day) alone was sufficient to cure a third woman of the same problem, again in one week.

Leishmaniasis

Urcuyo FG, Zaias N: Oral ketoconazole in the treatment of leishmaniasis. Int J Dermatol 21:414–416, 1982.

Six patients with mucocutaneous leishmaniasis due to *Leishmania braziliensis* were cured by administration of **ketoconazole** (400 mg/day for three months).

Nelson DA, Gustafson TL, Spielvogel RL: Clinical aspects of cutaneous leishmaniasis acquired in Texas. J Am Acad Dermatol 12:985–992, 1985.

Reports five patients: two showed spontaneous healing; one was cured by lesion excision; one was cured by applying an **antimony potassium tartrate** 10 per cent cream (bid for three weeks); and one was cured by two courses of **sodium stibogluconate** (IV for 10 days, each course).

The mainstay of therapy for severe forms of leishmaniasis is the pentavalent antimonials, **N-methylglucamine antimonate** (Glucantine IV 60 mg/kg/day for 12 days, repeat in 15 days) or **sodium stibogluconate** (IV 20 mg/kg bid for 30 days). Alternate treatments include **amphotericin B** and **pentamidine.** Drugs still under study include **trimethoprim-sulfamethoxazole, rifampin, metronidazole,** and **ketoconazole.**

All require long courses. Localized lesions usually respond to cryotherapy, curettage, or simple excision. There is no effective immunization other than having the disease. Preventive measures include elimination of insect and animal vectors.

Aram H, El-On J: Recurrent cutaneous leishmaniasis: Successful treatment with sodium antimony gluconate. Cutis 37:177–179, 1986.

A 15-year-old boy with a 10-year history of recurrent cutaneous leishmaniasis of the face had failed to respond to (1) oral rifampin (900 mg/day) combined with isoniazid (300 mg/day) for two months, and (2) oral ketoconazole (400 mg/day for four months, then 600 mg/day for one month).

Cure came with **sodium antimony gluconate** (800 mg IM daily for 10 days, followed 16 days later by 600 mg IM daily for 10 days). At the end of the second course, the lesions were completely healed clinically and parasitologically. There was no recurrence in four months.

Lipodystrophy

Rees TD, Coburn RJ: Silicone treatment of partial lipodystrophy. JAMA 230:868–870, 1974.

Soft-tissue contours were restored and absence of adipose tissue effectively masked in nine patients afflicted with the cadaverous or mask-like facies of lipodystrophy. The reversal was achieved in a period of one to two years and involved 8 to 15 office visits for percutaneous injections of **silicone** (1 to 2 ml of medical-grade, high-viscosity dimethicone fluid injected subcutaneously into various atrophic sites at one-month intervals to a total of 20 to 50 ml).

Valenta LJ, Elias AN: Insulin-induced lipodystrophy in diabetic patients resolved by treatment with human insulin. Ann Intern Med 102:790–791, 1985.

Intralesional injections of recombinant DNA **human insulin** (Humulin) completely eliminated within three months the fat atophy that had resulted from prior injections of conventional bovine-porcine insulin in five diabetics.

Hurwitz PJ, Sarel R: Facial reconstruction in partial lipodystrophy. Ann Plast Surg 8:253–257, 1982.

The hollow cheeks of a 16-year-old patient were restored to normal contour by dermal fat grafts from the buttocks.

Lymphomatoid Granulomatosis

Brodell RT, Miller CW, Eisen AZ: Cutaneous lesions of lymphomatoid granulomatosis. Arch Dermatol 122:303–306, 1986.

Complete resolution of skin lesions occurred within two months of starting **cyclophosphamide** (Cytoxan 2 mg/kg/day) and **prednisone** (1 mg/kg/day) in a 33-year-old man with lymphomatoid granulomatosis of seven months' duration. By three months the pulmonary infiltrates had completely involuted. At four months the prednisone dosage was tapered, and it was stopped at six months. The cyclophosphamide therapy was continued for an entire year, during which time the patient had been disease-free for nine months. Six months after stopping the cyclophosphamide the cutaneous and pulmonary infiltrates had returned. On resuming cyclophosphamide and prednisone in original dosage, all lesions again involuted within two months. The treatment has been reduced to cyclophosphamide (50 mg/day) and prednisone (15 mg/day) with no recurrence in 1.5 years.

Malignant Atrophic Papulosis

Degos R: Malignant atrophic papulosis. Br J Dermatol 100:21–35, 1979.

Anticoagulants are the most likely agents to inhibit the progress of this disease. Of these, **heparin** has pride of place and should be given in high doses intravenously if there is any sign of gastrointestinal involvement. Corticosteroids are contraindicated, having been associated with intestinal perforations.

Trials with antibiotics, chloroquine, immunosuppressants, and a score of other modalities had no success in this lethal disease of skin and gut.

Melasma

Kligman AM, Willis I: A new formula for depigmenting human skin. Arch Dermatol 111:40–48, 1975.

Although **hydroquine** (2 to 5 per cent applied bid for three months) may help some patients with hyperpigmentation, the majority of patients are disappointed. The authors recommend a formula of **tretinoin** 0.1 per cent, **hydroquinone** 5 per cent, and **dexamethasone** 0.1 per cent in hydrophilic ointment (applied once daily for five to seven weeks). This preparation produced satisfactory results in 14 of 16 patients with melasma.

Milstein HG: 5-Fluorouracil as an aid in the management of acne and melasma. J Am Acad Dermatol 4:97–98, 1981.

For treatment of melasma, use **5-fluorouracil** cream (Efudex once daily for two weeks) followed by a bleaching cream with **hydroquinone** (Eldoquin once daily for three to six months).

Mucous Cysts

Epstein E: A simple technique for managing digital mucous cysts. Arch Dermatol 115:1315–1316, 1979.

Needling the cyst with a 26-gauge hypodermic needle and expression of the cyst contents on a prn basis induced 29 of 40 digital mucous cysts to disappear permanently. This cure rate matches or exceeds that achieved with injection of steroids or with simple excision. This technique can be taught to the patient.

Sonnex TS, Leonard J, Ralfs I, Dawber RPR: Myxoid cysts of the finger: Treatment by liquid nitrogen spray cryosurgery. Br J Dermatol 107(Suppl 22):21–22, 1982.

Cryosurgery (two freeze times of 30 seconds of ice field with a four-minute thaw interval) cured 12 of 14 patients with myxoid cysts of the finger.

Mycetoma

Magana M: Mycetoma: A review. Int J Dermatol 23:221–236, 1984.

Among the drugs used for treatment are sulfones, sulfonamides, **tetracycline, isoniazid, streptomycin sulfate, rifampin, amphotericin B,** and **ketoconazole.**

Dapsone is a favorite, using high-dose and long-term routines (200 to 300 mg daily for up to two years); alternately, Bactrim DS (one tablet every 12 hours for months) is helpful. Tetracycline (2 gm/day for months) may be of value. Ketoconazole has not been helpful in treating mycetomas.

Neonatal Jaundice

Bracon AK, McDonagh AF: Phototherapy for neonatal hyperbilirubinemia: Efficacy, mechanism and toxicity. Adv Pediatr 27:341–389, 1980.

A definitive review with 230 references on the value of treating physiologically jaundiced neonates with natural sunlight or fluorescent light. Phototherapy should not be used in liver disease and is of limited value if the problem is of hemolytic origin.

Neonatal Pyoderma

Seeberg S, Brinkhoff B, John E, Kjellmer I: Prevention and control of neonatal pyoderma with chlorhexidine. Acta Paediatr Scand 73:498–504, 1984.

Chlorhexidine detergent solution 4 per cent (Hibiscrub) used daily in umbilical cord care decreased neonatal pyoderma due to *Staphylococcus aureus* from 0.7 to 0.1 per cent of infants in one hospital nursery. Continued use of chlorhexidine after discharge was recommended to prevent purulent omphalitis and other forms of neonatal pyoderma.

Neurotic Excoriations

Duke EE: Clinical experience with pimozide: Emphasis on its use in postherpetic neuralgia. J Am Acad Dermatol 8:845–850, 1983.

Two elderly patients with neurotic excoriations cleared within one month of **pimozide** administration (Orap 2 mg bid).

Nocardiosis

Kalb RE, Kaplan MH, Grossman ME: Cutaneous nocardiosis: Case reports and review. J Am Acad Dermatol 13:125–133, 1985.

The best therapy for treating these rare gram-positive, often acid-fast filamentous bacterial infections centers on **sulfadiazine, trimethoprim-sulfamethoxazole,** or **minocycline.** Treatment must be continued for many months. Severe cases of nocardiosis require hospitalization and intravenous trimethoprim-sulfamethoxazole or aminoglycosides (**amikacin**). Always, surgical drainage is necessary and may be curative in a large percentage of patients. The authors give a splendid, complete review of 107 references, stressing the clinical masks this infection may wear: cellulitis, lymphangitis, abscesses, pustules, nodules, ulcers, sinuses, granulomas, and adenopathy.

Boudoulas O, Camisa C: *Nocardia asteroides* infection with dissemination to skin and joints. Arch Dermatol 121:898–900, 1985.

Two weeks of intravenous **trimethoprim-sulfamethoxazole** (320 to 1600 mg IV q6h) resulted in clearing of cellulitis, bullae, ulcers, and tongue lesions in a 56-year-old woman with biopsy- and culture-proven nocardiosis.

During this period, the affected joints were aspirated daily for one week. To prevent relapse, Bactrim was given orally for the subsequent three months.

Onchocerciasis

Rozenman D, Kremer M, Zuckerman F: Onchocerciasis in Israel. Arch Dermatol 120:505–507, 1984.

A 15-year-old boy was successfully treated for onchocerciasis with **diethylcarbamazine citrate** (10 mg/kg/day using a lower starting dose during the first week). After three weeks the pruritus and lichenoid eruption had disappeared, and ocular microfilariae were no longer seen on ophthalmoscopic examination. The drug was then stopped, and there has been no recurrence in two years.

Suramin sodium (IV 1 gm/week for seven weeks) is used to rid patients of adult worms. On occasion, surgical excision is also used.

Onycholysis

Kechijian P: Onycholysis of the fingernails: Evaluation and management. J Am Acad Dermatol 12:552–560, 1985.

This definitive reference for therapy of a common complaint focuses on first finding and eliminating the cause. Most examples of onycholysis result from trauma, maceration, and contact with occupational chemicals or nail care products.

Recommendations:

- short length finger nails
- protective gloves (with inner cotton gloves)
- avoidance of all nail cosmetics
- avoidance of organic chemicals, as well as overhydration

The most common microbial pathogen is *Candida albicans.* For therapy:

1. Cut back unattached nail monthly
2. Wash less frequently
3. Frequent application of tincture of iodide diluted with equal parts of 70 per cent isopropyl alcohol
4. Apply **econazole, miconazole, clotrimazole, ciclopirox olamine**

5. Consider **ketoconazole** orally

If onychomycosis is present, treat with **griseofulvin** or ketoconazole.

For *Pseudomonas-* or *Corynebacterium*-induced onycholysis, apply Clorox (diluted 1 to 4 tid).

Drug-induced onycholysis usually arises on a phototoxic basis, so protection from ultraviolet light and sunlight is critical.

Onycholysis due to psoriasis or lichen planus requires potent local steroids applied tid to the nail bed after cutting the nail back. At times, intralesional **triamcinolone acetonide** (2.5 mg/ml) may be necessary, but precede this with local **xylocaine** (no epinephrine) anesthesia. Local PUVA is also helpful.

Be sure to rule out nail bed neoplasm, wart, or pyogenic granuloma as a curable cause.

Check for hypo- or hyperthyroidism, iron deficiency, pellagra, and peripheral circulatory disease.

Otitis Externa

Neu HC: Contemporary antibiotic therapy in otolaryngology. Otolaryngol Clin North Am 17:745–760, 1984.

Malignant necrotizing external otitis, occurring usually in elderly diabetics and due to *Pseudomonas aeruginosa*, can invade cartilage and bone and can be responsible for cranial nerve palsies, intense pain, brain abscess, and death. Its presence calls for surgical debridement, as well as massive doses of **penicillin** (18 to 24 gm/day) or intensive **piperacillin** and **tobramycin** therapy for at least six weeks.

Pachyonychia Congenita

Thomsen RJ, Zuehlke RL, Beckman BI: Pachyonychia congenita. Surgical management of the nail changes. J Dermatol Surg Oncol 8:24–28, 1982.

A comparative study of techniques of ablation of fingernails in a 37-year-old woman with pachyonychia congenita showed that the best results came from vigorous curettage and electrofulguration of the matrices and beds of the nails.

Panniculitis

Shelley WB: Chloroquine-induced remission of nodular panniculitis present for 15 years. J Am Acad Dermatol 5:168–170, 1981.

Chloroquine (250 mg/day) induced clearing of a nodular form of panniculitis within one month in a 62-year-old woman who had had lesions for 15 years. The dose was gradually tapered to 250 mg every fifth day, with complete suppression for over 1.5 years. Further reduction of dosage was associated with early signs of recrudescence.

The panniculitis previously had been unresponsive to nine different systemic antibiotics over a 15-year period, but was temporarily responsive to Kenalog (40 mg IM).

Papular Urticaria

Rustin MHA, Munro DD: Papular urticaria caused by *Dermestes maculatus degeer*. Clin Exp Dermatol 9:317–321, 1984.

This is the first report of larvae of this photophobic carpet beetle causing papular urticaria. Most patients are unaware of their presence in the home. Alert them to look in all window casements.

Heng MCY, Kloss SG, Haberfelde GC: Pathogenesis of papular urticaria. J Am Acad Dermatol 10:1030–1034, 1984.

Three adult patients with papular urticaria were cured after elimination of fleas from their apartments by professional insect exterminators.

Herwick RP: Lesions caused by canine ear mites. Arch Dermatol 114:130, 1978.

Canine ear mites (*Otodectes cynotis*) in a recently acquired cocker spaniel puppy proved to be the cause of an intensely pruritic papular eruption in the owner. Interestingly, the patient's husband was unaffected by these mites.

Paracoccidioidomycosis

Van Tyle JH: Ketoconazole: Mechanism of action, spectrum of activity, pharmacokinetics, drug interactions, adverse reactions and therapeutic use. Pharmacotherapy 4:343–373, 1984.

The literature reveals that 153 of 158 paracoccidioidomycosis (South American blastomycosis) patients treated with **ketoconazole** (200 to 400 mg/day for 6 to 12 months) were either cured or improved.

Ketoconazole (Nizoral) thus replaces both **sulfonamide** therapy (which required three to five years) and **amphotericin B,** which are less effective.

Paronychia

Wong E-SM, Hay RJ, Clayton YM, Noble WC: Comparison of the therapeutic effect of ketoconazole tablets and econazole lotion in the treatment of chronic paronychia. Clin Exp Dermatol 9:489–496, 1984.

Paronychia is etiologically multifactorial with micrococci, diphtheroids, and gram-negative organisms joining forces with *Candida albicans* to cause chronic inflammation.

Patients must be instructed to either avoid wet work or wear rubber gloves, avoid nail polish, and avoid manipulation of the cuticle.

In a study of 24 patients with positive candidal cultures, application of topical **econazole** (Spectazole lotion bid to the nail folds) was as effective as systemic **ketoconazole** (Nizoral 200 mg/day).

Pitted Keratolysis

Stanton RL, Schwartz RA, Aly R: Pitted keratolysis: A clinicopathologic review. J Am Podiatry Assoc 72:436–439, 1982.

Topical **erythromycin** (2 per cent solution applied bid) to the sole of a 31-year-old male with pitted keratolysis produced resolution of all pitting within four weeks.

Porokeratosis

Shelley WB, Shelley ED: Disseminated superficial porokeratosis: Rapid therapeutic response to 5-fluorouracil. Cutis 32:139–140, 1983.

Disseminated superficial porokeratosis, present for several years in a 50-year-old man, completely disappeared in three weeks after application of **5-fluorouracil** cream (Efudex 5 per cent cream once daily). There had been no recurrence one year later.

Puncture Wounds

Tunnessen WW Jr: Practical aspects of bacterial skin infections in children. Pediatr Dermatol 2:255–265, 1985.

Discusses puncture wounds of the foot, 98 per cent of which were caused by nails.

Treatment: soaking, elevation of the extremity, rest, and antimicrobial therapy, either oral or intravenous. If there is no response, incise, drain, and search for retained foreign body.

Pustular Eruptions of Palms and Soles

Baker H: Pustular psoriasis. Dermatol Clin 2:455–470, 1984.

A survey of the common treatment options for a handful of localized macroscopic pustular eruptions that answer to any of the following names:

- localized pustular psoriasis
- palmoplantar pustulosis
- acropustulosis
- acrodermatitis continua
- pustular acrodermatitis
- dermatitis repens

The author recommends trials of the following:

- **tetracycline** (250 mg tid)
- **etretinate** (0.5 to 1.0 mg/kg/day)
- **colchicine** (1 to 2 mg/day)
- **dapsone** (100 mg/day)
- **triamcinolone** (2 to 4 mg/day)
- PUVA—the best treatment of all (total dose 17 J/sq cm given in 14 to 22 sessions)

Halberg D, Neolin L: Remission of pustulosis palmaris et plantaris after intestinal shunt operation: Reports of three cases. Acta Derm Venereol 54:155–156, 1974.

Three patients with severe incapacitating pustular eruption of the palms and soles experienced dramatic improvement and clearing of their eruption within two weeks after having intestinal shunt operations for treatment of extreme obesity.

Lassus A, Lauharanta J, Eskelinen A: The effect of etretinate compared with different regimens of PUVA in the treatment of persistent palmo-plantar pustulosis. Br J Dermatol 112:455–459, 1985.

Etretinate wins hands down. Of 17 patients treated with etretinate (Tigason 1.0 mg/kg/day for two weeks, then maintenance 0.6 mg/kg/day for ten weeks), 14 completely cleared, whereas only 4 of 28 patients in the PUVA program cleared.

White SW: Palmoplantar pustular psoriasis provoked by lithium therapy. J Am Acad Dermatol 7:660–662, 1982.

After six months of **lithium carbonate** (1200 mg/day), a 49-year-old woman developed pustular psoriasis of the palms and soles. It was refractory to treatment but promptly cleared on stopping the lithium and recurred two weeks after resuming the lithium.

Goette DK, Morgan AM, Fox BJ, Horn RT: Treatment of palmoplantar pustulosis with intralesional triamcinolone injections. Arch Dermatol 120:319–323, 1984.

Five patients with chronic intermittent pustular eruption of the palms and soles promptly cleared and remained clear for three to six months after sublesional injections of **triamcinolone acetonide** (10 mg/ml diluted to 3.3 or 5.0 mg/ml by adding 2 per cent lidocaine hydrochloride, 30-gauge needle). A four-second liquid nitrogen freeze prior to needle entry reduced discomfort. By using a "fanning" technique for injection, 3 to 5 ml of suspension was adequate to cover 30 to 60 sq cm.

Raynaud's Phenomenon

Surwit RS, Gilgor RS, Allen LM, Duvic M: A double-blind study of prazosin in the treatment of Raynaud's phenomenon in scleroderma. Arch Dermatol 120:329–331, 1984.

Minipress (**prazosin hydrochloride,** 1 mg orally tid) effectively reduced the frequency and severity of vasospasm in 19 patients with Raynaud's phenomenon associated with progressive systemic sclerosis. There was a 50 per cent reduction in both within one week.

Reiter's Syndrome

Gerber RC: Diagnosis and management of Reiter's syndrome. Compr Ther 10(8):51–57, 1984.

Treatment is empiric and difficult. Try nonsteroidal anti-inflammatory drugs:

Methotrexate (10 to 50 mg/week IV, IM, or orally)
Azathioprine (Imuran 10 to 25 mg/kg/day)

Refer to ophthalmologist and rheumatologist.

Benoldi D, Alinovi A, Bianchi G, et al: Reiter's disease: Successful treatment of the skin manifestations with oral etretinate. Acta Derm Venereol 64:352–354, 1984.

Etretinate (Tigason 0.8 mg/kg/day) induced considerable clearing of skin lesions within three weeks in a 54-year-old man with Reiter's disease. His arthritis improved concurrently. Long-term maintenance (0.5 mg/kg every other day) has kept the disease in remission for over six months.

Lesher JL, Chalker DK: Response of the cutaneous lesions of Reiter's syndrome to ketoconazole. J Am Acad Dermatol 13:161–163, 1985.

Ketoconazole (Nizoral 200 mg/day for five weeks) resulted in striking improvement in the skin and joint manifestations of Reiter's disease in a 32-year-old man. Initially responsive but later intolerant to **methotrexate,** he showed 90 per cent clearing of all skin changes at the end of a five-week course of ketoconazole. There was no relapse upon stopping the drug.

Reticulohistiocytosis

Brandt F, Lipman M, Taylor JR, Halprin KM: Topical nitrogen mustard therapy in multicentric reticulohistiocytosis. J Am Acad Dermatol 6:260–262, 1982.

Topical **nitrogen mustard** (Mustargen 10 mg in 50 ml water applied daily for two weeks) cleared the skin papules and nodules of a 53-year-old black male with multicentric reticulohistiocytosis. Lesions recurred when the treatment was stopped but could be controlled when they occasionally appeared with resumption of nitrogen mustard on a daily or every-other-day schedule. Topical treatment produced no improvement in his arthritis, which was subsequently controlled with **cyclophosphamide** (Cytoxan 50 mg daily).

Zeale PJ, Miner D, Honig S, et al: Multicentric reticulohistiocytosis: A cause of dysphagia with response to corticosteroids. Arthritis Rheum 28:231–234, 1985.

A 38-year-old black woman with dysphagia, arthritis, and skin nodules improved dramatically with **prednisone** (30 mg bid, slowly tapered to 10 mg daily).

Scar

Amroliwalla FK: Vaccination scar with soft-tissue atrophy restored by local insulin treatment. Br Med J 1:1389–1390, 1977.

A 42-year-old woman with a deep scar on her left arm as a result of an influenza vaccination four years previously was successfully treated with intralesional insulin. Monocomponent porcine soluble **insulin** (4 U tid before meals) was injected subcutaneously in divided doses into each quadrant of the scar. The injections were given by her husband, and there was no evidence of hypoglycemia. By five weeks the deep 3-cm scar was reduced to the size of a dimple, and by the eighty-second day the treatment was discontinued since the skin was normal in contour and appearance. There was no loss of the regained tissue in the subsequent seven months.

Sporotrichosis

Dismukes WE, Stamm AM, Graybill JR, et al: Treatment of systemic mycoses with ketoconazole: Emphasis on toxicity and clinical response in 52 patients: National Institute of Allergy and Infectious Diseases Collaborative Antifungal Study. Ann Intern Med 98:13–20, 1983.

Score card for sporotrichosis:

1 cured
1 improved
2 relapsed
3 failed
7 total (4 of whom had bone and joint involvement)

Dosage—oral **ketoconazole** (200 to 400 mg/day).

Shelley WB, Sica PA: Disseminate sporotrichosis of skin and bone cured with 5-fluocytosine: Photosensitivity as a complication. J Am Acad Dermatol 8:229–235, 1983.

Oral **5-fluocytosine** (Ancobon 8 gm/day) with conjoint **amphotericin B** (50 mg IV daily for three weeks) produced clearing of skin lesions and bone pain within three weeks. The amphotericin was continued in reduced dosage for four months and the 5-fluocytosine (8 gm/day) was continued for six months, then reduced to 3 gm/day for a final six months. There was no relapse in the following three years.

The 39-year-old patient had previously been refractory to saturated solution of **potassium iodide** (45 drops qid for three months). A prior course of amphotericin (50 mg IV daily to a total of 2 gm) had produced improvement, but relapse occurred within one week of stopping the drug.

Alternate treatments to be considered in such refractory cases include **zinc, iron, cimetidine,** local heat, **trimethoprim-sulfamethoxazole, miconazole,** and **transfer factor.** (Today, ketoconazole in high dosage for many months is the treatment of choice if the classic treatment with saturated solution of potassium iodide [15 drops tid] fails.)

Stevens-Johnson Syndrome

Marvin JA, Heimbach DM, Engrev LH, et al: Improved treatment of the Stevens-Johnson syndrome. Arch Surg 119:601–605, 1984.

Standard treatment centers on systemic steroids, prophylactic antibiotics, topical antibacterials, and nutritional support.

The novel avenue used here on five patients with severe Stevens-Johnson syndrome was to approach the problem as a burn. In the burn center urgent operative debridement of the wounds was performed and followed by application of porcine xenografts immediately after admission. Steroids were not given and antibiotics were used only for culture-proven infections. All patients re-epithelialized within a mean of 18 days.

Sulzberger-Garbe Syndrome

Sulzberger MB: Distinctive exudative discoid and lichenoid chronic dermatosis (Sulzberger and Garbe) re-examined—1978. Br J Dermatol 100:13–20, 1979.

"In my experience, the best therapeutic measures are a complete change of environment and systemic administration of corticosteroids. The dermatosis often responds to quite small doses of corticosteroids by mouth. But this medication must be continued until self-healing occurs—the steroids are morbistatic, not curative."

Freeman K, Hewitt M, Warin AP: Two cases of distinctive exudative discoid and lichenoid chronic dermatosis of Sulzberger and Garbe responding to azathioprine. Br J Dermatol 111:215–220, 1984.

Two corticosteroid-resistant examples of Sulzberger-Garbe disease showed dramatic relief of pruritus and rapid clearing of the skin lesions in two weeks with **azathioprine** (Imuran 50 mg tid). The drug was continued for 7 and 12 months, respectively, with no relapse on stopping it.

Sweet's Syndrome

Horio T, Imamura S, Danno K, et al: Treatment of acute febrile neutrophilic dermatosis (Sweet's syndrome) with potassium iodide. Dermatologica 160:341–347, 1980.

Potassium iodide (900 mg/day for two weeks) was effective treatment for six patients with Sweet's syndrome. All became afebrile and symptom-free in 24 to 48 hours, and the cutaneous eruption was gone within three to five days. There were no recurrences.

Systemic corticosteroids are equally effective, but antibiotics to date have not helped.

Kibbi AG, Zaynoun ST, Kurban AK, et al: Acute febrile neutrophilic dermatosis (Sweet's syndrome): Case report and review of literature. Pediatr Dermatol 3:40–44, 1985.

Despite the clinical appearance of infection (fever, leukocytosis, and erythematous plaques and pustules), this eight-month-old infant showed no response to **cloxacillin** (900 mg q6h). By contrast, **prednisone** (2 mg/kg/day orally) produced prompt, dramatic improvement.

The prednisone (5 mg qid) at the time of discharge from the hospital was tapered and discontinued after three months. New lesions reappeared seven months later and were again responsive to prednisone.

Soderstrom RM: Sweet's syndrome and acute myelogenous leukemia: A case report and review of the literature. Cutis 28:255–258, 1981.

Look for evidence of a leukemic or preleukemic state, since 10 per cent of reported cases occur in association with acute myelogenous leukemia.

Su WPD, Liu HH: Diagnostic criteria for Sweet's syndrome. Cutis 37:167–170, 1986.

Five cases were temporally associated with the following:

- Bactrim therapy for vaginitis
- Venipuncture
- Diverticulitis
- Sinusitis
- Acute myelocytic leukemia

Each case responded well to oral **prednisone** (20 to 60 mg/day).

Syringomas

Maloney ME: An easy method for removal of syringoma. J Dermatol Surg Oncol 8:973–975, 1982.

Individual excision of these tumors using an ophthalmologic spring-action straight scissors (Vanna) gives an excellent cosmetic result.

Systemic Lupus Erythematosus

Hall RP, Lawley TJ, Smith HR, et al: Bullous eruption of systemic lupus erythematosus. Dramatic response to dapsone therapy. Ann Intern Med 97:165–170, 1982.

Dapsone (100 mg/day) immediately and completely suppressed the appearance of vesiculobullous lesions that were developing in four patients with systemic lupus erythematosus. Each of these patients' skin lesions had been unresponsive to steroids and to antimalarials. Stopping the dapsone was followed by the appearance of new vesicles within 48 hours. The dapsone had no effect on the systemic aspects of the disease.

Fenton DA, Black MM: Low-dose dapsone in the treatment of subacute cutaneous lupus erythematosus. Clin Exp Dermatol 11:102–103, 1986.

Dapsone (25 mg/day for three weeks) induced total involution of an eruption that had been indifferent to a systemic antimalarial drug and several potent topical corticosteroids for three years. The fading of the lesions was evident after one week, and at three weeks the eruption was gone. The dapsone was then stopped and there has been no recurrence.

Schur PH (ed): The Clinical Management of Systemic Lupus Erythematosus. In Decker JL: Systemic lupus erythematosus management. New York, Grune and Stratton, 1983, pp 259–281.

A valuable monograph on all aspects of treating a disease that produces not only rashes, but also nephritis, central nervous system episodes, pneumonitis, and thrombocytopenic purpura.

Recommendations:

- No treatment if patient is well and only evidence of disease is serologic or laboratory in nature.
- Nonsteroidal anti-inflammatory drugs (**aspirin** 3 to 6 gm/day) alone or with antimalarials (**chloroquine** 250 mg/day) if problem is fatigue, fever, arthritis, sinusitis, or a skin rash.
- Systemic steroids, ranging from oral **prednisone** (20 mg/day) to bolus IV **methylprednisolone** (1 gm/day) for more severe involvement.
- Immunosuppressants (**cyclophosphamide** 150 mg/day)
- Adjunctive drugs (antihypertensives, anticonvulsants, tranquilizers, sunscreens, topical steroids)
- Patient support: Spend time with patient, attend to details, regular office visits, telephone availability for emergencies, acquaint patients with available books, pamphlets, and support groups (appendix has five pages of citation on this facet).

Tuffanelli DL: Management of cutaneous lupus erythematosus. Clin Dermatol 3:123–130, 1985.

The dermatologist may act as the primary physician in patients with systemic lupus erythematosus whose major problem is cutaneous. All call for assessment of the extent of disease by doing a complete history and physical examination, as well as securing data on renal function, C_3 values, anti-nDNA antibodies. Referral to the appropriate specialist (nephrologist, hematologist, rheumatologist, neurologist) should be made.

Specific caveats for the patient:

- Avoid fatigue of a rat-race lifestyle.
- Avoid sun exposure if there is a history of general sun intolerance.
- Avoid oral contraceptives or estrogens.
- Avoid drugs known to induce LE, e.g., procainamide, hydralazine, isoniazid.
- Avoid photosensitizing drugs, e.g., tetracycline, Dyazide.
- Avoid ingestion of alfalfa.

Finally, inform the patient that flares may occur during pregnancy or the postpartum period. Furthermore, a low percentage of offspring may have or develop the disease.

Telangiectasia

Shelley WB, Fierer JA: Focal intravascular coagulation in progressive ascending telangiectasia: Ultrastructural studies of ketoconazole-induced involution of vessels. J Am Acad Dermatol 10:876–887, 1984.

Progressive ascending telangiectasia of nine years' duration in a 54-year-old woman was refractory to tetracycline. **Ketoconazole** (Nizoral 200 mg/day) eliminated much of the telangiectasia within three weeks, and by three months improvement was even more striking. Ketoconazole was continued for eight months, at which point new telangiectatic vessels suddenly appeared at the time of a severe episode of acute sinusitis.

Salabrasion (sodium chloride crystals rubbed into anesthetized skin to the point of vivid erythema) was also an effective local treatment of telangiectatic vessels.

Shelley WB: Essential progressive telangiectasia: Successful treatment with tetracycline. JAMA 216:1343–1344, 1971.

A 39-year-old woman had had progressive ascending telangiectasia of seven years' duration. **Tetracycline** (250 mg qid) induced nearly complete involution of the fine telangiectatic vessels within three months but did not affect associated varicose veins. Long-term maintenance dosage (tetracycline 250 mg bid) was necessary to prevent reappearance of the telangiectasia.

Bodian EL: Techniques of sclerotherapy for sunburst venous blemishes. J Dermatol Surg Oncol 11:696–704, 1985.

The treatment of choice: Use **hypertonic saline** (23.4 per cent sodium chlorine in water), a very fine needle (No. 30, 31, or 33), and a magnifier.

Laser surgery is unsatisfactory.

Alternate method is electrodesiccation (treat entire length with bursts at low intensity every 2 to 3 mm).

Trichomycosis

Bargman H: Trichomycosis of the scrotal hair. Arch Dermatol 120:299–300, 1984.

One per cent **clindamycin** hydrochloride lotion (Cleocin T applied bid) produced a cure within two weeks.

Note: All cases of trichomycosis axillaris can be cured with any of a variety of topical antibiotic lotions, so that the older recommendations of shaving, or applying 3 per cent sulfur ointment, 2 per cent formaldehyde in alcohol, or 1 per cent bichloride of mercury in 70 per cent alcohol are only of historical interest.

Wegener's Granulomatosis

DeRemee RA, McDonald TJ, Weiland LH: Wegener's granulomatosis: Observations on treatment with antimicrobial agents. Mayo Clin Proc 60:27–32, 1985.

Of 12 patients with Wegener's granulomatosis, 11 improved following treatment with antimicrobial agents, chiefly **trimethoprim-sulfamethoxazole** (Bactrim DS 1 per day, long-term).

In their study of 100 patients with this disease, however, **cyclophosphamide** (Cytoxan) is currently the drug of choice. Glucocorticoids may cause temporary subsidence of lesions, but recrudescence often follows discontinuation of the steroid.

Xeroderma Pigmentosum

Epstein EH Jr, Burk PG, Cohen IK, et al: Dermatome shaving in the treatment of xeroderma pigmentosum. Arch Dermatol 105:589–590, 1972.

Dermabrasion as well as excision of the superficial dermis and epidermis (0.017 inch thick) with a dermatome retarded the development of malignant tumors in a 26-year-old woman with xeroderma pigmentosum.

Zinc Deficiency Dermatitis

Bye AME, Goodfellow A, Atherton DJ: Transient zinc deficiency in a full-term breast-fed infant of normal birth weight. Pediatr Dermatol 2:308–311, 1985.

Oral **zinc sulfate** syrup (30 mg tid) produced dramatic improvement within one week in a five-month-old boy with dermatitis of the face, groin, and feet for three months. The initial plasma zinc level was 4.2 μmol/liter (normal range 9.2–29.1). At age one year the zinc therapy was stopped, with no relapse in the ensuing year.

Zoon's Balanitis

Sonnex TS, Dawber RPR, Ryan TJ, Ralfs IG: Zoon's (plasma-cell) balanitis: Treatment by circumcision. Br J Dermatol 106:585–588, 1982.

This plasma-cell balanitis was cured in two patients by simple circumcision. It is the treatment of choice for a chronic problem that othewise requires years of sequential topical steroids and antifungal and antibacterial creams.

In the pitchblende of your daily practice, look for the radium.

The young physician starts life with twenty drugs for each disease,
and the old physician ends life with one drug for twenty diseases.
William Osler

L'envoi

And so gentle reader, we bid adieu, with the fond hope that our book has given you a therapeutic brain lift.

Our current literature is brimming with facts, but many, I am afraid, are no longer available.

ERWIN CHARGAFF

Postscript

The library has been our daily haunt for the two years of writing this book. Our indebtedness to the many authors we have cited is very real and best illustrated by our colleague Ervin Epstein's story. Many years ago when he was writing his textbook *Regional Dermatology*, he had open journals and books spread all around his typewriter. His mother-in-law came by, looked at the scene, and remarked, "You call that writing a book? I call it copying."

Patients know more than you think, and think more than you know.

A Limerick Duet

There once was a doctor perplexed
Who didn't know what to do next
So he opened this book
For just one little look
And the answer was there in the text.

With new access to ideas and pills
Used for treating cutaneous ills
He has patients galore
Beating paths to his door
To seek out his new spectrum of skills.

When instructing patients, make the implicit explicit.

Le traitement? C'est moi.
HENRI GOUGEROT

Index

Advice For Your Patient's Lawyer

1. Don't equate patient dissatisfaction with physician malpractice.
2. Make the patient bear some responsibility for taking the risks of medical treatment.
3. Eschew contingency fee gambling on trivial patient complaints.
4. Hindsight doesn't make the unexpected become commonplace.
5. Malpractice insurance is for the physician, not the patient.
6. The fault may be of metabolic rather than of physician origin.
7. A sick person has no risk-free options.
8. Listen to the counsel of expert physician panels.
9. Medicine is no more of an exact science than law.
10. Ignore the above and I'll see you in court.

Advice From Your Patient's Lawyer

1. Make the correct diagnosis.
2. Recommend safe, appropriate treatment.
3. Keep legible, accurate records at each visit.
4. Know and respect your patient's drug allergies.
5. Avoid unnecessary surgery.
6. Limit your care to your expertise.
7. Never guarantee results or cure.
8. Refer when appropriate—even within your own specialty.
9. Keep yourself and your patient well informed.
10. Ignore the above and I'll see you in court.